Lecture Notes in Artificial Intelligence   8266

Subseries of Lecture Notes in Computer Science

LNAI Series Editors

Randy Goebel
  University of Alberta, Edmonton, Canada
Yuzuru Tanaka
  Hokkaido University, Sapporo, Japan
Wolfgang Wahlster
  DFKI and Saarland University, Saarbrücken, Germany

LNAI Founding Series Editor

Joerg Siekmann
  DFKI and Saarland University, Saarbrücken, Germany

Félix Castro   Alexander Gelbukh
Miguel González (Eds.)

Advances in Soft Computing and Its Applications

12th Mexican International Conference
on Artificial Intelligence, MICAI 2013
Mexico City, Mexico, November 24-30, 2013
Proceedings, Part II

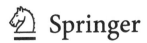 Springer

Volume Editors

Félix Castro
Universidad Autónoma del Estado de Hidalgo
Hidalgo, Mexico
E-mail: fcastro@uaeh.reduaeh.mx

Alexander Gelbukh
Centro de Investigación en Computación
Instituto Politécnico Nacional
Mexico City, Mexico
E-mail: gelbukh@gelbukh.com

Miguel González
Tecnológico de Monterrey
Estado de México, Mexico
E-mail: mgonza@itesm.mx

ISSN 0302-9743　　　　　　　　　　e-ISSN 1611-3349
ISBN 978-3-642-45110-2　　　　　　e-ISBN 978-3-642-45111-9
DOI 10.1007/978-3-642-45111-9
Springer Heidelberg New York Dordrecht London

Library of Congress Control Number: 2013953898

CR Subject Classification (1998): I.2.1, I.2.3-11, I.4, I.5.1-4, J.3, H.4.1-3, F.2.2, H.3.3-5, H.5.3

LNCS Sublibrary: SL 7 – Artificial Intelligence

Typesetting: Camera-ready by author, data conversion by Scientific Publishing Services, Chennai, India

Printed on acid-free paper

Springer is part of Springer Science+Business Media (www.springer.com)

Preface

The Mexican International Conference on Artificial Intelligence (MICAI) is a yearly international conference series organized by the Mexican Society of Artificial Intelligence (SMIA) since 2000. MICAI is a major international AI forum and the main event in the academic life of the country's growing AI community.

MICAI conferences publish high-quality papers in all areas of AI and its applications. The proceedings of the previous MICAI events have been published by Springer in its *Lecture Notes in Artificial Intelligence* (LNAI) series, vols. 1793, 2313, 2972, 3789, 4293, 4827, 5317, 5845, 6437, 6438, 7094, 7095, 7629, and 7630. Since its foundation in 2000, the conference has been growing in popularity and improving in quality.

The proceedings of MICAI 2013 are published in two volumes. The first volume, *Advances in Artificial Intelligence and Its Applications*, contains 45 papers structured into five sections:

- Logic and Reasoning
- Knowledge-Based Systems and Multi-Agent Systems
- Natural Language Processing
- Machine Translation
- Bioinformatics and Medical Applications

The second volume, *Advances in Soft Computing and Its Applications*, contains 45 papers structured into eight sections:

- Evolutionary and Nature-Inspired Metaheuristic Algorithms
- Neural Networks and Hybrid Intelligent Systems
- Fuzzy Systems
- Machine Learning and Pattern Recognition
- Data Mining
- Computer Vision and Image Processing
- Robotics, Planning and Scheduling
- Emotion Detection, Sentiment Analysis, and Opinion Mining

The books will be of interest for researchers in all areas of AI, students specializing in related topics, and for the general public interested in recent developments in AI.

The conference received 284 submissions by 678 authors from 45 countries: Algeria, Argentina, Australia, Austria, Bangladesh, Belgium, Brazil, Bulgaria, Canada, Chile, China, Colombia, Cuba, Czech Republic, Egypt, Finland, France, Germany, Hungary, India, Iran, Ireland, Italy, Japan, Mauritius, Mexico, Morocco, Pakistan, Peru, Poland, Portugal, Russia, Singapore, South Africa, South Korea, Spain, Sweden, Switzerland, Thailand, Tunisia, Turkey, UK, Ukraine,

Uruguay, and USA. Of these submissions, 85 papers were selected for publication in these two volumes after a peer-reviewing process carried out by the international Program Committee. In particular, the acceptance rate was 29.9%.

MICAI 2013 was honored by the presence of such renowned experts as Ildar Batyrshin of the IMP, Mexico; Erik Cambria of the National University of Singapore; Amir Hussain, University of Stirling, UK; Newton Howard, Massachusetts Institute of Technology, USA; and Maria Vargas-Vera, Universidad Adolfo Ibáñez, Chile, who gave excellent keynote lectures. The technical program of the conference also featured tutorials presented by Roman Barták (Czech Republic), Ildar Batyrshin (Mexico), Erik Cambria (Singapore), Alexander Garcia Castro (Germany), Alexander Gelbukh (Mexico), Newton Howard (USA), Ted Pedersen (USA), Obdulia Pichardo and Grigori Sidorov (Mexico), Nelishia Pillay (South Africa), and Maria Vargas-Vera (Chile). Four workshops were held jointly with the conference: the First Workshop on Hispanic Opinion Mining and Sentiment Analysis, the 6th Workshop on Hybrid Intelligent Systems, the 6th Workshop on Intelligent Learning Environments, and the First International Workshop on Semantic Web Technologies for PLM.

In particular, in addition to regular papers, the volumes contain five invited papers by keynote speakers and their collaborators:

- "Association Measures and Aggregation Functions," by Ildar Batyrshin
- "An Introduction to Concept-Level Sentiment Analysis," by Erik Cambria
- "The Twin Hypotheses. Brain Code and the Fundamental Code Unit: Towards Understanding the Computational Primitive Elements of Cortical Computing," by Newton Howard
- "Towards Reduced EEG Based Brain-Computer Interfacing for Mobile Robot Navigation," by Mufti Mahmud and Amir Hussain
- "Challenges in Ontology Alignment and Solution to the Contradictory Evidence Problem," by Maria Vargas-Vera and Miklos Nagy

The authors of the following papers received the Best Paper Award on the basis of the paper's overall quality, significance, and originality of the reported results:

1st place: "A Bayesian and Minimum Variance Technique for Arterial Lumen Segmentation in Ultrasound Imaging," by Sergio Rogelio Tinoco-Martínez, Felix Calderon, Carlos Lara-Alvarez, and Jaime Carranza-Madrigal (Mexico)

2nd place: "The Best Genetic Algorithm I. A Comparative Study of Structurally Different Genetic Algorithms," by Angel Kuri-Morales and Edwin Aldana-Bobadilla (Mexico)
"The Best Genetic Algorithm II. A Comparative Study of Structurally Different Genetic Algorithms," by Angel Kuri-Morales, Edwin Aldana-Bobadilla, and Ignacio López-Peña (Mexico)

3rd place: "A POS Tagger for Social Media Texts Trained on Web Comments,"
by Melanie Neunerdt, Michael Reyer, and Rudolf Mathar (Germany)[1]

The authors of the following paper selected among all papers of which the first author was a full-time student, excluding the papers listed above, received the Best Student Paper Award:

1st place: "A Massive Parallel Cellular GPU Implementation of Neural Network to Large Scale Euclidean TSP," by Hongjian Wang, Naiyu Zhang, and Jean-Charles Créput (France)

We want to thank all the people involved in the organization of this conference. In the first place, the authors of the papers published in this book: It is their research work that gives value to the book and to the work of the organizers. We thank the track chairs for their hard work, and the Program Committee members and additional reviewers for their great effort spent on reviewing the submissions.

We are grateful to Dr. Salvador Vega y León, the Rector General of the Universidad Autónoma Metropolitana (UAM), Dr. Romualdo López Zárate, the Rector of the UAM Azcapotzalco, Dr. Luis Enrique Noreña Franco, Director of the Fundamental Science and Engineering Division, M.Sc. Rafaela Blanca Silva López, Head of the Systems Department, M.Sc. Roberto Alcántara Ramírez, Head of the Electronics Department, and Dr. David Elizarraraz Martínez, Head of the Fundamental Science Department, for their invaluable support of MICAI and for providing the infrastructure for the keynote talks, tutorials and workshops. We are also grateful to the personnel of UAM Azcapotzalco for their warm hospitality and hard work, as well as for their active participation in the organization of this conference. We greatly appreciate the generous sponsorship provided by the Mexican Government via the Museo Nacional de Antropología, Instituto Nacional de Antropología e Historia (INAH).

We are deeply grateful to the conference staff and to all members of the local Organizing Committee headed by Dr. Oscar Herrera Alcántara. We gratefully acknowledge the support received from the following projects: WIQ-EI (Web Information Quality Evaluation Initiative, European project 269180), PICCO10-120 (ICYT, Mexico City Government), and CONACYT-DST (India) project "Answer Validation through Textual Entailment." The entire submission, reviewing, and selection process, as well as preparation of the proceedings, was supported for free by the EasyChair system (www.easychair.org). Last but not least, we are grateful to the staff at Springer for their patience and help in the preparation of this volume.

October 2013   Félix Castro
                                                Alexander Gelbukh
                                          Miguel González Mendoza

---

[1] This paper is published in a special issue of the journal *Polibits* and not in this set of books.

Conference Organization

MICAI 2013 was organized by the Mexican Society of Artificial Intelligence (SMIA, Sociedad Mexicana de Inteligencia Artificial) in collaboration with the Universidad Autónoma Metropolitana Azcapotzalco (UAM Azcapotzalco), Universidad Autónoma del Estado de Hidalgo (UAEH), Centro de Investigación en Computación del Instituto Politécnico Nacional (CIC-IPN), and Tecnológico de Monterrey (ITESM).

The MICAI series website is at: www.MICAI.org. The website of the Mexican Society of Artificial Intelligence, SMIA, is at: www.SMIA.org.mx. Contact options and additional information can be found on these websites.

Conference Committee

General Chairs:	Alexander Gelbukh, Grigori Sidorov, and Raúl Monroy
Program Chairs:	Félix Castro, Alexander Gelbukh, and Miguel González Mendoza
Workshop Chair:	Alexander Gelbukh
Tutorials Chair:	Félix Castro
Doctoral Consortium Chairs:	Miguel Gonzalez Mendoza and Antonio Marín Hernandez
Keynote Talks Chair:	Jesus A. Gonzalez
Publication Chair:	Ildar Batyrshin
Financial Chair:	Grigori Sidorov
Grant Chairs:	Grigori Sidorov and Miguel González Mendoza
Organizing Committee Chair:	Oscar Herrera Alcántara

Track Chairs

Natural Language Processing	Sofia N. Galicia-Haro
Machine Learning and Pattern Recognition	Alexander Gelbukh
Data Mining	Félix Castro
Intelligent Tutoring Systems	Alexander Gelbukh
Evolutionary and Nature-Inspired Metaheuristic Algorithms	Oliver Schütze, Jaime Mora Vargas
Computer Vision and Image Processing	Oscar Herrera Alcántara
Robotics, Planning and Scheduling	Fernando Martin Montes-Gonzalez
Neural Networks and Hybrid Applications Intelligent Systems	Sergio Ledesma-Orozco

Logic, Knowledge-Based Systems,
Multi-Agent Systems and
Distributed AI
: Mauricio Osorio, Jose Raymundo
Marcial Romero

Fuzzy Systems and Probabilistic
Models in Decision Making
: Ildar Batyrshin

Bioinformatics and Medical
Applications
: Jesus A. Gonzalez, Felipe
Orihuela-Espina

Program Committee

Ashraf Abdelraouf
Juan-Carlos Acosta
Teresa Alarcón
Alfonso Alba
Fernando Aldana
Rafik Aliev
Javad Alirezaie
Oscar Alonso Ramírez
Leopoldo Altamirano
Jose Amparo Andrade Lucio
Jesus Angulo
Annalisa Appice
Alfredo Arias-Montaño
García Gamboa Ariel Lucien
Jose Arrazola
Gustavo Arroyo
Serge Autexier
Gideon Avigad
Juan Gabriel Aviña Cervantes
Victor Ayala Ramirez
Sivaji Bandyopadhyay
Maria Lucia Barrón-Estrada
Ildar Batyrshin
Albert Bifet
Bert Bredeweg
Ivo Buzon
Eduardo Cabal
Felix Calderon
Hiram Calvo
Nicoletta Calzolari
Oscar Camacho Nieto
Sergio Daniel Cano Ortiz
Jose Luis Carballido
Mario Castelán
Oscar Castillo

Félix Castro
Martine Ceberio
Michele Ceccarelli
Gustavo Cerda Villafana
Niladri Chatterjee
Edgar Chavez
Zhe Chen
David Claudio Gonzalez
Maria Guadalupe Cortina Januchs
Stefania Costantini
Nicandro Cruz-Ramirez
Heriberto Cuayahuitl
Erik Cuevas
Iria Da Cunha
Oscar Dalmau
Justin Dauwels
Enrique De La Rosa
Maria De Marsico
Beatrice Duval
Asif Ekbal
Michael Emmerich
Hugo Jair Escalante
Ponciano Jorge Escamilla-Ambrosio
Vlad Estivill-Castro
Gibran Etcheverry
Eugene Ezin
Denis Filatov
Juan J. Flores
Pedro Flores
Andrea Formisano
Anilu Franco
Claude Frasson
Juan Frausto-Solis
Alfredo Gabaldon
Ruslan Gabbasov

Sofia N. Galicia-Haro
Ana Gabriela Gallardo-Hernández
Carlos Hugo Garcia Capulin
Ma. de Guadalupe Garcia Hernandez
Arturo Garcia Perez
Alexander Gelbukh
Onofrio Gigliotta
Pilar Gomez-Gil
Eduardo Gomez-Ramirez
Arturo Gonzalez
Jesus A. Gonzalez
Miguel Gonzalez
José Joel González Barbosa
Miguel Gonzalez Mendoza
Felix F. Gonzalez-Navarro
Efren Gorrostieta
Carlos Gracios
Monique Grandbastien
Christian Grimme
De Ita Luna Guillermo
Joaquin Gutierrez
D. Gutiérrez
Rafael Guzman Cabrera
Hartmut Haehnel
Dongfeng Han
Jin-Kao Hao
Yasunari Harada
Antonio Hernandez
Donato Hernandez Fusilier
Eva Hernandez Gress
J.A. Hernandez Servin
Oscar Herrera
Dieter Hutter
Pablo H. Ibarguengoytia
Mario Alberto Ibarra Manzano
Oscar Gerardo Ibarra Manzano
Rodolfo Ibarra-Orozco
Berend Jan Van Der Zwaag
Héctor Jiménez Salazar
W. Lewis Johnson
Laetitia Jourdan
Pinar Karagoz
Timoleon Kipouros
Olga Kolesnikova
Konstantinos Koutroumbas

Vladik Kreinovich
Angel Kuri-Morales
James Lam
Ricardo Landa
Dario Landa-Silva
Reinhard Langmann
Adriana Lara
Bruno Lara
Yulia Ledeneva
Sergio Ledesma Orozco
Yoel Ledo
Juan Carlos Leyva Lopez
Derong Liu
Rocio Alfonsina Lizarraga Morales
Aurelio Lopez
Omar Lopez
Virgilio Lopez
Juan Manuel Lopez Hernandez
Gladys Maestre
Tanja Magoc
Claudia Manfredi
Stephane Marchand-Maillet
Jose Raymundo Marcial Romero
Antonio Marin Hernandez
Luis Martí
Ricardo Martinez
Rene Alfredo Martinez Celorio
Francisco Martínez-Álvarez
José Fco. Martínez-Trinidad
Jerzy Martyna
Ruth Ivonne Mata Chavez
María Auxilio Medina Nieto
R. Carolina Medina-Ramirez
Jorn Mehnen
Patricia Melin
Ivan Vladimir Meza Ruiz
Efren Mezura
Mikhail Mikhailov
Vicente Milanés
Sabino Miranda-Jiménez
Dieter Mitsche
Joseph Modayil
Luís Moniz Pereira
Raul Monroy
Fernando Montes

Héctor A. Montes
Fernando Martin Montes-Gonzalez
Manuel Montes-y-Gómez
Carlos Rubín Montoro Sanjose
Jaime Mora Vargas
Marco Antonio Morales Aguirre
Guillermo Morales-Luna
Masaki Murata
Michele Nappi
Juan Antonio Navarro Perez
Jesús Emeterio Navarro-Barrientos
Juan Carlos Nieves
Juan Arturo Nolazco Flores
Leszek Nowak
C. Alberto Ochoa-Zezatti
Ivan Olmos
Felipe Orihuela-Espina
Eber Enrique Orozco Guillén
Magdalena Ortiz
Mauricio Osorio
Helen Pain
Rodrigo Edgar Palacios Leyva
Vicente Parra
Mario Pavone
Ted Pedersen
Hayde Peregrina-Barreto
Héctor Pérez-Urbina
Alexey Petrovsky
Obdulia Pichardo-Lagunas
David Pinto
Carlos Adolfo Piña-García
Natalia Ponomareva
Volodymyr Ponomaryov
Joel Quintanilla Dominguez
Marco Antonio Ramos Corchado
Risto Rangel-Kuoppa
Luis Lorenzo Rascon Perez
Carolina Reta
Alberto Reyes
Orion Fausto Reyes-Galaviz
Carlos A. Reyes-Garcia
Bernardete Ribeiro
Alessandro Ricci
François Rioult
Erik Rodner

Arles Rodriguez
Horacio Rodriguez
Katia Rodriguez
Eduardo Rodriguez-Tello
Leandro Fermín Rojas Peña
Alejandro Rosales
Paolo Rosso
Horacio Rostro Gonzalez
Samuel Rota Bulò
Imre Rudas
Salvador Ruiz Correa
Marta Ruiz Costa-Jussa
Jose Ruiz Pinales
Leszek Rutkowski
Klempous Ryszard
Andriy Sadovnychyy
Abraham Sánchez López
Raul Enrique Sanchez Yañez
Guillermo Sanchez-Diaz
Antonio-José Sánchez-Salmerón
Jose Santos
Paul Scheunders
Oliver Schütze
Friedhelm Schwenker
J.C. Seck-Tuoh
Nikolay Semenov
Shahnaz Shahbazova
Oleksiy Shulika
Patrick Siarry
Grigori Sidorov
Gerardo Sierra
Bogdan Smolka
Jorge Solís
Elliot Soloway
Peter Sosnin
Humberto Sossa Azuela
Mu-Chun Su
Luis Enrique Sucar
Shiliang Sun
Salvatore Tabbone
Atsuhiro Takasu
Hugo Terashima
Miguel Torres Cisneros
Luz Abril Torres-Méndez
Genny Tortora

Gregorio Toscano-Pulido
Leonardo Trujillo
Fevrier Valdez
Edgar Vallejo
Antonio Vega Corona
Josue Velazquez
Francois Vialatte
Javier Vigueras
Manuel Vilares Ferro
Jordi Vitrià

Panagiotis Vlamos
Zhanshan Wang
Qinglai Wei
Cornelio Yáñez-Márquez
Iryna Yevseyeva
Alla Zaboleeva-Zotova
Ramon Zatarain
Zhigang Zeng
Claudia Zepeda Cortes

Additional Reviewers

Roberto Alonso
Miguel Ballesteros
Somnath Banerjee
Jared Bernstein
Veronica Borja
Ulises Castro Peñaloza
Ning Chen
Santiago E. Conant-Pablos
Joana Costa
Victor Darriba
Agostino Dovier
Milagros Fernández Gavilanes
Santiago Fernández Lanza
Samuel González López
Braja Gopal Patra
Esteban Guerrero
Daniela Inclezan
Yusuf Kavurucu
Anup Kolya
Kow Kuroda
Pintu Lohar
Maricarmen Martinez

Alfonso Medina Urrea
Alev Mutlu
Fernando Orduña Cabrera
Santanu Pal
Yan Pengfei
Soujanya Poria
Gerardo Presbitero
Francisco Rangel
Juan Carlo Rivera Dueñas
Edgar Rodriguez
Mark Rosenstein
Nayat Sanchez-Pi
Alejandro Santoyo
Yasushi Tsubota
Nestor Velasco
Darnes Vilariño
Esaú Villatoro-Tello
Francisco Viveros Jiménez
Shiping Wen
Xiong Yang
Daisuke Yokomori

Organizing Committee

Local Chair:
Local Arrangements Chair:
Finance Chair:
Logistics Chair:
Student Chair:
International Liaison Chair:

Oscar Herrera Alcántara
R. Blanca Silva López
Elena Cruz M.
Iris Iddaly Méndez Gurrola
Eric Rincón
Dr. Antonin Sebastien P.

Table of Contents – Part II

Evolutionary and Nature-Inspired Metaheuristic Algorithms

Neural Networks and Hybrid Intelligent Systems

Best Student Paper Award:

Fuzzy Systems

Invited Paper:

Machine Learning and Pattern Recognition

Data Mining

Computer Vision and Image Processing

Robotics, Planning and Scheduling

Invited Paper:

Emotion Detection, Sentiment Analysis, and Opinion Mining

Invited Paper:

Table of Contents – Part I

Logic and Reasoning

Knowledge-Based Systems and Multi-Agent Systems

Natural Language Processing

Invited Paper:

Machine Translation

Bioinformatics and Medical Applications

Invited Paper:

Best Paper Award, First Place:

The Best Genetic Algorithm I

A Comparative Study of Structurally Different Genetic Algorithms

Angel Fernando Kuri-Morales[1] and Edwin Aldana-Bobadilla[2]

[1] Instituto Tecnológico Autónomo de México
Río Hondo No. 1
México 01000, D.F.
México
akuri@itam.mx

[2] Universidad Nacional Autónoma de México
IIMAS
México 04510, D.F.
México
edwynjavier@yahoo.es

Abstract. Genetic Algorithms (GAs) have long been recognized as powerful tools for optimization of complex problems where traditional techniques do not apply. However, although the convergence of elitist GAs to a global optimum has been mathematically proven, the number of iterations remains a case-by-case parameter. We address the problem of determining the best GA out of a family of structurally different evolutionary algorithms by solving a large set of unconstrained functions. We selected 4 structurally different genetic algorithms and a non-evolutionary one (NEA). A schemata analysis was conducted further supporting our claims. As the problems become more demanding, the GAs significantly and consistently outperform the NEA. A particular breed of GA (the Eclectic GA) is superior to all other, in all cases.

Keywords: Global optimization, Genetic algorithms, Unconstrained functions, Schemata analysis.

1 Introduction

Optimization is an all pervading problem in engineering and the sciences. It is, therefore, important to rely on an optimization tool of proven efficiency and reliability. In this paper we analyze a set of optimization algorithms which have not been analyzed exhaustively before and achieve interesting conclusions which allow us to recommend one such algorithm as applicable to a large number complex problems. When attempting to assess the relative efficiency of a set of optimization algorithms one may take one of two paths: a) Either one obtains closed models for the algorithms thus allowing their parametric characterization [1], [2], [3] or b) One selects a set of problems considered to be of interest and compares the performance of the algorithms

F. Castro, A. Gelbukh, and M. González (Eds.): MICAI 2013, Part II, LNAI 8266, pp. 1–15, 2013.

when measured vs. such a set. Modeling an algorithm is frequently a complex task and, more importantly, even slight changes in the algorithm lead to basically different models [4], thus making the purported characterization impractical. The second option, therefore, seems better suited for practical purposes. However, although there are many examples of such an approach (for instance see [5], [6], [7]) it is always true that a) The nature of the algorithms under study and their number are necessarily limited and b) The selection of the benchmarking functions obeys to subjective criteria. In this paper we choose to establish the relative efficiency of a set of genetic algorithms (GAs) which are structurally different from one another as will be discussed in the sequel. We have selected a set of such GAs and, for completeness, we have also included a particular non-evolutionary algorithm (the Random Mutation Hill Climber or RMH) whose efficiency has been reported in previous works [8], [9]. Many GAs are variations (i.e. different selection criteria [10], crossover strategies [11], population size [12], 13] relationship between Pc and Pm, [14], [15], etc.) of the initial one proposed by Holland (the so-called "Simple" or "Canonical" Genetic Algorithm [CGA] [16]) which do not significantly improve on CGA's overall performance. For benchmarking purposes the mentioned variations are not useful since they all share the same basic algorithmic structure. However there are GAs where the strategies to a) select, b) identify and c) recombine candidate solutions differ from the CGA's substantially. The purported changes impose structural differences between these algorithms which have resulted in remarkable performance implications. We have selected four GAs with this kind of diverse characteristics. We begin, in Section 2, by introducing the necessary notation; then presenting some concepts and definitions. In Section 3 we describe the five algorithms in our work. In section 4 we present the functions and results for a suite of problems that traditionally have been used for benchmarking purposes of optimization algorithms [17] [18]. In Section 5 we present our general conclusions.

2   Preliminaries

Throughout we use the following notation and definitions: A: Set of selected optimization algorithms; A_i: The i-th optimization algorithm (i.e. $A_i \in A$); $\vec{x}$: Vector in $\mathfrak{R}^n$; Ω: Feasibility region of the space $\mathfrak{R}^n$; B: Set defined as $B = \{0,1\}$; t: Iteration number such that $1 \le t \le G; t \in \mathcal{N}$; G: Upper bound on the number of iterations of A_i. Without loss of generality our discussion will be focused on numerical optimization problems. One such problem f is defined as:

$$Minimize \quad f(x)$$
$$Subject\ to \quad h_i(\vec{x}) = 0 \quad i = 1,...m \quad\quad (1)$$
$$g_i(\vec{x}) \le 0 \quad i = m+1,...p$$

where $f(x): \mathfrak{R}^n \to \mathfrak{R}$ is the objective function, $h_i(\vec{x}) = 0$ and $g_i(\vec{x}) \le 0$ are constraint functions defining Ω. This means that if a vector $\vec{x}$ complies with all constraints it belongs to Ω. In a problem without constraints, such as the ones discussed here, all vectors $\bar{x}$ lie within Ω.

We briefly pause to define what we understand as a genetic algorithm. Elsewhere [20], it has been argued that an algorithm is "genetic" when it exhibits implicit parallelism. Instead, we list the characteristics an iterative algorithm must have to be considered "genetic". Implicit parallelism is a consequence of these.

Definition 1:

A genetic algorithm is one which satisfies the following conditions:

1. It works on an n-dimensional discrete space D defined in $\mathbb{N}^n$ rather than in $\mathbb{R}^n$.
2. It traverses D searching an approximation of the optimum vector $\bar{x}$ of (1) by simultaneously analyzing a finite set $S(t) \in D$ of candidate solutions.
3. The elements of $S(t) = \{s_1(t), s_2(t), ..., s_n(t)\}$ are explicitly encoded in some suitable way.
4. The information regarding the partial adequacy of the elements in $S(t)$ is extracted by solving the optimization problem for all $s_i(t)$.
5. The qualified elements of $S(t)$ are analyzed to select an appropriate subset in order to improve the search in the problem's space.
6. Selected sections of the codes of $s_i(t)$ are periodically combined.
7. Selected elements of the codes of the $s_i(t)$ are periodically and randomly altered.
8. A subset of the best solutions of $S(t)$ is preserved for all the future steps of the algorithms.
9. The algorithm cycles through steps 4-8 until a stopping condition is met.

The algorithms selected for this study satisfy all of the characteristics above and, therefore, may be aptly considered to be genetic in a broader sense then the one implied by the frequently cited "bio-inspired" analogy. In fact, this analogy, attractive as it may seem, frequently distracts the attention of the user from the basic efficiency elements which any optimization algorithm should incorporate. These issues must supersede other considerations when determining the desirability of one algorithm over others.

Consequently, set A includes the following GAs:

a) An elitist canonical GA (in what follows referred to as TGA [eliTist GA]) [21].
b) A Cross generational elitist selection, Heterogeneous recombination, and Cataclysmic mutation algorithm (CHC algorithm) [22].
c) An Eclectic Genetic Algorithm (EGA) [23].
d) A Statistical GA (SGA) [24] [25].

3   Selected Genetic Algorithms

It is frequent to cite the variations of the GAs by their "popular name". However, in so doing one incurs in the risk of not being precise on the details of the algorithm. One of the basic tenets of this paper is that even small variations lead to potentially important differences in their behaviors. For this reason, we now include the pseudo-codes of the algorithms in our study. Keep in mind that our results refer to their precise implementation and no others. As a case in point, when discussing SGA (the Statistical GA) it may be easy to confuse it with EDA (Estimation of Distribution Algorithm). However, in EDA no mutation is explicitly included, whereas in SGA it is (see the code below)

In the description of the algorithms which follows a) We denote the arguments $\vec{x} = (x_1,...,x_k)$ with x_i and the corresponding fitness function $f(x) = f(x_1,...,x_k)$ with $f(x_i)$, b) The function $f(x_i)$ to be optimized is numerical, c) We aim to minimize $f(x_i)$, and d) The arguments x_i of the fitness function $f(x_i)$ are encoded in binary.

Let $G \equiv$ number of generations; $n \equiv$ number of individuals; $I(n) \equiv$ *the n-th individual;* $L \equiv$ length of the chromosome; $P_C \equiv$ probability of crossover; $P_M \equiv$ probability of mutation.

By "*Generation of a random population*" we mean that, for a population of n individuals each of whose chromosome's length is L we make

> *for i = 1 to n*
>> *for j=1 to L*
>>> Generate a uniform random number $0 \le \rho < 1$.
>>> If $\rho < 0.5$ make $bit_j \leftarrow 0$; else make $bit_j \leftarrow 1$.
>> *endfor*
> *endfor*

3.1   Elitist Canonical GA (TGA)

This is the classical CGA with two provisions: a) The best individual is kept along the whole process forming part of the evolving population and b) In step 3 of the algorithm

$$\varphi(x_i) = f(x_i) + |min(f(x_i))| + avg(|f(x_i)|) \qquad (A.1)$$

is used. These two steps ensure that no fitness value is negative making the proportional selection scheme always feasible (see [28, 29, 30]).

0. Make $k \leftarrow 1$.
1. Generate a random population
2. Select randomly an individual from the population (call it *best*).
   Make $f(best) \leftarrow \infty$.

3. Evaluate.

> for i=1 to n
>> Evaluate $f(x_i)$.
>>
>> Make $f(x_i) \leftarrow \varphi(f(x_i))$.
>>
>> If $f(x_i) < f(best)$ make $best \leftarrow x_i$ and $f(best) \leftarrow f(x_i)$
>
> endfor

4. If $k = G$ return $best$ and stop.

5. Selection

> Make $F = \sum_{i=1}^{n} f(x_i)$
>
> for $i = 1$ to n; $PS_i = \dfrac{f(x_i)}{F}$; Endfor
>
> for $i = 1$ to n; Select $I(i)$ with probability PS_i; endfor

6. Crossover

for $i = 1$ to n step 2

> Randomly select two individuals (say $I(X)$ and $I(Y)$) with probabilities PS_X and PS_Y, respectively.
>
> Generate a uniform random number $0 \leq \rho < 1$.
>
> If $\rho \leq P_C$ do
>
> - Randomly select a locus ℓ of the chromosome; Pick the leftmost L-ℓ bits of $I(X)$ and the rightmost ℓ bits of $I(Y)$ and concatenate them to form the new chromosome of $I(X)$. Pick the leftmost L-ℓ bits of $I(Y)$ and the rightmost ℓ bits of the previous $I(X)$ and concatenate them to form the new chromosome of $I(Y)$
>
> Make $I(i) \leftarrow I(X)$; $I(i+1) \leftarrow I(Y)$.

endfor

7. Mutation

for $i = 1$ to n

> Select $I(i)$
>
> for $j=1$ to L
>> Generate a uniform random number $0 \leq \rho < 1$.
>>
>> If $\rho \leq P_M$ make $bit_j \leftarrow \overline{bit_j}$.
>
> endfor

endfor

8. Make $k \leftarrow k+1$ and go to step 3.

3.2   Cross Generational Elitist Selection, Heterogeneous Recombination and Cataclysmic Mutation GA (CHC)

This algorithm focuses on maintaining diversity while retaining the characteristics of the best individuals. Inter-generational survival-of-the-fittest is attempted by unbiased parent selection. Furthermore it tries to maintain diversity implementing the so-called HUX crossover (Half, Uniform X-over) and introducing cataclysmic mutations when the population's diversity falls below a pre-defined threshold (see [20]).

0. Make
  $\ell \leftarrow 0$
  threshold $\leftarrow L / 4$
1. Generate a random population.
2. Evaluate $f(x_i)$ $\forall i$
3. $f(best) \leftarrow min(f(x_i))$ $\forall i$
  $best \leftarrow I(i \mid f(x_i)$ is best$)$
4. $\ell \leftarrow \ell + 1$
  If $\ell = G$ return *best* and stop.
5. *Copy all individuals from population P into set C*
6. [HUX Crossover]
Let Bit_{xy} denote the y-th bit of individual x
for i=1 to n/2
    Randomly select individuals I_X and I_Y from C
    hammingXY $\leftarrow 0$
    for $j \leftarrow 1$ to L
        if bit j $(I_X) \neq$ bit j(I_Y); DiffXY[j]=true;
            hammingXY $\leftarrow$ hammingXY+1; else DiffXY[j]=false; f
    endfor
    if (hammingXY/2 $\leq$ threshold)
            eliminate C(X) and C(Y) from C
    else
            mutated $\leftarrow 0$
            while (mutated<hammingXY/2)
                    j $\leftarrow$ random number between 1 and L
                    if DiffXY[j]
                            Interchange the j-th bit of I_X and I_Y
                            mutated $\leftarrow$ mutated+1; DiffXY[j] $\leftarrow$ false
            endwhile
endfor
Evaluate $f(x_i)$ in C(i) $\forall i$
Make P'= P $\cup$ C
Sort P' from best to worst
P' $\leftarrow$ Best n individuals from P'; f (best) $\leftarrow$ f(x_1); best $\leftarrow P_1'$
if P = P'
    threshold $\leftarrow$ threshold-1
    if threshold=0
        for i=2 to n
            Select the i-th individual

for j=1 to L

    Generate a uniform random number $0 \leq \rho < 1$

    If $\rho \leq 0.35$ *make* $bit_j \leftarrow \overline{bit}_j$

threshold $\leftarrow L/4$

$P \leftarrow P'$; *go to 4*

3.3   Eclectic GA (EGA)

This algorithm uses deterministic selection, annular crossover, uniform mutation and full elitism (a strategy akin to $\mu + \lambda$ selection of evolutionary strategies [31]). The probabilistic nature of EGA is restricted to parameters P_C and P_M. In EGA avoidance of premature convergence is achieved by a two-fold strategy. First, the $2n$ individuals from the last two generations are ordered from best to worst and only the best n are allowed to survive. Then the individuals are deterministically selected for crossover by mixing the best with the worst (*1* with n), the second with the second worst (*2* and n-1, . . .,), and so on. In this way n new individuals are generated. As the iterations proceed, the surviving individuals become the top elite of size n of the whole process. Annular crossover (equivalent to two-point crossover) is preferred because it makes the process less dependent on a particular encodings. This algorithm was first reported in [26] and included self-adaptation and periodic cataclysmic mutation. Later studies [27] showed that neither of the two mechanisms was necessary. EGA is relatively simple, fast and easy to program.

0. $B2M \leftarrow \lceil nL \times P_M \rceil$ (Expected number of mutations per generation)

1. $i \leftarrow 1$

2. Generate a random population

3. Evaluate the population.

4. [Duplicate Population]

for j = 1 to n

    $I(n+j) \leftarrow I(j)$

    fitness(n+j) $\leftarrow$ *fitness(j)*

endfor

5. [Deterministic Selection Annular Crossover]

for j=1 to n/2

    Generate a uniform random number $0 \leq \rho < 1$

    If $\rho \leq P_c$

        Generate a random number $1 \leq \rho < L/2$

        Interchange the semi-ring starting at locus ρ *between I(j)*

            and I(n-j-1)

    endif

endfor

5. [Mutation]

for j=1 to B2M

Generate uniform random numbers $0 \leq \rho_1, \rho_2 < 1$

Mutate Bit $\lceil \rho_2 L \rceil$ *of* $I(\lceil \rho_1 n \rceil)$

endFor

6. [Evaluate the New Individuals]

Calculate fitness(x_i) for i=1,...,n

7. [$\mu + \lambda$ Selection]

Sort the 2n individuals by their fitness, ascending

8. $i \leftarrow i+1$

    if $i = G$ *return* $I(1)$ *and stop*

    Go to 3

3.4   Statistical GA (SGA)

In this case the algorithm takes advantage of the fact that the average behavior of traditional TGA may be achieved without actually applying the genetic operators but, rather, statistically simulating their behavior [24]. SGA starts by generating the initial population's (P_0) individuals randomly. The fitness for each individual is calculated as per (A.1). It is then easy to determine its relative fitness $\Phi(x) \leftarrow f(x_j)/\sum_j f(x_j)$

which, immediately, induces a partial ordering in the population according to the value of $\Phi(x)$. Once this is done, the so-called *probabilistic genome* (PG) is calculated. In this genome, the probability that the *k-th* bit of a genome attains a value of 1 is derived from

$$P_k = \sum_j \Phi_j b_{jk} \quad k = 1, ..., L \tag{A.2}$$

where b_{jk} denotes the *k-th* bit of the *j-th* individual. Notice that P_k actually represents the weighted expected number of times that bit k will take the value *1* as a function of the fitness of the *i-th* population. This is equivalent to defining a set of probability distribution functions (*pdfs*); one for each of the L bits in the genome. These *pdfs* are Bernoulli distributed and, initially, may have rather large variances (σ^2). Every new population is generated by sampling from the *j-th* distribution to compose its new N individuals. The *i-th* population consists of individuals that respond to the average behavior of the *(i-1)-th*. Every new population is also Bernoulli distributed but with an increasingly small σ. Eventually the *pdfs* of the final population will have a Bernoulli distribution with $\sigma \approx 0$, implying approximate convergence. In a strict sense, the SGA avoids the need to include explicit mutation provisions. Preliminary tests showed that premature convergence is avoided if such provisions are made. The whole process may be seen as a search for a crisp encoding of the solution with a set of fuzzy bits. Each bit is progressively de-fuzzyfied in consecutive generations.

0. Make $k \leftarrow 1$;

$B2M \leftarrow \lceil nL \times P_M \rceil$ (Expected number of mutations per generation)

1. Generate a random population

2. Select randomly an individual from the population (call it *best*). Make *f(best)* $\leftarrow \infty$.

3. [Get probabilistic genome]

> *PopFit* $\leftarrow 0$
>
> *for i=1 to n*
>
> > *Evaluate f(x_i)*
> >
> > *If f(x_i)<f(best)*
> >
> > > *best* $\leftarrow I(i); f(best) \leftarrow f(x_i)$
> >
> > *endif*
> >
> > *Make* $f(x_i) \leftarrow \varphi(f(x_i))$; *PopFit* $\leftarrow PopFit + f(x_i)$
>
> *Endfor*
>
> *for i=1 to n*
>
> > *RelFit_i* $\leftarrow f(x_i)/PopFit$;
>
> *endfor*
>
> *for i=1 to L*
>
> > *PG_i* $\leftarrow 0$;
> >
> > *for j=1 to n*
> >
> > > if $bit_{ji} = 1 \rightarrow PG_i \leftarrow PG_i + RelFit_j$
> >
> > *endFor*
>
> *endFor*

4. [Get new population]

> [Probabilistic Individuals]
>
> *for i = 1 to n*
>
> > *for j = 1 to L*
> >
> > > *Generate a uniform random number* $0 \leq \rho < 1$
> > >
> > > if $\rho \leq PG_j \rightarrow Bit_{ij} \leftarrow 1$; else $Bit_{ij} \leftarrow 0$
> >
> > *endFor*
>
> *endFor*
>
> [Mutate Individuals]
>
> *for i=1 to B2M*
>
> > *Generate uniform random numbers* $0 \leq \rho_1, \rho_2 < 1$
> >
> > *Mutate Bit* $\lceil \rho_2 L \rceil$ *of* $I(\lceil \rho_1 n \rceil)$
>
> *endFor*

5. $k \leftarrow k+1$

> If $k = G$ return *best* and stop; else *Go to step 3*

3.5   Random Mutation Hill-Climber (RMH)

This algorithm is the only non-evolutionary one considered in this study. In general, a "hill-climber" is an algorithm which attempts, iteratively, to improve on its best found value by refining the last attempt.

1. [Generate the individual]
for i=1 to L

       Generate a uniform random number $0 \leq \rho < 1$.

  If $\rho < 0.5$ make $bit_i \leftarrow 0$; else make $bit_i \leftarrow 1$.

endfor
Make *best* $\leftarrow$ I(0)

    BestFit $\leftarrow$ ∞

2. [Iterate]
for i = 1 to G

    [Evaluate the individual]

    f(i) $\leftarrow$ *fitness (x_i)*

    if *fitness(i)<BestFit* $\rightarrow$ *best* $\leftarrow$ I(x_i); *BestFit* $\leftarrow$ *fitness(x_i)*

    [Mutate]

      Generate a uniform random number $1 \leq k \leq L$; Make $bit_k \leftarrow \overline{bit_k}$

endfor

For the case of RMH, $S(t)$ is a unitary set such that $S(t) = \{s(t)\}$ where $s(t)$ is also a binary encoded candidate solution which is chosen at random and whose fitness is evaluated. We explored the behavior of the A_i's taking snapshots of their progress in steps of 50 generations up to 800. A GA works with several candidate solutions that allow it to explore different regions of Ω in parallel. On the other hand, the RMH works with a single candidate solution that allows it to explore a single region of Ω. The number of iterations of RMH needed for convergence, for this reason, differs significantly from that of a GA. For benchmarking purposes, therefore, we established the following standard.

1) Let M be the number of candidate solutions for a GA. Thus, for A_i it holds that $|S(t)| = M$

2) The upper bound on the number of iterations of a RMH is set to $M \times G$.

3) The upper bound on the number of iterations of any GA is set to G.

Any A_i will, therefore, approach the solution to a problem f in at most G iterations. For a detailed discussion of the algorithms see Appendix A.

4   Selected Functions

In this section we discuss the behavior of the algorithms for selected functions whose minima are known and, therefore, allow us to establish a measure of effectiveness relative to the best value found by the algorithm. The evaluation of all algorithms in A is based on a set of unconstrained functions (UF) which have some properties (multimodality, non-convexity, non-linearity, etc.) that make them good choices for benchmarking purposes,

For reasons of space we may only succinctly present 6 of the 23 functions considered in this study. 1) **Hansen Function**. Unimodal; it is defined in a n-dimensional space $\forall n \in N$:

$$f(n,x) = \sum_{i=0}^{4}(i+1)\cos(ix_0 + i + 1)\sum_{j=0}^{4}(j+1)\cos((j+2)x_1 + j + 1).$$ Ω is $|x_i| \leq 10$;

the known minimum is -176.54. 2) **De Jong's Function**. Continuous, convex and unimodal: $f(x) = \sum_{i=1}^{n} x_i^2$. Ω is $-5.12 \leq x_i \leq 5.12$, $i = 1,...,n$; the known minimum is 0: 3) **Rotated hyper-ellipsoid function**. Continuous, convex and unimodal:

$$f(x) = \sum_{i=1}^{n}\left(\sum_{j=1}^{i} x_j\right)^2 ;$$ Ω is $-65536 <= x_i <= 65536$; the known minimum is 0.

4) **Rosenbrock's valley function.** The global optimum lies inside a long, narrow, parabolic shaped flat valley. To find the valley is trivial. However convergence to the global optimum is difficult and hence this problem has been frequently used to test the performance of optimization algorithms: $f(x) = \sum_{i=1}^{n-1}[100(x_{i+1} - x_i^2)^2 + (1 - x_i)^2$.

Ω is $-2.048 \leq x_i \leq 2.048$, $i = 1,...,n$; the known minimum is 0. 5) **Rastrigin's function.** It is based on the function of De Jong with the addition of cosine modulation in order to produce frequent local minima. The function is highly multimodal: $f(x) = 10n + \sum_{i=1}^{n}[x_i^2 - 10\cos(2\pi x_i)$. Ω is $-5.12 \leq x_i \leq 5.12$, $i = 1,...,n$; the known minimum is 0. 6) **Schwefel's function.** It is deceptive in that the global minimum is geometrically distant, over the parameter space, from the next best local minima. Therefore, the search algorithms are potentially prone to convergence in the wrong direction: $f(x) = \sum_{i=1}^{n}[-x_i \sin(\sqrt{|x_i|}]$. Ω is $-500 \leq x_i \leq 500$, $i = 1,...,n$; the known minimum is -418.9828n.

All 23 functions have known optima. This allows us to define a relative measure of performance for A_i as follows:

$$Q(A_i, f_j) = \frac{y_j^* - y_j}{y_j^*} \tag{2}$$

where y_j^* is the known optimum of f_j and y_j is the best value found by A_i. We ran every algorithm 100 times for every problem and obtained its average performance. We obtained this average performance for all A_i with $G = 800$. We got snapshots of the process every 50 generations. In Figure 1 we show the corresponding results.

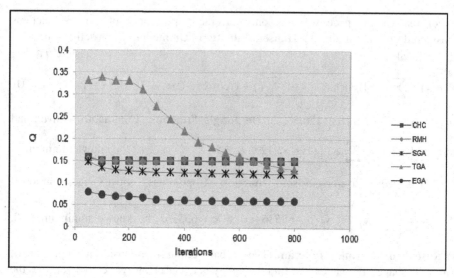

Fig. 1. Average Performance for UF

Notice that in these functions all of the GAs outperform the RMH only marginally, with the exception of EGA which is considerably better. Also notice that TGA (the canonical GA) is able to reach an acceptable value only after a large number of generations. From a further analysis we determined how the algorithms identify larger order schemata. We indicate that A_i is better than A_j when the order of the schemata of A_i is larger than the order of the schemata of A_j. (see Fig. 2). Consistent with the previous results, TGA is the slowest algorithm to identify schemata of higher order. That is, the sluggish nature of TGA is due to the fact that it spends many more generations in identifying the better individuals in terms of their schemata order.

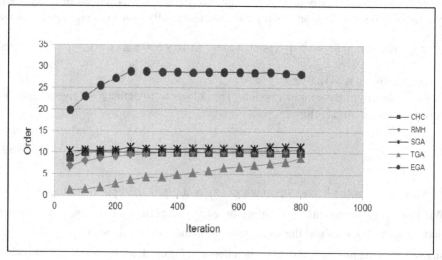

Fig. 2. Average order of the schemata for UF

5   Conclusions

The table for the suite of unconstrained problems (see Table 1) show that EGA outperforms the rest of the algorithms; in this case, notably so. TGA is, by far, the worst of the algorithms. Again RMH's behavior is close to SGA's and CHC's.

Table 1. Average minimum for the suite of unconstrained problems

Algorithm	Average Minimum	Relative Efficiency
EGA	0.0635	100.00%
SGA	0.1260	50.43%
RMH	0.1491	42.60%
CHC	0.1501	42.32%
TGA	0.2272	27.96%

The best algorithm is EGA. Considering the wide size and variety of the set of problems we can say that, with high probability, the EGA is the best global optimization algorithm in our study.

In concluding:

1. In all experiments, the EGA exhibited the best performance. We know that EGA is a good alternative in problems with hard search spaces (e.g. non-convex, constrained or highly dimensional spaces).
2. From a large set of runs it is possible to obtain a practical estimate of the schemata found by the algorithms.
3. The analysis of schemata order of the algorithms leads to results consistent with the previous one.
4. A similar analysis including other optimization techniques (e.g. Simulated annealing, Evolution strategies, Ant colony optimization, Particle swarm optimization, Differential evolution, etc.) may be easily implemented.

References

1. MacKay, B.: Mathematics and Statistics Models, http://serc.carleton.edu/introgeo/mathstatmodels/index.html
2. Mooney, D., Swift, R., Mooney, D.: A Course in Mathematical Modeling. Cambridge University Press (1999)
3. Kolesárová, A., Mesiar, R.: Parametric characterization of aggregation functions. Fuzzy Sets Syst. 160(6), 816–831 (2009)
4. Back, T.: Evolutionary algorithms in theory and practice: evolution strategies, evolutionary programming, genetic algorithms, ch. 4, pp. 149–159 (1996)
5. Coello, C.: A comprehensive survey of evolutionary-based multiobjective optimization techniques. Knowledge and Information Systems 1, 269–308 (1998)
6. De Jong, K.: An analysis of the behavior of a class of genetic adaptive systems, Diss. PhD thesis, Dept. of Computer and Comm. Sciences, Univ. of Michigan, Ann Arbor, MI (1975)

7. Endre, A., Hinterding, R., Michalewicz, Z.: Parameter control in evolutionary algorithms. IEEE Transactions on Evolutionary Computation 3(2), 124–141 (1999)
8. Mitchell, M.: An Introduction to Genetic Algorithms. MIT Press (1996)
9. Mitchell, M., Holland, J., Forrest, S.: When Will a Genetic Algorithm Outperform Hill Climbing? In: Advances of Neural Information Processing Systems, vol. 6, pp. 51–58. Morgan Kaufmann (1994)
10. Baker, J.: Adaptive selection methods for genetic algorithms. In: Grefenstette, J. (ed.) Proceedings of the 1st International Conference on Genetic Algorithms and their Applications, pp. 101–111. Lawrence Earlbaum Associates, N.J. (1985)
11. Spears, W.M., Anand, V.: A Study of Crossover Operators in Genetic Programming. In: Raś, Z.W., Zemankova, M. (eds.) ISMIS 1991. LNCS, vol. 542, pp. 409–418. Springer, Heidelberg (1991)
12. Bäck, T.: Self-Adaptation in Genetic Algorithms. In: Varela, F., Bourgine, P. (eds.) Toward a Practice of Autonomous Systems: Proceedings of the First European Conference on Artificial Life, pp. 263–271. MIT Press (1991)
13. Bäck, T.: Evolutionary Algorithms in Theory and Practice. Oxford University Press (1996)
14. De Jong, K.: An Analysis of the Behavior of a Class of Genetic Adaptive Systems. Doctoral Dissertation, University of Michigan (1975)
15. De Jong, K.A., Spears, W.M.: An Analysis of the Interacting Roles of Population Size and Crossover in Genetic Algorithms. In: Schwefel, H.-P., Männer, R. (eds.) PPSN 1990. LNCS, vol. 496, pp. 38–47. Springer, Heidelberg (1991)
16. Holland, J.: Adaptation in Natural and Artificial Systems. University of Michigan Press, Ann Arbor (1975)
17. Pohlheim, H.: GEATbx: Genetic and Evolutionary Algorithm Toolbox for use with MATLAB Documentation, Version 3.80 (released December 2006), http://www.geatbx.com/docu/index.html
18. Digalakis, J., Margaritis, K.: An experimental study of Benchmarking functions for genetic algorithms. Intern. J. Computer Math. 79(4), 403–416 (2002)
19. Vose, D.: Generalizing the notion of schema in genetic algorithms. Artificial Intelligence 50(3), 385–396 (1991)
20. Eshelman, L.: The CHC Adaptive Search Algorithm. How to Have Safe Search When Engaging in Nontraditional Genetic Recombination. In: Rawlins, G. (ed.) FOGA-1, pp. 265–283. Morgan Kaufmann (1991)
21. Rudolph, G.: Convergence Analysis of Canonical Genetic Algorithms. IEEE Transactions on Neural Networks 5(1), 96–101 (1994)
22. Eshelman: Op. cit. (1991)
23. Rezaee Jordehi, A., Hashemi, N., Nilsaz Dezfouli, H.: Analysis of the Strategies in Heuristic Techniques for Solving Constrained Optimisation Problems. Journal of American Science 8(10) (2012)
24. Sánchez-Ferrero, G.V., Arribas, J.I.: A Statistical-Genetic Algorithm to Select the Most Significant Features in Mammograms. In: Kropatsch, W.G., Kampel, M., Hanbury, A. (eds.) CAIP 2007. LNCS, vol. 4673, pp. 189–196. Springer, Heidelberg (2007)
25. Kuri-Morales, A.: A statistical genetic algorithm. In: Proc. of the 3rd National Computing Meeting, ENC 1999, Hgo., México, pp. 215–228 (1999)
26. Kuri-Morales, A., Villegas-Quezada, C.: A universal eclectic genetic algorithm for constrained optimization. In: Proceedings of the 6th European Congress on Intelligent Techniques and Soft Computing, vol. 1 (1998)

27. Kuri-Morales, A.F.: A methodology for the statistical characterization of genetic algorithms. In: Coello Coello, C.A., de Albornoz, Á., Sucar, L.E., Battistutti, O.C. (eds.) MICAI 2002. LNCS (LNAI), vol. 2313, pp. 79–88. Springer, Heidelberg (2002)
28. Back, T.: Evolutionary algorithms in theory and pactice: evolution strategies, evolutionary programming, genetic algorithms, ch. 4, pp. 149–159 (1996)
29. Mitchell, M.: An Introduction to Genetic Algorithms. MIT Press (1996)
30. Vose, D.: The Walsh Transform and the Theory of the Simple Genetic Algorithm. In: Pal, S., Wang, P. (eds.) Genetic Algorithms for Pattern Recognition. CRC Press (1996)
31. Rowhanimanesh, A., Sohrab, E.: A Novel Approach to Improve the Performance of Evolutionary Methods for Nonlinear Constrained Optimization. Advances in Artificial Intelligence (2012)

The Best Genetic Algorithm II

A Comparative Study of Structurally Different Genetic Algorithms

Angel Fernando Kuri-Morales[1], Edwin Aldana-Bobadilla[2], and Ignacio López-Peña[3]

[1] Instituto Tecnológico Autónomo de México
Río Hondo No. 1
México 01000, D.F.
México
akuri@itam.mx

[2] Universidad Nacional Autónoma de México
IIMAS
México 04510, D.F.
México
edwynjavier@yahoo.es

[3] Universidad Nacional Autónoma de México
IIMAS
México 04510, D.F.
México
ignalp@gmail.com

Abstract. Genetic Algorithms (GAs) have long been recognized as powerful tools for optimization of complex problems where traditional techniques do not apply. In [1] we reported the superior behavior, out of 4 evolutionary algorithms and a hill climber, of a particular breed: the so-called Eclectic Genetic Algorithm (EGA). EGA was tested vs. a set (TS) consisting of large number of selected problems most of which have been used in previous works as an experimental testbed. However, the conclusions of the said benchmark are restricted to the functions in TS. In this work we extend the previous results to a much larger set (U) consisting of $\zeta \approx \sum_{i=1}^{31} (2^{64})^i \approx 11 \times 10^{50}$ unconstrained functions. Randomly selected functions in U were minimized for 800 generations each; the minima were averaged in batches of 36 each yielding $\overline{X}_i$ for the i-th batch. This process was repeated until the $\overline{X}_i$'s displayed a Gaussian distribution with parameters $\mu_{\overline{x}}$ and $\sigma_{\overline{x}}$. From these, the parameters μ and σ describing the probabilistic behavior of each of the algorithms for U were calculated with 95% reliability. We give a sketch of the proof of the convergence of an elitist GA to the global optimum of any given function. We describe the methods to: a) Generate the functions; b) Calculate μ and σ for U and c) Evaluate the relative efficiency of all algorithms in our study. EGA's behavior was the best of all algorithms.

Keywords: Genetic algorithms, Unbiased functions, Statistical validation.

F. Castro, A. Gelbukh, and M. González (Eds.): MICAI 2013, Part II, LNAI 8266, pp. 16–29, 2013.

1   Introduction

Optimization is an all pervading problem in engineering and the sciences. It is, therefore, important to rely on an optimization tool of proven efficiency and reliability. In this paper we compare a set of optimization algorithms which were analyzed in [1] over a set of unconstrained selected functions in $\Re \times \Re$. Here we extend our study in two ways: First, we consider a, for all practical purposes, unlimited reservoir of unconstrained functions. Second, we use the same basic reservoir so that the functions correspond to $\Re \times \Re$, $\Re \times \Re^2$ and $\Re \times \Re^3$. The results may be generalized for $\Re \times \Re^n$. In analogous comparative studies in the past (for instance see [2], [3], [4]) it is always true that a) The nature of the algorithms under study and their number are necessarily limited and b) The selection of the benchmarking functions obeys to subjective criteria. We know that any elitist GA will find the global optimum. The time (iterations) the GA has to spend is, however, not bounded. Therefore it seems appropriate to seek the fastest GA, in general. We analyze a set whose functions are a) Representative , b) Large enough, c) Automatically generated and d) Randomly selected. We may apply statistical methodologies to extract the probabilistic behavior of the algorithms under study with arbitrary reliability. The results from an analysis following the previous guidelines will enable us to ascertain which of the GAs is fastest, i.e. the best, for most functions likely to be found in practice.

In [5] it is shown that elitist GAs always converge to a global optimum. The basic idea hinges on the following: a) Because GAs perform the search in a discrete space, the number of possible points to examine is finite; b) Any combination of individuals in the population may be thought of as a state in a Markov chain (MC), c) Via mutation, there is a non-zero probability that the GA will reach all possible states in the MC and d) If the best individual is retained throughout the process, when the GA is stopped, the best individual will correspond to the best possible solution to the problem. This is true iff there is no sink state (i.e. if there is always a non-zero probability of exiting a given state of the MC). Holland's original GA [6] did not include elitism. But most practical implementations do. In fact, any elitist algorithm, even if it is not evolutionary, satisfying the condition of exhaustive visits to all possible states, will, by the same token, reach a global optimum. A case in point is the so-called Random Mutation Hill Climber or RMH (for which see [1, 7, 8]). If we keep track of the best value, however, the behavior of the algorithm may be illustrated as in Figure 1. In this case, even if the process looses its aim in the final stages of the evolutionary search, the best value is retained and, eventually, the best overall value will be reached.

It is easy to see that, given the above, the only basic difference in speed between a RMH (for example) and a GA has to reside in the crossover operator. The crossover component of a GA is actually responsible for the convergence speed of the process. Because of this we want to analyze several possible alternative GAs in trying to determine which is most effective. The GAs considered were the following:

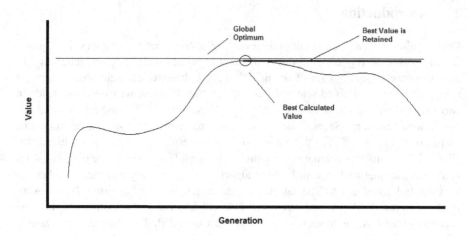

Fig. 1. Convergence with Elitism

- a) An elitist canonical GA (in what follows referred to as TGA [eliTist GA]) [7].
- b) A Cross generational elitist selection, Heterogeneous recombination, and Cataclysmic mutation algorithm (CHC algorithm) [9].
- c) An Eclectic Genetic Algorithm (EGA) [12].
- d) A Statistical GA (SGA) [10] [11].

For a detailed description and the pseudo-code of all the algorithms see [1]. Because we found that EGA was the best, we consider of interest to reproduce it here. When this algorithm was first reported it included self-adaptation and periodic cataclysmic mutation. Later studies [13] showed that neither of the two mechanisms was compulsory. EGA is relatively simple, fast and easy to program. In what follows, the next variables are used: $n \rightarrow$ number of individuals; $L \rightarrow$ length of the chromosome in bits; $P_M \rightarrow$ Probability of mutation; $Pc \rightarrow$ probability of crossover; $I(i) \rightarrow$ the i-th individual; $G \rightarrow$ number of generations.

Pseudo-Code of the Eclectic GA (EGA)
0. $B2M \leftarrow \lceil nL \times P_M \rceil$ (Expected number of mutations per generation)
1. $i \leftarrow 1$
2. Generate a random population
3. Evaluate the population.
4. [Duplicate Population]
for j = 1 to n
    $I(n+j) \leftarrow I(j)$
    fitness(n+j) $\leftarrow$ fitness(j)
endfor

5. [Deterministic Selection Annular Crossover]

for j=1 to n/2

    Generate a uniform random number $0 \le \rho < 1$

    If $\rho \le P_c$

        Generate a random number $1 \le \rho < L/2$

        Interchange the semi-ring starting at locus ρ between I(j)

        and I(n-j-1)

    endif

endfor

5. [Mutation]

for j=1 to B2M

    Generate uniform random numbers $0 \le \rho_1, \rho_2 < 1$

    Mutate Bit $\lceil \rho_2 L \rceil$ of $I(\lceil \rho_1 n \rceil)$

endFor

6. [Evaluate the New Individuals]

Calculate fitness(x_i) for i=1,...,n

7. [$\mu + \lambda$ Selection]

Sort the 2n individuals by their fitness, ascending

8. *i $\leftarrow$ i+1*

  if i = G return I(1) and stop

  Go to 3

The rest of the paper is organized as follows: in Section 2 we show how to extract the mean value μ and the standard deviation σ from the minima of the functions in U.

In Section 3 we describe how the functions in U may be generated and evaluated in $\Re \times \Re$, $\Re \times \Re^2$ and $\Re \times \Re^3$. In Section 4 we present our conclusions.

2   Statistical Determination of the Best Algorithm in U

A thorough experimental test of a given set of algorithms (A) implies running a large series of minimization trials. The probability that A_i reaches some minimum value (which we denote by κ) is unknown. These κ will vary for every problem and will distribute with mean μ and standard deviation σ which are also unknown. We shall approximate these values by sampling U. It is, therefore, of utmost importance that we select sample S adequately; both in its nature and its size. Typically, the size of S is determined from assumptions (directly or indirectly) depending on the form of the population's (κ's distribution). We followed a method which does not necessitate from such assumptions. It relies on the knowledge that any sampling distribution of means (sdom) will eventually become Gaussian. Therefore, we generate a succession of problems to optimize (i.e. minimizing, every time, 36 problems of U) and calculate the corresponding mean $\overline{X}$. The iterations will be stopped only after the κ's are distributed normally. Normality was considered to have been reached after dividing the results in deciles when a) $\chi^2 \leq 3.28$ and b) O_i, the number of observations in the *i-th* decil, is 5 or more. We rely on the following theorems.

Theorem 1

Any sampling distribution of means (*sdom*) is distributed normally for a large enough sample size n. [The Central Limit Theorem].

Remark: It is considered that any $n>20$ is satisfactory. We have chosen $n=36$.

Theorem 2

In a normal distribution (with mean $\mu_{\bar{X}}$ and standard deviation $\sigma_{\bar{X}}$) approximately one tenth of the observations lie in the intervals: $\mu_{\bar{X}}-5\sigma_{\bar{X}}$ to $\mu_{\bar{X}}-1.29\sigma_{\bar{X}}$; $\mu_{\bar{X}}-1.29\sigma_{\bar{X}}$ to $\mu_{\bar{X}}-0.85\sigma_{\bar{X}}$; $\mu_{\bar{X}}-0.85\sigma_{\bar{X}}$ to $\mu_{\bar{X}}-0.53\sigma_{\bar{X}}$; $\mu_{\bar{X}}-0.53\sigma_{\bar{X}}$ to $\mu_{\bar{X}}-0.26\sigma_{\bar{X}}$; $\mu_{\bar{X}}-0.26\sigma_{\bar{X}}$ to $\mu_{\bar{X}}$ and the positive symmetrical.

Remark: These deciles divide the area under the normal curve in 10 unequally spaced intervals where the expected number of observed events will be one tenth.

Theorem 3

The relation between the population distribution's parameters μ and σ and the *sdom*'s parameters $\mu_{\bar{X}}$ and $\sigma_{\bar{X}}$ is given by $\mu = \mu_{\bar{X}}$ and $\sigma = \sqrt{n} \cdot \sigma_{\bar{X}}$.

Theorem 4

The proportion of any distribution found within k standard deviations of the mean is, at least, $1-1/k^2$. That is, $p(\mu - k\sigma \leq y_i \leq \mu + k\sigma) \geq 1 - 1/k^2$.

We selected $k = 3.1623$, which guarantees that our observations will lie within the selected interval with $p \geq 0.90$.

The question we want to answer is: How small should χ^2 be in order for us to ascertain normality? Remember the χ^2 test is designed to verify whether two distributions *differ* significantly so that one may reject the null hypothesis, i.e. the two populations are statistically NOT equivalent. This corresponds to large values of χ^2 and is a function of the degrees of freedom. In this case, if we wanted to be 95% certain that the observed $\bar{x}_i$'s were NOT normally distributed, we would demand that $\chi^2 \geq 14.0671$. However, this case is different. We want to ensure the likelihood that the observed behavior of the $\bar{x}_i$'s IS normal. In order to do this we performed the following Monte Carlo experiment. We set a desired probability P that the $\bar{x}_i$'s are normal. We establish a best desired value of χ^2 which we will call χ_{best}. We make $NS \leftarrow 50$. We then generate NS instances of $N(0,1)$ and count the number of times the value of the instance is in every decile. We calculate the value of the corresponding χ^2 and store it. We thusly calculate 100,000 combinations of size NS. Out of these combinations we count those for which $\chi^2 \leq \chi_{best}$ AND there are at least $o_{min} = 5$ observations per decile. This number divided by 100,000 (which we shall call p) is the experimental probability that, for NS observations, χ^2 "performs" as required.

We repeat this process increasing *NS* up to 100. In every instance we test whether $p >$ *P*. If such is the case we decrement the value of χ_{best} and re-start the process. Only when $p \leq P$ does the process end. The probability that χ^2 exceeds χ_{best} as a function of the number of problems being minimized (M) is shown in Figure 2. Every point represents the proportion of combinations satisfying the required conditions per 100,000 trials. For this experiment, $\chi_{best} = 3.28$. We obtained an approximation to a Gompertz model with *S=0.0023* and *r=0.9926*. It has the form $p = ae^{-e^{b-cM}}$; where $a = 0.046213555$, $b = 12.40231200$, $c = 0.195221110$. From this expression we solve for M, to get $M = \{b - \ln[\ln(a / p)]\} / c$. As may be observed, *p<0.05* for $M \geq 85$, which says that the probability of obtaining $\chi^2 \leq 3.28$ by chance alone is less than five in one hundred. Therefore, it is enough to obtain 85 or more $\overline{x_i}$'s to calculate μ and σ with 95% reliability.

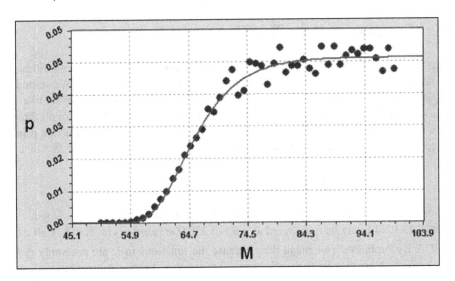

Fig. 2. Probability of χ^2 and $O_i>5$ as a function of the number of problems solved

In what follows we describe the algorithm which results from all the foregoing considerations.

Algorithm for the Determination of the Distribution's Parameters
Select an optimization algorithm *A*.
1. Make $G \leftarrow$ number of generations.
2. Generate a random binary string. This is one possible $f_i(x)$.
3. Minimize $f_i(x)$ iterating *A*, *G* times.
4. Store the best minimum value κ_i.
5. Repeat steps (2-4) 36 times.

6. Calculate the average best value $\overline{K}_j = (1/36) \sum_{i=1}^{36} \kappa_i$.

7. Repeat steps (5-6) 50 times.

8. Calculate $\mu_{\overline{\kappa}}$ and $\sigma_{\overline{\kappa}}$.

9. Repeat step (7) 85 times. The *sdom*'s distribution is normal with $p=0.95$.

10. Calculate $\mu = \mu_{\overline{\kappa}}$ and $\sigma = 6\sigma_{\overline{\kappa}}$. We have inferred the expected best value κ and the standard deviation for this algorithm.

From T4:

$$P(\mu - 3.1623\sigma \leq \kappa \leq \mu + 3.1623\sigma) \geq 0.90 \tag{1}$$

We have found a quantitative, unbiased measure of A_i's performance in $\Re \times \Re$. These values for the different A_i's allow us to make a fair unbiased assessment of their behavior.

3   Generation of U for $\Re \times \Re^n$

Once we have determined how to extract the parameters of the *pdf* for the algorithms we need an unbiased and automated way to obtain the problems to solve. We started by using Walsh's polynomials for $\Re \times \Re$. Next we used a monomial basis to, likewise, do so for $\Re \times \Re$, $\Re \times \Re^2$, $\Re \times \Re^3$. The behavior of the algorithms for all three cases was analyzed. The distributions were statistically equivalent. An induction principle leads to the conclusion that the observed behavior will be similar for $\Re \times \Re^n$.

3.1   Generation of Unbiased Functions Using Walsh Polynomials

A reservoir of 250,000 randomly generated binary strings of length L ($32 \leq |L| \leq 1024$) may be interpreted as a set of 250,000 functions in $\Re \times \Re$. Call this set "U". By "unbiased" we mean that, because the functions in U are randomly generated, there is no bias in their selection. To generate functions automatically we resort to Walsh functions $\psi_j(x)$ which form an orthogonal basis for real-valued functions defined on $(0,1)^\ell$, where x is a bit string and ℓ is its length. Henceforth, any function $f(x)$ thusly defined can be written as a linear combination of the ψ_j's yielding a Walsh polynomial.

$$f(x) = \sum_{j=0}^{31} \omega_j \psi_j(x) \tag{2}$$

where
$$\psi_j(x) = \begin{cases} +1 & \text{if } \pi(x \wedge j) = 0 \\ -1 & \text{if } \pi(x \wedge j) = 1 \end{cases} \tag{3}$$

$x \wedge j$ is the bitwise AND of x and j; $\pi(x)$ denotes the parity of x; and $\omega_j \in \Re$. Therefore, the index j and argument x of $\psi_j(x)$ must be expressed in comparable binary. We, therefore, used 16 bits to represent x in a $P_{0,15}(x)$ format. This means that we used one sign bit, 0 integers and 15 bits in a fixed point format for every term in the x's of (2). Consequently, we also used 16 bits for the indices j of (2). That implies that $-0.999969482421875 \leq x \leq +0.999969482421875$ and $0 \leq j \leq 65,535$. For example, consider $\psi_{61,680}(0.00048828125) = -1$. To see why, notice that $j=61,680$, in binary, is 1111000011110000. Also, $x= 0.00048828125$ (with $P_{0,15}(x)$ format), corresponds to 0000000000010000. And $x \wedge j = 0000000000010000$ for which $\pi(0000000000010000) = 1$. The length of the binary strings for the coefficients was also made 16 and, hence, $-0.999969482421875 \leq \omega_j \leq +0.999969482421875$. Therefore, any Walsh monomial $\omega_j \psi_j$ is uniquely represented by a binary string of length 32. Finally, we allow at least one but no more than 32 non-zero terms in (2). This last conditions is mathematically expressed by including an α_j term which may only take two values (1 or 0) depending on whether the term appears. Given this, we have

$$\gamma(x) = \sum_{j=1}^{32} \alpha_j \omega_j \psi_j(x)$$

(3)

where $\qquad \alpha_j = \begin{cases} 1 & \textit{if the } j-\textit{th term is present} \\ 0 & \textit{if the } j-\textit{th term is not present} \end{cases}$

Denoting with τ the number of non-zero terms in 3 we see that a full ($\tau = 32$) function's binary representation is 1,024 bits long. We denote the space of all possible functions defined by (3) with U and its cardinality with ξ. It is easy to see that $\xi \approx \sum_{i=1}^{31} (2^{64})^i \approx 11 \times 10^{50}$. The method outlined provides us with an unlimited reservoir of functions in $\Re \times \Re$. Equally importantly, the random selection of a number τ and the further random selection of τ different indices and τ different ω_j's yields a uniquely identifiable function from such reservoir. The pool of Walsh functions was randomly generated at the beginning; the $f(x)$'s which the algorithms were required to minimize were all gotten from the same pool, thus allowing us to test the algorithms in a homogeneous functional environment.

3.2   Generation of Unbiased Functions from a Monomial Basis

Although it is possible to extend Walsh polynomials to higher dimensions, we found it more convenient to appeal to a monomial basis for the remaining cases, as follows.

3.2.1   The Case y=f(x)

For the same functions in U we generated 150 random values $0 \le x_i < 1$ and calcu-lated $y_i = f(x_i)$ for $i=1,...,150$. The sample consists of 150 binary strings of length 16. We stored these binary strings in a set we shall call **B**. Likewise, we stored the resulting y_i's in a set we shall call **F**. Notice that $x_i, y_i \in \mathfrak{R}$. Then we obtained the least squares approximating polynomial of degree 7. We will denote this set of ap-proximated polynomial functions as U_2.

We minimized enough polynomials in U_2 for the distribution of the means to be normal. We did this for each of the algorithms in our study. The results of the mini-mization process are shown in Figure 3.

A χ^2 goodness-of-fit test did not justify us to reject the null hypothesis H0: "The distributions of the Walsh basis functions (WBF) and the monomial basis functions (MBF) are similar". Hence, we conclude that the statistical behaviors of the algorithms when faced with problems defined with WBF and MBF are analogous. A quality index Q = *mean value of the minima* with $p = 0.95$ was defined for all the algorithms in our study. To visually enhance the difference between algorithms, we represent the values of Q in a logarithmic scale. Since some of the Q's are negative, we first scaled them into the interval $[\delta ,1)$, where $\delta << 1$. $Q*$ is defined as follows:

$$Q*= log_{10}\{[Q_i-min(Q)]/[max(Q)-min(Q)](1-\delta)+\delta\}$$

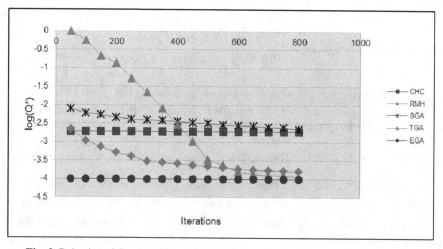

Fig. 3. Behavior of the algorithms minimizing unbiased polynomial *y=f(x)* functions

3.2.2   The Case z=f(x,y)

In this case we considered the binary strings of set **B**. They were split into two binary string sets of length 8 each, with $P_{0.7}$. Then the leftmost 8 bits were mapped into $\mathfrak{R}$ (which we now call x) and the rightmost 8 bits were also mapped into $\mathfrak{R}$ (which we shall call y). These (x_i,y_i) pairs were stored in matrix XY. The values of the indepen-dent variable z were those of set **F**. Our aim is to find polynomials of the form

$z=f(x,y)$. In general, the problem is to find a set of (m) coefficients on a set of (n) independent variables expressed as a linear combination of monomials of the n variables of degree up to $d_1,...,d_n$ such that the absolute difference between an approximating function and the observed data is minimized. This problem is considerably more complex than the case $y=f(x)$. Furthermore, m grows exponentially as n and d_i do. For instance, if $n=2$ and $d_1=d_2=7$, $m=64$; likewise, for $n=3$, $d_1 = d_2 = d_3 = 7$ we have that $m=512$. This is the so-called called *curse of dimensionality*. Both problems were circumvented by applying the Ascent Algorithm (AA) [14]. The purpose of this algorithm is to express the behavior of a dependent variable (y) as a function of a set of n independent variables (v).

$$y = f(v_1, v_2,..., v_n)$$
$$y = f(\mathbf{v})$$
(4)

The approximant is <u>defined</u> to have the following form:

$$y = c_1 X_1 + c_2 X_2 + ... + c_m X_m$$
(5)

X_i denotes a combination of the independent variables. That is, $X_i = f_i(v)$. According to the way these combinations are defined one may obtain different approximants. Now, from the universal approximation theorem [15], any function of n variables may be approximated with at most

$$T = \sum_{i=1}^{k} \left[\frac{\left(2i-1+\left(\sum_{j=1}^{k} \frac{(2j-1+n)!}{(2j-1)!n!}\right)\right)!}{(2i-1)!\left(\left[\sum_{j=1}^{k} \frac{(2j-1+n)!}{(2j-1)!n!}\right]\right)!} \right]$$
(6)

terms of degree k. The expression of T yields numbers of the order of 10^{12} even for small n. Obviously it makes no sense to try to approximate any function with a polynomial of these many terms. Therefore, we use a GA to select the best subset of the terms we decide to consider to make the problem reasonably expressible.

Genetic Polynomials
The basic reason to choose AA is that it is not dependent on the origin of the X_i in (5). We decided them to be the monomials of a full polynomial

$$y = \sum_{i_1=0}^{d_1}...\sum_{i_n}^{d_n} c_{i1}...c_{in} v_1^{i1}...v_n^{in}$$. But it makes no difference to the AA whether the X_i

are gotten from a set of monomials or they are elements of arbitrary data vectors. To avoid the problem of the coefficient's explosion we define the number (say β) of desired monomials of the approximant and then focus on slecting which of the p possible ones these will be. There are $C(p, \beta)$ possible combinations of monomials and even for modest values of p and β an exhaustive search is out of the question. This optimization problem may be tackled using a genetic algorithm (GA), as follows.

The genome is a binary string of size p. Every bit in it represents a monomial. These monomials are ordered as per the sequence of the consecutive powers of the variables. If the bit is '1' it means that the corresponding monomial remains while if it is a '0' it means that such monomial is not to be considered. All one has to ensure is that the number of 1's is equal to β. Assume, for example, that $y = f(v_1, v_2, v_3)$ and that $d_1=1$, $d_2=d_3=2$. In such case the powers assigned to the $2 \times 3 \times 3 = 18$ positions of the genome are

000,001,002,010,011,012,020,021,022,100,101,102,110,111,112,120,121,122.

For the case where $\beta=6$ the genome 110000101010000001 corresponds to the polynomial in (7).

$$P(v_1,v_2,v_3) = c_{000} + c_{001}v_3 + c_{020}v_2{}^2 + c_{022}v_2{}^2v_3{}^2 + c_{101}v_1v_3 + c_{122}v_1v_2{}^2v_3{}^2 \qquad (7)$$

The initial population of the GA consists of a set of binary strings of length p in which there are only β 1's. The RMS error

$$\varepsilon_{RMS} = \sqrt{\frac{1}{N}\sum_{i=1}^{N}(f_i - y_i)^2} \qquad (8)$$

is calculated for each tested polynomial and, at the end of the process, the one exhibiting the smallest such error is selected as the best approximant for the original data set. That is, for every genome the terms corresponding to the 1's are calculated. These take the place of the X in (5). Then the AA is applied to get the corresponding coefficients. To each combination of β 1's there corresponds a set of β coefficients minimizing $\varepsilon_{MAX} = max(|f_i - y_i|) \; \forall i$. For this set of coefficients ε_{RMS} is calculated. This is the fitness function for the GA. In the end, we retain the coefficients which best minimize ε_{RMS} (from the GA) out of those which best minimize ε_{MAX} (from the AA).

In our experiments, we set $d_1=d_2=4$ and $\beta=6$. We obtained an expression of the form:

$$z = c_1 X_1 + c_2 X_2 + c_3 X_3 + c_4 X_4 + c_5 X_5 + c_6 X_6 \qquad (9)$$

where ς_{ij}'s value is either 0 or 1 as determined by the GA and

$$X_i = \sum_{i=0}^{4}\sum_{j=0}^{4}\varsigma_{ij}c_{ij}x^i y^j \qquad (10)$$

Following the above procedure we found a polynomial for each of the functions in xyz. We denote this new set of approximated polynomial functions as U_3. Once the distribution of the means is normal, as before, we inferred the mean μ and the standard deviation σ of the *pdf* of the minimum values reached by each of the algorithms in our study. The results of the minimization process are shown in Figure 4.

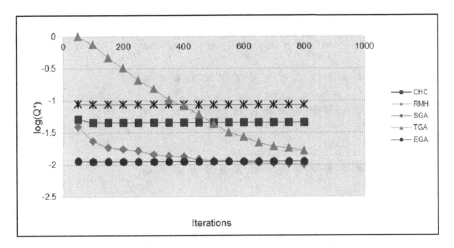

Fig. 4. Behavior of algorithms minimizing unbiased polynomial $z=f(x,y)$ functions

3.2.3   The Case w=f(x,y,z)

In this case we considered the binary strings of set **B** but they were now split into three binary sets of lengths 5-5-6 with $P_{0,4}$, $P_{0,4}$, $P_{0,5,}$ respectively. Then the leftmost 5 bits, the middle 5 bits and the rightmost 6 bits were, likewise, mapped into $\Re$. We call the corresponding variables x, y and z. These (x_i, y_i, z_i) triples were stored in matrix *XYZ*. The values of the independent variable w were those of set **F**. Our aim is to find a polynomial of the form $w=f(x,y,z)$. Following a process entirely similar to the one described above, we now defined $d1=d2=d3=4$ with $\beta=6$ and obtained

$$w = c_1 X_1 + c_2 X_2 + c_3 X_3 + c_4 X_4 + c_5 X_5 + c_6 X_6 \tag{11}$$

but now

$$X_i = \sum_{i=0}^{4} \sum_{j=0}^{4} \sum_{k=0}^{4} \varsigma_{ij} c_{ij} x^i y^j z^k \tag{12}$$

Again we found a polynomial for each of the functions now in *wxyz*. We denote this new set of approximated polynomial functions with U_4. We minimized enough polynomials in U_4 for the distribution of the means to be normal. Again we inferred the mean μ and the standard deviation σ of the *pdf* of the minimum values reached by each of the algorithms. The results of the minimization process are shown in Figure 5.

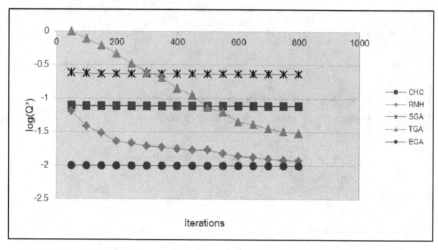

Fig. 5. Behavior of algorithms minimizing unbiased polynomial $w=f(x,y,z)$ functions

4   Conclusions and Future Work

The results of our study show:

1) All the algorithms have a very similar behavior. We had to use a logarithmic scale on the quality (Q*) of the results to make them apparent.

2) Remarkably, the RMH turns out to be as efficient as any of the GAs except for EGA.

3) Their behavior as the search space grows from $\Re \times \Re$, to $\Re \times \Re^2$ to $\Re \times \Re^3$ is statistically indistinguishable.

4) We may expect, from an induction principle, that the algorithms behave similarly in $\Re \times \Re^n$.

5) Even though all algorithms eventually approach similar minima, they do so with evidently different rates. For example, TGA does not reach adequate values until the very last generations.

6) SGA turns out to be the worst algorithm albeit it is the fastest (in CPU time) of all the A_i.

7) As in [1], where the minimized functions were hand-picked, EGA is the best algorithm of all.

8) EGA reaches its best minima in a relatively short number of generations. Therefore, it is guaranteed to reach the best solution without having to specify a large G.

In a paper to appear soon, we show that EGA works above par even when faced with constrained problems. Intuitively this should be the case since even constrained problems have to be, somehow, transformed into unconstrained ones. In the end, it appears that, for very simple problems, RMH is enough to reach acceptable solutions given enough time. However, when faced with more demanding ones, EGA seems to be the best alternative: it is better and faster.

References

1. Kuri-Morales, A., Aldana-Bobadilla, E.: The Best Genetic Algorithm I: A Comparative Study of Structurally Different Genetic Algorithms (sent for publication)
2. De Jong, K.: An analysis of the behavior of a class of genetic adaptive systems., Diss. PhD thesis, Dept. of Computer and Comm. Sciences, Univ. of Michigan, Ann Arbor, MI (1975)
3. Endre, A., Hinterding, R., Michalewicz, Z.: Parameter control in evolutionary algorithms. IEEE Transactions on Evolutionary Computation 3(2), 124–141 (1999)
4. Molga, M., Smutnicki, C.: Test functions for optimization needs, http://www.zsd.ict.pwr.wroc.pl/files/docs/functions.pdf (retrieved March 11, 2012)
5. Rudolph, G.: Convergence Analysis of Canonical Genetic Algorithms. IEEE Transactions on Neural Networks 5(1), 96–101 (1994)
6. Holland, J.: Adaptation in Natural and Artificial Systems. University of Michigan Press, Ann Arbor (1975)
7. Mitchell, M.: An Introduction to Genetic Algorithms. MIT Press (1996)
8. Mitchell, M., Holland, J., Forrest, S.: When Will a Genetic Algorithm Outperform Hill Climbing? In: Advances of Neural Information Processing Systems, vol. 6, pp. 51–58. Morgan Kaufmann (1994)
9. Eshelman, L.: The CHC Adaptive Search Algorithm. How to Have Safe Search When Engaging in Nontraditional Genetic Recombination. In: Rawlins, G. (ed.) FOGA-1, pp. 265–283. Morgan Kaufmann (1991)
10. Sánchez-Ferrero, G.V., Arribas, J.I.: A Statistical-Genetic Algorithm to Select the Most Significant Features in Mammograms. In: Kropatsch, W.G., Kampel, M., Hanbury, A. (eds.) CAIP 2007. LNCS, vol. 4673, pp. 189–196. Springer, Heidelberg (2007)
11. Kuri-Morales, A.: A statistical genetic algorithm. In: Proc. of the 3rd National Computing Meeting, ENC 1999, Hgo., México, pp. 215–228 (1999)
12. Kuri-Morales, A., Villegas-Quezada, C.: A universal eclectic genetic algorithm for constrained optimization. In: Proceedings of the 6th European Congress on Intelligent Techniques and Soft Computing, vol. 1 (1998)
13. Kuri-Morales, A.: A methodology for the statistical characterization of genetic algorithms. In: Coello Coello, C.A., de Albornoz, Á., Sucar, L.E., Battistutti, O.C. (eds.) MICAI 2002. LNCS (LNAI), vol. 2313, pp. 79–88. Springer, Heidelberg (2002)
14. Ugowski, H.: Remarks on the Ascent Algorithm for the Linear Minimax Problem. COMPEL: The International Journal for Computation and Mathematics in Electrical and Electronic Engineering 8(3), 181–184 (1989)
15. Cybenko, G.: Approximations by superpositions of sigmoidal functions. Mathematics of Control, Signals, and Systems 2(4), 303–314 (1989)

The Concept of Confidence
for Inheritance-Based Genetic Algorithms

Rubén Aguilar-Rivera[1], Manuel Valenzuela-Rendón[2],
and José Rodríguez-Ortiz[3]

[1] Doctorado Tecnologías de Información y Comunicaciones
ITESM Campus Monterrey
ra.aguilar.phd@itesm.mx
[2] Depto. Ciencias Computacionales
ITESM Campus Monterrey
valenzuela@itesm.mx
[3] Depto. Mecatrónica y Automatización
ITESM Campus Monterrey
jjrodriguez@itesm.mx

Abstract. In this article the possibility of saving evaluations during
the running of the genetic algorithm is investigated. The study begins
with the presentation of the concept on inheritance, already proposed
in literature. The article develops further this idea with the addition of
the concept of confidence, enabling the possibility of new schemes of inheritance, such as dynamic ones. The intuition of this enhancement is
mathematically explored. The performance of the new schemes is compared via experimentation, leading to some interesting results.

1 Introduction

The genetic algorithm (GA) can be used as a powerful optimization technique
suitable for a wide range of applications. A brief description follows: Several solutions are proposed as a population of candidates; these are efficiently recombined
using suitable operators to make the population converge into the optimal solution. Schemata theorem provides an explanation to GA dynamics, establishing
landmark concepts such as "building-blocks" or "Implied parallelism".

The properties which are the foundations of GA advantages are also the base
of their hindrances. Assuming a population of N individuals evolved along M
generations, a total of MN evaluations should be needed to find the optimal
solution. Some of them can be avoided with little effort. For example, if the new
individual is identical to some of the parents, its evaluation is not necessary. The
possibility of further savings implies an interesting question.

The literature describes some of the efforts taken into the direction of an
answer. For example, Goldberg [2] provides useful guidelines to determine population size and number of generations. Although it is true the proper selection of
GA parameters is essential to good performance, these approaches do not take
into account the possibility "to do more with less." It is the objective of this

F. Castro, A. Gelbukh, and M. González (Eds.): MICAI 2013, Part II, LNAI 8266, pp. 30–40, 2013.

article the exploration of promising ways to make an efficient search with some given MN computation time.

This work is organized in the following manner: In the first part, the concept of inheritance is introduced. Then the concept of confidence is proposed as a way to improve inheritance performance. Then, confidence-based schemes are presented. In the second part, the GA and the inheritance-based algorithms are compared with the use of benchmark problems. Finally, the results are discussed in the conclusion.

2   About Inheritance

In the direction of improving the efficiency of GA, the work of Smith [6] is found. In that report, the concept of inheritance is explained for the first time. From the ideas of Goldberg ([2] and [3]), it is clear that noise is inherent to the operation of GAs. The idea behind inheritance is that noise can be purposely induced into the run of GA for the sake of evaluation-saving. In the work of Grefenstette [4], the possibility to use approximate function evaluations instead of the real objective functions is investigated.

The key idea of inheritance sustains that parent fitness can be used to compute a good enough estimation of child fitness value. Recalling the schemata theorem, it is clear an individual contains several schemata (according to Goldberg [1], around the order of $O(N^3)$ in an entire population), when crossover takes place, parents common schemata will pass unmodified to the child. Therefore, an approximation based on parents evaluation will be an estimation of common schemata average fitness. When the parents are more alike, the estimation will be a better approximation of the child's real fitness value. At the light of this idea, parents not common schemata passed down to the child will be a source of noise. Then, the use of approximate evaluation will induce a source of noise besides the ones already present in the GA dynamics.

The original idea is to estimate a fraction of the population each generation. For the sake of this article, let α be the fraction of the population that is estimated, therefore, randomly chosen αN individuals will inherit their evaluations from their parents. In the work of Smith [6], the average of parents fitness is proposed as a good estimator of child fitness. Also, the weighted sum of fitness, based on cross-point, is proposed in that report. Expressions for both ways of inheritance estimation appear in equations 1 and 2.

$$\hat{f} = \left(\frac{f_{p1} + f_{p2}}{2} \right), \tag{1}$$

$$\hat{f} = (k c_{p1} + (1 - k) c_{p2}). \tag{2}$$

In equation 2, k represents the normalized crossover point. From Smith [6], an expression of the evolution of schemata fitness over time when inheritance is applied can be found to be

$$f_{e(t+1)}(H_i) = \left[\frac{f_{e(t)} + \bar{f}}{2}\right]\alpha + (1 - \alpha)f_t(H_i). \tag{3}$$

Equation 3 means the overall effect of inheritance is to drift estimations to the mean value of common schemata present in population. From this equation, the use of equation 1 as a way to compute inheritance seems reasonable. For the sake to remain supported over the developed theory, this work will use equation 1 to compute inheritance.

3   About Confidence

It should be clear the use of inheritance makes the GA work under uncertainty. Since crossover is a stochastic operator, there is the possibility an individual inherits its fitness from parents who are heirs themselves. As more ancestors are selected to inherit evaluation, there is less certitude about the child's fitness estimation. It seems reasonable to think there is a trade-off among uncertainty and the quality of the solution. Besides, it is clear there is a relationship among uncertainty and speed. To achieve higher evaluation savings, a higher α value is needed, and this will cause higher uncertainty in the evaluations which could be harmful if not handled properly.

There could be several ways to compute confidence. Basically, confidence should be a quantity which decreases when inheritance takes places and should be a function of parents confidence. Following the same ideas of inheritance an analogous expression for confidence can be proposed

$$c_c = \beta\left(\frac{c_{p1} + c_{p2}}{2}\right). \tag{4}$$

In equation 4, the parameter $\beta \in (0, 1)$ and can be understood as a decay factor. This expression implies confidence is inherited in a similar way as estimations do.

Although the precision of estimation is not directly computed by confidence, some correlation between confidence and estimation error is expected. In figure 1, this relationship is shown for the case of inheritance-based GA. The feature of confidence was added to the GA, even the information provided is not used at the moment. Figure 1 suggests the existence of negative correlation between error and population mean-confidence. Therefore, confidence can be used someway to lead the algorithm into better performance.

It could be hypothesized, as correlation becomes higher, the performance of a confidence-based GA will improve. In the ideal case, where real evaluations could be obtained without computation, inheritance-based GA would behave as a GA with variable population. It is not the case for regular inheritance-based GA, as estimations induce noise into the algorithm, making it harder to find the optimal solution. A good estimation of confidence would lead inheritance-based GA into the direction of a variable-population GA.

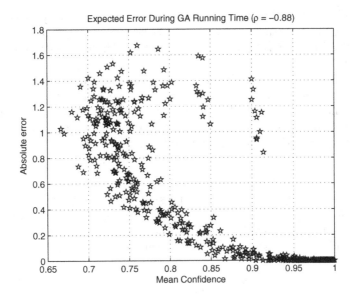

Fig. 1. An example of expected relationship between absolute-mean error and mean confidence for a inheritance-based GA. The samples are taken from the results of 10 different runs. From the graph can be inferred some negative relationship between the variables. The correlation coefficient $\rho = -0.88$.

3.1   A Model of Confidence

It is possible to modify an inheritance-based GA to perform confidence estimation and then investigate the effects of uncertainty, even if confidence itself is not used in someway to control the process. It is possible to derive an equation of the evolution of mean population confidence during runtime by realizing the following facts:

- Evaluated individual have a confidence of 1.
- There are $(1 - \alpha)N$ individuals in the population which are evaluated.
- Estimated individuals will have a confidence computed by equation 4.
- Individuals not selected to crossover ($p_c < 1$) will retain their original confidence value.
- There is the possibility for the crossover of identical parents. In this case, their children will be also identical to their parents. These individuals will retain their original confidence value.

All these effects can be summarized in the following equation

$$\bar{C}_t = \left[p_{c1}\beta\bar{C}_{t-1} + p_{c2}\bar{C}_{t-1} + (1 - p_c)\bar{C}_{t-1} \right] \alpha + (1 - \alpha). \tag{5}$$

In equation 5, $\bar{C}_t$ is the mean population confidence value for time t. p_{c1} represents the probability of crossover which lead to children who are different to their parents. On the other hand, p_{c2} represents the probability of crossover which lead to children identical to parents. Therefore, $p_c = p_{c1} + p_{c2}$. The exact values of p_{c1} and p_{c2} are a function of the quantity of individuals in population that share the same schemata.

Although equation 5 is not so difficult to solve under certain conditions, empirical observations made clear that the final state and the steady-state are actually the ones of some interest. In the final state of the algorithm the population converges to the (hopefully) optimal solution. In this case, $p_{c1} \to 0$ and $p_{c2} \to p_c$. Performing the required operations leads to the result

$$\bar{C}_M = 1. \tag{6}$$

On the other hand, the steady-state expression can be found by realizing the steady-state happens early during runtime and it is broken when population converges to a single solution. At that moment $p_{c1} \to p_c$, $p_{c2} \to 0$ and $\bar{C}_{ss} = \bar{C}_t = \bar{C}_{t-1}$. Under these assumptions the $\bar{C}_{ss}$ can be expressed as

$$\bar{C}_{ss} = \frac{1 - \alpha}{1 - \alpha(1 - p_c(1 - \beta))}. \tag{7}$$

From equations 6 and 7, it can be concluded the algorithm begins with absolute certainty of evaluations (every individual is evaluated as a first step) and then confidence will drop until some stable value. As good building-blocks dominate the population, individuals start to be more alike with each generation. This causes the confidence of new individuals to raise, as individuals identical to their parents do not suffer confidence degradation. Eventually the new offspring will be identical to the final solution and they will preserve their confidence value of 1. If the GA is given enough time to converge completely, all individuals in the populations will be identical with confidence value of 1.

4   Applying Confidence to Inheritance

The information about uncertainty provided by confidence can be used to control inheritance. Several schemes could be devised. In this article the possibility to use the mean population confidence $\bar{C}_t$ as the proportion of estimated individuals, α, will be explored. This is reasonable because of the correlation between error and mean population confidence. Also, both confidence and α are defined in the range $[0, 1]$. If the value of mean confidence is high, this will imply uncertainty is low and there is room for more estimations. In the other case, if confidence is too low, this will imply an urgency for more evaluations.

The effect on this scheme can be analyzed in the manner shown in the past section. In this case, $\bar{C}_{ss}$ and α can be used interchangeably. The analysis of the final state leads again to a final confidence of 1. For this new case, equation 5 should be modified to

$$\bar{C}_t = \left[p_{c1}\beta\bar{C}_{t-1} + p_{c2}\bar{C}_{t-1} + (1 - p_c)\bar{C}_{t-1}\right]\bar{C}_{t-1} + (1 - \bar{C}_{t-1}). \qquad (8)$$

Under the same assumptions applied for equation 5, the steady-state mean confidence value can be found to be

$$\bar{C}_{ss} = \frac{1}{1 + \sqrt{p_c(1 - \beta)}}. \qquad (9)$$

It could be useful to see the plots of equations 7 and 9. As an example, let us take the values of $\alpha = 0.5$ and $p_c = 1$. The plot is shown in figure 2. There is no intersection different from the cases when $\beta = 0$ and $\beta = 1$. In this case, it is clear the confidence-controlled GA will work with higher confidence than a regular inheritance-based GA. It is possible to choose any value of β to outperform the inheritance GA and to enjoy higher confidence level. The same applies for lower values of α.

As another example, the plot for the case of $\alpha = 0.7$ and $p_c = 1$ is presented in figure 3. In this case, there is an intersection when $\beta \approx 0.81$. It is possible to outperform the inheritance GA by choosing a higher value of β, although, the algorithm will work with lower confidence than the inheritance GA. Is it possible for the confidence GA to outperform inheritance GA while working with lower confidence level? This will be clarified in the experiments section.

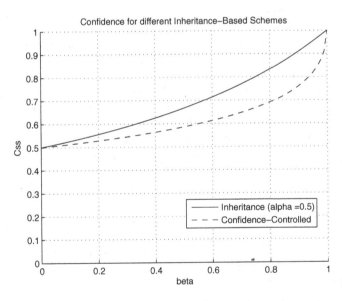

Fig. 2. Mean Confidence plots for $\alpha = 0.5$ and $p_c = 1$

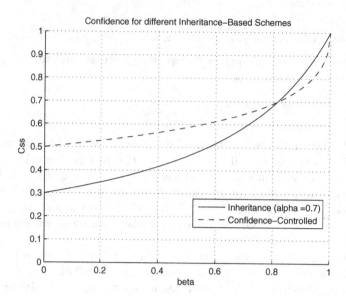

Fig. 3. Mean Confidence plots for $\alpha = 0.7$ and $p_c = 1$

5 Experiments

To make a fair comparison, the following experiment is suggested: After a common test problem is selected, the algorithms to compare should be selected. In this case, the GA, and inheritance-based GA and the confidence-controlled GA will be tested. The base of comparison will be the GA. The population size and number of generations will be configured in order to make them able to complete the test successfully, finding the optimal solution every run. The test consist in running each algorithm a fixed amount of times (100 times for these experiments) to compute the best-so-far curve based in the average of these tests. Crossover probability p_c and mutation probability p_m will be selected as 1 and 0, respectively. The particular parameters of each algorithm (α for inheritance-based GA and β for confidence-controlled GA) will be adjusted in order to make the respective algorithm able to find the optimum in every single run. The common parameters will be the same for the three algorithms.

The benchmark problems selected are the following: The onemax problem, which has been an important benchmark in several publications, as the report of Smith [6] or Sastry [5]. Looking for another problem, one with inherent non-linear nature, the sphere problem (found among others in the compendium by Tang [7]) is proposed. This can be defined as

$$f(x) = \sum_{i=1}^{D} x_i^2. \tag{10}$$

In equation 10, D is the quantity of dimensions considered in space. Considering a string of ℓ bits, the problem would have ℓ/D bits per dimension.

6   Results

In figures 4, 5, and 6, the results of the proposed experiments can be found. The final configuration of parameters for each algorithm can be found in tables 1, 2, and 3. The purpose of the values of p_c and p_m is to analyze the effects of confidence and inheritance without disturbances from other sources. The values of quantity of generations M and population size N were selected to enable the GA to find the optimum in every run. The standard deviation of the final value of each best-so-far curve shown is 0.

Table 1. Parameters Configuration for 20-bits Onemax Problem

Algorithm	p_c	p_m	M	N	Parameter	$p - value$
GA	1	0	50	60	NA	0
Inheritance-Based	1	0	50	60	$\alpha = 0.5$	2.59×10^{-13}
Confidence-Controlled	1	0	50	60	$\beta = 0.6$	NA

Table 2. Parameters Configuration for 40-bits Onemax Problem

Algorithm	p_c	p_m	M	N	Parameter	$p - value$
GA	1	0	120	120	NA	0
Inheritance-Based	1	0	120	120	$\alpha = 0.4$	0
Confidence-Controlled	1	0	120	120	$\beta = 0.6$	NA

Table 3. Parameters Configuration for 8 dimensions, 32-bits Sphere Problem

Algorithm	p_c	p_m	M	N	Parameter	$p - value$
GA	1	0	80	200	NA	0
Inheritance-Based	1	0	80	200	$\alpha = 0.7$	2.91×10^{-8}
Confidence-Controlled	1	0	80	200	$\beta = 0.8$	NA

Under the described conditions both inheritance-based GA and confidence-controlled GA performed better than the simple GA, as expected. In all the experiments the performance of the confidence GA was higher than the other ones. The best-so-far curve of the confidence GA practically dominates along the whole run. Due to the conditions of the test, even a small difference is significant.

It can be said all these algorithms can be configured to work faster. For example, it is possible to configure the inheritance GA for higher estimation levels, making it able to achieve the promised performance saving of 70% (Smith [6]). Nevertheless, that configuration would make the inheritance GA unable to abide to the conditions of the proposed experiments. The results suggest the use of confidence leads to a more robust algorithm. Under these conditions, the performance is more in accordance with the results reported by Sastry [5], which are more conservative.

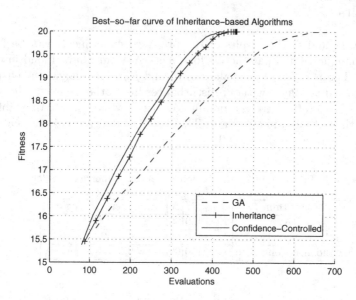

Fig. 4. Best-so-far curves of algorithms for the 20 bits onemax problem

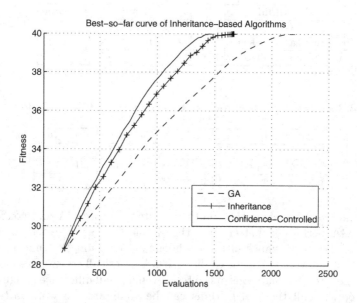

Fig. 5. Best-so-far curves of algorithms for the 40 bits onemax problem

An important fact is that the values of α and β allowed the confidence GA to work with higher confidence than the inheritance GA for every test presented. It should be noted the parameters were not chosen to attain a higher confidence beforehand, but to allow the algorithms to abide to experiment conditions. The

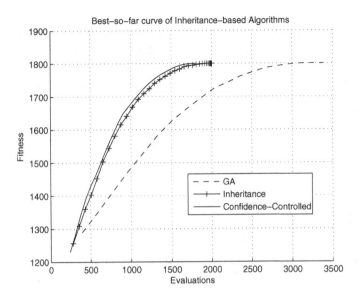

Fig. 6. Best-so-far curves of algorithms for the 32 bits sphere problem

cases of $\alpha = 0.4$ and $\alpha = 0.5$ are clear. In the case of $\alpha = 0.7$, the difference is small, although undeniable. This could explain why the best-so-far curves of confidence GA are clearly better for the onemax problem but tighter for the sphere problem. In the sphere problem, the trade-off between working with higher α value (faster algorithm) and working with higher confidence difference (better estimation precision) is more critical.

Finally, in tables 1 to 3, the p-value of a statistical t-test is presented. The null hypothesis H_0 holds the mean value of the best-so-far curve stabilization time (the moment the curve reaches its maximum) of the confidence-controlled algorithm is the same than the other algorithms (not real improvement). H_1 holds the other algorithms have higher stabilization time, therefore, confidence-controlled savings are significant. It is considered a significance value $\alpha_{test} = 0.05$. From the results, it is clear the statistical evidence is enough to say the other algorithms have higher stabilization time, then, they are slower. It can be said the confidence-controlled scheme actually helps to save unnecessary evaluations.

7 Conclusions

In this article, the concept of inheritance in GA was extended by considering the concept of confidence. Confidence was conceived as a measurement of the uncertainty caused by the estimation of ancestral lines along the GA run. It was shown that population average confidence is related to estimation error. The hypothesis of a highly correlated confidence measurements can lead to a variable population GA was stated. Some mathematical results about the proposed scheme performance were found. The experimental results suggest the proposed confidence-controlled GA is a more robust approach than regular inheritance-based GA. The results were object of statistical testing, showing the results are significant.

The possibility of better definitions of confidence and their use are still open questions. The conjecture about how high correlation between error and confidence can lead to better performance is remarked. There is still room for future work and development.

References

1. Goldberg, D.E.: Genetic Algorithms in Search, Optimization and Machine Learning. Addison Wesley (1989)
2. Goldberg, D.E., Deb, K., Clark, J.H.: Genetic algorithms, noise, and the sizing of populations. Complex Systems 6, 333–362 (1991)
3. Goldberg, D.E., Rudnick, M.: Genetic algorithms and the variance of fitness. Complex Systems 5(3), 265–278 (1991)
4. Grefenstette, J.J., Michael Fitzpatrick, J.: Genetic search with approximate function evaluation. In: Proceedings of the 1st International Conference on Genetic Algorithms, pp. 112–120. L. Erlbaum Associates Inc. (1985)
5. Sastry, K., Goldberg, D.E., Pelikan, M.: Don't evaluate, inherit. In: Proceedings of the Genetic and Evolutionary Computation Conference, pp. 551–558. Morgan Kaufmann, San Francisco (2001)
6. Smith, R.E., Dike, B.A., Stegmann, S.A.: Fitness inheritance in genetic algorithms. In: Proceedings of the 1995 ACM Symposium on Applied Computing, pp. 345–350. ACM (1995)
7. Tang, K., Yao, X., Suganthan, P.N., MacNish, C., Chen, Y.-P., Chen, C.-M., Yang, Z.: Benchmark functions for the congress on evolutionary computation 2008 special session and competition on large scale global optimization. In: Nature Inspired Computation and Applications Laboratory, USTC, China (2007)

WIGA: Wolbachia Infection Genetic Algorithm for Solving Multi-Objective Optimization Problems

Mauricio Guevara-Souza and Edgar E. Vallejo

ITESM, Campus Estado de México, Computer Science Department,
Carretera a Lago de Guadalupe km 3.5, Atizapán de Zaragoza,
Estado de México, México
{A00456476,vallejo}@itesm.mx

Abstract. This paper introduces a new evolutionary algorithm for solving multi-objective optimization problems. The proposed algorithm simulates the infection of the endosymbiotic bacteria *Wolbachia* to improve the evolutionary search. We conducted a series of experiments to compare the results of the proposed algorithm to those obtained by state of the art multi-objective evolutionary algorithms (MOEAs) at solving the ZDT test suite. Our experimental results show that the proposed model outperforms established MOEAs at solving most of the test problems.

Keywords: Evolutionary Algorithms, Genetic Algorithms, Multi-Objective Optimization, *Wolbachia*.

1   Introduction

Over the last few years, our research efforts have been directed towards the construction of computational simulation models that would be useful to increase our knowledge on the dynamics of populations of disease vectors and its potential application to the control of vector borne diseases such as malaria and dengue [6]. A promising biological strategy for the control of such diseases is the release of mosquitoes infected with the *Wolbachia* bacteria into wild populations for controlling the dengue disease [12] [5]. The *Wolbachia* bacteria comprises a collection of fitness and reproduction altering mechanisms that can induce the rapid establishment of immune populations replacing the native ones [4]. The *Wolbachia* bacteria infection is considered a safer approach than the use of transgenic mosquitoes for population replacement because no DNA modification is involved[7].

As part of our results, we have implemented and tested a collection of computer simulation models for a variety of gene drive mechanisms such as transposable genes and the maternal effect dominant embryonic arrest (MEDEA) in order to explore the conditions required to the replacement of a wild population with a transgenic one for disease control purposes [8] [9]. So far, these computational tools have proven to be useful for understanding the dynamics of the interacting populations and posses several advantages over experimental approaches.

F. Castro, A. Colbukh, and M. González (Eds.): MICAI 2013, Part II, LNAI 8266, pp. 41–51, 2013.
© Springer-Verlag Berlin Heidelberg 2013

Conversely, we believe that these biological mechanisms could be simulated to improve the efficiency of evolutionary algorithms. So far, we have developed a genetic algorithm that incorporates *Wolbachia* infection and tested its performance on the optimization of a collection of continuous functions. Our preliminary experimental results suggested that *Wolbachia* infection could prevent evolving populations from sticking in local optima [10].

In this work, we explore how the proposed model performs at solving complex multi-objective optimization problems. Our prediction is that the *Wolbachia* infection could help to improve the performance of the evolutionary algorithm by infecting the non-dominated solutions among the entire population and thus improving the dynamics of convergence to the Pareto front. In this paper, we present a collection of experiments with the most widely used benchmark of multi-objective functions (ZDT) using the proposed model [3]. The results are then compared with those yielded by the state of the art multi-objective evolutionary algorithms (MOEAs) NSGAII, SPEA2, MOEA/D and MODE-LD+SS. The results presented here suggest that *Wolbachia* infection improves the performance of the MOEAs in terms of the Pareto front obtained.

2   Background

2.1   *Wolbachia*

Wolbachia pipientis is a bacteria that is pervasive among insect species. It is estimated that about half of the insect species are infected by this bacteria.

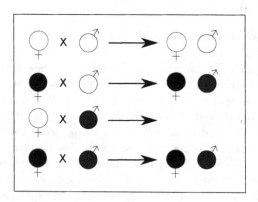

Fig. 1. Cytoplasmic incompatibility in *Wolbachia*. Filled circles correspond to individuals infected with *Wolbachia*.

Wolbachia possess the capability of spreading rapidly in an uninfected population due to the induction of an specific biological mechanism known as cytoplasmic incompatibility [5]. This mechanism causes the death of the offspring when an uninfected female mates with an infected male. In all other cases the

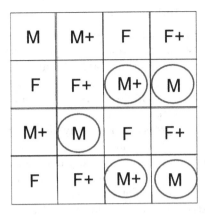

Fig. 2. Geographic distribution of males and females in the population. Circles indicate the possible mates of the female in the center of its neighborhood. Individuals with the plus sign are infected with *Wolbachia*.

offspring will survive but the infection status of the progeny is determined by the infection status of their parents(See figure 1).

Wolbachia bacteria provides the infected host with some advantages such as immunity to virus infection that contributes to increase the host's fitness. This attribute contributes to the rapid invasion of the host population. Similar biological mechanisms have been embedded into evolutionary algorithms to assist them achieve better results. In the evolutionary algorithms literature, several mating restrictions have been proposed to help maintain the genetic variability in the population an thereby favoring the balance between exploration and exploitation of the solution space. However, despite of its usefulness in natural organisms, the cytoplasmic incompatibility mechanism has not been explored within genetic algorithms until recently [10].

3   Materials and Methods

The computer model we propose here is a MOEA but we introduce several variations that make it resemble more to natural populations. The first one is the structure of the population that mimics in a more realistic way the spread of the individuals of the population in the environment. In our MOEA, the population is located on a two dimensional grid array so as to model geographic proximity. The second is related with the individual itself. The reproduction process we are introducing is a little different from the reproduction in a canonical MOEA. We incorporated the cytoplasmic incompatibility caused by the *Wolbachia* bacteria in the reproduction process when generating each new population. Finally, we simulated a *Wolbachia* infection during reproduction in the population to allow us to achieve better solutions and in some cases, in less generations.

3.1   Representation of Individuals

Each individual of the population was represented by a set of attributes that try to resemble the *Wolbachia* infection process. In particular, we represented the chromosome as an array of floating point numbers of the same length as the dimensions of the problem we want to optimize. Each one of the numbers in the chromosome was forced to lie within a desired range in order for the individual to remain a feasible solution. It is important to point out that all of the genetic operators used enforce this property. Probably the most important difference between how we modeled the individuals of the population in contrast to a canonical MOEA is that in our algorithm every individual has a gender: male or female. We wanted to emulate a natural population as close as possible not only in its structure, but in the reproduction process so we decided to include this important feature to restrict sexual reproduction between individuals of different gender.

In our model, location of the individuals is very important especially in the reproduction process so we maintain a record of the position of every individual within the population using two variables. The *Wolbachia* infection is simulated by a boolean variable that indicates whether the individual is infected or not; once the individual is infected it cannot be disinfected. The fitness of the individual is maintained in a vector of variables that represent the evaluation of the functions we want to optimize using the values in the chromosome of the individual. Finally, for selection purposes, two variables are used to determine if an individual belongs to the Pareto front. The first variable represents the number for individuals of the population that dominates it. The second variable represents the number of individuals that it dominates.

3.2   Population Structure

The structure of the population was modeled by a two dimensional symmetric toroidal array similar to those used in cellular genetic algorithms [1] (See figure 2). The position of the individuals in the grid is relevant because we are not only restricting reproduction between individuals by gender. We are also restricting the possible mates within a neighborhood.

We are proposing the neighborhood restriction to favor the exploration of the search space. It is known that MOEAs not possessing a proper balance between exploration and exploitation tend to get stuck in local optima or to diverge from optima. It is important to mention that the composition of the initial population is about half males and half females. The composition can vary randomly generation by generation but the proportion of females and males remains approximately even along the whole simulation.

As with the gender, we used this population structure to keep the reproduction process as close as possible of how it occurs in natural populations where the geographic location of the individuals poses spatial constraints on the reproduction of individuals. It is known that the best adapted individuals of a population are often clustered together in the center of the population while the less favored ones segregate from the optimal clusters.

3.3 Wolbachia Infection

Every generation, a portion of the population is infected with the *Wolbachia* bacteria. To select these individuals from the rest of the population we use a very well known criteria in multi-objective optimization called non-dominance. In particular, we are using weak non-dominance. Those individuals in the Pareto front are the ones that become infected. We selected these individuals because they are the best solutions found hitherto so we want them to produce more offspring than the less favored ones. Overall, we tried to move towards an equilibrium between exploration and exploitation. The gender and neighborhood mating restrictions were used to enforce exploration. By using *Wolbachia* infection we are encouraging the spread of the best solutions to assert exploitation as well.

3.4 Genetic Operators

Selection. As mentioned previously, we used two restrictions in the selection process. The first one is the gender restriction and the second one is the neighborhood restriction. These restrictions are enforced as follows. To produce offspring, it is required to mate individuals with different gender. The first parent we selected from the population was the female. The selection is done randomly so each female had the same chance to be selected.

After we have selected the female, we selected the male. The neighborhood restriction took place at this point. Only males that are within the neighborhood of the female could be eligible for reproduction(See figure 2). The size of the neighborhood depends on the benchmark function and can be consulted in table 1. We used a tournament between the males to pick the best of them based on two criteria. The first one was its Pareto ranking –the number of individuals that strongly dominated it. If two or more males were tied on this criteria we chose the one that strongly dominated more individuals of the population. If two or more males tied on these criteria, one of these male was selected randomly.

Crossover. The first step before performing the crossover was to verify if the parents were infected with *Wolbachia*. As described before, if the male was infected but the female did not, crossover is not needed since cytoplasmic incompatibility would kill all of the offspring. If the offspring is feasible, we used a one-point crossover operation. After the chromosome is obtained, the infection attribute of the offspring is set according to the parent's infection status. The canonical MOEA usually recombines parents with a probability around 60% to 75%. In our algorithm, we performed crossover with a 100% of probability. We did that to increase exploration during the evolutionary search.

Mutation. We implemented a single point mutation for our computer model [11]. Given that our chromosome is not binary but an array of floating point numbers, the mutation was a little different. First, we generated a random number for every position in the chromosome. If this number was above a certain threshold, the chromosome was mutated at that locus. To perform the mutation we generated a random number between 0 and 0.1. Then, this number was added or subtracted from the number at the position of the chromosome depending on a bit flip. If the mutated number fell off the feasible range of the function, we changed it to the closest valid number possible. The range of the random number generated for the mutation was obtained empirically so we used the values that produced the best results in our experiments.

3.5   Pareto Front

To calculate the Pareto front we used the criterion of weak non-dominance. At every generation, the non-dominated solutions were saved in a one-dimensional array separated from the population. The individuals in the Pareto front were infected with *Wolbachia* and included in the population so that they can partici-pate in the reproduction process. After the reproduction, the new non-dominated solutions were added to the Pareto front array. If one of the individuals that were already in the Pareto front resulted to be dominated by a newcomer, the domi-nated one was taken out of the Pareto front array. At the end of the simulation, the hyper-volume was calculated using the current Pareto front individuals [3].

4   Experiments and Results

In this section, we present the results we obtained by testing our algorithm with the ZDT benchmark functions; ZDT1, ZDT2, ZDT3, ZDT4 and ZDT6. We decided to use this suite because it has proven to be a very useful and reliable tool to measure the effectiveness and efficiency of evolutionary algorithms for multi-objective optimization [3]. To measure the quality of the solutions we are using the S-metric –also known as hyper-volume. This quality indicator is wide used because it measures in a single value how good a Pareto front is [14]. At the end of the section, we compare our algorithm against state of the art MOEAs: SPEA2, NSGAII, MOEA and MODE-LD+SS [3]. A general algorithm used in all the experiments is described in Algorithm 1:

4.1   ZDT Test Suite

Originally proposed by Zitzler, Deb and Thiele, this suite comprises six functions, all of them are bi-objective. The functions do not scale with the number of objectives [13]. For this paper, we tested our algorithm with five out of the six functions. We left out function ZDT5 because it defines a boolean function over binary strings and for this study we are not using binary encoded solutions. In all of the experiments, we used the same parameters that can be found in table 1, unless otherwise specified.

Algorithm 1.

1 - Create Initial Population
2 - Calculate Pareto Ranking
3 - Store Pareto Front
4 - Infect Individuals of Pareto Front with *Wolbachia*
while *Generations* $\leq$ 100 **do**
   5 - Mix Individuals in Pareto Front with Population
   while *Mosquitoes* $\leq$ *PopulationSize* **do**
     6 - Select parents
     if Offspring is feasible **then**
       7 - Calculate number of offspring
       while $N \leq Numberofoffspring$ **do**
         8 - Perform crossover
         9 - Perform mutation
         10 - Calculate fitness of the offspring
       end while
     end if
     11 - Calculate Pareto Ranking
     12 - Store Pareto Front
     13 - Infect Individuals of Pareto Front with *Wolbachia*
   end while
end while

Table 1. ZDT test suite parameters

Parameter	Value
Population	100
Generations	150
Mutation Probability	10%
Tournament Size	15
Maximum Offspring	1
Neighborhood Size	5
Crossover Probability	100%
Hyper-Volume Reference Point	(1.05,1.05)

ZDT1. This function possesses a convex Pareto-optimal front. We employed a chromosome length of 30. Each value in the chromosome was restricted in the range of [0,1]. Figure 3(a) shows the Pareto front obtained at the end of the simulation. As can be seen in the figure, the solutions are well distributed among the Pareto front.

ZDT2. This function possesses a non-convex Pareto-optimal front. In this experiment, we used again a chromosome length of 30 and a range of [0,1] for the values in the chromosome as the experiment above. Figure 3(b) shows the Pareto front obtained after the simulation. The individuals are relatively well distributed in the Pareto front but a bit of crowding can be observed near the beginning.

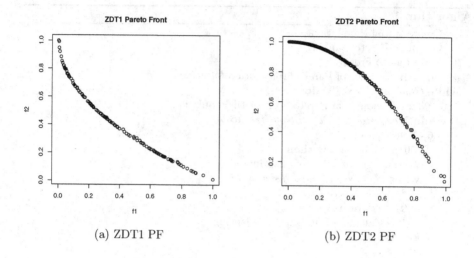

(a) ZDT1 PF   (b) ZDT2 PF

Fig. 3. ZDT Results

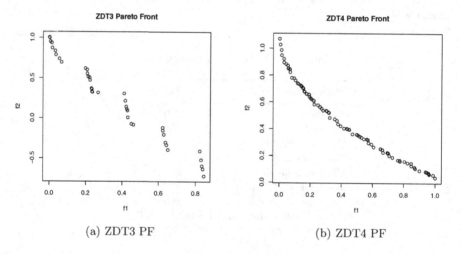

(a) ZDT3 PF   (b) ZDT4 PF

Fig. 4. ZDT Results

ZDT3. The Pareto-optimal front of this function is convex, disconnected and have five segments in total. As with the other two experiments, the chromosome length is 30 and the range of the values in the chromosome is [0,1]. As can be seen in figure 4(a), our algorithm was able to find the five segments of the Pareto-optimal and the spread of the solutions is good. Although, the algorithm found just a few individuals of the Pareto-optimal.

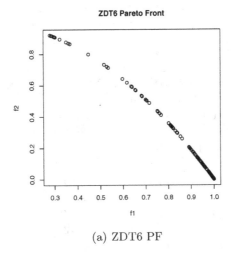

(a) ZDT6 PF

Fig. 5. ZDT Results

ZDT4. This function possesses a Pareto-optimal front that is identical in shape to that of the ZDT1 but is a much more complicated function because the solution space contains 21^9 local Pareto fronts. The chromosome length used for this problem is 10. The ranges of the values within the chromosome are [0,1] for the first variable and [-5,5] for the rest. Additionally, in contrast with the other functions of the test suite, we are using 200 generations. The increase in the number of generations is due to the difficulty of this particular problem. All the other parameters are the same(See table 1). Figure 4(b) shows the Pareto front obtained by our algorithm. The spread of the solutions is good but they are a little bit far from the Pareto-optimal front.

ZDT6. This function is very similar to ZDT2. It possesses a non-convex Pareto-optimal front. It has two major complications though: The first one is a deformity in the search space. The second one is a difference in the density of the solutions in the function fitness landscape. The number of variables in the chromosome is 10 and the values it can take vary between [0,1]. As shown in figure 5(a) our algorithm could surpass the difficulties and find solutions very near or in the Pareto-optimal front. The solutions are well spread, although there are some empty spaces between the solutions.

4.2   Summary of Results

Table 2 shows a summary of the results of the functions used in this paper. The results for the NSGAII, SPEA2, MOEA/D and MODE-LD+SS algorithms were reported in [2]. The upper value is the average hyper-volume of 30 independent runs. The lower value is the standard deviation. The values in bold highlight the

Table 2. The values in the table represent the average hyper-volume obtained by all the algorithms after 30 runs with their respective standard deviation

Summary of Results

Function	NSGAII	SPEA2	MOEA/D	MODE-LD+SS	WIGA
ZDT1	0.757357	0.761644	0.749964	0.763442	**0.8305106**
	0.000928	0.000556	0.009777	0.000112	0.0303432
ZDT2	0.422221	0.321971	0.387237	0.430358	**0.4422294**
	0.001263	0.171286	0.061361	0.000141	0.0376425
ZDT3	0.61148	0.615533	0.608377	0.616381	**0.703495**
	0.008038	0.000416	0.015638	0.00015	0.104415
ZDT4	0.217626	0.287359	**0.745887**	0.74177	0.6537009
	0.192914	0.188726	0.009983	0.058697	0.0803251
ZDT6	0.345949	0.392697	0.39772	0.411054	**0.5091942**
	0.008772	0.002336	0.002886	0.000003	0.1084696

best result of every test function. As can bee seen, our algorithm produced the best results in 4 out of the 5 test problems. The standard deviation is a little higher in most cases due to the difference between runs, sometimes the algorithm got very superior results and in the rest of the runs, the results were just above or the same as the other algorithms.

5   Conclusion

This paper shows how the simulated infection of the *Wolbachia* bacteria contributes to improve the performance of genetic algorithms for solving multi-objective problems. The proposed mechanism seems to produce a synergic interaction with the proposed mating restriction mechanism to provide an appropriate balance between exploration and exploration during the evolutionary search. To test our algorithm we used the ZDT test suite that is the the most used in the literature. The computer model proposed, in fact, provided better hyper-volume values in most cases. Sometimes, these results were achieved in less generations than the other MOEAs presented here.

Given the good results obtained in our experiments, the next step is to test our algorithm with more benchmark functions like the DTLZ test suite, the WFG test suite and the Okabe functions [3]. This will help us determine in what kind of problems our algorithm would be a good alternative. Further, these additional experiments would contribute to understand the capabilities and limitations of the proposed approach at solving multi-objective problems generally.

Another avenue we are considering to explore is to apply the proposed model in real life problems. Also, additional comparisons between our algorithm and other state of the art MOEAs, would be valuable to continue to asses the effectiveness and efficiency of the proposed *Wolbachia* infection mechanism.

In addition, we believe that formal statistical analyses would be needed to support the validity of the results shown here and to corroborate the robustness of the computer model proposed.

All in all, we believe that population replacement strategies that have been proven its effectiveness in controlling vector borne diseases are a promising alternative worth to consider in order to improve the performance of the evolutionary algorithms for solving multi-objective optimization problems, in general.

References

[1] Alba, B., Dorronsoro, B.: Cellular Genetic Algorithms. Springer (2010)

[2] Arias-Montano, A., Coello, C.A.C., Mezura-Montes, E.: Multi-objective airfoil shape optimization using a multiple-surrogate approach. In: IEEE Congress on Evolutionary Computation (CEC 2012), pp. 1188–1195. IEEE Press (June 2012)

[3] Coello, C.A.C., Lamont, G.B., van Veldhuizen, V.A.: Evolutionary Algorithms for Solving Multi-Objective Problems. Springer (2007)

[4] Crain, P., Mains, J., Suh, E.: Wolbachia infections that reduce immature insect survival: Predicted impacts on population replacement. BMC Evolutionary Biology 11(290) (2011)

[5] Presgraves, D.C.: A genetic test of the mechanism of wolbachia-induced cytoplasmic incompatibility in drosophila. Genetics (154), 771–776 (2000)

[6] Guevara-Souza, M., Vallejo, E.E.: Computer simulation on disease vector population replacement driven by the maternal effect dominant embryonic arrest(medea). In: Software Tools and Algorithms for Biological Systems, pp. 335–344. Springer (April 2011)

[7] Hoffman, A., Montgomery, B., Popovici, J.: Successful establishment of wolbachia in *aedes* populations to suppress dengue transmission. Nature (476), 454–459 (2011)

[8] Guevara, M., Vallejo, E.: A computer simulation model of gene replacement in vector populations. In: 8th IEEE International Conference on BioInformatics and BioEngineering Proceedings, pp. 1–6. IEEE (October 2008)

[9] Guevara, M., Vallejo, E.: Computer simulation on the maternal effect dominant embryonic arrest (medea) for disease vector population replacement. In: 11th Annual Conference on Genetic and Evolutionary Computation Proceedings, pp. 1787–1788. ACM (July 2009)

[10] Guevara-Souza, M., Vallejo, E.E.: Wolbachia infection improves genetic algorithms as optimization procedure. In: Dediu, A.-H., Martín-Vide, C., Truthe, B. (eds.) TPNC 2012. LNCS, vol. 7505, pp. 161–173. Springer, Heidelberg (2012)

[11] Michalewicz, Z.: Genetic Algorithms + Data Structures = Evolution Programs. Artificial intelligence. Springer (1998)

[12] Dobsonl, S.L., Fox, W., Jiggins, F.: The effect of wolbachia-induced cytoplasmic incompatibility on host population size in natural and manipulated systems. Proc. Biol. Sci. 269(1490), 437–445 (2002)

[13] Zitzler, E., Deb, K., Thiele, L.: Comparison of multiobjective evolutionary algorithms: Empirical results. Evolutionary Computation 8(2), 173–195 (2000)

[14] Zitzler, E., Thiele, L., Laumanns, M., Fonseca, C.M., da Fonseca, V.G.: Performance assessment of multiobjective optimizers: an analysis and review. Trans. Evol. Comp. 7(2), 117–132 (2003)

B-spline Surface Approximation
Using Hierarchical Genetic Algorithm

G. Trejo-Caballero[1,2], C.H. Garcia-Capulin[2], O.G. Ibarra-Manzano[1],
J.G. Avina-Cervantes[1], L.M. Burgara-Lopez[2], and H. Rostro-Gonzalez[1]

[1] DICIS - Universidad de Guanajuato, Department of Electronics,
Com. Palo Blanco s/n, Salamanca 36885, Guanajuato, México
trejocg@ugto.mx
[2] Instituto Tecnológico Superior de Irapuato, Department of Mechatronics,
Carr. Irapuato-Silao Km. 12.5, Irapuato 36821, Guanajuato, México
cagarcia@itesi.edu.mx

Abstract. Surface approximation using splines has been widely used in
geometric modeling and image analysis. One of the main problems associated with surface approximation by splines is the adequate selection
of the number and location of the knots, as well as, the solution of the
system of equations generated by tensor product spline surfaces. In this
work, we use a hierarchical genetic algorithm (HGA) to tackle the B-
spline surface approximation problem. The proposed approach is based
on a novel hierarchical gene structure for the chromosomal representation, which allows us to determine the number and location of the knots
for each surface dimension, and the B-spline coefficients simultaneously.
Our approach is able to find solutions with fewest parameters within of
the B-spline basis functions. The method is fully based on genetic algorithms and does not require subjective parameters like smooth factor or
knot locations to perform the solution. In order to validate the efficacy of
the proposed approach, simulation results from several tests on smooth
surfaces have been included.

1 Introduction

Surface approximation is a recurrent problem in geometric modeling, data analysis, image processing and many other engineering applications. In this regard,
surface approximation aims to construct a surface that represents the best estimation of an unknown function from given a data set of noisy values. To tackle
this problem, several methods have been proposed in the literature. For instance,
the Shepard's method [1], the finite element methods [2, 3] and the tensor product spline [4–7] are the most widely used and successful methods.

The Shepard's method, also known as the original inverse distance weighted
interpolation method deals with this issue through a continuous interpolation
function from the weighted average of the data. The finite element method is
a numerical approach for solving differential equations. This method consists of
assuming the piecewise continuous function for the solution and obtaining the

F. Castro, A. Gelbukh, and M. González (Eds.): MICAI 2013, Part II, LNAI 8266, pp. 52–63, 2013.

parameters of the functions in a manner that reduces the error in the solution. The tensor product spline is another method commonly used to approximate surfaces. It is a generalization of the spline approximations, which aims to get smooth functions from scattered points.

Since we consider a spline based approach, we remark the fact that the main issue associated with the surface approximation through splines is to find the best set of knots, where the term "best" implies an adequate choice in the number and location of the knots. To perform this task, in [4], the author provides a survey on the main algorithms used to carry out this task, which are based on regression spline methods and their respective optimizations.

Unlike the authors mentioned above, we tackle the B-spline surface approximation problem by using the hierarchical genetic algorithm. To be more specific, we consider a hierarchical structure to represent both, the model structure (number and knots location) as a binary encoding and the model parameters (spline coefficients) as a real encoding. Thus, we search for the best B-spline based surface model using a novel fitness function. As a result, our method can simultaneously determine the number and position of the knots as well as B-spline coefficients. In addition, our approach is able to find solutions with fewest parameters within the B-spline basis functions.

This paper is organised as follows: the notation and description of B-spline surfaces are presented in section 2, followed by the description of our approach in section 3. In section 4 we present some numerical results and we conclude in section 5.

2   Surface Approximation by Tensor Product Splines

We can describe the problem of surface approximation as follows: given a set of noisy measurements in a rectangular domain described as $z_{i,j}$, $i = 1, \ldots, N_x$, $j = 1, \ldots, N_y$ and expressed in the following form:

$$z_{i,j} = f(x_i, y_j) + \epsilon_{i,j} \tag{1}$$

where f is an unknown functional relationship that we wish to estimate, the term $\epsilon_{i,j}$ represents the zero-mean random errors and $z_{i,j}$ is a sample at (x_i, y_i). Therefore, the goal is to find the best estimation of the function f.

In this study, we assume that f is a smooth surface that can be well approximated in the interval $[a, b] \times [c, d]$ by a B-spline surface. The B-spline surfaces are constructed as a tensor product of univariate B-spline basis functions. The B-spline surface is modeled using the following considerations: let us define $\{u_1, \ldots, u_m\}$ as a set of m points placed along the domain of the variable x and $\{v_1, \ldots, v_n\}$ be a set of n points placed along the domain of the variable y, which are called interior knots. Thus, the knot vectors are defined as follow:

$$\mathbf{u} : u_{1-k} =, \ldots, = u_0 = a < u_1 < \ldots < u_m < b = u_{m+1} = \ldots = u_{m+k}$$
$$\mathbf{v} : v_{1-l} =, \ldots, = v_0 = c < v_1 < \ldots < v_n < d = v_{n+1} = \ldots = v_{n+l} \tag{2}$$

with these assumptions, the function f can be now written as a tensor product:

$$f(x,y) = \sum_{i=1}^{m+k} \sum_{j=1}^{n+l} P_{i,j} B_{i,k}(x) B_{j,l}(y) \tag{3}$$

where $P_{i,j}$ are the B-spline coefficients and $B_{i,k}(x), B_{j,l}(y)$ are the B-spline basis functions of order k and l respectively defined over the knot vectors $\mathbf{u}$ and $\mathbf{v}$. The B-spline basis functions are denoted by the following recurrence relations:

$$B_{i,1}(x) = \begin{cases} 1, \text{ if } t_i \le x < t_{i+1} \\ 0, \text{ otherwise} \end{cases} \tag{4}$$

and

$$B_{i,k}(x) = \frac{x - t_i}{t_{i+k-1} - t_i} B_{i,k-1}(x) + \frac{t_{i+k} - x}{t_{i+k} - t_{i+1}} B_{i+1,k-1}(x) \tag{5}$$

If k and l are specified beforehand, f can be completely specified by $\theta = \{\mathbf{u}, \mathbf{v}, P\}$, where $\mathbf{u}$ and $\mathbf{v}$ are the knot vectors and P is the coefficient matrix. Now, the problem is to find the number and location of the interior knots $\{u_1, \ldots, u_m, v_1, \ldots, v_n\}$ and then estimate the coefficients $P_{i,j}$. This problem cannot be solved with simple standard methods due to fact that is a high-dimensional nonlinear optimization problem. A more detailed discussion about B-splines can be found in [8, 9].

3 B-spline Surface Approximation Using HGA

Compared to conventional GA [10], the main difference with the HGA is the structure of the chromosome. From the biological viewpoint, the genetic structure of a chromosome is formed by a number of gene variations arranged in a hierarchical manner. In the light of this issue, Man et. al. [11] proposed a hierarchical structure of chromosome to emulate the formulation of a biological DNA structure. The computational chromosome in an HGA consists of two types of genes, which are known as control genes and parametric genes.

Typically, control genes are represented as a binary encoding, while parametric genes are coded as real numbers. The purpose of control genes is to enable or to disable the parametric genes, which is particularly important to determine the genetic structure of the chromosome.

In this paper, we use an HGA to determine simultaneously the number and positions of the knots (model structure) and the B-spline coefficients (model parameters) by minimizing a fitness function. In this approach, the main characteristics to consider are: (1) the chromosome encoding of potential solutions, (2) the fitness function, to evaluate the fitness of the chromosomes and (3) the operators to evolve the individuals.

3.1 Chromosome Encoding

We use a fixed length binary string to represent the number and the locations of the interior knots $\{u_1, \ldots, u_m, v_1, \ldots, v_n\}$, and real numbers to represent the P B-spline coefficients. We represent the chromosome of an individual as:

$$\theta = \{b_1, \ldots, b_m, b_{m+1}, \ldots, b_{m+n}, r_{1-k/2, 1-l/2}, \ldots, r_{1-k/2, n+l/2},$$
$$\ldots, r_{m+k/2, 1-l/2}, \ldots, r_{m+k/2, n+l/2}\}$$

where each b_i is a control bit and $r_{i,j}$ is a real value (coefficient).

Here, each control bit enables or disables one of the interior knots and one of the coefficients simultaneously. We establish one-to-one correspondences between the interior knots and the coefficients to be activated at the same time. The real values represent the coefficients of the B-spline. The general structure of a chromosome is graphically shown in Figure 1.

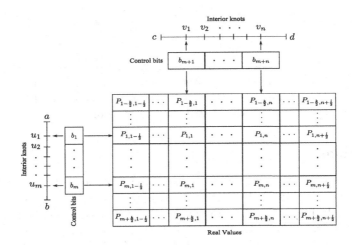

Fig. 1. General structure of a chromosome

This representation scheme does not allows us to duplicate knots, it because our interest is on smooth functions. However, it can be extended to handle discontinuous functions if we introduce an additional type of gene.

3.2   Fitness Function

To evaluate the fitness of each individual θ, the fitness function F is formulated as a sum of three terms and is given by the following equation:

$$F(\theta) = \omega_1 RSS + \omega_2 SSD + \omega_3 PKS \tag{6}$$

where each term of the equation is described as follows:

(a) The first term is the residual sum of squares (RSS). It is used as a measure of the deviation between the observed data set and the estimated function $\hat{f}$. The RSS is calculated as follows:

$$RSS = \sum_{i=1}^{N_x} \sum_{j=1}^{N_y} \left\{ z_{i,j} - \hat{f}(x_i, y_j) \right\}^2 \tag{7}$$

(b) The second term is the sum of the squared differences (SSD), which is the discrete approximation of the gradient. This term is used to penalize high sums of gradients to generate smooth solutions. The SSD is given by the next equation:

$$SSD = \sum_{i=1}^{N_x} \sum_{j=1}^{N_y} \left\{ [\hat{f}(x_i, y_j) - \hat{f}(x_{i-1}, y_j)]^2 + [\hat{f}(x_i, y_j) - \hat{f}(x_i, y_{j-1})]^2 \right\} \quad (8)$$

(c) The last term is a penalty function for knot structure (PKS). It is computed as follows:

$$PKS = \sum_{i=0}^{m} \frac{b - a}{(u_{i+1} - u_i)^2} + \sum_{i=0}^{n} \frac{d - c}{(v_{i+1} - v_i)^2} \quad (9)$$

In equation 9, PKS tries to favor solutions with uniform distributions of knots for each dimension. In other words, it penalizes solutions with knots very close, which generates over fitting of the function. Therefore, the individuals with fewest knots and better distribution are favoured.

3.3   Operators

Selection Operator. The roulette wheel method is used as a selection operator. In this method, each individual is assigned to one of the slices in the roulette wheel. This selection strategy favors best fitted individuals but also gives a chance to the less fitted individuals to survive. To prevent premature convergence, the sigma scaling method [12] is used. This method tries to keep the selection pressure relatively constant over all evolution process, and it is calculated according to:

$$F_{new} = \begin{cases} F_{act} - (\bar{F} - c \cdot \sigma) & \text{if } (F_{act} > \bar{F} - c \cdot \sigma) \\ 0 & \text{otherwise} \end{cases} \quad (10)$$

where F_{new} is the new scaled fitness value, F_{act} is the current fitness value, $\bar{F}$ is the average fitness, σ is the standard deviation of the population and c is a constant to control the selection pressure. In addition, elitism is used in order to keep elite individuals in the next population to prevent losing the best solution found.

Crossover Operators. The uniform crossover operator is used for the binary-valued chromosome and the simulated binary crossover operator (SBX) is used for the real-valued chromosome [13]. These crossover operators are applied with the same crossover probability. In the uniform crossover method, two parents are chosen to be recombine into a new individual. Each bit of the new individual is selected from one of the parents depending on a fixed probability. On the other hand, in SBX method, two new individuals c_1 and c_2 are generated from the parents p_1 and p_2 using a probability distribution.

The procedure used in SBX is the following: first, a random number u between 0 and 1 is generated. Then the probability distribution β is calculated as:

$$\beta = \begin{cases} (2u)^{\frac{1}{\eta+1}} & \text{if } u \leq 0.5 \\ \left(\frac{1}{2(1-u)}\right)^{\frac{1}{\eta+1}} & \text{otherwise} \end{cases} \tag{11}$$

where η is a non-negative real number that controls the distance between parents and the new individuals generated. After obtaining β, new individuals are calculated according to:

$$c_1 = 0.5[(1+\beta)p_1 + (1-\beta)p_2]$$
$$c_2 = 0.5[(1-\beta)p_1 + (1+\beta)p_2] \tag{12}$$

Mutation Operators. For the binary-valued chromosome, the bit mutation method is used. In this method, each bit is inverted or not depending on a mutation probability. For the real-valued chromosome each numeric value γ is changed depending on the same mutation probability according to:

$$\gamma_i = \gamma_i + \delta(\text{rand} - 0.5) \tag{13}$$

where δ is the maximum increment or decrement of the real value and $rand$ is a function that generates a random value between 0 and 1.

4   Numerical Results

We carried out numerical simulations to evaluate the performance of our approach. Thus, in order to perform these tests, we defined an experimental set of five bivariate functions, whose equations are given in Table 1 and graphically shown in Figure 2. These test functions were taken from previous works [14, 15, 4] as a reference to validate our method.

Table 1. Experimental set of five bivariate functions

Function 1:	$f(x,y) = 10.391\{(x - 0.4)(y - 0.6) + 0.36\}$
Function 2:	$f(x,y) = 24.234\{r^2(0.75 - r^2)\}, r^2 = (x - 0.5)^2 + (y - 0.5)^2$
Function 3:	$f(x,y) = 42.659\{0.1 + \hat{x}(0.05 + \hat{x}^4 - 10\hat{x}^2\hat{y}^2 + 5\hat{y}^4)\}, \hat{x} = x - 0.5, \hat{y} = y - 0.5$
Function 4:	$f(x,y) = 1.3356[1.5(1 - x) + e^{(2x-1)}sin\{3\pi(x - 0.6)^2\} + e^{(3(y-0.5))}sin\{4\pi(y - 0.9)^2\}]$
Function 5:	$f(x,y) = 1.9[1.35 + e^x sin\{13(x - 0.6)^2\}e^{-y}sin(7y)])$

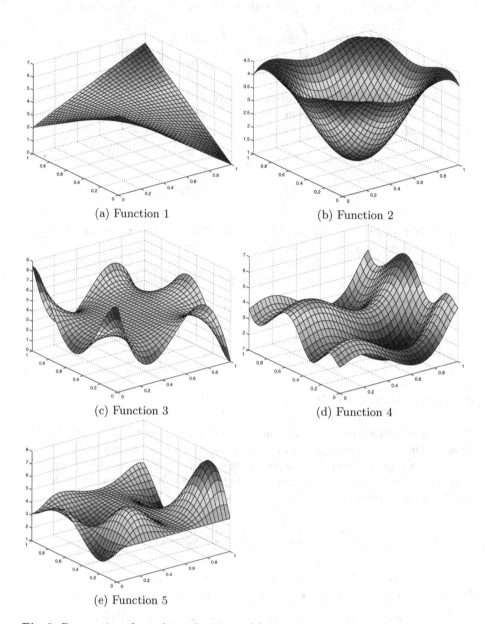

(a) Function 1

(b) Function 2

(c) Function 3

(d) Function 4

(e) Function 5

Fig. 2. Perspective plots of test functions: (a) simple interaction function, (b) radial function, (c) harmonic function, (d) additive function and (e) complicated interaction function

4.1 Simulation

A data set of 1024 noisy points was generated for each function in a uniform grid. The functions were evaluated over the interval $[0, 1] \times [0, 1]$ and translated to make the range non-negative in order to facilitate comparisons among them. The noisy data sets were generated according to 1, with a zero-mean normal noise and σ known. The signal noise ratio (SNR) is defined as $SD(f)/\sigma$ and it was set in 3. Note that the SNR is roughly equal to 3, it because we considered a small number of samples. The generated noisy data for the five functions are shown in Figures 3(a), 3(c), 3(e), 4(a) and 4(c).

In the numerical tests, our approach was configured as follows: we used cubic B-spline functions, i.e. $k = 4$, $l = 4$ and interior knots as a subset of design points. The population was randomly initialized at the beginning. Each control gene b_i was randomly selected from $[0, 1]$ and each real gene r_i was considered as a random real number defined over the range $[min(z_{i,j}), max(z_{i,j})]$ of the measurements $z_{i,j}$.

Table 2. Parameters used for the HGA

Parameter	Value
Population size	90
Crossover probability	0.85
Mutation probability	0.008
Number of elite individuals	9

The HGA parameters were experimentally tunned and they are presented in Table 2. The population was evolved during 3000 generations in all cases.

4.2 Results

To evaluate the performance of our approach, we used the mean square error (MSE) given by:

$$MSE = \frac{1}{n} \sum_{i=1}^{n} \{\hat{f}(x_i) - f(x_i)\}^2 \qquad (14)$$

where f is the real function and $\hat{f}$ is the estimated function given by the proposed method. For each test function, the MSE is calculated and the results are summarized in Table 3. The test and the obtained functions are graphically shown in Figures 3(b), 3(d), 3(f), 4(b) and 4(d).

In order to compare the obtained results, we performed a comparison against the LOWESS (Locally Weighted Scatter Smoothing) method [16]. For this, we made use of the Curve Fitting Toolbox provided by MATLAB. In this simulation (the Matlab one), the default parameters were considered.

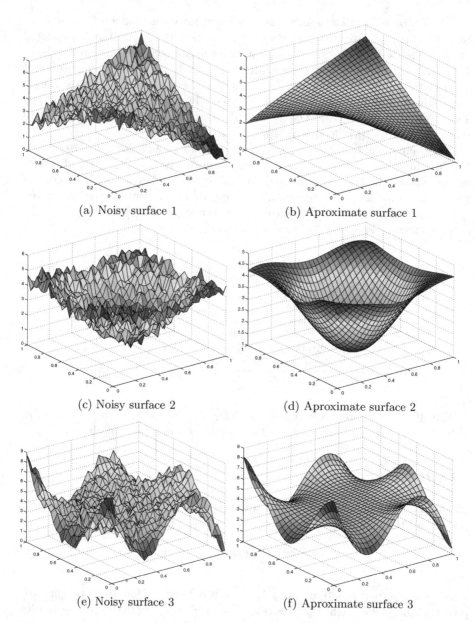

(a) Noisy surface 1   (b) Aproximate surface 1

(c) Noisy surface 2   (d) Aproximate surface 2

(e) Noisy surface 3   (f) Aproximate surface 3

Fig. 3. Numerical results for test functions 1, 2 and 3. On the left side, the figures show the noisy data used as inputs. The figures in the right side show the approximate surfaces (outputs) by HGA.

Table 3. Mean-squared error (MSE) for test functions

Test Function	LOWESS	HGA
1	0.0032	0.0022
2	0.0049	0.0038
3	0.0470	0.0134
4	0.0237	0.0122
5	0.0345	0.0188

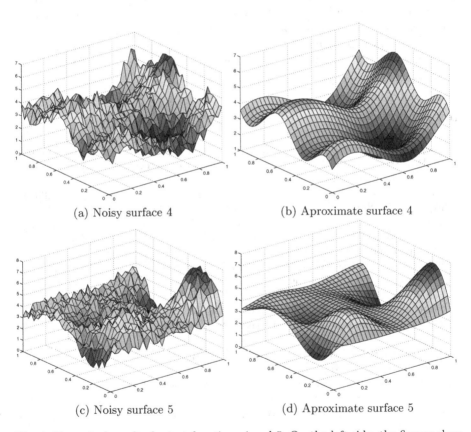

(a) Noisy surface 4   (b) Aproximate surface 4

(c) Noisy surface 5   (d) Aproximate surface 5

Fig. 4. Numerical results for test functions 4 and 5. On the left side, the figures show the noisy data used as inputs. The figures in the right side show the approximate surfaces (outputs) by HGA.

5   Conclusions

In this paper, we proposed an efficient hierarchical genetic algorithm to tackle the B-spline surface approximation problem. The method introduced a novel hierarchical gene structure for the chromosomal representation, thus allowing us to find simultaneously the best model with fewest knots, optimal knot locations and coefficients of the B-spline surface. It is important to highlight the fact that the method does not require subjective parameters like smooth factor or knot locations to perform the solution.

To test our method, we performed several tests on benchmark functions as well as a comparison with the LOWESS method, which is provided with the Matlab Curve Fitting Toolbox. Numerical results show that our method responds successfully to the problem of surface approximation. In terms of visualization (qualitatively), the obtained results are comparable to the original surfaces. Comparative tests demonstrated a better performance of our method than the LOWESS method over all the proposed tests. Given the performance characteristics of the proposed approach, our future work will be to apply this method over an experimental data set. We are interesting on extending our approach to experiment with variable length chromosome and different basis functions.

References

1. Shepard, D.: A two-dimensional interpolation function for irregularly-spaced data. In: Proceedings of the 1968 23rd ACM National Conference, ACM 1968, pp. 517–524. ACM, New York (1968)
2. Olshanskii, M.A., Reusken, A., Grande, J.: A Finite Element Method for Elliptic Equations on Surfaces. SIAM Journal on Numerical Analysis 47, 3339–3358 (2009)
3. Cohen, L.D., Cohen, I.: Finite-element methods for active contour models and balloons for 2-D and 3-D images. IEEE Transactions on Pattern Analysis and Machine Intelligence 15, 1131–1147 (1993)
4. Lee, T.C.M.: On algorithms for ordinary least squares regression spline fitting: a comparative study. Journal of Statistical Computation and Simulation 72, 647–663 (2002)
5. Mazroui, A., Mraoui, H., Sbibih, D., Tijini, A.: A new method for smoothing surfaces and computing hermite interpolants. BIT Numerical Mathematics 47, 613–635 (2007)
6. Schütze, T., Schwetlick, H.: Bivariate free knot splines. BIT Numerical Mathematics 43, 153–178 (2003)
7. Yoshimoto, F., Moriyama, M., Harada,T.: Automatic knot placement by a genetic algorithm for data fitting with a spline. In: Proceedings of the International Conference on Shape Modeling and Applications, SMI 1999, p. 162. IEEE Computer Society, Washington, DC (1999)
8. De Boor, C.: On calculating with b-spline. Journal of Approximation Theory 6, 50–62 (1972)
9. De Boor, C.: A Practical Guide to Splines. Springer, New York (1978)

10. Holland, J.H.: Adaptation in Natural and Artificial Systems: An Introductory Analysis with Applications to Biology, Control, and Artificial Intelligence. The MIT Press (1992)
11. Man, K.F., Tang, K.S., Kwong, S.: Genetic Algorithms: Concepts and Designs with Disk. Springer-Verlag New York, Inc., Secaucus (1999)
12. Goldberg, D.E.: Genetic Algorithms in Search, Optimization, and Machine Learning. Addison-Wesley Professional (1989)
13. Deb, K., Agrawal, R.B.: Simulated binary crossover for continuous search space. Complex Systems 9, 115–148 (1995)
14. Hwang, J.N., Lay, S.R., Maechler, M., Martin, R., Schimert, J.: Regression modeling in back-propagation and projection pursuit learning. IEEE Transactions on Neural Networks 5, 342–353 (1994)
15. Denison, D.G.T., Mallick, B.K., Smith, A.F.M.: Bayesian mars. Statistics and Computing 8, 337–346 (1998)
16. Cleveland, W.S.: Robust Locally Weighted Regression and Smoothing Scatterplots. Journal of the American Statistical Association 74, 829–836 (1979)

A Study of Genetic Algorithms
to Solve the School Timetabling Problem

Rushil Raghavjee and Nelishia Pillay

School of Mathematics, Statistics and Computer Science, University of KwaZulu-Natal,
Pietermaritzburg Campus, KwaZulu-Natal, South Africa
{raghavjee,pillayn32}@ukzn.ac.za

Abstract. This paper examines the use of genetic algorithms (GAs) to solve the
school timetabling problem. The school timetabling problem falls into the category of NP-hard problems. Instances of this problem vary drastically from
school to school and country to country. Previous work in this area has used
genetic algorithms to solve a particular school timetabling problem and has not
evaluated the performance of a GA on different problems. Furthermore, GAs
have not previously been applied to solving the South African primary or high
school timetabling problem. The paper presents a two-phased genetic algorithm
approach to solving the school timetabling problem and provides an analysis of
the effect of different low-level construction heuristics, selection methods and
genetic operators on the success of the GA approach in solving these problems
with respect to feasibility and timetable quality. The GA approach is tested on
a benchmark set of "hard" school timetabling problems, the Greek high school
timetabling problem and a South African primary and high school timetabling
problem. The performance of the GA approach was found to be comparable to
other methods applied to the same problems. This study has also revealed that
different combinations of low-level construction heuristics, selection methods
and genetic operators are needed to produce feasible timetables of good quality
for the different school timetabling problems. Future work will investigate methods for the automatic configuration of GA architectures of both phases.

Keywords: Timetabling, genetic algorithms, combinatorial optimization, evolutionary computation.

1   Introduction

Genetic algorithms have been successfully applied to solving combinatorial optimization problems such as university course and examination timetabling problems[1], the
travelling salesman problem [2], and the bin packing problem [3] amongst others.
Given the success in these domains, this paper presents an investigation of genetic
algorithms in solving the school timetabling problem.

The school timetabling problem (STP) involves the scheduling of resources, or
combinations of resources, to timetable slots in such a manner that the hard constraints of the problem are met and the soft constraints minimized [4]. Resources for
this problem include classes, teachers and venues, amongst others. The requirements

F. Castro, A. Gelbukh, and M. González (Eds.): MICAI 2013, Part II, LNAI 8266, pp. 64–80, 2013.
© Springer-Verlag Berlin Heidelberg 2013

of the problem include a specification of the number of times a particular teacher must meet a class. Some versions of the problem do not require venue allocations to be made while others include this constraint. Resources are allocated as class-teacher (or class-teacher-venue) tuples to the different timetable periods. The hard constraints of a problem are constraints that must be satisfied by a timetable in order for it to be operable. A timetable meeting all the hard constraints of the problem is said to be feasible. Examples of hard constraints include all class-teacher meetings must be scheduled the required number of times in the specified venue; no clashes, i.e. a resource, namely, a teacher, class, or venue, must not be scheduled more than once in a timetable period. The soft constraints on the other hand measure the quality of the timetable. These constraints define characteristics that we would like the timetable to possess but which may not always be possible. The aim is to minimize the number of soft constraints violated and this value is a measure of the quality of the timetable, i.e. the fewer soft constraints violated the better the timetable quality. A common soft constraint is daily limits on the number of lessons taken by a class on a particular subject and the number of lessons taught by a particular teacher. The hard and soft constraints differ from one timetabling problem to the next to such an extent that in some cases what may be defined as a hard constraint for one problem is a soft constraint for another and vice versa.

Genetic algorithms take an analogy from Darwin's theory of evolution. The standard genetic algorithm presented by Goldberg [5] implements the processes of initial population, evaluation, selection and regeneration by means of genetic operators. Elements of the population are represented as binary strings and each element, called a chromosome, is randomly created. A measure of how close a chromosome is to the solution is referred to as the fitness of a chromosome. The fitness is used to select parents to create offspring of the successive generation. Fitness proportionate or roulette wheel selection is traditionally used to choose parents. The reproduction, mutation and crossover operators are usually used to create the offspring of each generation. As the field has developed, variations of the standard genetic algorithm have emanated. These include the representation of chromosomes which now range from binary strings and character strings to matrices, depending on the problem domain. The effectiveness of tournament selection over fitness proportionate selection has also been established. In addition to this, instead of probabilities of each genetic operator being attached to each chromosome, application rates are set globally and applied in the creation of each generation, e.g. 40% of each generation will be created using mutation and 60% by means of crossover. Furthermore, implementation of genetic algorithms with just mutation has also proven to be effective [6].

Various methods have been applied to solving different versions of the school timetabling problem including tabu search, integer programming, constraint programming and constraint satisfaction methods, simulated annealing, neural networks, GRASP, tiling algorithms, the walk down jump up algorithm, bee algorithms and the cyclic transfer algorithm [4]. Hybrid approaches have also been applied to solving the school timetabling problem. Successful combinations of methods include randomized non-ascendant search (RNA) and tabu search, tabu search and the Floyd-Warshall algorithm, tabu search and graph colouring algorithms, beam search and branch and bound techniques, simulated annealing and very large neighbourhood search [4].

The school timetabling problem differs from school to school and country to country. However previous work has used genetic algorithms to find a solution to a specific school timetabling problem. The study presented in this paper evaluates genetic algorithms over different types of school timetabling problems. A two-phased approach, employing a GA in the first phase to evolve feasible timetables and a GA in the second phase to improve the quality of timetables generated in the first phase, is evaluated in solving the school timetabling problem.

The GA approach was tested on four different types of school timetabling problems, namely, the set of "hard" artificial timetabling problems made available by [6], the Greek high school timetabling problem, a South African primary and high school timetabling problem. It was found that combinations of different construction heuristics, selection methods and mutation operators were needed to generate feasible timetables of good quality for different problems. Hence, there appears to be a need for the automatic configuration of the GA architectures of both phases for the school timetabling problem. This will be examined as part of future work.

The contributions made by the study presented in the paper are: an evaluation of genetic algorithms over a set of different problems with varying characteristics, the identification and evaluation of low-level construction heuristics for this domain, and an evaluation of GAs in solving the South African school timetabling problems. The following section provides an overview of previous work using evolutionary algorithms to solve the school timetabling problem. The two-phased GA approach is presented in section 3. The methodology used to evaluate this approach is outlined in section 4 and section 5 discusses the performance of this approach in solving the different school timetabling problems. A summary of the findings of the study and future extensions of this work are presented in section 6.

2   Genetic Algorithms and School Timetabling

There has been a fair amount of research into using genetic algorithms to solve different types of school timetabling problems including generated problems [7, 8, 9], the Italian [10], Brazilian [11], German [12], Turkish [13], Greek [14] and Bosnian [15] school timetabling problem. Each element of the population is generally a two-dimensional array representing the timetable [8, 10, 13]. The fitness of an individual is the number of constraint violations [15] or the weighted sum of the constraint violations [10, 14]. Either fitness proportionate selection [8, 9, 12, 14] or tournament selection [15] is used to choose parents for each generation. The genetic operators applied to create the offspring of each generation are reproduction, mutation and crossover.

GAs have also been used in combination with other techniques to obtain solutions to school timetabling problems. The h-HCCA genetic algorithm is used by Nurmi et al. [16] to evolve timetables for Finnish schools. This GA incorporates the use of hill-climbing in the mutation operator and simulated annealing to select timetable periods to allocate tuples to. The GA implemented by Zuters et al. [17] uses a neural network to calculate the fitness of the population. A combination of genetic algorithms and a non-random ascent method (RNA) produced better results in solving a set of high school timetabling problems than applications of these methods separately [18].

3   The Two-Phased GA Approach

A two-phased approach is taken in solving the school timetabling problem. The first phase uses a genetic algorithm to produce feasible timetables (Phase I), the quality of which is improved in the second phase by a second genetic algorithm (Phase II). Trial runs conducted revealed that a two-phased approach, with different GAs dealing with hard and soft constraints, was more effective than using a single GA to evolve both feasible and good quality timetables. Previous work [1] applying genetic algorithms to solving the examination timetabling problem has also revealed the effectiveness of a two-phased approach, with each phase employing different GAs to optimize hard and soft constraints.

Both GAs begin by creating an initial population of individuals, i.e. timetables, which are iteratively improved over successive generations with respect to either feasibility or quality. The number of individuals remains constant over all generations. Each successive generation involves evaluation of the population, selecting parents and applying mutation operators to the parents to create the next generation. The stopping criterion for both GAs is a set number of generations. The processes of initial population generation, evaluation, selection and regeneration are described in the following subsections.

3.1   Initial Population Generation

A majority of the studies in section 2 have used a matrix representation for each chromosome. Thus, in this study each element of the population is also a matrix representing a school timetable with each row corresponding to a timetable period and each column a class to be taught. The teacher teaching the class in the particular period (and the venue in which the lesson is to be taught if venue allocation is part of the problem) is stored at the intersection of each row and column.

The requirements, i.e. class-teacher meetings of a problem are defined in terms of class-teacher or class-teacher-venue (if venue allocation is included) tuples. For example, (C1,T4) is a tuple indicating that teacher T4 must teach class C1 and (C3,T1,V1) specifies that class C3 must be taught by teacher T1 in venue V1. If teacher T4 has to meet with class C1 five times in the school week, (C1, T4) will occur five times in the list of tuples to be allocated.

Initially, the timetables of the population of the first generation of the GA for Phase I were created by randomly allocating tuples to timetable periods. However, this is not very effective as the search space represented by the initial population was too large. This led to the derivation of a sequential construction method (SCM) to create each element of the initial population. The SCM creates n timetables. The most appropriate value for n is problem dependant. Each timetable is created by sorting the tuples to be allocated to the timetable according to the difficulty of scheduling the tuple. Low-level construction heuristics are used to assess this difficulty. Each tuple is scheduled in a feasible timetable period, i.e. a period to which the tuple can be allocated without resulting in any hard constraint violations. If there is more than one feasible period available the tuple is allocated to the minimal penalty period, i.e. the period which produces the lowest soft constraint cost. If more than one minimal penalty period exists, a period is randomly selected from these. If there are no feasible periods available the tuple is scheduled in a randomly selected slot. Each timetable is evaluated and its fitness is determined. In Phase I the fitness is the number of hard constraints violated. The SCM returns the fittest of the n timetables. If there is more than one timetable with the same fitness, the soft constraint cost is used as a secondary measure.

One of the contributions of this work is the identification of a set of low-level construction heuristics that can be used to measure the difficulty of scheduling a tuple. Low-level construction heuristics generally used for the university examination and course timetabling problems are the graph colouring heuristics largest degree, largest colour degree, largest weighted degree, largest enrollment and saturation degree [1]. Due to the differences in these problems and the school timetabling problem the largest colour degree, largest weighted degree and largest enrollment are not relevant to the STP. The largest degree and saturation degree have been adapted for the STP and other low-level construction heuristics have been identified for this domain. The following low-level heuristics have been defined for this purpose:

- Random – In this case a construction heuristic is not used and tuples to be allocated are randomly chosen from the list of unscheduled tuples.
- Largest degree – Tuples with a larger number of class-teacher meetings are scheduled first. Once a tuple is allocated the largest degree of the remaining tuples with the same class and teacher (and venue if applicable) is reduced by one. For example, suppose that teacher T3 is required to meet class C1 in venue V4 four times a week. There will be four occurrences of the tuple (C1, T3, V4) in the list of tuples to be allocated and all four occurrences will have a largest degree of 4. Suppose one occurrence is scheduled, leaving three occurrences in the list of unscheduled tuples. The largest degree of three remaining tuples will be reduced by one giving each occurrence a largest degree of 3.
- Saturation degree – The saturation degree of a tuple is the number of feasible, i.e. a period that will not result in hard constraint violations if the tuple is scheduled in it, timetable periods which the tuple can be scheduled in at the current point of the construction process. Tuples with a lower saturation degree are given priority. At the beginning of the timetable construction process all tuples have the same saturation degree, i.e. the number of timetable periods for the problem. For example, suppose that the tuple (C1,T3) has been allocated. The saturation degree of all tuples containing either C1 and/or T3 will be reduced by one.
- Class degree – Tuples containing a class that is involved in the most class-teacher meetings is given priority.
- Teacher degree – Tuples containing the teacher involved in the most number of class-teacher meetings are given priority.
- Consecutive periods – Tuples that need to be scheduled in consecutive periods, i.e. doubles and triples, are given priority and scheduled first.
- Sublclass/co-teaching degree – Tuples that have co-teaching or subclass requirements are given priority and allocated to the timetable before the other tuples.

- Period preferences – Tuples that have to be scheduled in specific periods are scheduled first and hence given priority over the other tuples. For example, if all Mathematics lessons must be scheduled within the first four periods for certain grades all the tuples for these lessons will be given priority.
- Teacher availability – Tuples containing teachers that are available for the least number of days are given priority.

One of these low-level heuristics is usually used to sort tuples. Alternatively, a combination of low-level heuristics can be applied to sort the list of tuples. In this case a primary heuristic and one or more secondary heuristics can be used for sorting purposes. For example, if saturation degree is employed as a primary heuristic and period preferences as a secondary heuristic, the tuples will firstly be sorted in ascending order according to the saturation degree. If two tuples have the same saturation degree, the tuples with a larger number of period preferences will be scheduled first. The initial population of the GA in Phase II is the population of the last generation of Phase I. All the timetables in this population are usually feasible.

3.2   Evaluation and Selection

Evaluation of the population on each generation involves calculating a fitness measure for each individual, i.e. timetable. The fitness of a timetable is the number of hard constraint violations in Phase I and the number of soft constraint violations in Phase II. Thus, in both phases we aim to minimize the fitness of an individual. The fitness of the elements of the population is used by the selection method to choose the parents of the next generation.

The tournament selection method is used to select parents. This method randomly selects t elements of the population where t is referred to as the tournament size. The element of the tournament with the best fitness, i.e. the lowest fitness measure, is returned as a parent.

During trial runs a variation of the tournament selection method, called a sports tournament method, proved to be more effective in the evolution of solutions to the school timetabling problem than the standard tournament selection method. The pseudo code for the sports tournament selection is depicted in Figure 3. The selection method takes an analogy from sport such as cricket where the best team may not always win. Instead of always returning the fittest element of the   tournament this method firstly randomly selects the first element of the tournament and in comparing the successive elements of the tournament randomly decides to leave the *current_champion* unchanged, replace the *current_champion* with the contender, even if the contender is not fitter, or replace the *current_champion* with the contender if the contender is fitter (standard tournament selection). The two-phased GA approach will use either the tournament or sports tournament selection for both GAs of both phases and the choice of selection method is problem dependant.

3.3   Regeneration

One or more mutation operators are applied to chosen parents to create the offspring for each generation. Section 3.3.1 presents the mutation operators used by the GA in

Phase 1 and section 3.3.2 those used by the GA in Phase 2. A certain percentage of mutation operations are usually reduced to reproduction, i.e. the offspring is a copy of the parent. Thus the reproduction operator is not used to reduce the possibilities of cloning. Previous studies have found the use of a crossover operator usually results in violation of the problem requirements, e.g. allocation of the same tuple to the same period. Thus, application of the crossover operator is usually followed by a repair mechanism being applied to rectify the side effects [7, 9]. This is time consuming and results in an increase in runtimes. Hence, Bedoya et al. [8] do not implement a crossover operator. The same approach is taken in this study.

3.3.1 Phase 1 Operators

The following three mutation operators are available for the GA for Phase 1:

- Double violation mutation (2V) – This operator locates two tuples assigned to periods which have resulted in hard constraint violations and swaps these tuples. This swap may result in no change in the fitness of the timetable, i.e. the swap has not removed the violations or may improve the fitness by resulting in one or both of the violations being eliminated.
- Single violation mutation (1V) – This mutation operator selects a tuple causing a hard constraint violation and swaps it with a randomly selected tuple. This could result in a further violation worsening the fitness. Alternatively, the swap may remove the constraint violation improving the fitness of the timetable or have no effect.
- Random swap – This operator selects two tuples or two sets of consecutive tuples randomly and swaps the locations of the tuples or sets in the timetable.

Each of these operators performs s swaps and the best value for s is problem dependant. Versions of these operators incorporating hill-climbing is also available. The hill-climbing versions of these operators continue mutating the parent until an offspring fitter than the parent is produced. In order to prevent premature convergence of the GA and long runtimes, a limit l is set on the number of attempts at producing a fitter individual. If this limit is reached the last offspring created is returned as the result of the operation. The performance of the different mutation operators with and without the incorporation of hill-climbing will be tested for the different school timetabling problems. This is discussed in section 4.

3.3.2 Phase 2 Operators

This section describes the four mutation operators that are used by the GA in Phase 2 of the approach. As in the first phase, each mutation operator performs s swaps, with the best value for s being problem dependant. Swaps producing hard constraint violations are not allowed. The four mutation operators for Phase 2 are:

- Random swap – This operator randomly selects two tuples and swaps their positions in the timetable.
- Row swap - Two rows in the timetable are randomly selected and swapped, changing the period that the tuples in both the rows are scheduled in.
- Double violation mutation – Two tuples causing soft constraint violations are chosen and swapped. This can have no effect on the fitness or improve the fitness by eliminating one or both of the violations.

- Single violation mutation – The position of a tuple causing a soft constraint violation is swapped with that of a randomly selected tuple. As in the first phase this could result in a further violation, have no effect or remove the soft constraint violation.
- Subclass+co - teaching row swap (1VSRS) – The row containing a tuple that is violating a subclass or co-teaching constraints is swapped with another row.

As in the first phase, versions of these operators including the use of hill-climbing are also implemented. In this case the mutation operator is applied until an offspring at least as fit as the parent is produced. Again to prevent premature convergence and lengthy runtimes a limit is set on the number of attempts at producing such an offspring.

4   Experimental Setup

This section describes the school timetabling problems that the GA approach presented in the previous section is evaluated on, the genetic parameter values used and the technical specifications of the machines the simulations were run on.

4.1   School Timetabling Problems

The school timetabling problem varies from school to school due to the different educational systems adopted by different countries. Thus, there are different versions of the school timetabling problem. In order to thoroughly test the two-phased GA approach and to evaluate it in a South African context, the approach was applied to four school timetabling problems:

- A set of hard benchmark school timetabling problems
- The Greek high school timetabling problem
- A South African primary school timetabling problem
- A South African high school timetabling problem

Each of these problems is described in the following subsections.

4.1.1 Benchmark Timetabling Problems
Abramson [7] has made available five artificial timetabling problems [19]. These problems are "hard" timetabling problems (hence the *hdtt*) as all periods must be utilized with very little or no options for each allocation. The characteristics of the problems are listed in Table 1. Each school week is comprised of five days with six periods a day with a total of 30 timetable periods.

Table 1. Characteristics of the artificial school timetabling problems

Problem	Number of teachers	Number of Venues	Number of Classes
hdtt4	4	4	4
hdtt5	5	5	5
hdtt6	6	6	6
hdtt7	7	7	7
hdtt8	8	8	8

All five problems have the following hard constraints:

- All class-teacher-venue tuples must be scheduled the required number of times.
- There must be no class clashes, i.e. a class must not be scheduled more than once in a period.
- There must be no teacher clashes, i.e. a teacher must not be scheduled more than once in a period.
- There must be no venue clashes, i.e. a venue must not be allocated more than once to a timetable period.

4.1.2 The Greek School Timetabling Problem

The GA approach is applied to two Greek school timetabling problems, namely, that made available by Valouxis et al. [20] and Beligiannis et al. [21]. The problem presented by Valouxis et al. involves 15 teachers and 6 classes. There are 35 weekly timetable periods, i.e. 5 days with 7 periods per day. The hard constraints of the problem are:

- All class-teacher meetings must be scheduled.
- There must be no class or teacher clashes.
- Class free/idle periods must be scheduled in the last period of the day.
- Each teacher's workload limit for a day must not be exceeded.
- Class-teacher meetings must be uniformly distributed over the school week.

The soft constraints for the problem are:

- The number of free periods in the class timetable must be minimized.
- Teacher period preferences must satisfied if possible.

The GA approach is also tested on six of the problems made available by Beligiannis et al. [21]. The characteristics of these problems are depicted in Table 2. There are 35 timetable periods per week.

Table 2. Characteristic of the Beligiannis Problem Set

Problem	Number of Teachers	Number of Classes	Number of Co-Teaching/Sublcass Requirements
HS1	11	34	18
HS2	11	35	24
HS3	6	19	0
HS4	7	19	12
HS5	6	18	0
HS6	13	35	20

The hard constraints for the problem are:

- All class-teacher meetings must be scheduled.
- There must be no class or teacher clashes.
- Teachers must not be scheduled to teach when they are not available.

- Class free/idle periods must be scheduled in the last period of the day.
- Co-teaching and subclass requirements must be met.

The problem soft constraints are:

- The number of idle/free periods for teachers must be minimized.
- Free periods must be equally distributed amongst teachers.
- The workload for a teacher must be uniformly distributed over the week.
- Classes should not be taught the same subject in consecutive periods or more than once in a day if possible.

4.1.3 South African Primary School Problem

This problem involves 19 teachers, 16 classes and 14 subjects. There are a maximum of 11 weekly timetable periods. However, different grades have a different number of daily periods ranging from 9 to 11. The hard constraints for the problem are:

- All required class-teacher meetings must be scheduled.
- There must be no class or teacher clashes.
- Certain subjects must be taught in specialized venues, e.g. Technology in the computer laboratory.
- Mathematics must be taught in the mornings (specified in terms of valid periods).
- All co-teaching requirements must be met.
- All double period requirements must be met.

The problem has one soft constraint, namely, the lessons per class must be uniformly distributed throughout the school week.

4.1.4 South African High School

The South African high school problem that the GA approach is applied to involves 30 classes, 40 teachers and 44 subjects. The hard constraints for the problem are:

- All required class-teacher meetings must be scheduled.
- There must be no class or teacher clashes.
- All sub-class and co-teaching requirements must be met.

The soft constraints for the problem are:

- Teacher period preferences must be met if possible.
- Period preferences for classes must be met if possible.

4.2 Genetic Parameter Values

Trials runs were conducted to determine the most appropriate values for the following genetic parameters:

- SCM population size (*n*) – The SCM is used to create each element of the population. It creates *n* timetables, the fittest of which is included in the GA population of Phase I.
- GA population size
- Number of generations
- Tournament size
- Number of mutation swaps
- Number of generations

Table 3 lists the values tested for each of these parameters.

Table 3. Ranges for each parameter value

Parameter	Tested range	Note:
SCM size	1 to 100	Only applicable in Phase 1
Population size	200 to 1000	Constant population size adopted for every generation
Tournament size	5 to 20	Applicable to tournament selection for Phase 1 and Phase 2
Swaps	20 to 200	Applicable to mutation operators for Phase 1 and Phase 2
Generations	20 to 75	Applicable to Phase 1 and Phase 2

When testing each parameter value, 30 runs were performed. In order to test the impact that each parameter has on the performance of the genetic algorithm, all other parameter values, construction heuristics, selection methods and genetic operators were kept constant. The most appropriate values found for each problem are listed in Table 4.

Table 4. Parameter values for each data set

Problem	SCM	Population Size	Tournament Size	Swaps per Mutation	Genera- tions
HDTT4	50	1000	10	200	50
HDTT5	50	1000	10	200	50
HDTT6	50	1000	10	200	50
HDTT7	50	1000	10	200	50
HDTT8	50	1000	10	200	50
Valouxis	50	1000	10	100	50
HS1 – HS4, HS6	25	750	15	200	50
HS5	50	750	10	20	75
Lewitt	20	500	10	200	50
Woodlands	20	750	10	150	75

4.3   Technical Specifications

The GA system was developed using Visual C++ 2008. The random number generator function available in C++ is used to generate random numbers. A different seed is used for each run of the genetic algorithm approach. Simulations (trial and final) were run on several machines:

- Intel Core 2 Duo CPU @ 2.40 GHz, 2.00 GB RAM, Windows XP, Windows 7 Enterprise OS.
- Intel Core I7 870 CPU @ 2.93 GHz, 4.00 GB RAM, Windows 7 64-bit OS.
- Intel Core I7 860 CPU @ 2.80 GHZ, 4.00 GB RAM (3.49 Usable), Windows 7 32-bit OS.
- Pentium Dual Core @ 2GHZ, 2.00 GB RAM, Windows XP.

5   Results and Discussion

The two-phased genetic algorithm approach was able to evolve feasible solutions of good quality for all problems. Different combinations of construction heuristics, selection method and genetic operators were found to produce the best quality solution for each problem. The GA approach was run using different combinations of these components. In order to test the impact that each component has on the performance of each genetic algorithm, all other genetic algorithm components and parameter values are kept constant. Thirty runs were performed for each component. The statistical significance of the performance of the different construction heuristics, selection methods and genetic operators was ascertained using hypothesis tests[1] (tested at the 1%, 5% and 10% levels of significance). The combination producing the best result for each problem is listed Table 5. Note that if hill-climbing was used with the genetic operator this is indicated by HC and if it was not used by NH.

The use of saturation degree as a primary heuristic produced the best results for all except one problem. A secondary heuristic was needed for all of the real world problems especially problems involving subclass and co-teaching constraints. For the Abramson data set double violation mutation without hill-climbing appears to be the most effective during Phase 1. For the real world problems single violation mutation with hill-climbing produced the best results for a majority of the problems. Hill-climbing was not needed in Phase 2 to produce the best soft constraint cost for any of the problems with single violation mutation proving to be the most effective for a majority of the problems. The sports tournament selection method appears to be effective in the GA implemented in Phase 1 focused on optimizing the hard constraint costs while the standard tournament selection appears to have produced better results in Phase 2, which improves the quality of timetables, for most of the problems. It is evident from Table 5 that different combinations of low-level constructive heuristics, selection method and mutation operators is needed to solve each problem. Future work will investigate whether there is a correlation between the architecture of the GAs of each phase and the characteristics of the different problems as well as methods for the automatic configuration of the GA architectures of both phases for the school timetabling problem.

---

[1] Throughout the paper hypothesis tests conducted test that the means are equal and the Z test is used.

Table 5. Summary of best heuristics, methods and operators for each data set

Problem	PHASE 1				PHASE 2	
	Primary Heuristic	Secondary Heuristics	Selection Method	Genetic Operators	Selection Method	Genetic Operator
HDTT4	Saturation Degree	None	Std/Sports	2VNH	N/A	N/A
HDTT5	Saturation Degree	None	Sports	2VNH	N/A	N/A
HDTT6	Saturation Degree	None	Sports	2VNH	N/A	N/A
HDTT7	Saturation Degree	None	Sports	2VNH	N/A	N/A
HDTT8	Saturation Degree	None	Standard	2VNH	N/A	N/A
Valouxis	Saturation Degree	Teacher Degree Teacher availability	Sports	1VHC	Sports	Random Swap
HS1	Saturation Degree	SubClass/Co-Teaching degree	Sports	1VHC	Standard	Single Violation
HS2	Saturation Degree	SubClass/Co-Teaching degree	Sports	1VHC	Standard	Single Violation
HS3	Saturation Degree	SubClass/Co-Teaching degree	Sports	1VHC	Standard	Single Violation
HS4	Saturation Degree	SubClass/Co-Teaching	Sports	1VHC	Sports	Single Violation
HS5	Largest Degree	SubClass/Co-Teaching degree	Sports	1VNH	Standard	Random Swap
HS7	Saturation Degree	SubClass/Co-Teaching degree	Sports	1VHC	Standard	Single Violation
Lewitt	Saturation Degree	Consecutive Periods	Standard	Hybrid (2VHC, 1VHC, Random Swap)	Sports	Random Swap
Woodlands	Saturation Degree	SubClass/Co-Teaching degree	Standard	1VHC	Standard	1VSRS

The performance of the GA approach was compared to other methods applied to the same set of problems. For the first set of problems, namely, the benchmark hard problems made available by Abramson [7], the GA approach was compared to the following:

- SA1 – A simulated annealing method implemented by Abramson et al. [22].
- SA2 – A simulated annealing algorithm implemented by Randall [23].
- TS – A tabu search employed by Randall [23].
- GS – The greedy search method used by Randall [23].
- NN-T2 – A neural network employed by Smith et al. [24].
- NN-T3 – A second neural network employed by Smith et al. [24].

The hard constraints for this set of problems are listed in section 4. The minimum (best cost - BC) and average (average cost – AC) hard constraint costs for each of these methods and the GA approach is listed in Table 6. In this study the average is taken over thirty runs. The best results are highlighted in bold. The GA approach has produced the minimum for all of the problems and the best average for three of the problems. For the remaining two problems, the average obtained is very close to the best results.

Table 6. Comparison for the Abramson Data Set

Method	HDTT4	HDTT5	HDTT6	HDTT7	HDTT8
SA1	BC: Unknown AC: Unknown	BC: 0 AC: 0.67	BC: 0 AC: 2.5	BC: 2 AC: 2.5	BC: 2 AC: 8.23
SA2	**BC: 0** **AC: 0**	BC: 0 AC: 0.3	BC: 0 AC: 0.8	BC: 0 AC: 1.2	BC: 0 AC: 1.9
TS	BC: 0 AC: 0.2	BC: 0 AC: 2.2	BC: 3 AC: 5.6	BC: 4 AC: 10.9	BC: 13 AC: 17.2
GS	BC: 5 AC: 8.5	BC: 11 AC: 16.2	BC: 19 AC: 22.2	BC: 26 AC: 30.9	BC: 29 AC: 35.4
HNN1	BC: 0 AC: 0.1	BC: 0 AC: 0.5	BC: 0 AC: 0.8	BC: 0 AC: 1.1	BC: 0 AC: 1.4
HNN2	BC: 0 AC: 0.5	BC: 0 AC: 0.5	BC: 0 AC: 0.7	**BC: 0** **AC: 1**	**BC: 0** **AC: 1.2**
GA approach	**BC: 0** **AC: 0**	**BC: 0** **AC: 0**	**BC: 0** **AC: 0**	BC: 0 AC: 1.067	BC: 0 AC: 1.733

The GA approach was also applied to the school timetabling problem presented by Valouxis et al. [20]. In the study conducted by Valouxis et al. constraint programming was used to solve this problem. The timetables induced by both methods were run through an evaluator developed by the authors which assessed the hard and soft constraint costs. Feasible timetables were produced by both methods. The timetable produced by constraint programming had 45 soft constraint violations while that produced by the GA approach had 35.

The timetables generated by the evolutionary algorithm implemented by Beligiannis et al. [21] are compared to those produced by the GA approach. Again an evaluator developed by the authors was used to assess the hard and soft constraint cost of all timetables for comparison purposes. Both methods produced feasible timetables for the 6 problems tested. The soft constraint costs of the timetables are listed in Table 7.

Table 7. Comparison with the Beligannis data set [21]

Problem	Evolutionary Algorithm	GA Approach
HS1	139	96
HS2	175	99
HS3	61	34
HS4	102	59
HS5	43	40
HS6	226	117

The timetable used by the South African primary school is induced by a package. The timetable produced by the package is manually changed to meet the hard and soft constraints. The current timetable used by the school does not meet all the double period requirements while the best timetable evolved by the GA approach satisfies these. The best timetable produced by the GA for the South African high school problem is a feasible timetable and has the same soft constraint cost, namely a cost of two, as the timetable currently being used by the school. From the above comparisons it is evident that the performance of the GA approach is comparable and in some cases better, than other methodologies applied to the same problems.

6   Conclusion and Future Work

This study has presented a two-phased genetic algorithm approach for solving the school timetabling problem. In previous work a genetic algorithm was developed to solve a particular problem whereas this study has evaluated genetic algorithms as a means of solving different school timetabling problems. The paper has also defined low-level construction heuristics for this domain. The performance of a methodology on a variety of problems is important as the school timetabling problem varies drastically from one school to the next. The two-phased genetic programming approach was tested on four different types of problem sets involving a total of 13 different problems. This approach was able to produce feasible timetables for all problems. The soft constraint cost of these timetables were found to be comparable to and in some cases better than other methodologies applied to the same problems. Different combinations of genetic algorithm components, namely, construction heuristics, selection methods and genetic operators were needed to produce the best results for the different problems. Thus, future work will focus on identifying the correlation between different combinations and problem characteristics and methods for the automatic configuration of the GA architecture for both phases of the GA approach in solving the school timetabling problem. This research will investigate the use of case-based reasoning and an evolutionary algorithm, to explore a space of strings representing the GA components to find the optimal combination, as options for automatic GA architecture configuration. The study has also revealed that GAs can successful solve both the South African primary and high school timetabling.

References

1. Pillay, N., Banzhaf, W.: An Informed Genetic Algorithm for the Uncapacitated Examination Timetabling Problem. Applied Soft Computing 10, 45–67 (2010)
2. Larranaga, P., Kuijpers, C.M.H., Murga, R.H., Inza, I., Dizdarevic, S.: Genetic Algorithms for the Travelling Salesman Problem: A Review of Representations and Operators. Artificial Intelligence Review 11(2), 129–170 (1999)
3. Ponce-Perez, A., Perez-Garcia, A., Ayala-Ramirez, V.: Bin-Packing Using Genetic Algorithms. In: Proceedings of CONIELECOMP 2005: 15th International Conference on Electronics, Communications and Computers, pp. 311–314. IEEE Press (2005)
4. Pillay, N.: A Survey of School Timetabling. Annals of Operations Research (February 2013), doi:10.1007/s10479-013-1321-8
5. Goldberg, D., Genetic Algorithms in Search, Optimization and Machine Learning. Addison-Wesley Longman Publishing Co. (1989).
6. Beasley, D., Bull, D.R., Martin, R.R.: An Overview of Genetic Algorithms: Part 1 and Part 2, Research Topics. University Computing 15(4), 170–181 (1993)
7. Abramson, D., Abela, J.: A Parallel Genetic Algorithm for the Solving the School Timetabling Problem. In: Proceedings of the Fifteenth Australian Conference: Division of Information Technology, C.S.I.R.O. pp. 1–11 (1991)
8. Bedoya, C.F., Santos, M.: A Non-Standard Genetic Algorithm Approach to Solve Constrained School Timetabling Problems. Eurocast, 26–37 (2003)
9. Calderia, J.P., Ross, A.C.: School Timetabling Using Genetic Search. In: The Proceedings of the International Conference on the Practice and Theory of Automated Timetabling (PATAT 1997) pp. 115-122 (1997)
10. Colorni, A., Dorigo, M., Maniezzo, V.: Metaheuristics for High School Timetabling. In: Computational Optimization and Applications, vol. 9, pp. 275–298. Kluwer Academic Publishers (1998)
11. Filho, G.R., Lorena, L.A.N.: A Constructive Evolutionary Approach to School Timetabling. In: Boers, E.J.W., Gottlieb, J., Lanzi, P.L., Smith, R.E., Cagnoni, S., Hart, E., Raidl, G.R., Tijink, H. (eds.) EvoWorkshop 2001. LNCS, vol. 2037, pp. 130–139. Springer, Heidelberg (2001)
12. Wilke, P., Gröbner, M., Oster, N.: A Hybrid Genetic Algorithm for School Timetabling. In: McKay, B., Slaney, J.K. (eds.) AI 2002. LNCS (LNAI), vol. 2557, pp. 455–464. Springer, Heidelberg (2002)
13. Yigit, T.: Constraint-Based School Timetabling Using Hybrid Genetic Algorithms. In: Basili, R., Pazienza, M.T. (eds.) AI*IA 2007. LNCS (LNAI), vol. 4733, pp. 848–855. Springer, Heidelberg (2007)
14. Beligiannis, G.N., Moschopoulos, C.N., Likothanassis, S.D.: A Genetic Algorithm Approach to School Timetabling. Journal of the Operational Research Society 60(1), 23–42 (2009)
15. Srndic, N., Dervisevic, M., Pandzo, E., Konjicija, S.: The Application of a Parallel Genetic Algorithm to Timetabling of Elementary School Classes: A Coarse Grained Approach. In: Proceedings of ICAT 2009 -2009 22nd International Symposium on Information, Communication and Automation Technologies, pp. 1–5. IEEE (2009)
16. Nurmi, K., Kyngas, J.: A Framework for School Timetabling Problem. In: Proceedings of the 3rd Multidisciplinary International Scheduling Conference: Theory and Application (2007)

17. Zuters, J.: Neural Networks to Enrich Fitness Function in a GA-Based School Timetabling Model. Proceedings of WSEAS Transactions on Information Science and Application 4(2), 346–353 (2007)
18. Cedeira-Pena, A., Carpente, L., Farina, A., Seco, D.: New Approaches for the School Timetabling Problem. In: Proceedings of the 7th Mexican Conference on Artificial Intelligence (MICAI 2008), pp. 261–267 (2008)
19. Beasley, J.F.: OR Library, http://people.brunel.ac.uk/mastjjb/jeb/orlib/tableinfo.html (accessed May 25, 2011)
20. Valouxis, C., Housos, E.: Constraint Programming Approach for School Timetabling. Computers and Operations Research 30, 1555–1572 (2003)
21. Beligiannis, G.N., Moschopoulos, C.N., Kaperonis, G.P., Likothanassis, S.D.: Applying Evolutionary Computation to the School Timetabling Problem: The Greek Case. Computers and Operations Research 35, 1265–1280 (2008)
22. Abramson, D., Dang, H.: School Timetable: A Case Study in Simulated Annealing. In: Applied Simulated Annealing Lecture Notes in Economics and Mathematical Systems, ch. 5, pp. 103–124 (1993)
23. Randall, M.: A General Meta-Heuristic Based Solver for Combinatorial Optimization Problems. Computational Optimization and Applications 20(2), 185–210 (2000)
24. Smith, K.A., Abramson, D., Duke, D.: Hopfield Neural Networks for Timetabling: Formulations, Methods, and Comparative Results. Computers and Industrial Engineering 44, 285–305 (2003)

Explicit Exploration in Estimation of Distribution Algorithms

Rogelio Salinas-Gutiérrez[1], Ángel Eduardo Muñoz-Zavala[1],
Arturo Hernández-Aguirre[2], and Manuel Alonso Castillo-Galván[1]

[1] Universidad Autónoma de Aguascalientes, Aguascalientes, México
{rsalinas,aemz}@correo.uaa.mx, gerber.heelflip@gmail.com
[2] Center for Research in Mathematics (CIMAT), Guanajuato, México
artha@cimat.mx

Abstract. This work proposes an Estimation of Distribution Algorithm (EDA) that incorporates an explicit separation between the exploration stage and the exploitation stage. For each stage a probabilistic model is required. The proposed EDA uses a mixture of distributions in the exploration stage whereas a multivariate Gaussian distribution is used in the exploitation stage. The benefits of using an explicit exploration stage are shown through numerical experiments.

Keywords: Estimation of Distribution Algorithm, Exploration stage, Exploitation stage.

1 Introduction

Estimation of Distribution Algorithms (EDAs) [10] are metaheuristics designed for searching good solutions in optimization problems. Similar to other metaheuristics of Evolutionary Computation (EC), EDAs are iterative algorithms based on the use of populations. However, an important characteristic of EDAs is the incorporation of probabilistic models in order to represent the dependencies among the decision variables of selected individuals. Once a probabilistic model is learnt by an EDA, it is possible to replicate dependencies in the new population by sampling from the model.

Algorithm 1 shows a pseudocode for EDAs. According to step 4, the dependencies among decision variables are taken into account by means of the probabilistic distribution $\mathcal{M}_t$. Step 5 shows how the dependence structure of the selected individuals is transferred to the new population, which greatly modifies the performance of an EDA.

As shown in Algorithm 1, step 4 involves an important and critical procedure in EDAs. For this reason, much of the research in EDAs has been focused precisely on proposing and enhancing new probabilistic models with many contributions in discrete and continuous domains [9,12,3]. Some of these probabilistic models are based on Bayesian and Markov networks [14,5,11]. Other EDAs have

F. Castro, A. Gelbukh, and M. González (Eds.): MICAI 2013, Part II, LNAI 8266, pp. 81–92, 2013.

Algorithm 1. Pseudocode for EDAs

1: Initialize the generation counter $t \longleftarrow 0$
   Generate the initial population $\mathcal{P}_0$ with N individuals at random.
2: Evaluate population $\mathcal{P}_t$ using the cost function.
3: Select a subset $\mathcal{S}_t$ from $\mathcal{P}_t$ according to the selection method.
4: Estimate a probabilistic model $\mathcal{M}_t$ from $\mathcal{S}_t$.
5: Generate the new population $\mathcal{P}_{t+1}$ by sampling from the model $\mathcal{M}_t$
   Assign $t \longleftarrow t + 1$.
6: If stopping criteria are not reached go to step 2.

---

used Gaussian assumptions [6,7,1,2], such as Gaussian kernels, Gaussian mixture models and the multivariate Gaussian distribution. The interested reader is referred to [8,4] for knowing more about the probabilistic models used in EDAs.

Although the active research in EDAs has been oriented to model adequately dependencies among decision variables [13], the generation of individuals in the exploration stage has not been investigated. This observation gives an opportunity for proposing a new exploration procedure and for studying its effects in EDAs.

The structure of the paper is the following: Section 2 describes the proposal of this work, Section 3 shows some preliminary results of the implementation of the exploration stage, Section 4 presents the experimental setting to solve five test global optimization problems, and Section 5 resumes the conclusions.

2   The Exploration Stage

According to Algorithm 1, the initial population is generated at random. This means that the first population is generated by sampling from the uniform distribution. However, once the first population is generated, the following populations are generated by sampling from a probabilistic model $\mathcal{M}_t$ which is in general different than the uniform distribution. A common practice in EDAs is that the probabilistic model $\mathcal{M}_t$ is selected beforehand from a family of probabilistic distributions. Therefore, the immediate transition between the uniform distribution and the probabilistic model $\mathcal{M}_t$ could affect the performance of the exploration stage. This work investigates the effects of having an explicit separation between the exploration stage and the exploitation stage.

The proposal of incorporating an explicit exploration stage in EDAs requires the support of an adequate estrategy. Firstly, the number of generations for the exploration stage must be defined in advance. For example, the number of generations can be given by a fixed number. Secondly, a probabilistic model is needed in order to generate populations in the exploration stage. The natural choice for exploration purposes is a probabilistic distribution with high variance. However, the progress of the exploration stage must be reflected in the variance of the probabilistic model.

This work proposes the incorporation of a mixture of distributions for the exploration stage. The mixture is formed with the uniform distribution and with a distribution based on a modified histogram. The uniform distribution allows to generate individuals with high variance. The histogram is a statistics tool for density estimation and its implementation is well known. The histogram is used as a model for the selected individuals in each generation within the exploration stage. However, in order to favor the generation of individuals with high variance, we propose the use of a histogram with similar height for all bars. Figure 1 illustrates this idea. The total area of each histogram, (a) and (b), is normalized to 1.

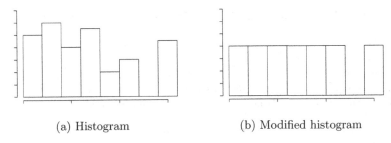

(a) Histogram   (b) Modified histogram

Fig. 1. The modified histogram (b) is based on the initial histogram (a) and its rectangles have the same height

The expression for the proposed mixture of distributions is given by:

$$\mathcal{E}_t = w_t \cdot \mathcal{U} + (1 - w_t) \cdot \mathcal{H} \ , \text{with } w_t \in [0, 1]. \tag{1}$$

The mixture (1) offers the following characteristics:

1. The initial weight of the uniform distribution $\mathcal{U}$ is the highest possible whereas the weight of the modified histogram $\mathcal{H}$ is the lowest. This allows to start the exploration stage with individuals sampled from a distribution of high variance.
2. According to the advance of the exploration stage, the weight of the uniform distribution $\mathcal{U}$ is decreased whereas the weight of the modified histogram $\mathcal{H}$ is increased.

Algorithm 2 shows the inclusion of a procedure for the exploration stage in EDAs. It can be noted that the number of 100 generations (step 2) and the rule for decreasing the weight w_t (step 7) are defined in this way to indicate the extension of the exploration stage. Both the number of generations and the expression for the weight can be changed by other values. On the other hand, it can be also note that the exploitation stage has elitism whereas the exploration stage has not elitism. However, the best individuals found during the process of the exploration stage are used as the initial population for the exploitation stage.

Algorithm 2. Pseudocode for EDA with explicit exploration

1: Exploration stage
   Initialize the weight $w_t \longleftarrow 1$
2: **for** $t = 1 \rightarrow 100$ **do**
3:     Generate the population $\mathcal{P}_t$ with N individuals by sampling from the model $\mathcal{E}_t$
       (see Eq. (1))
4:     Evaluate population $\mathcal{P}_t$ using the cost function.
5:     Select a subset $\mathcal{S}_t$ from $\mathcal{P}_t$ according to the selection method.
6:     Estimate a modified histogram $\mathcal{H}$ from $\mathcal{S}_t$.
7:     Assign $w_t \longleftarrow 1 - (t/100)$.
8:     Select the best N individuals from all the previous generations and record them
       in $\mathcal{B}$.
9: **end for**
10: Exploitation stage
    Assign $\mathcal{P}_t \longleftarrow \mathcal{B}$.
11: Evaluate population $\mathcal{P}_t$ using the cost function.
12: Select a subset $\mathcal{S}_t$ from $\mathcal{P}_t$ according to the selection method.
13: Estimate a probabilistic model $\mathcal{M}_t$ from $\mathcal{S}_t$.
14: Generate the new population $\mathcal{P}_{t+1}$ by sampling from the model $\mathcal{M}_t$
15: Set $\mathcal{P}_{t+1}$ with the best N individuals from $\mathcal{P}_{t+1} \cup \mathcal{P}_t$
    Assign $t \longleftarrow t + 1$.
16: If stopping criteria are not reached go to step 2.

---

3   Preliminary Results

In order to gain some insight about how the inclusion of the exploration stage modifies the performance of an EDA, we compare two EDAs in two test problems. The comparison is done through the Estimation of Multivariate Normal Algorithm (EMNA) and the EMNA with the exploration stage (EMNA+E). The test problems are the Rosenbrock and Sphere functions. These test functions are described in Fig. 2.

The benchmark test suite includes separable functions and non-separable functions, from which there are unimodal and multimodal functions. In addition, the search domain is asymmetric. All test functions are scalable. We use test problems in 10 dimensions. Each algorithm is run 30 times for each problem. The population size is 100 and the maximum number of generations is 150.

A graphical comparison between EMNA and EMNA+E is shown in Figure 3. According to these graphical results, the EMNA has a better performance than the EMNA+E in the first 100 generations. However, after the exploration stage is done, the performance of the EMNA+E outperforms the performance of the EMNA.

4   Experiments

Five test problems are used to compare an EDA with exploration against a typical EDA without explicit exploration. These algorithms are, respectively, the

Description
Ackley

$$-20 \cdot \exp\left(-0.2\sqrt{\frac{1}{d} \cdot \sum_{i=1}^{d} x_i^2}\right) - \exp\left(\frac{1}{d} \cdot \sum_{i=1}^{d} \cos(2\pi x_i)\right) + 20 + \exp(1)$$

$$\boldsymbol{x} \in [-10, 30]^d$$

Properties: Multimodal, Non-separable   Global Minimum: $f(\mathbf{0}) = 0$

Griewangk

$$1 + \sum_{i=1}^{d} \frac{x_i^2}{4000} - \prod_{i=1}^{d} \cos\left(\frac{x_i}{\sqrt{i}}\right) \; ; \quad \boldsymbol{x} \in [-200, 1000]^d$$

Properties: Multimodal, Non-separable   Global Minimum: $f(\mathbf{0}) = 0$

Rastrigin

$$\sum_{i=1}^{d} (x_i^2 - 10\cos(2\pi x_i) + 10) \; ; \quad \boldsymbol{x} \in [-10, 30]^d$$

Properties: Multimodal, Separable   Global Minimum: $f(\mathbf{0}) = 0$

Rosenbrock

$$\sum_{i=1}^{d-1}[100 \cdot (x_{i+1} - x_i^2)^2 + (1 - x_i)^2] \; ; \quad \boldsymbol{x} \in [-10, 30]^d$$

Properties: Unimodal, Non-separable   Global Minimum: $f(\mathbf{1}) = 0$

Sphere Model

$$\sum_{i=1}^{d} x_i^2 \; ; \quad \boldsymbol{x} \in [-200, 1000]^d$$

Properties: Unimodal, Separable   Global Minimum: $f(\mathbf{0}) = 0$

Fig. 2. Names, mathematical definition, search domains, global minimum and properties of the test functions

EMNA+E and the EMNA. The multivariate Gaussian distribution is incorporated as probabilistic model to the EMNA and the same distribution is used for the exploitation stage in the EMNA+E. Algorithm 1 is the basis for the EMNA whereas Algorithm 2 is the corresponding basis for the EMNA+E. In order to make a fair comparison, the elitism in the exploitation stage of EMNA+E is also included in the EMNA.

The test problems used in the experiments are the Ackley, Griewangk, Rastrigin, Rosenbrock, and Sphere functions. Fig. 2 describe the test functions. The algorithms are tested in different dimensions and asymmetric search domain. Each algorithm is run 30 times for each problem. The population size is ten times the dimension $(10 * d)$. The maximum number of evaluations is 100,000. However, when convergence to a local minimum is detected the run is stopped. Any improvement less than 1×10^{-6} in 25 iterations is considered as convergence. The goal is to reach the optimum with an error less than 1×10^{-4}.

The results in dimensions 4, 6, 8, 10, 15 and 20 for non-separable functions are reported in Table 1, whereas the results for separable functions are reported

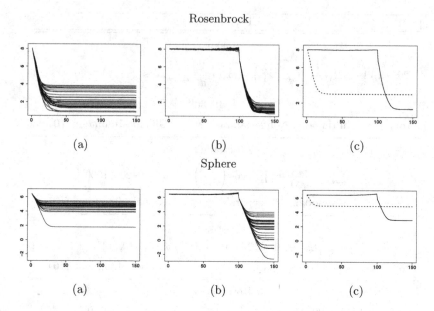

Fig. 3. The horizontal axis represents the generation and the vertical axis represents the fitness in logarithmic scale (base 10). (a) The fitness performance of EMNA. (b) The fitness performance of EMNA+E. (c) The dashed line is used for the average performance of EMNA and the solid line is used for the average performance of EMNA+E.

in Table 2. Both tables report descriptive statistics for the fitness values reached in the all runs. The fitness value corresponds to the value of a test problem. For each algorithm and dimension, the minimum, median, mean, maximum, standard deviation and success rate are shown. The minimum (maximum) value reached is labelled best (worst). The success rate is the proportion of runs in which an algorithm found the global optimum.

Besides the descriptive results shown in Tables 1 and 2, a hypothesis test is conducted to properly compare the performance of EMNA+E against EMNA. The statistical comparisons are for the algorithms with the same test problem and the same dimension. The t-test is employed to compare the fitness average between EMNA+E and EMNA. When a hypothesis test indicates that EMNA+E is significantly better than the EMNA, the corresponding average in in Tables 1 and 2 is marked with an asterix (*).

Another measure that can help in the comparisons of the algorithms is the success rate. Tables 1 and 2 show respectively the success rate in each dimension for non-separable and separable functions. If the success rate of EMNA+E is greater than the success rate of EMNA, it is marked with a dagger (†).

Table 1. Descriptive results of the fitness for non-separable functions

Algorithm	d	Best	Mean	Median	Worst	Std. Dev.	Success Rate
Ackley							
EMNA	4	1.86E-7	5.28E-1	1.42E-3	4.30E+0	1.11E+0	0.40
	6	5.01E-5	1.57E+0	8.50E-1	5.60E+0	1.72E+0	0.00
	8	1.65E-2	3.20E+0	3.22E+0	9.14E+0	2.41E+0	0.00
	10	6.86E-1	3.85E+0	3.12E+0	8.53E+0	1.97E+0	0.00
	15	1.34E+0	5.21E+0	5.54E+0	8.36E+0	1.60E+0	0.00
	20	4.81E+0	7.09E+0	7.34E+0	1.00E+1	1.33E+0	0.00
EMNA + E	4	2.71E-7	6.29E-3**	9.24E-7	1.49E-1	2.77E-2	0.60 †
	6	6.46E-7	4.57E-2**	2.22E-3	5.76E-1	1.14E-1	0.23 †
	8	7.26E-7	1.57E-1**	2.69E-2	1.32E+0	3.11E-1	0.03 †
	10	7.12E-6	3.59E-1**	1.60E-1	1.59E+0	4.42E-1	0.00
	15	2.15E-2	1.96E+0**	1.81E+0	3.25E+0	8.35E-1	0.00
	20	2.10E+0	3.84E+0**	3.66E+0	6.44E+0	1.23E+0	0.00
Griewangk							
EMNA	4	5.26E-2	1.64E+0	1.68E-1	1.28E+1	3.31E+0	0.00
	6	9.41E-2	3.58E+0	4.67E-1	3.39E+1	7.25E+0	0.00
	8	2.49E-1	9.65E+0	5.24E+0	9.45E+1	1.73E+1	0.00
	10	9.86E-1	1.33E+1	8.47E+0	5.01E+1	1.36E+1	0.00
	15	7.46E+0	5.97E+1	5.46E+1	1.21E+2	2.44E+1	0.00
	20	6.36E+1	1.08E+2	1.06E+2	2.03E+2	3.05E+1	0.00
EMNA + E	4	4.95E-2	1.27E-1**	1.23E-1	2.43E-1	5.09E-2	0.00
	6	1.49E-1	2.86E-1**	3.01E-1	4.10E-1	7.07E-2	0.00
	8	3.36E-5	3.59E-1**	3.53E-1	6.70E-1	1.96E-1	0.00
	10	1.37E-3	5.08E-1**	1.89E-1	2.90E+0	7.50E-1	0.00
	15	1.54E+0	9.27E+0**	7.03E+0	2.73E+1	7.28E+0	0.00
	20	4.32E+0	2.97E+1**	3.04E+1	6.46E+1	1.49E+1	0.00
Rosenbrock							
EMNA	4	3.32E-7	3.01E+0	1.23E+0	4.32E+1	7.76E+0	0.03
	6	3.26E-5	1.24E+1	4.28E+0	1.19E+2	2.34E+1	0.00
	8	1.26E-1	7.82E+2	4.61E+1	1.22E+4	2.31E+3	0.00
	10	7.24E+0	3.24E+3	1.28E+2	3.71E+4	8.25E+3	0.00
	15	4.36E+2	3.14E+4	1.47E+4	1.64E+5	4.50E+4	0.00
	20	7.12E+2	1.05E+5	6.40E+4	5.45E+5	1.30E+5	0.00
EMNA + E	4	4.13E-5	1.77E+0	1.37E+0	9.71E+0	2.01E+0	0.00
	6	1.01E+0	4.53E+0*	4.01E+0	1.32E+1	2.12E+0	0.00
	8	2.05E+0	1.56E+1*	8.20E+0	4.44E+1	1.38E+1	0.00
	10	7.03E+0	3.51E+1*	1.29E+1	2.72E+2	5.09E+1	0.00
	15	1.46E+1	1.35E+2**	7.45E+1	1.31E+3	2.37E+2	0.00
	20	7.73E+1	8.23E+2**	4.00E+2	4.26E+3	8.83E+2	0.00

* denotes EMNA+E is significantly better than the EMNA, at $\alpha = 0.05$
** denotes EMNA+E is significantly better than the EMNA, at $\alpha = 0.01$
† denotes that the EMNA+E has greater success rate than the EMNA

Table 2. Descriptive results of the fitness for separable functions

Algorithm	d	Best	Mean	Median	Worst	Std. Dev.	Success Rate
				Rastrigin			
EMNA	4	3.57E-7	4.74E+0	3.69E+0	2.09E+1	4.86E+0	0.07
	6	1.99E+0	1.24E+1	1.04E+1	3.32E+1	6.76E+0	0.00
	8	9.95E+0	3.10E+1	2.72E+1	8.77E+1	1.63E+1	0.00
	10	2.17E+1	5.01E+1	4.81E+1	1.01E+2	1.94E+1	0.00
	15	6.45E+1	1.15E+2	1.07E+2	2.16E+2	3.83E+1	0.00
	20	1.35E+2	2.37E+2	2.27E+2	4.58E+2	7.26E+1	0.00
EMNA + E	4	1.30E+0	3.91E+0	3.92E+0	7.91E+0	1.36E+0	0.00
	6	4.79E-7	1.08E+1	1.04E+1	1.57E+1	3.30E+0	0.03 †
	8	1.30E+1	1.99E+1**	1.92E+1	2.75E+1	4.15E+0	0.00
	10	8.26E-2	3.27E+1**	3.39E+1	4.58E+1	8.23E+0	0.00
	15	5.16E+1	7.22E+1**	7.38E+1	8.48E+1	9.23E+0	0.00
	20	8.67E+1	1.20E+2**	1.22E+2	1.54E+2	1.45E+1	0.00
				Sphere			
EMNA	4	4.46E-7	3.70E+3	3.13E+1	4.83E+4	9.38E+3	0.17
	6	9.20E-7	1.27E+4	4.76E+3	1.02E+5	2.08E+4	0.03
	8	1.16E-2	3.66E+4	2.90E+4	2.02E+5	4.52E+4	0.00
	10	1.14E+4	9.86E+4	7.30E+4	3.09E+5	8.14E+4	0.00
	15	9.27E+4	2.04E+5	1.94E+5	3.65E+5	7.13E+4	0.00
	20	1.43E+5	3.94E+5	3.80E+5	6.51E+5	1.42E+5	0.00
EMNA + E	4	7.18E-8	6.21E-3*	8.64E-7	1.61E-1	2.94E-2	0.53 †
	6	2.08E-7	1.25E+0**	3.66E-4	2.58E+1	4.70E+0	0.33 †
	8	4.99E-7	9.94E+1**	6.34E+0	2.11E+3	3.83E+2	0.03 †
	10	3.29E-2	9.01E+2**	1.24E+2	7.68E+3	1.82E+3	0.00
	15	1.16E+3	3.25E+4**	3.12E+4	8.48E+4	2.22E+4	0.00
	20	7.24E+3	1.26E+5**	1.20E+5	2.28E+5	6.04E+4	0.00

* denotes EMNA+E is significantly better than the EMNA, at $\alpha = 0.05$
** denotes EMNA+E is significantly better than the EMNA, at $\alpha = 0.01$
† denotes that the EMNA+E has greater success rate than the EMNA

Tables 1 and 2 show a total of 30 comparisons. Out of the 18 comparisons for the non-separable functions, the EMNA+E excels in 17 cases. Similarly, out of the 12 comparisons for the separable functions, the EMNA+E excels in 10 cases. These results give an evidence of the benefits achieved by the incorporation of the exploration stage in EDAs. However, regarding the number of evaluations, Tables 3 and 4 show that EMNA+E requires more function evaluations than the EMNA.

Table 3. Descriptive results of the number of evaluations for non-separable functions

Algorithm	d	Best	Mean	Median	Worst	Std. Dev.
Ackley						
EMNA	4	1.52E+3	2.07E+3	2.20E+3	2.56E+3	3.78E+2
	6	3.42E+3	4.11E+3	4.02E+3	5.58E+3	4.19E+2
	8	5.52E+3	6.34E+3	6.12E+3	8.48E+3	6.95E+2
	10	7.60E+3	8.80E+3	8.35E+3	1.54E+4	1.56E+3
	15	1.17E+4	1.52E+4	1.46E+4	2.16E+4	1.93E+3
	20	2.02E+4	2.37E+4	2.33E+4	2.94E+4	2.22E+3
EMNA + E	4	5.04E+3	5.46E+3	5.20E+3	6.00E+3	4.00E+2
	6	8.64E+3	9.45E+3	9.60E+3	9.90E+3	3.94E+2
	8	1.24E+4	1.34E+4	1.34E+4	1.38E+4	2.52E+2
	10	1.69E+4	1.73E+4	1.72E+4	1.80E+4	2.31E+2
	15	2.73E+4	2.81E+4	2.78E+4	2.99E+4	6.78E+2
	20	3.86E+4	4.01E+4	4.00E+4	4.22E+4	9.20E+2
Griewangk						
EMNA	4	1.40E+3	2.64E+3	2.52E+3	5.32E+3	9.65E+2
	6	2.34E+3	4.64E+3	3.90E+3	1.01E+4	1.85E+3
	8	4.00E+3	8.52E+3	8.92E+3	1.17E+4	2.22E+3
	10	5.20E+3	1.01E+4	1.03E+4	1.38E+4	1.93E+3
	15	8.40E+3	1.33E+4	1.43E+4	1.56E+4	2.00E+3
	20	1.28E+4	1.81E+4	1.78E+4	2.38E+4	2.15E+3
EMNA + E	4	5.00E+3	5.95E+3	5.64E+3	8.92E+3	9.07E+2
	6	7.98E+3	9.30E+3	9.15E+3	1.20E+4	1.00E+3
	8	1.10E+4	1.39E+4	1.29E+4	2.04E+4	2.96E+3
	10	1.42E+4	2.11E+4	2.11E+4	2.58E+4	2.54E+3
	15	2.25E+4	2.75E+4	2.81E+4	3.08E+4	2.32E+3
	20	3.64E+4	3.75E+4	3.70E+4	4.04E+4	1.22E+3
Rosenbrock						
EMNA	4	1.64E+3	2.70E+3	2.60E+3	3.52E+3	3.73E+2
	6	3.84E+3	4.71E+3	4.47E+3	6.30E+3	6.22E+2
	8	3.52E+3	6.91E+3	6.68E+3	9.92E+3	1.11E+3
	10	7.80E+3	1.05E+4	1.01E+4	1.71E+4	1.84E+3
	15	1.25E+4	1.69E+4	1.66E+4	2.42E+4	2.31E+3
	20	1.60E+4	2.45E+4	2.46E+4	2.88E+4	2.49E+3
EMNA + E	4	5.48E+3	6.19E+3	6.16E+3	7.04E+3	2.64E+2
	6	9.78E+3	1.02E+4	1.00E+4	1.14E+4	4.09E+2
	8	1.37E+4	1.44E+4	1.44E+4	1.57E+4	5.07E+2
	10	1.79E+4	1.90E+4	1.88E+4	2.11E+4	9.03E+2
	15	2.49E+4	3.13E+4	3.14E+4	3.47E+4	1.85E+3
	20	3.64E+4	4.39E+4	4.29E+4	5.38E+4	4.02E+3

Table 4. Descriptive results of the number of evaluations for separable functions

Algorithm	d	Best	Mean	Median	Worst	Std. Dev.
			Rastrigin			
EMNA	4	1.44E+3	2.49E+3	2.26E+3	5.80E+3	9.40E+2
	6	2.46E+3	4.27E+3	3.93E+3	8.64E+3	1.42E+3
	8	2.96E+3	5.50E+3	5.40E+3	1.16E+4	1.96E+3
	10	4.30E+3	7.18E+3	6.90E+3	1.37E+4	2.44E+3
	15	7.05E+3	1.11E+4	1.03E+4	2.58E+4	3.91E+3
	20	8.60E+3	1.65E+4	1.49E+4	2.64E+4	5.04E+3
EMNA + E	4	5.00E+3	5.73E+3	5.60E+3	8.80E+3	8.19E+2
	6	7.62E+3	9.21E+3	8.82E+3	1.51E+4	1.53E+3
	8	1.08E+4	1.28E+4	1.28E+4	1.45E+4	1.07E+3
	10	1.33E+4	1.58E+4	1.51E+4	2.65E+4	2.54E+3
	15	2.01E+4	2.37E+4	2.34E+4	2.96E+4	2.43E+3
	20	2.84E+4	3.36E+4	3.38E+4	4.04E+4	3.16E+3
			Sphere			
EMNA	4	1.24E+3	2.51E+3	2.82E+3	3.32E+3	6.04E+2
	6	2.46E+3	4.68E+3	4.80E+3	5.16E+3	5.30E+2
	8	6.32E+3	7.07E+3	7.12E+3	7.44E+3	2.51E+2
	10	9.00E+3	9.48E+3	9.50E+3	9.90E+3	2.05E+2
	15	1.49E+4	1.60E+4	1.61E+4	1.64E+4	2.78E+2
	20	2.28E+4	2.34E+4	2.34E+4	2.40E+4	2.73E+2
EMNA + E	4	4.60E+3	5.21E+3	4.76E+3	6.08E+3	5.54E+2
	6	7.86E+3	9.19E+3	9.60E+3	1.02E+4	9.05E+2
	8	1.14E+4	1.40E+4	1.42E+4	1.46E+4	5.57E+2
	10	1.77E+4	1.85E+4	1.86E+4	1.90E+4	3.72E+2
	15	3.00E+4	3.04E+4	3.05E+4	3.11E+4	2.39E+2
	20	4.22E+4	4.27E+4	4.26E+4	4.32E+4	2.98E+2

5   Conclusions

This work has introduced an explicit exploration stage for EDAs. In particular, the numerical implementation of the exploration stage has been done with continuous decision variables in a well known EDA (EMNA). According to the numerical experiments, the explicit separation between the exploration stage and the exploitation stage (EMNA+E) can help achieving better fitness values. Nonetheless, the benefit of including an exploration stage requires an increase of function evaluations.

An important contribution of this paper is the design of a probabilistic model for the exploration stage. The goal of the proposed model in the exploration stage is to provide a new tool for finding an set of individuals that can be used as initial population in the exploitation stage.

Although the statistical comparisons clearly indicate that the EDA with the exploration stage has better performance than the typical EDA, the success rate shows that more experiments are necessary in order to identify where the exploration stage have a positive impact in EDAs.

Acknowledgments. The first author acknowledges financial support from the Programa de Mejoramiento del Profesorado (PROMEP) of México.

References

1. Bosman, P.: Design and Application of Iterated Density-Estimation Evolutionary Algorithms. Ph.D. thesis, University of Utrecht, Utrecht, The Netherlands (2003)
2. Bosman, P., Grahl, J., Thierens, D.: AMaLGaM IDEAs in Noiseless Black-Box Optimization Benchmarking. In: Proceedings of the 11th Annual Conference Companion on Genetic and Evolutionary Computation Conference: Late Breaking Papers, GECCO 2009, pp. 2247–2254. ACM (2009)
3. De Bonet, J., Isbell, C., Viola, P.: MIMIC: Finding Optima by Estimating Probability Densities. In: Advances in Neural Information Processing Systems, vol. 9, pp. 424–430. The MIT Press (1997)
4. Hauschild, M., Pelikan, M.: An introduction and survey of estimation of distribution algorithms. Swarm and Evolutionary Computation 1(3), 111–128 (2011)
5. Larrañaga, P., Etxeberria, R., Lozano, J., Peña, J.: Combinatorial optimization by learning and simulation of Bayesian networks. In: Proceedings of the Sixteenth Conference on Uncertainty in Artificial Intelligence, pp. 343–352 (2000)
6. Larrañaga, P., Etxeberria, R., Lozano, J., Peña, J.: Optimization in continuous domains by learning and simulation of Gaussian networks. In: Proceedings of the Optimization by Building and Using Probabilistic Models OBUPM Workshop at the Genetic and Evolutionary Computation Conference, GECCO 2000, pp. 201–204 (2000)
7. Larrañaga, P., Lozano, J., Bengoetxea, E.: Estimation of Distribution Algorithm based on multivariate normal and Gaussian networks. Tech. Rep. EHU-KZAA-IK-1/01, Department of Computer Science and Artificial Intelligence, University of the Basque Country (2001)
8. Larrañaga, P., Lozano, J. (eds.): Estimation of Distribution Algorithms: A New Tool for Evolutionary Computation. Genetic Algorithms and Evolutionary Computation. Kluwer Academic Publishers (2002)
9. Mühlenbein, H.: The Equation for Response to Selection and its Use for Prediction. Evolutionary Computation 5(3), 303–346 (1998)
10. Mühlenbein, H., Paaß, G.: From recombination of genes to the estimation of distributions I. Binary parameters. In: Voigt, H.-M., Ebeling, W., Rechenberg, I., Schwefel, H. (eds.) PPSN 1996. LNCS, vol. 1141, pp. 178–187. Springer, Heidelberg (1996)
11. Pelikan, M., Goldberg, D., Cantú-Paz, E.: BOA: The Bayesian Optimization Algorithm. In: Banzhaf, W., Daida, J., Eiben, A., Garzon, M., Honavar, V., Jakiela, M., Smith, R. (eds.) Proceedings of the Genetic and Evolutionary Computation Conference, GECCO 1999, vol. 1, pp. 525–532. Morgan Kaufmann Publishers (1999)
12. Pelikan, M., Mühlenbein, H.: The Bivariate Marginal Distribution Algorithm. In: Roy, R., Furuhashi, T., Chawdhry, P. (eds.) Advances in Soft Computing - Engineering Design and Manufacturing, pp. 521–535. Springer, London (1999)

13. Salinas-Gutiérrez, R., Hernández-Aguirre, A., Villa-Diharce, E.: Estimation of Distribution Algorithms based on Copula Functions. In: GECCO 2011: Proceedings of the 13th Annual Conference on Genetic and Evolutionary Computation, Graduate Students Workshop, pp. 795–798. ACM (2011)
14. Soto, M., Ochoa, A., Acid, S., de Campos, L.: Introducing the polytree approximation of distribution algorithm. In: Ochoa, A., Soto, M., Santana, R. (eds.) Second International Symposium on Artificial Intelligence. Adaptive Systems, CIMAF 1999, pp. 360–367, Academia, La Habana (1999)

An Ant Colony Algorithm for Improving Ship Stability in the Containership Stowage Problem

Paula Hernández Hernández[1], Laura Cruz-Reyes[1], Patricia Melin[2],
Julio Mar-Ortiz[3], Héctor Joaquín Fraire Huacuja[1],
Héctor José Puga Soberanes[4] and Juan Javier González Barbosa[1]

[1] Instituto Tecnológico de Ciudad Madero, México
[2] Tijuana Institute of Technology, México
[3] Universidad Autónoma de Tamaulipas, México
[4] Instituto Tecnológico de León, México
paulahdz314@hotmail.com, {lcruzr,hfraire}@prodigy.net.mx,
jjgonzalezbarbosa@hotmail.com
pmelin@tectijuana.mx, jmar@uat.edu.mx,
pugahector@yahoo.com

Abstract. This paper approaches the containership stowage problem. It is an NP-hard minimization problem whose goal is to find optimal plans for stowing containers into a containership with low operational costs, subject to a set of structural and operational constraints. In this work, we apply to this problem an ant-based hyperheuristic algorithm for the first time, according to our literature review. Ant colony and hyperheuristic algorithms have been successfully used in others application domains. We start from the initial solution, based in relaxed ILP model; then, we look for the global ship stability of the overall stowage plan by using a hyperheuristic approach. Besides, we reduce the handling time of the containers to be loaded on the ship. The validation of the proposed approach is performed by solving some pseudo-randomly generated instances constructed through ranges based in real-life values obtained from the literature.

Keywords: Containership Stowage Problem, Ant Colony Optimization, Hyperheuristic Approach.

1 Introduction and Problem Description

The containership stowage problem, denoted in the literature as the Master Bay Planning Problem (MBPP) [1], is one of the relevant problems involves in the efficient operation of ports.

MBPP is an NP-hard minimization problem and can be to define as follows: Given a set C of n containers of different types to be loaded on the ship and a set S of m available locations on the containership. We have to determine the assignment of each container to a location of the ship, such that, all the given structural and operational constraints are satisfied, and the total stowage time is minimized.

F. Castro, A. Gelbukh, and M. González (Eds.): MICAI 2013, Part II, LNAI 8266, pp. 93–104, 2013.
© Springer-Verlag Berlin Heidelberg 2013

In MBPP each container $c \in C$ must be stowed in a location $l \in S$ of the ship. The l-th location is actually addressed by the indices i, j, k representing, respectively: the bay (i), the row (j), and the tier (k). We denote by I, J and K, respectively, the set of bays, rows and tiers of the ship, and by b, r and s their corresponding cardinality.

The objective function is expressed in terms of the sum of the time t_{lc} required for loading a container $c, \forall c \in C$, in location $l, \forall l \in S$, such that $L = \sum_{lc} t_{lc}$. However, when two or more quay cranes are used for the loading operations the objective function is given by the maximum over the minimum loading time (L_q) for handling all containers in the corresponding ship partition by each quay crane q, that is $L = \max_{QC}\{L_q\}$, where QC, is the set of available quay cranes.

The main constraints that must be considered for the stowage planning process for an individual port are related to the structure of the ship and focused on the size, type, weight, destination and distribution of the containers to be loaded. For a detailed description of such constraints, the reader is referred to [2].

In order to optimize a stowage planning, we decompose the problem hierarchically like in current approaches [3, 4]. The problem is divided into two phases: the first one consist of generating a relaxed solution, that is, we remove the constraints of stability; and the second phase is intended to make this solution feasible through simple heuristics handled by the hyperheuristic, in less time. This hyperheuristic was designed with online learning [5].

A hyperheuristic is a high-level algorithm that acts as a planner over a set of heuristics, which can be selected in a deterministic or nondeterministic form [6]. Hyperheuristic does not operate on the problem directly, that is, it does not have domain knowledge of the problem over which it operates. They aim to be apply to an even problem domains, such as to be tackled in this work.

This paper is organized into four parts. Section 2 describes our proposed hyperheuristic. Section 3 presents the experimental results. Finally, the last section shows the conclusions and future work.

2   Proposed Algorithm

We propose a hyperheuristic algorithm to optimize the global ship stability of the overall stowage plan, and at the same time it minimizes the containers loading time on the ship.

The proposed hyperheuristic approach (*Ant Colony Optimization Hyperheuristic*, ACOHH) uses an ant colony optimization (ACO) algorithm [7] as a high-level metaheuristic and seven low level heuristics that interact directly with *the solutions* of the problem. An important characteristic to be pointed out is that ACO can only interact with the low level heuristics.

ACOHH starts with an initial solution S_0, which is obtained by solving its associated relaxed 0/1 LP model up to the first feasible solution reached by the commercial software Gurobi. Relaxed 0/1 LP model is composed by the complete 0/1 LP model proposed in [1] but removing the constraints of horizontal and cross equilibrium. Once obtained the initial solution, ACOHH applies to it a heuristic, which generates a new candidate solution. This solution is feasible if satisfies the assignment, weight and destination constraints (8)-(15) of the MBPP problem formulation [1].

In order to evaluate the heuristic performance, like in [4], we consider the objective function $Z(x) = M\big(\sigma_1(x) + \sigma_2(x)\big) + L(x)$, where $\sigma_1(x)$ and $\sigma_2(x)$ are the horizontal and cross equilibrium stability violation functions, respectively. M is a coefficient, such that $M \gg 0$, to strongly penalize, the stability violation functions, in such a way that we give a high priority to the generation of feasible solutions.

2.1   Low Level Heuristics

The seven low level heuristics (LLH) used in ACOHH was inspired by Ambrosino, et. al. [4] and are detailed as follows:

1. Anterior-Posterior exchange of location's contents: This kind of move exchanges the current content assigned to the locations $l \in A \cap X$ and $l' \in P \cap X$, X being a fixed side of the ship (L or R). Note that this change may affect the cross equilibrium but does not modify the horizontal equilibrium of the ship.
2. Left-Right exchange of location's contents: This kind of move exchanges the current content assigned to the locations $l \in L \cap X$ and $l' \in R \cap X$, X being a fixed side of the ship (A or P). This move may affect the horizontal equilibrium whereas it does not modify the cross one.
3. Cross exchange of location's contents: This kind of move exchanges the current content assigned to the locations $l \in A \cap L$ and $l' \in P \cap R$ (or $l \in A \cap R$ and $l' \in P \cap L$). This move affects both the horizontal and the cross equilibrium.
4. Anterior-Posterior exchange of stacks: This move exchanges the positions of two whole stacks of containers, s and s', where $s = \{l\colon l \in A \cap X, l = (i,j,k)$ with i and j fixed$\}$ and $s' = \{l'\colon l' \in P \cap X, l = (i',j',k)$ with i' and j' fixed$\}$, X being a fixed side of the ship (L or R). Like heuristic 1, this move may affect only the cross equilibrium.
5. Left-Right exchange of stacks: This move exchanges the positions of two whole stacks of containers, s and s', where $s = \{l\colon l \in L \cap X, l = (i,j,k)$ with i and j fixed$\}$ and $s' = \{l'\colon l' \in R \cap X, l = (i',j',k)$ with i' and j' fixed$\}$, X being a fixed side of the ship (A or P). Like heuristic 2, with this move only horizontal equilibrium may be affected.
6. Cross exchange of stacks: This move exchanges the positions of two whole stacks of containers, s and s', where $s = \{l\colon l \in A \cap L, l = (i,j,k)$ with i and j fixed$\}$ and $s' = \{l'\colon l' \in P \cap R, l = (i',j',k)$ with i' and j' fixed$\}$ (or $s = \{l\colon l \in A \cap R, l = (i,j,k)$ with i and j fixed$\}$ and $s' = \{l'\colon l' \in P \cap L, l = (i',j',k)$ with i' and j' fixed$\}$). Like heuristic 3, both the horizontal and cross equilibrium might be affected.
7. Anterior-Posterior exchange of bays: This move exchanges all locations in two bays i and i' located in A and P, respectively, without changing the original row and tier positions of the containers, for this reason, this move may affect only the cross equilibrium.

In the LLH description, we used the following additional notation:

E and O: sets of even and odd bays, respectively, such that $E \subset I$, $O \subset I$ and $E \cup O \equiv I$; A and P: sets of anterior and posterior bays, respectively, such that $A \subset I$, $P \subset I$ and $A \cup P \equiv I$; R and L: sets of right side and left side rows, respectively, such that $R \subset J$, $L \subset J$ and $R \cup L \equiv J$.

In the heuristics 1 to 3, l or l' could be both: empty or assigned. In order to apply some of these heuristics, l and l' must be assigned, that is, when l and l' are empty, the current solution will not improve, so it is not necessary to apply them. For the heuristics 4 to 6, if two whole stacks of containers s and s' are empty, that is, they do not have anything assigned, these heuristics will not be applied. This is the case for heuristic 7, but applied to the bays. For any LLH, two bays i and i' must be the same type (E or O).

Since the choice of the containers to be exchanged is performed randomly, it might be not satisfy the criteria previously established to apply the heuristic move. In order to overcome the possible infeasibility, ACOHH allows a certain number of attempts to choose an item. The items are single location's contents, stacks and bays.

2.2   Graph Description

In ACOHH, the graph G is complete (network), directed and self-directed, that is, for any pair of vertices i and j, including the case where $j = i$, there exists a directed edge from i to j. The set of vertices V of graph $G = (V, E)$, represents the set of low level heuristics, i.e., $V = H = \{h_1, h_2, h_3, ..., h_{|H|}\}$, and the set of directed edges E joins every heuristic to each other $E = \{(h_1, h_1), (h_1, h_2), (h_1, h_3), ..., (h_{|H|}, h_{|H|})\}$. ACOHH uses a certain number of ants $HHA = \{a_1, a_2, a_3, ..., a_{|A|}\}$, which in the literature are known as *hyperheuristic agents*, to construct paths on the graph by traversing it (see Fig. 1). In this study we fix $|HHA| = |H| = 7$, which means that there are the same number of ants and heuristics. A *path* P_k constructed by an ant k is a sequence of LLH to be applied to a solution of the problem, the length of any P_k is $|H|$.

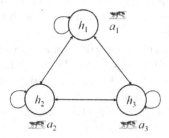

Fig. 1. Example of a complete, directed and self-directed graph G traversed by the hyperheuristic agents

At each vertex, each ant selects the next vertex to be visited, traverses the edge to that vertex, and applies the heuristic represented by the selected vertex to the current solution of the problem. Vertices and edges could be selected more than once in the path of any ant. After that, each ant evaluates its generated route (compute the objective value of the constructed solution), and lays a pheromone trail, which is proportional to the solution quality, on those edges crossed by the ant in its path.

2.3   Data Structures

In ACO, the artificial ants used are stochastic solution construction procedures that probabilistically build a solution by iteratively adding solution components to partial solutions. For that, the ants take into account: heuristic information on the problem instance being solved, if available, and (artificial) pheromone trails which change dynamically at run-time to reflect the agents' acquired search experience [8,9].

Unlike ACO, our hyperheuristic approach has no domain knowledge. The domain is LLH and their ability to improve an initial solution. When ACOHH chooses the following low level heuristic through Equation 1, it is based on the following tables:

1. Visibility table η has a size of $|H|$ and stores information that represents the uniformly distributed current confidence that heuristic $h_j \in H$ will lead to a good solution. Visibility table is initially impartial and continually adaptive, due to the hyperheuristic approach has no knowledge of each low-level heuristic's potential in advance, and this potential varies as the colony traverses the solution space [10].
2. Pheromone table τ has a size of $|H| \times |H|$ and is a dynamic memory structure containing information on the quality of previously obtained result. The pheromone trails are associated with arcs and therefore τ_{ij} refers to the desirability of applying heuristic j directly after heuristic i. ACOHH algorithm initializes the pheromone trails with low values, $\forall(i,j), \tau_{ij} = \tau_0 = 0.009$ [11].

2.4   Algorithmic Description

Algorithm 1 shows the ant hyperheuristic process, which is performed by the *hyperheuristic agents* supplied with an initial solution S_0. This process is performed until a maximal number of cycles is reached. A *cycle* is the period of time between all ants beginning their paths and all ants completing their paths. The operation of the algorithm can be divided into three phases.

In the first phase (lines 1-13), so-called *initialization*, visibility table does not have information and all pheromone table is initialized with a low value named τ_0. First, the ants are located uniformly among the vertices of the network (line 4), that is, a_1 in the vertex 1 (heuristic 1), a_2 in the vertex 2, and so on. After that, they are provided with an initial solution $S = S_0$ (line 7) and each ant applies to its copy of S, the heuristic i (corresponding to its location) to provide an initial visibility value (line 12). Besides, each ant adds its first heuristic i to its respective path (line 9).

Subsequently, the next phase is the *construction process* (lines 15-24), which is a basic ingredient of any ACO algorithm [12]. The ants then construct a path (sequence of heuristics) by traversing the network. The choice of the next vertex (heuristic) to be added is done probabilistically according to Equation 1 at each construction step (line

17). Later, each ant traverses the arc to the selected vertex, and applies the heuristic represented by that vertex to its current solution (line 18). When all ants have completed one construction step of the path, visibility table is updated through Equation 4. This updating process is done until all ants construct their paths completely.

Algorithm 1. ACOHH $(G = (V, E), S_0)$

1. Initialize: $S \leftarrow S_0$, $S_{bc} \leftarrow S_0$, $S_g \leftarrow S_0$, $h_{bc} \leftarrow 0$
2. for each vertex i set an initial value $\eta_i \leftarrow 0$
3. for each edge (i, j) set an initial value $\tau_{ij} \leftarrow \tau_0$
4. Scatter the ants uniformly on the $|H|$ vertices
5. for each ant k do
6.   Initialize the path $P_k \leftarrow \{\emptyset\}$
7.   Provide a copy of initial solution $S_k \leftarrow S$
8.   Apply heuristic i to solution S_k to produce S_k'
9.   Add to path $P_k \leftarrow P_k \cup i$
10.   Update S_{bc} and h_{bc}
11.   if S_k' is better than S_{bc}, then $S_{bc} \leftarrow S_k'$ and $h_{bc} \leftarrow i$
12.   Update η_i according to the Equation 4
13. end for
14. for each cycle c do
15.   for each step s do
16.   for each ant k do
17.   Apply the selection rule: $j = f(\{p_{k,i,j} | j \in H\})$
18.   Apply heuristic j to solution S_k to produce S_k'
19.   Add to path $P_k \leftarrow P_k \cup j$
20.   Update S_{bc} and h_{bc}
21.   if S_k' is better than S_{bc}, then $S_{bc} \leftarrow S_k'$ and $h_{bc} \leftarrow j$
22.   end for
23.   Update η_j according to the Equation 4
24.   end for
25.   Update $\tau_{i,j}$ according to the Equation 5
26.   for each ant k do
27. $S \leftarrow S_{bc}$
28.   Provide a copy of best solution of the cycle $S_k \leftarrow S$
29. $i \leftarrow h_{bc}$
30. $i_k \leftarrow i$
31.   end for
32.   Update S_g //S_g is the output of the algorithm
33.   if S_{bc} is better than S_g, then $S_g \leftarrow S_{bc}$
34. end for

In the final phase, named *update process*, of the algorithm ACOHH (lines 25-33) the ants evaluate their generated solution, this rule is formalized in Equation 5. Additionally each ant deposits the pheromone trail on the traveled path (line 25), that is, the sequence of low level heuristics selected for it. At the end of each cycle all of the ants are relocated in region of the solution space where the best solution of that cycle was found. Then, in the next cycle the ants start their paths at the vertex of the network whose associated heuristic discovered the best solution of the previous cycle (lines 26-31). ACOHH returns the best solution S_g found during all cycles.

2.5   Behavior Rules

ACOHH has three rules of behavior: the selection, visibility update and pheromone update. These rules update the data structures introduced in Section 3.2. We now describe them in the following paragraphs.

Selection Rule

The selection process of the current ant requires combining the visibility (η table) and pheromone (τ table) values for each arc. At each construction step, ant k applies a probabilistic action choice rule, called *random proportional rule*, to decide which heuristic to apply next. This rule is based on the ant system formulation [13].

In particular, the probability with which ant k, currently at vertex (heuristic) i, chooses to visit vertex j is:

$$p_{k,i,j} = \frac{(\phi_{i,j})^\alpha (\delta_j)^\beta}{\sum_{l \in H}(\phi_{i,j})^\alpha (\delta_j)^\beta} \tag{1}$$

where α and β are two parameters which determine the relative influence of the heuristic information and the pheromone trail, and H is the set of low level heuristics. When one or more heuristics find a solution of poorer quality than the current solution, the heuristic j will not have possibility to be selected, as stated in Equation 2.

$$\delta_j = \begin{cases} \eta_j, & \text{if } \eta_j > 0 \\ 0, & otherwise \end{cases} . \tag{2}$$

Like η, when one or more arcs have pheromone trails with a large penalization, none of them will have a possibility to be selected, this is given by:

$$\phi_{i,j} = \begin{cases} \tau_{i,j}, & \text{if } \tau_{i,j} > 0 \\ 0, & otherwise \end{cases} . \tag{3}$$

In the case that all heuristics have negative performance, we choose one heuristic randomly. This is with the finality of encourage a diverse search of the solution space. Initially, beginning the first cycle ($c = 1$), the ants are scattered uniformly among the vertices of the network with a copy of an initial solution S. In the first step of this cycle, each ant applies the heuristic to its copy of S corresponding to its location, and adds the first heuristic in its path. That is, in this step the ants do not apply the Equation 1. Besides, the ants provide an initial visibility value, according to Equation 4.

After the first cycle, the ants adopt the best solution found of the previous cycle, which will be the new S in current cycle. For the example of Fig. 1, assuming the best solution S_{bc} of the previous cycle was discovered by the ant a_3 applying heuristic h_3, the ants will adopt this best solution in current cycle ($S = S_{bc}$) [10].

Visibility Update Rule

Like in [10], in this paper visibility function η_j is adaptive and corresponding to individual performance of the heuristic h_j, this value is updated after all ants have completed each step s of their paths:

$$\eta_j(s) = \gamma\eta_j(s - 1) + \sum_{k \in \text{HHA}} \frac{I_{k,j}(s)}{T_{k,j}(s)} \qquad (4)$$

where HHA is the set of ants in the colony, $I_{k,j}(t)$ is the improvement (which could be negative) produced by heuristic h_j on ant k-th current solution at decision point s (step), $T_{k,j}(s)$ is the running time spent by heuristic h_j at decision point s, this value is given in CPU nanosecond, and γ is the decreasing rate of visibility (number between zero and one). The parameter γ is used to avoid unlimited accumulation of the heuristic information and it enables the algorithm to "forget" older preferences previously taken.

Pheromone Update Rule

This rule is based on the ant system formulation [13] and the hyperheuristic pheromone function [10].

Once all the ants have constructed their paths, the pheromone trails are updated. This is done by first lowering the pheromone value on all arcs by a constant factor, and then adding a determined amount of pheromone on the arcs where the ants have crossed in their paths. In fact, if an arc is not chosen by the ants, its associated pheromone value decreases exponentially with respect to the number of cycles.

The amount of pheromone on each arc $\tau_{i,j}$ between heuristic i and heuristic j at cycle c is adjusted as follows:

$$\tau_{k,i,j}(c) = (1 - \rho)\tau_{i,j}(c - 1) + \sum_{k \in \text{HHA}} \frac{TN_{i,j}(P_k(c))I_k(P_k(c))}{T_k(P_k(c))} \qquad (5)$$

where ρ is a parameter called *evaporation coefficient* (number between zero and one), $P_k(c)$ is the path that ant k traversed during the final cycle, $TN_{i,j}(P_k(c))$ is the number of times the arc (i,j) was traversed by the ant during path $P_k(c)$. The improvement produced by ant k used during its last path is $I_k(P_k(c))$, this is the difference between the best solution quality found during this path and the best solution quality found at the end of the previous cycle, and $T_k(P_k(c))$ is the running time in CPU nanoseconds. Thus, arcs that are used by many ants and which have high quality of the solutions achieved receive more pheromone and are therefore more likely to be chosen by ants in future cycles of the ACOHH algorithm.

3   Experimental Results

In this section the performance of the ACOHH algorithm is tested. In the following subsections we describe the test instances, experimental environment and the performance analysis.

3.1   Test Cases

In order to validate our hyperheuristic approach, we generate a set of pseudo-random instances (test cases) according to the format and conditions defined in [2].

The dataset is formed by small-sized instances. Table 1 reports the containers characteristics of the considered 10 instances, showing the total number of containers, in TEU and absolute number (n), the number of containers of types 20' (T) and 40' (F), the number of containers for three classes of weight (L: low, M: medium, H: high) and the partition of containers for each destination. Three classes of weight are considered, namely low (from 5 to 15 tons), medium (from 16 to 25 tons) and high containers (from 26 to 32 tons).

Table 1. Containers for the set of small-sized instances

Instance	TEU	n	Type (n)		Weight (n)			Destination (n)		
			T	F	L	M	H	D_1	D_2	D_3
1	69	50	31	19	23	25	2	23	27	0
2	83	60	37	23	26	32	2	27	33	0
3	85	65	45	20	30	33	2	31	34	0
4	88	65	42	23	29	34	2	31	34	0
5	90	70	50	20	31	37	2	30	40	0
6	90	75	60	15	35	38	2	32	43	0
7	93	65	37	28	30	33	2	31	34	0
8	93	70	47	23	29	39	2	32	38	0
9	93	70	47	23	31	36	3	25	20	25
10	94	74	54	20	34	38	2	25	25	24

These instances concerns a small size containership, with a maximum capacity of 240 TEU, composed of 12 odd bays, 4 rows and 5 tiers (3 in the hold and 2 in the upper deck, respectively). Table 2 shows the loading times for the small containership. The maximum horizontal weight tolerance (Q_1) was fixed to 18% of the total weight of the all containers to load. While the maximum cross weight tolerance (Q_2) was fixed to 9% of the total weight, expressed in tons. Respecting MT, that is, the maximum stack weight tolerance of three containers of 20', was fixed to 45 tons and MF (the maximum stack weight tolerance of three containers of 40') was fixed to 66 tons.

Pseudo-random instances were generated for the purpose of their reproduction in a reasonable time, because the initial solution is found by an exact method. Each row in the Table 1 is associated to each instance. This row represents the characteristics of the containers set C to be loaded on the containership. In each instance, the first |T| containers of set C are of 20' and the following |F| containers are of 40'. In relation to the characteristic of *Weight*, the first |L| containers of the set C are light, the next |M| are medium weight and the last |H| are heavy. Finally, the characteristic of *Destination* of the containers of the set C, are established of the same sequence that *Weight* characteristic.

Table 2. Loading times for the set of small-sized instances, the times are expressed in 1/100 of minute, taken from [4]

Tier	Row			
	3	1	2	4
2	240	250	260	270
4	230	240	250	260
6	220	230	240	250
82	210	220	230	240
84	200	210	220	230

3.2 Infrastructure

The following configuration corresponds to the experimental conditions:

- *Software:* Operating system Microsoft Windows 7 Home Premium; Java programming language, Java Platform, JDK 1.6; and integrated development, NetBeans 7.2. Solver Gurobi 5.0.1.
- *Hardware:* Computer equipment with processor Intel (R) Core (TM) i5 CPU M430 2.27 GHz and RAM memory of 4 GB.

3.3 Performance Analysis

Table 3 shows the comparison of the results obtained by three solution methods for the set of small-sized instances. The objective values are given in 1/100 of minute (Obj) and CPU time, expressed in seconds (Time). The results are divided into three relevant columns according to solutions found by: complete 0/1 LP model [1]; relaxed 0/1 LP model; and ACOHH algorithm. The computational execution of complete 0/1 LP model and relaxed 0/1 LP model were stopped when the first feasible solution is reached by the commercial software Gurobi.

ACOHH algorithm was executed thirty times per instance with the following configuration: ants number, LLH number, and the length of each path was fixed to 7, the number of cycles was fixed to 1000 , $\tau_0 = 0.009$, $\alpha = 1.0$, $\beta = 2.0$ and $\gamma = \rho = 0.5$. The *Avg Obj* column reports the average of total loading time reported by ACOHH, *Avg Time* column shows its running time (CPU time) and the last column *Tot Time* indicates the total (average) CPU time needed by the relaxed 0/1 LP model and ACOHH phases.

It is observed that the ACOHH algorithm outperforms the first solutions produced by the complete model for the MBPP. ACOHH algorithm achieved an average performance of 158.727 minutes for total loading time, in an average total CPU time of 33.888 seconds; while the performance achieved by complete 0/1 LP model was of 160.12 minutes of total loading time, in a CPU time of 57.497.

Additionally, to validate the results, non-parametric statistical test of Wilcoxon [14] was performed through the VisTHAA tool [15]. The results of this test reveals that the performance of the algorithm ACOHH shows a significant improvement over the solutions found by complete 0/1 LP model, on the set of the 10 test instances, at a confidence level 95%. Besides, ACOHH reduced the CPU time in 41.06% with respect CPU time spent by 0/1 LP Model.

Table 3. Comparison of the computational results for the small-sized instances

Inst.	0/1 LP Model*		Relaxed 0/1 LP Model* (Initial solution for ACOHH)				ACOHH		
	Obj_1	Time	Obj_2	Time	σ_1	σ_2	Avg Obj	Avg Time	Tot Time
1	11930	13.357	11970	4.081	77	283	11996.666	7.359	11.440
2	14290	23.825	14590	23.975	77	200	14363	8.733	32.708
3	15840	47.987	15610	14.723	79	398	15544.666	9.852	24.576
4	15440	30.897	15650	19.874	26	110	15523.666	10.374	30.248
5	17050	68.121	16790	29.659	238	22	16743.666	9.554	39.213
6	18020	62.720	18000	31.245	126	110	17949.333	11.112	42.358
7	15650	53.697	15200	8.505	457	0	15389	10.441	18.946
8	16910	71.581	16760	25.651	62	183	16712	11.165	36.817
9	16990	95.706	16820	36.064	50	59	16746.666	14.205	50.269
10	18000	107.077	17980	40.735	0	84	17758.666	11.565	52.301
Avg	16012	57.497	15937	23.451			15872.733	10.436	33.888

*It was stopped when the first feasible solution is reached by the commercial software Gurobi.

4   Conclusions and Future Work

In this paper, we apply an ant-based hyperheuristic algorithm, so-called ACOHH, for the first time, according to our literature review, for the Containership Stowage Problem. The hyperheuristic algorithm optimizes the global ship stability of the overall stowage plan, and also at the same time it reduces the handling time of the containers to be loaded on the ship.

Additionally, we proposed a dataset of pseudo-random instances to validate the proposed approach. On this dataset instances, ACOHH algorithm outperformed the first solutions produced by the exact complete model for the MBPP taken from the literature, and reduced the CPU time in 41.06% too.

According to the experimental results we can conclude that our proposed hyperheuristic is competitive regards to other alternatives from the current state of the art. ACOHH can produce feasible solutions in a short running time, and this approach could be applied to solve real instances. Moreover, as a future work it is considered to test other initial solutions for ACOHH, for example a variety of heuristic methods. It could be interesting to compare ACO against some other metaheuristic approaches, such as Genetic Algorithms, Simulated Annealing, among others.

References

1. Ambrosino, D., Sciomachen, A., Tanfani, E.: Stowing a containership: the master bay plan problem. Transportation Research Part A: Policy and Practice 38, 81–99 (2004)
2. Cruz-Reyes, L., Paula Hernández, H., Melin, P., Fraire H., H.J., Mar O., J.: Constructive algorithm for a benchmark in ship stowage planning. In: Castillo, O., Melin, P., Kacprzyk, J. (eds.) Recent Advances on Hybrid Intelligent Systems. SCI, vol. 451, pp. 393–408. Springer, Heidelberg (2013)

3. Delgado, A., Jensen, R.M., Janstrup, K., Rose, T.H., Andersen, K.H.: A Constraint Programming Model for Fast Optimal Stowage of Container Vessel Bays. European Journal of Operational Research (2012)

4. Ambrosino, D., Anghinolfi, D., Paolucci, M., Sciomachen, A.: A new three-stepheuristic for the master bay plan problem. Maritime Economics & Logistics 11, 98–120 (2009)

5. Burke, E.K., Hyde, M.R., Kendall, G., Ochoa, G., Ozcan, E., Woodward, J.R.: Exploring Hyper-heuristic Methodologies with Genetic Programming. In: Mumford, C.L., Jain, L.C. (eds.) Computational Intelligence. ISRL, vol. 1, pp. 177–201. Springer, Heidelberg (2009)

6. Özcan, E., Bilgin, B., Korkmaz, E.: A Comprehensive Analysis of Hyper-heuristics. Journal Intelligent Data Analysis. Computer & Communication Sciences 12(1), 3–23 (2008)

7. Maniezzo, V., Carbonaro, A.: Ant colony optimization: an overview. In: Essays and Surveys in Metaheuristics, pp. 469–492. Springer (2002)

8. Dorigo, M., Stützle, T.: Ant colony optimization: overview and recent advances. In: Handbook of Metaheuristics, pp. 227–263. Springer (2010)

9. Dorigo, M., Stützle, T.: The ant colony optimization metaheuristic: Algorithms, applications, and advances. In: Handbook of Metaheuristics, pp. 250–285. Springer (2003)

10. Burke, E., Kendall, G., Landa Silva, D., O'Brien, R., Soubeiga, E.: An ant algorithm hyperheuristic for the project presentation scheduling problem. In: The 2005 IEEE Congress on Evolutionary Computation, vol. 3, pp. 2263–2270. IEEE (2005)

11. Hernández, P., Gómez, C., Cruz, L., Ochoa, A., Castillo, N., Rivera, G.: Hyperheuristic for the parameter tuning of a bio-inspired algorithm of query routing in P2P networks. In: Batyrshin, I., Sidorov, G. (eds.) MICAI 2011, Part II. LNCS, vol. 7095, pp. 119–130. Springer, Heidelberg (2011)

12. Dorigo, M., Blum, C.: Ant colony optimization theory: A survey. Theoretical Computer Science 344, 243–278 (2005)

13. Dorigo, M., Maniezzo, V., Colorni, A.: Ant system: optimization by a colony of cooperating agents. IEEE Transactions on Systems, Man, and Cybernetics, Part B: Cybernetics 26, 29–41 (1996)

14. García, S., Molina, D., Lozano, F., Herrera, F.: A study on the use of non-parametric testsfor analyzing the evolutionary algorithms' behaviour: a case study on the CEC 2005 Special Session on Real Parameter Optimization. Journal of Heuristics (2008)

15. Cruz-Reyes, L., Gómez-Santillán, C., Castillo-García, N., Quiroz, M., Ochoa, A., Hernández-Hernández, P.: A visualization tool for heuristic algorithms analysis. In: Uden, L., Herrera, F., Bajo, J., Corchado, J.M. (eds.) 7th International Conference on KMO. AISC, vol. 172, pp. 515–524. Springer, Heidelberg (2013)

Including Modal Improvisation and Music-Inspired Components to Improve Harmony Search*

Nicolás Rojas and María-Cristina Riff

Departamento de Informática
Universidad Técnica Federico Santa María, Valparaíso, Chile,
{nerojas,Maria-Cristina.Riff}@inf.utfsm.cl

Abstract. In this paper we present new components to be included in harmony search algorithms. These components are inspired from music improvisation. The Modal improvisation uses musical modes rather than chord progressions as a harmonic framework. We also include the notion of tone scales that allows the algorithm to visit different parts of the search space. We evaluate our approach solving instances of the Multidimensional Knapsack Problem instances. We compare our results with those obtained by the former harmony search algorithm, and with the well-known state-of-the-art results.

Keywords: Harmony Search, Discrete Optimization.

1 Introduction

Harmony Search has been introduced as a new metaheuristic inspired from jazz music improvisation to solve hard problems, [1]. This technique has been successfully applied to solve various well-known problems, [2]. Because the idea of using a technique based on music looks very promising, we propose in this paper to include components inspired from music into harmony search algorithms. These components allow the search of the standard harmony search algorithm to improve. Moreover, because of the great presence of musical components, our approach is much different from classical metaheuristics. The goal of our research is to improve the search of harmony search algorithms by including new inspired musical components. We find the best parameter values for our algorithms using EVOCA [3], a recently proposed tuner for metaheuristics. We also report a statistical analysis for comparison. In the next section, we briefly describe the classical harmony search algorithm. This is followed by a description of the Multidimensional Knapsack Problem (MKP), which we use to evaluate our approach. The musical based components and mechanisms incorporated on the harmony search structure are introduced in Section 5. Section 6 presents the experimentation, statistical analysis and comparison using well-known MKP instances, and finally, Section 7 gives the conclusions of our work and ideas for future work.

---

* This work is partially supported by FONDECYT Project 1120781 and Centro Científico Tecnológico de Valparaíso (CCT-Val) FB0821.

F. Castro, A. Gelbukh, and M. González (Eds.): MICAI 2013, Part II, LNAI 8266, pp. 105–117, 2013.

2   Standard Harmony Search Algorithm

[4] introduces the Harmony Search (HS) metaheuristic inspired in the jazz music improvisation. Roughly speaking, the idea comes from musicians who search to improve harmonies in order to obtain aesthetic melodies. Thus, HS is a population-based metaheuristic. From the optimization point of view, each harmony represents a candidate solution which is evaluated using an evaluation function. The changes are inspired by music improvisation that are randomly applied to previous candidate solutions in memory. The HS algorithm uses a population of candidate solutions or Harmony Memory (HM). At the beginning a HM is randomly generated. At each iteration a new solution is either generated from memory information, or randomly. Two parameters guide the generation of the new solution. The Harmony memory considering rate (HMCR) and Pitch adjusting rate (PAR) correspond to the rate of randomly updated solutions. For each variable, its value in the new solution is either obtained from a direct copy of a selected value in the memory, or from a selected value from the memory that goes through a small perturbation, or randomly generated. The new solution is evaluated and replaces the worst candidate solution in the population if it obtains a better evaluation value. This process is repeated, until a termination criterion is reached. The pseudocode is presented in algorithm 1. At step (5) in this figure, the variable value comes from the memory. Different strategies can be applied. The most popular are to randomly select a value for this variable from the memory. Another strategy is to select the value from the best evaluated harmony the memory. At step (7) a little perturbation using equation 1 is made to the previously selected value using a bandwidth (BW) value. When the algorithm does not use the value in memory (step (10)), a new value belonging to the variable domain is randomly generated. Finally, after the evaluation, if the new solution is better than the worst one, it takes its place in the memory (step(15)).

$$new\_solution[i] = new\_solution[i] + random(0, 1) * BW \tag{1}$$

This algorithm has been applied to solve various problems with continuous domains, [5]. Some modifications have been proposed to solve discrete problems, [6] , [7], as well as to include an on-line tuning strategy in order to control the parameters HCMR and PAR during the search, [8].

Before describing the new musical inspired components, we briefly present the Multidimensional Knapsack Problem (MKP) in the following section. We use MKP to illustrate our new components, and also to evaluate the algorithm in the experiments section.

3   Multidimensional Knapsack Problem

The 0-1 Multidimensional Knapsack Problem (MKP), defined as a knapsack with multiple resource constraints. It consists in selecting a subset of n objects or items in such a way that the total profit of the selected objects is maximized while a set of m knapsack constraints are satisfied.

Algorithm 1. Standard Harmony Search

```
1:  Generate Randomly Initial Population HM of size HMS
2:  while (max − number − iterations) do
3:     for i = 1 to N do
4:        if (HMCR < rnd(0,1)) then
5:           new-solution[i] from HM
6:           if (PAR < rnd(0,1)) then
7:              new-solution[i] ← perturbed(new-solution[i])
8:           end if
9:        else
10:          new-solution[i] ← randomly generated
11:       end if
12:    end for
13:    Fitness-new-solution ← Evaluate(new-solution)
14:    if (Fitness-new-solution better Worst memory solution) then
15:       Replace Worst memory solution
16:    end if
17: end while
```

Formally, given

$$X_i = \begin{cases} 1 & \text{if object } i \text{ is in knapsack} \\ 0 & \text{other case} \end{cases} \tag{2}$$

$$\text{Maximize } Z = \sum_i^n p_i X_i \tag{3}$$

Subject to:
- Knapsack Constraints

$$\sum_i^n X_i w_{ij} \leq c_j, \forall j = 1, \ldots, m \tag{4}$$

where p_i is the profit of the object i. MKP is an NP-hard optimization problem that can formulate many practical problems such as capital budgeting where project i has profit p_i and consume w_{ij} units of resource j. The goal is to determine a subset of n projects such that the total profit is maximized and all resource constraints are satisfied. We have choosen this problem because many approaches already exist to solve it, and because there are well-known benchmarks that can be used to evaluate our work.

4   Adaptive Binary Harmony Search

Adaptive Binary Harmony Search (ABHS) has been proposed in [6] to solve applications with binary domains. Thus, this algorithm can solve MKP. In this algorithm the classical equation 1 is replaced by a bit assignment from the best solution found. Pseudocode is presented in algorithm 2. Initially, $ABHS$ sets the values for PAR (Pitch

Adjusting Rate), $HMCR$ (Harmony Memory Considerating Rate), HMS (Harmony Memory Size) and NI (Number of Iterations). Then the population is randomly generated in $InitHarmonyMemory()$. $ABHS$ uses a binary representation and the algorithm selects only feasible solutions. $ABHS$ creates a new harmony called NH in $ImproviseNewHarmony()$ and if it's better than the worst solution in memory, $UpdateHarmonyMemory()$ replaces the worst with NH. Finally, $SetBestHarmony()$ identifies the best solution in memory.

Algorithm 3 shows the procedure $ImproviseNewHarmony()$. A new solution is constructed by selecting a bit either from $HarmonyMemory$ or at random according to the HMCR parameter value. The procedure $ImproviseNewHarmony$ is focused on improving NH by including some bits from the best solution ($BestGlobalSolution$). For this, it uses the PAR parameter.

Algorithm 2. ABHS

Set $PAR, HCMR, HMS, NI$
InitHarmonyMemory();
while ($current\_iteration < NI$) **do**
  ImproviseNewHarmony();
  UpdateHarmonyMemory();
  SetBestHarmony();
  $current\_iteration + +$;
end while

---

5 Our Approach

In this section, we introduce modifications and different components to use in harmony search inspired algorithms. To explain our approach we use ABHS and MKP. We introduce in the following sections four algorithms that use different musical concepts named $ABHS^*$, HS_wHC, HS_wTones and HS_wModes. These algorithms use the same procedure to create the initial harmony as well as the perturbation criteria.

Initial Harmony: All of the previous algorithms use a binary representation and generate the initial harmony as follows.: In the classical HS the initial harmony memory or population is randomly generated. However, when a musician begins to play a given piece of music, he/she actually has an initial knowledge about the different harmonies and which combinations sound good or not. Thus, for MKP, we generate the initial population using the following three heuristics:

  – A random generation
  – Weight decreasing order: This heuristic is used to first consider the light objects with the idea of obtaining a greater profit.
  – Efficiency increasing order: This heuristic takes into account both the weight and the profit of the object to be included. It uses a rate computed as $\frac{p_i}{w_i}$, to measure the contribution related to the reduction of the knapsack free-capacity .

Algorithm 3. ImproviseNewHarmony()

$NH \leftarrow ZeroVector$ of n size (n: number of objects)
for Each bit k of the Vector of NH **do**
    $ran_1 \leftarrow$ Random number between 0 and 1
    if $(ran_1 \leq HMCR)$ **then**
        $i \leftarrow$ Random number between 0 and HMS-1
        $NH[k] \leftarrow HM[k][i]$
        if (!CheckFeasibleSolution()) **then**
            $NH[k] \leftarrow 0$
        end if
    else
        $ran_2 \leftarrow$ Random number between 0 and 1
        if $(ran_2 > 0.5)$ **then**
            $NH[k] \leftarrow 1$
        else
            $NH[k] \leftarrow 0$
        end if
    end if
end for

for Each bit k of the Vector NH **do**
    $ran_2 \leftarrow$ Random number between 0 and 1
    if $(ran_3 \leq PAR)$ **then**
        $NH[k] \leftarrow BestGlobalSolution[k]$
        if (!CheckFeasibleSolution()) **then**
            $NH[k] \leftarrow 0$
        end if
    end if
end for

The heuristics are used by a greedy procedure. We have made special attention in the diversity of the initial population. For this, all the candidate solutions in memory are checked to be different. Algorithm 4 shows the procedure. Init Harmony Memory is a greedy procedure which takes the objects from an ordered list. This list can be randomly ordered or drawn up either in weight decreasing order or in efficiency increasing order.

Perturbation Criteria: Some decisions made in the classical HS implementation do not take into account the quality of the intermediate solution obtained. For instance, it can use a value from memory, and decide to apply a perturbation to this value. The algorithm will apply this perturbation whether or not it improves the current solution. Doing that, the algorithm can loose some good solutions without remembering that they were already generated. Therefore, in all of our algorithms, perturbations are only accepted when the current solution is improved.

5.1 $ABHS^*$

The algorithm $ABHS^*$ is similar to ABHS, but it generates the initial harmony and includes the perturbation criteria described above.

Algorithm 4. InitHarmonyMemory()

 1: RandomList ← OrderRandomly();
 2: WeightList ← OrderByWeight();
 3: EfficiencyList ← OrderByEfficiency();
 4: *option* ← 0
 5: **while** (!completed population) **do**
 6:    **switch** (*option*)
 7:    **case 0:**
 8:       GenerateSolutions(RandomList);
 9:    **case 1:**
10:       GenerateSolutions(WeightList);
11:    **case 2:**
12:       GenerateSolutions(EfficiencyList);
13:    **default:**
14:       break;
15:    **end switch**
16:    (*option* + 1)%3;
17: **end while**
18: SelectBestHMSSolutions();

5.2   HS_wHC

The essential of the human improvisation task is oriented to improve musical aesthetics. Thus, in our the HS_wHC algorithm, when it constructs a new harmony, it follows a local search procedure that uses a first-improvement strategy with a swap move, before being evaluated to be included in memory. Algorithm 5 shows this procedure. The algorithm only allows feasible candidate solutions.

Algorithm 5. HS_wHC

 1: Set $PAR, HCMR, HMS, NI, RAN$
 2: InitHarmonyMemory();
 3: **while** ($current\_iteration < NI$) **do**
 4:    ImproviseNewHarmony();
 5:    HC();
 6:    UpdateHarmonyMemory();
 7:    SetBestHarmony();
 8:    $current\_iteration + +$;
 9: **end while**

5.3   HS_wTones

In order to do a good improvisation, a musician knows the tones to use. Different tonal changes are done during the improvisation task. An experienced musician knows the most suitable tone to be used to produce a better harmony. Using this idea, we include a new component whose goal is to modify the tone before harmony improvisation. It is translated by modifying the seed before the improvisation of each harmony, such that

Algorithm 6. HC()

1: $Aux\_NH \leftarrow NH$
2: **for** N times (N: size of the Vectors Aux_NH and NH) **do**
3:     $i \leftarrow$ Random number between 0 and $N-1$
4:     $j \leftarrow$ Random number between 0 and $N-1$
5:     Swap($Aux\_NH[i], Aux\_NH[j]$);
6:     **if** (!CheckFeasibleSolution()) **then**
7:         Swap($Aux\_NH[j], Aux\_NH[i]$)
8:     **else**
9:         **if** ($Fitness\_Aux\_NH > Fitness\_NH$) **then**
10:            $NH \leftarrow Aux\_NH$
11:            break;
12:         **end if**
13:     **end if**
14: **end for**

each harmony follows different patterns according to the associated seed. Algorithm 7 shows the pseudocode with the tonal modifications. The algorithm, before trying to include the new solution in memory, uses the same hill climbing procedure as in the previous algorithm.

Algorithm 7. HS_wTones

1: Set $PAR, HCMR, HMS, NI, RAN$
2: InitHarmonyMemory();
3: **while** ($current\_iteration < NI$) **do**
4:     srand(seed);
5:     ImproviseNewHarmony();
6:     HC();
7:     UpdateHarmonyMemory();
8:     SetBestHarmony();
9:     $current\_iteration + +$;
10:     seed $+ =$ current_iteration;
11: **end while**

5.4 HS_wModes

Instead of focusing on the chord sequence of the song, modal jazz is all about scales and modes. This gives more freedom. The accompanying instruments don't have to follow the chords, the soloist can create melodies of his own instead of arpeggiating, on and on the same chord sequence. Thus, to create jazz improvisations it is also possible to use various scales beginning from the same tone. It gives the option of changing the melody colour during scale changes by doing variations in the interval sequences, which allows the space of new harmonies to increase. This is known as musical modes and comes from Greek musical theory, but they were only incorporated in the sixties by Miles Davis and John Coltrane [9]. The seven modes are organized from each step of the scale, thus the modes that have no sharps and no flats are: C Ionian/Major, D Dorian, E Phrygian, F Lydian, G Mixolydian, A Aeolian/Minor and B Locrian [10]. In our implementation, this theory is included by generating seven new harmonies beginning at a fixed tone at each iteration. The idea is to apply the tones modification and to select the best harmony from the seven choices which have previously followed a hill climbing procedure. Algorithms 8 and 9 show the details of the procedure. The difference between HS_wTones and HS_wModes is a new procedure called $Modes()$, which includes $ImproviseNewHarmony$ (for creating all the new harmonies) and $HC()$ (to improve them). HS_wModes includes the HS_wTones tonal variation, modifying the seed at each iteration. At the end of each iteration in Algorithm 9, $Modes()$ creates one solution per Mode with $ImproviseNewHarmony$, then HC tries to improve it. The best of the seven harmonies is selected.

Algorithm 8. HS_wModes

1: Set $PAR, HCMR, HMS, NI, RAN$
2: InitHarmonyMemory();
3: **while** $(current\_iteration < NI)$ **do**
4:     srand(seed);
5:     Modes();
6:     UpdateHarmonyMemory();
7:     SetBestHarmony();
8:     $current\_iteration + +$;
9:     seed $+$ = current_iteration;
10: **end while**

Algorithm 9. Modes()

1: **for** Each of Seven Modes **do**
2:     ImproviseNewHarmony();
3:     HC();
4:     $Vector_{Modes} \leftarrow Push\_back(NH)$;
5: **end for**
6: NH $\leftarrow$ BestSolution($Vector_{Modes}$);

---

6   Experimental Evaluation

In this section we report the results obtained by the algorithms when solving MKP instances. The goal of the tests are:

1. To evaluate the ability of harmony search algorithms to find good values for MKP.
2. To compare the performance of the different algorithms and to evaluate the contribution of the new components and musical inspired ideas to improve the search.

To compare the approaches here presented, we only used MKP instances involving 20 objects or more. The MKP benchmarks can be found on the website[1].

---

[1] http://people.brunel.ac.uk/ mastjjb/jeb/orlib/mknapinfo.html
   http://www.cs.nott.ac.uk/ jqd/mkp/index.html

6.1   Comparing different Versions of HS

At this point it is important to remark that the goal of these tests is to evaluate if HS inspired techniques can solve MKP instances more than to find the best algorithm for solving MKP. Our ideas are focused on improving the Harmony Search metaheuristic. The tests are carried out on our four algorithms:

- the first one is the version $ABHS^*$,
- the second one includes the hill-climbing first-improvement procedure,
- the third algorithm incorporates the idea of Tones to the second algorithm, and
- finally, the approach which includes the Modal improvisation idea

Tuning Results. In order to do a good comparison, all algorithms have been fine-tuned using EVOCA, which is a new tuner recently proposed for metaheuristics, [3]. EVOCA and the tests are available on our webpage **comet.informaticae.org**[2]. The parameters tuned are the size of the harmony population, HMCR, PAR and RAN. Parameter RAN corresponds to the probability of taking a random value for a variable, instead one value from the memory which has been perturbed. The algorithms are independent from EVOCA. We can use any tuner like ParamILS, REVAC or another one. We use EVOCA because it strongly reduces the initial parameters values setting effort. Table 1 shows the parameter's values.

Table 1. EVOCA results

Algorithm	HMS	HMCR	PAR	RAN
$ABHS^*$	44	0.892	0.3	0.1
HS_wHC	44	0.871	0.5	0.1
HS_wTones	13	0.9	0.297	0.464
HS_wModes	26	0.2	0.3	0.1

Comparing ABHS to $ABHS^*$ The first set of tests is to contrast the results obtained using ABHS and $ABHS^*$. We have used 50 different seeds to run each algorithm for a maximum of 100000 iterations. The ABHS parameter's values are those reported by the authors: HMS 20, HMCR 0.6, PAR 0.4 and RAN 0.5.

Table 2 shows the results for each instance tested and reports the best value as well as the average of the best solutions obtained for each algorithm. The results show in black when $ABHS^*$ obtain better or equal results than ABHS. Thus, given these results in the following sections the algorithms are compared with respect to $ABHS^*$.

6.2   Instances Results

Table 3 shows the gap between the best value obtained by each algorithm and the best-known value for the MKP instances. HS_wModes shows a better performance than the other algorithms.

---

[2] The hardware platform adopted for the experiments was a PC with an Intel Corei7-920, having 4GB of RAM, and using the Linux Mandriva 2010 operating system.

Table 2. Comparison between ABHS and $ABHS^*$

Instance	ABHS		$ABHS^*$	
	Best	Avg	Best	Avg
HP 1	3418	3399.66	**3418**	3374.7
HP 2	3186	3112.8	**3168**	3070.62
MKNAP1.5	12400	12393.8	**12400**	**12397.8**
MKNAP1.6	10618	10583.98	10604	**10558.98**
MKNAP1.7	16537	16482.3	16519	16445.06
SENTO 1	7772	7704.04	**7772**	**7731.78**
SENTO 2	8711	8675.84	**8722**	**8710.86**
PB 5	2139	2117.6	**2139**	2093.24
PB 6	776	774.6	**776**	771.56
PB 7	1035	1034.6	**1035**	1022.82
WEISH 1	4554	4554.0	**4554**	4549.38
WEISH 6	5557	5545.8	**5557**	5538.44
WEISH 10	6339	6317.52	**6339**	6302.84
WEISH 15	7486	7421.84	**7486**	**7479.22**
WEISH 18	9533	9427.42	**9548**	**9525.62**
WEISH 22	8901	8595.4	**8929**	**8907.06**
WEING 1	141278	141278.0	**141278**	141258.0
WEING 2	130883	130883.0	**130883**	130879.8
WEING 3	95677	95677.0	**95677**	95665.0
WEING 4	119337	119337.0	**119337**	119317.08

Table 3. MKP instances results - %Gap best-known optimal value

Instance	n	m	ABHS	$ABHS^*$	HS_wHC	HS_wTones	HS_wModes
HP 1	28	4	0.0	1.42	0.0	0.0	0.0
HP 2	35	4	0.0	0.0	3.17	2.31	0.0
MKNAP1.5	28	10	0.0	0.0	0.0	0.0	0.0
MKNAP1.6	39	5	0.0	0.13	0.0	0.13	0.0
MKNAP1.7	50	5	0.0	0.0	0.0	0.0	0.0
SENTO 1	60	30	0.0	0.0	0.0	0.0	0.0
SENTO 2	60	30	0.13	0.0	0.0	0.01	0.08
PB 5	20	10	0.0	0.0	0.0	0.0	0.0
PB 6	40	30	0.0	0.0	0.0	0.0	0.0
PB 7	37	30	0.0	0.0	0.0	0.0	0.0
WEISH 1	30	5	0.0	0.0	0.0	0.0	0.0
WEISH 6	40	5	0.0	0.0	0.0	0.0	0.0
WEISH 10	50	5	0.0	0.0	0.0	0.0	0.0
WEISH 15	60	5	0.0	0.0	0.0	0.0	0.0
WEISH 18	70	5	0.49	0.0	0.0	0.0	0.0
WEISH 22	80	5	0.52	0.0	0.0	0.0	0.37
WEING 1	28	2	0.0	0.0	0.0	0.0	0.0
WEING 2	28	2	0.0	0.0	0.0	0.0	0.0
WEING 3	28	2	0.0	0.0	0.0	0.0	0.0
WEING 4	28	2	0.0	0.0	0.0	0.0	0.0

Table 4. Wilcoxon Test

Comparison	P-value
$ABHS^*$ vs HS_wHC	1.46E-002
$ABHS^*$ vs HS_wModes	2.20E-016
$ABHS^*$ vs HS_wTones	6.90E-005

Table 5. Comparison with the best known solutions and times to reach the results

Instance	n	m	Best Known	HS_wModes	AVG Execution Time[s]	AVG Optimal Time[s]
HP 1	28	4	3148	3148	136.06	15.14
HP 2	35	4	3186	3186	193.18	25.20
MKNAP1.5	28	10	12400	12400	300.84	0.02
MKNAP1.6	39	5	10618	10618	302.68	183.71
MKNAP1.7	50	5	16537	16537	445.84	421
SENTO 1	60	30	7772	7772	1764.38	1086.60
SENTO 2	60	30	8722	8715*	2059.96	–
PB 5	20	10	2139	2139	120.52	3.78
PB 6	40	30	776	776	1143.7	2.12
PB 7	37	30	1035	1035	1276.12	27.80
WEISH 1	30	5	4554	4554	97.72	7.14
WEISH 6	40	5	5557	5557	179.12	17.72
WEISH 10	50	5	6339	6339	292.3	68.78
WEISH 15	60	5	7486	7486	353.88	121.10
WEISH 18	70	5	9580	9580	2136.58	1734.00
WEISH 22	80	5	8947	8914*	639.44	–
WEING 1	28	2	141278	141278	47.52	8.92
WEING 2	28	2	130883	130883	44.56	17.02
WEING 3	28	2	95677	95677	44.7	4.30
WEING 4	28	2	119337	119337	46.72	0.04

Statistical Analysis: To better analyze these results, we have done a statistical comparison previously used in Ref. [11] to compare the performance of the algorithms proposed with $ABHS^*$. Using the information of the distance from the best-known solution obtained by the algorithms, we performed the well-known pair-wise Wilcoxon non-parametric test [12]. The results are shown in Table 4 for each pair comparison. All the computations have been done using the statistical software package R. The null-hypothesis tested is that each pair of algorithms are similar. Table 4 indicates that $ABHS^*$ is statistically significantly different to the other algorithms. Moreover, HS_wModes has the most remarkable performance.

Comparison with the Best Known Solutions. Compared to other approaches, the results provided in this paper were produced using small execution times. Table 5 shows a comparison of the best solution found by our algorithm HS_wModes with respect to the best known solution for each instance of the benchmarks. HS_wModes can not find the best-known value for just two of the evaluated instances (we mark this with $*$).

Table 6. CB and GK instances results - %Gap best-known optimal value

Instance	$n x m$	ABHS	HS_wModes
CB5x100-0.25-10	100 x 5	3.99	3.23
CB5x100-0.50-10	100 x 5	3.55	1.86
CB5x100-0.75-10	100 x 5	1.46	0.53
CB5x250-0.25-10	250 x 5	14.28	6.15
CB10x100-0.25-10	100 x 10	7.91	3.74
CB10x100-0.50-10	100 x 10	3.32	2.62
CB10x100-0.75-10	100 x 10	1.84	0.60
CB10x250-0.25-10	250 x 10	15.26	4.84
CB30x100-0.25-10	100 x 30	7.73	4.65
GK01	100 x 15	2.06	1.95
GK02	100 x 25	1.88	1.70
GK03	150 x 25	2.28	2.78

Comparing ABHS to HS_wModes. From table 3 the best results are obtained using HS_wModes. In order to do a better evaluation we have included some tests using bigger MKP instances proposed by Glover & Kochenberger (GK) and Chu & Beasley (CB). HS_wModes shows a better performace than ABHS in 91% of cases. Table 6 shows the results.

7   Conclusions

We have presented new ideas from the music domain, to be included into harmony search based algorithms to improve its search. Ideas that also allow to differentiate this metaheuristic from classical evolutionary algorithms. The simplest modification to the standard harmony search algorithm is related to the premise that good solutions must not be lost during the search. On the other hand, a musician searches for aesthetic improvisation, thus our algorithms are based on the key idea that the musician is focused on improving his performance. All of our algorithms use notions of local search improvement. The idea of Tones allows for a better diversification of the search. The idea of Modes allows more diversification with a higher level of intensification given its selection procedure. In a future work, we will evaluate our technique with other kinds of problems using dynamic parameter control.

References

1. Geem, Z.W., Kim, J.H., Loganathan, G.: A new heuristic optimization algorithm: harmony search. Simulation 76(2), 60–68 (2001)
2. Geem, Z.W. (ed.): Music-Inspired Harmony Search Algorithm. Studies in Computational Intelligence, vol. 191. Springer, Heidelberg (2009)
3. Riff, M.C., Montero, E.: A new algorithm for reducing metaheuristic design effort. In: Proceedings of the IEEE Congress on Evolutionary Computation (CEC 2013), pp. 3283–3290 (2013)

4. Yang, X.-S.: Harmony search as a metaheuristic algorithm. In: Geem, Z.W. (ed.) Music-Inspired Harmony Search Algorithm. Studies in Computational Intelligence, vol. 191, pp. 1–14. Springer, Heidelberg (2009)

5. Lee, K.S., Geem, Z.W.: A new meta-heuristic algorithm for continuous engineering optimization: harmony search theory and practice. Computer Methods in Applied Mechanics and Engineering 194(36), 3902–3933 (2005)

6. Wang, L., Yang, R., Xu, Y., Niu, Q., Pardalos, P.M., Fei, M.: An improved adaptive binary harmony search algorithm. Information Sciences 232, 58–87 (2013)

7. Wang, L., Xu, Y., Mao, Y., Fei, M.: A discrete harmony search algorithm. In: Li, K., Li, X., Ma, S., Irwin, G.W. (eds.) LSMS 2010. CCIS, vol. 98, pp. 37–43. Springer, Heidelberg (2010)

8. Alia, O., Mandava, R.: The variants of the harmony search algorithm: an overview. Artificial Intelligence Review 36(1), 49–68 (2011)

9. Monson, I.: Oh freedom: George russell, john coltrane, and modal jazz. The Course of Performance: Studies in the World of Musical Improvisation, 149–68 (1998)

10. Pease, F., Mattingly, R.: Jazz composition: theory and practice. Berklee Press (2003)

11. Rossi-Doria, O., et al.: A Comparison of the Performance of Different Metaheuristics on the Timetabling Problem. In: Burke, E.K., De Causmaecker, P. (eds.) PATAT 2002. LNCS, vol. 2740, pp. 329–351. Springer, Heidelberg (2003)

12. Bartz-Beielstein, T.: Experimental research in evolutionary computation. Springer, Berlin (2006)

A Massive Parallel Cellular GPU Implementation of Neural Network to Large Scale Euclidean TSP

Hongjian Wang, Naiyu Zhang, and Jean-Charles Créput

IRTES-SeT, Université de Technologie de Belfort-Montbéliard, 90010 Belfort, France
{hongjian.wang,naiyu.zhang,jean-charles.creput}@utbm.fr

Abstract. This paper proposes a parallel model of the self-organizing map (SOM) neural network applied to the Euclidean traveling salesman problem (TSP) and intended for implementation on the graphics processing unit (GPU) platform. The plane is partitioned into an appropriate number of cellular units, that are each responsible of a certain part of the data and network. The advantage of the parallel algorithm is that it is decentralized and based on data decomposition, rather than based on data duplication, or mixed sequential/parallel solving, as often with GPU implementation of optimization metaheuristics. The processing units and the required memory are with linear increasing relationship to the problem size, which makes the model able to deal with very large scale problems in a massively parallel way. The approach is applied to Euclidean TSPLIB problems and National TSPs with up to 33708 cities on both GPU and CPU, and these two types of implementation are compared and discussed.

Keywords: Neural network, Self-organizing map, Euclidean traveling salesman problem, Parallel cellular model, Graphics processing unit.

1 Introduction

A classical and widely studied combinatorial optimization problem is the Euclidean traveling salesman problem (TSP). The problem is NP-complete [1]. The self-organizing map (SOM), originally proposed by Kohonen [2], is a particular kind of artificial neural network (ANN) model. When applied in the plane, SOM is a visual pattern that adapts and modifies its shape according to some underlying distribution. The SOM has been applied to the TSP since a long time [3–5] and it was shown that this artificial neural network model is promising to tackle large size instances since it uses $O(N)$ memory size, where N is the instance size, i.e. the number of cities. In the light of its natural parallelism, we propose a parallel cellular-based SOM model to solve the Euclidean TSP and implement it on the graphics processing units (GPU) platform. From our knowledge, we did not find such type of SOM application to the Euclidean plane and implementation on GPU in the literature.

In recent years, the graphic hardware performance is improved rapidly and GPU vendors make it easier and easier for developers to harness the computation

F. Castro, A. Gelbukh, and M. González (Eds.): MICAI 2013, Part II, LNAI 8266, pp. 118–129, 2013.

power of GPU. Some methods for computing SOM on GPU have been proposed [6,7]. All these methods accelerate SOM process by parallelizing the inner steps in each basic iteration, of which mainly focus on two aspects as follows, firstly, to find out the winner neuron in parallel, secondly, to move the winner neuron and its neighbors in parallel. In our model, we use each parallel processing unit to do SOM iterations independently in parallel to a constant part of the data, instead of using many parallel processing units to cooperatively accelerate a sequential SOM procedure iteration by iteration. The processing units and the required memory are with linear increasing relationship to the problem size, which makes the model able to deal with very large scale problems in a massively parallel way. The theoretical computation time of our model is based on a parallel execution of many spiral search of closest points, each one having a time complexity in $O(1)$ in average when dealing with a uniform, or at most a bounded data distribution [8]. Then, one of the main interests of the proposed approach is to allow the execution of approximately N spiral searches in parallel, where N is the problem size. Thus, what would be done in $O(N)$ computation time in average for a sequential spiral search able to find N closest points, is performed in constant time $O(1)$ theoretical complexity for a parallel algorithm in the average case, for bounded distributions. This is what we intend by "massive parallelism", the theoretical possibility to reduce average computation time by factor N, when solving a Euclidean NP-hard optimization problem.

The rest of this paper is organized as follows. We briefly introduce the Euclidean traveling salesman problem and the self-organizing map in Section 2. After that, we present our parallel cellular-based model in Section 3 and give the detailed GPU implementation in Section 4. Our experimental analysis on both small and large scale problems is outlined in Section 5, before we summarize our work and conclude with suggestions for future study.

2 Background

2.1 Traveling Salesman Problem

The travelling salesman problem (TSP) can be simply defined as a complete weighted graph $G = (V, E, d)$ where $V = \{1, 2, \cdots, n\}$ is a set of vertices (cities), $E = \{(i, j)|(i, j) \in V \times V\}$ is a set of edges, and d is a function assigning a weight (distance) d_{ij} to every edge (i, j). The objective is to find a minimum weight cycle in G which visits each vertex exactly once. The Euclidean TSP, or planar TSP, is the TSP with the distance being the ordinary Euclidean distance. It consists, correspondingly, of finding the shortest tour that visits N cities where the cities are points in the plane and where the distance between cities is given by the Euclidean metric.

2.2 The Kohonen's Self-organizing Map

The standard self-organizing map [2] is a non directed graph $G = (V, E)$, called the network, where each vertex $v \in V$ is a neuron having a synaptic weight vector

$w_v = (x, y) \in \Re^2$, where $\Re^2$ is the two-dimensional Euclidean space. Synaptic weight vector corresponds to the vertex location in the plane. The set of neurons N is provided with the d_G induced canonical metric $d_G(v, v') = 1$ if and only if $(v, v') \in E$, and with the usual Euclidean distance $d(v, v')$.

In the training procedure, a fixed amount of T_{max} iterations are applied to a graph network (a ring network in TSP applications), the vertex coordinates of which being randomly initialized into an area delimiting the data set. Here, the data set is the set of cities. Each iteration follows three basic steps. At each iteration t, a point $p(t) \in \Re^2$ is randomly extracted from the data set (extraction step). Then, a competition between neurons against the input point $p(t)$ is performed to select the winner neuron n^* (competition step). Usually, it is the nearest neuron to $p(t)$. Finally, the learning law (triggering step) presented in Equation 1 is applied to n^* and to the neurons within a finite neighborhood of n^* of radius σ_t, in the sense of the topological distance d_G, using learning rate $\alpha(t)$ and function profile h_t. The function profile is given by the Gaussian in Equation 2. Here, learning rate $\alpha(t)$ and radius σ_t are geometric decreasing functions of time. To perform a decreasing run within T_{max} iterations, in each iteration t, coeffients $\alpha(t)$ and σ_t are multiplied by $exp(ln(\chi_{final}/\chi_{init})/T_{max})$ with respectively $\chi = \alpha$ and $\chi = \sigma$, χ_{init} and χ_{final} being respectively the values in starting and final iteration. Examples of a basic iteration with different learning rates and neighborhood sizes are shown in Fig.1.

$$w_n(t+1) = w_n(t) + \alpha(t) \times h_t(n^*, n) \times (p(t) - w_n(t)) . \qquad (1)$$

$$h_t(n^*, n) = exp(-d_G(n^*, n)^2/\sigma_t^2) . \qquad (2)$$

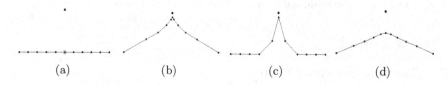

(a)   (b)   (c)   (d)

Fig. 1. A single SOM iteration with learning rate α and radius σ. (a) Initial configuration. (b) $\alpha = 0.9, \sigma = 4$. (c) $\alpha = 0.9, \sigma = 1$. (d) $\alpha = 0.5, \sigma = 4$.

3   Parallel Cellular Model

3.1   Cell Partition

It is intuitive that TSP and SOM can be connected by sharing the same Euclidean space. As a result, the input data distribution of SOM is the set of cities of TSP. The application consists of applying iterations to a ring structure with a fixed number of vertices (neurons) M. Specifically, M is set to $2N$, N being the number of cities. After training procedure, the ring transforms into a possible solution for the TSP along which a determined tour of cities can be obtained.

Fig.2 illustrates an example of training procedure on the $pr124$ instance from TSPLIB [9] at different steps of a long simulation run. Black dots are the city points of TSP. Small red circles and the black lines that connect them constitute the ring network of neurons. Execution starts with solutions having randomly generated neuron coordinates into a rectangular area containing cities, as shown in Fig.2(a). After 100 iterations, the ring network as shown in Fig.2(b) has roughly deployed towards cities. After 10000 iterations, the ring network has almost completely been mapped onto cities, as shown in Fig.2(c).

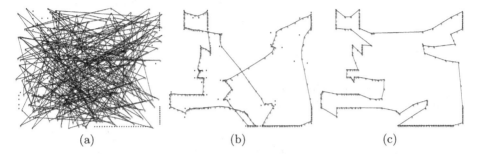

(a)   (b)   (c)

Fig. 2. Different steps of training procedure on the $pr124$ instance

In order to implement the parallel level at which parallel execution will take place, we introduce a supplementary level of decomposition of the ring network plane and input data. We uniformly partition the Euclidean space into small cells with the same size that constitute a two-dimensional cellular matrix. The scale of cell partition is decided by the number of cities. Specifically, the size of each dimension is set to $\lceil \sqrt{N \times \lambda} \rceil$, where N is the number of cities and parameter λ, which we set to 1.1 in the later experiments, is used to adjustment. The three main data structures of the parallel model are illustrated in Fig.3. This intermediate cellular matrix is in linear relationship to the input size. Its role will be to memorize the ring network in a distributed fashion and authorize many parallel closest neuron searches in the plane by a spiral search algorithm [8]. Each cell is then viewed as a basic training unit and will be executed in parallel. Thus, in each parallel iteration we conduct a number of parallel training procedures instead of carrying out one only. Each cell corresponds to a processing unit or GPU thread.

Each processing unit, that corresponds to a cell, will have to perform the different steps of the sequential SOM iteration in parallel. A problem that arises is then to allow many data points extracted at first step by the processing units, at a given parallel iteration, to reflect the input data density distribution. As a solution to this problem, we propose a particular cell activation formula stated in Equation 3 to choose those cells that will execute or not the iteration. Here, p_i is the probability that the cell i will be activated, q_i is the number of cities in the cell i, and num is the number of cells. The empirical preset parameter δ is used to adjust the degree of activity of cells/processing units. As a result, the more cities a cell contains, the higher is the probability this cell to be activated to carry out

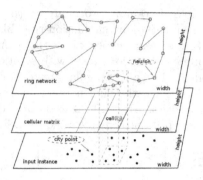

Fig. 3. Parallel cellular model

the SOM execution at each parallel iteration. In this way, the cell activation depends on a random choice based on the input data density distribution.

$$p_i = \frac{q_i}{\max\{q_1, q_2, \ldots, q_{num}\}} \times \delta .$$ (3)

3.2 Cellular-Based Parallel SOM

Based on the cell partition, the parallelized SOM training procedure carries out four parallel steps: cell activation step, extraction step, competition step and triggering step. Then, this parallel process is repeated T_{max} times. Note that T_{max} now represents the number of parallel iterations.

For each processing unit which is associated to a single cell, a cell is activated or not depending on the activation probability. If the cell is activated, the processing unit will continue to perform the next three parallel operations, otherwise it does nothing and directly skips to the end of the current iteration.

In the parallel extraction step, the processing unit randomly chooses a city from its own cell, unlikely the original sequential SOM which randomly extracts a point from the entire input data set.

In the competition step, the processing unit carries out a spiral search [8] based on the cell partition model to find the nearest neuron to the extracted city point. The cell in which this point lies will be searched first. If this cell is empty of neuron (ring node), then the cells surrounding it are searched one by one in a spiral-like pattern until a neuron is found. Once one neuron is found, it is guaranteed that only the cells that intersect a particular circle, which is centered at the extracted point and with the radius equal to the distance between the first found neuron and the extracted point, have to be checked before finishing searching. When performed on a uniform data distribution, or bounded density distribution [8], a single spiral search process takes $O(1)$ computation time according to the instance size. Then, one of the main interests of the method would be to perform $O(N)$ (the cell number) spiral searches in parallel, then in a theoretical constant time $O(1)$ for bounded density distribution, if $O(N)$ physical cores were available. This is what we call "massive parallelism".

In the triggering step, each processing unit moves its closest neuron and several neurons within a finite neighborhood toward the extracted city, according to the rule of Equation 1. All the processing units share one unique ring network of neurons in the Euclidean space. The coordinates of neurons are therefore stored into a shared buffer which is simultaneously accessed by all the parallel processing units.

After all the parallel processing units have finished their jobs in one single iteration, the learning rate α and radius σ are decreased, getting ready for the next parallel iteration.

To establish our cellular-based parallel SOM model, the scale of cell partition is $\lceil \sqrt{N \times \lambda} \rceil^2$, with N the number of cities. Hence, the number of parallel processors needed is $O(N)$. Since only one ring network is stored in memory, the memory complexity is also $O(N)$. Moreover, the parallel spiral search by every processor takes constant time $O(1)$ theoretically for bounded density distribution. For T_{max} parallel iterations, the maximum number of single SOM iterations is $T_{max} \times \lceil \sqrt{N \times \lambda} \rceil^2$, which corresponds to the extreme case where all the processing units are activated at the same time.

4   GPU Implementation

4.1   Platform Background

We use GPU to implement our parallel model with the compute unified device architecture (CUDA) programming interface. In the CUDA programming model, the GPU works as a SIMT co-processor of a conventional CPU. It is based on the concept of kernels which are functions written in C executed in parallel by a given number of CUDA threads. These threads will be launched onto GPU's streaming multi-processors and executed in parallel [10]. Hence, we apply CUDA threads as the parallel processing units in our model.

All CUDA threads are organized into a two level concepts: CUDA grid and CUDA block. A kernel has one grid which contains multiple blocks. Every block is formed of multiple threads. The dimension of grid and block can be one-dimension, two-dimension or three-dimension. Each thread has a *threadId* and a *blockId* which are built-in variables defined by the CUDA runtime to help user locate the thread's position in its block as well as its block's position in the grid [10, 11].

4.2   CUDA Code Design

In the CUDA program flow in Algorithm 1, Lines 2, 4, 7, 8, 11, and 13 are implemented with CUDA kernel functions that will be executed by GPU threads in parallel. The kernel function in Line 2 is used for calculating each cell's density value, i.e. the number of city points in each cell. After all the cells' density values are obtained, the maximum one is found. This last work in Line 3 is done on CPU since it is done only one time and does not directly concern the main behavior.

Note that computing a maximum value is a trivial job even when done on GPU. Then, the cells' activation probabilities are computed according to the activation formula of equation 3 by the kernel function of Line 4. In each iteration of the program, each cell needs two random numbers: one is used for cell activation and the other is used to extract input point in the activated cell. With respect to the large scale input instances with huge cellular matrix and numerous iterations, the random numbers generated via kernel functions shown in Line 7 and Line 8 are stored in a fixed size area due to the limited GPU global memory. Every time these random numbers are used out, a new set of random numbers are generated at the beginning of the next iteration, depending on a constant rate factor called *memory_reuse_set_rate*. The random number generators we use in Line 7 and Line 8 are from Nvidia CURAND library [10]. Line 10 and Line 11 concern the cell refreshing. Each cell has data structures where to deposit information of the number and indexes, in the neuron ring, of the neurons it contains. This information may change during each iteration, but it appears that it can be sufficient to make the refreshing based on a refresh rate coefficient called *cell_refresh_rate*. The cell contains are refreshed via kernel function in Line 11. Note that neurons' locations are moved in the plane at each single iteration, whereas the indexes in cells are refreshed based on a lower rate. Then, the parallel SOM process takes place with kernel function of Line 13 (see below). After the parallel SOM process is done, the SOM parameters will be modified getting prepared to do the next iteration.

Algorithm 1. CUDA program flow

1: Initialize data;
2: Calculate cells' density values;
3: Find the max cell density value;
4: Calculate cells' activated probabilities;
5: **for** $ite \leftarrow 0$ to max_ite **do**
6:     **if** $ite \% memory\_reuse\_set\_rate == 0$ **then**
7:         Set seeds for random number generators;
8:         Generate random numbers;
9:     **end if**
10:    **if** $ite == 0 \parallel ite \% cell\_refresh\_rate == 0$ **then**
11:        Refresh cells;
12:    **end if**
13:    Parallel SOM process;
14:    Modify SOM parameters;
15: **end for**
16: Save results;

Overall, the host code (CPU side) of the program is mainly used for flow control and the entire GPU threads synchronization by sequentially calling separate kernel functions. For all the kernel functions, one thread handles one cell and the number of threads launched by each kernel is no less than the number of cells.

The parallel SOM kernel function of Line 13 of Algorithm 1 is further illustrated by Algorithm 2. Firstly, it locates the cell's position by its *threadId* and *blockId*. Then, the thread checks if the cell is activated or not, by comparing the cell's activated probability to a random number with value between 0 and 1. If the cell is activated, the thread randomly selects a city point in the cell by using a second random number with value between 0 and the cell's density value (number of cities in that cell). After that, the thread performs a spiral search within a certain range on the grid for finding the closest neuron to the selected city point. The maximum number of cells a thread has to search equals $(range \times 2 + 1)^2$. After finding the winner neuron, the thread carries out learning process via modifying positions of the winner neuron and its neighbors. All the neurons' locations are stored in GPU global memory which is accessible to all the threads. Like all the multi-threaded applications, different threads may try to modify one same neuron's location at the same time, which causes race conditions. In order to guarantee a coherent memory update, we use the CUDA atomic function which performs a read-modify-write atomic operation without interference from any other threads [10].

Algorithm 2. GPU parallel SOM kernel flow

1: Locate cell position associated to current thread
2: Check if the cell is activated;
3: **if** the cell is activated **then**
4:    Randomly select a city point in the cell;
5:    Perform a spiral search within a certain range;
6:    Modify positions of the winner neuron and its neighbors;
7: **end if**

---

5 Experimental Analysis

5.1 Warp Divergence Analysis

In the CUDA architecture, a warp refers to a collection of 32 threads that are "woven together" and get executed in lockstep [11]. At every line in kernel function, each thread in a warp executes the same instruction on different data. When some of the threads in a warp need to execute an instruction while others in the same warp do not, this situation is known as warp divergence or thread divergence. Under normal circumstances, divergent branches simply result in performance degradation with some threads remaining idle while the other threads actually execute the instructions in the branch. The execution of threads in a warp with divergent branches are therefore carried out sequentially, resulting in performance degradation.

According to our trial tests, the most time consuming kernel function is the parallel SOM kernel. One of the reasons is that there exists warp divergence when this kernel is being executed because it has an unpredictable spiral search process in it. The spiral search is carried out in each cell of the search range, one by one, and it stops immediately when the thread finds a nearest neuron. As a result, different threads may stop at different times. Also, the more cells each thread is going to search in, the severer this problem gets. Hence, different search range settings have different influences on warp divergence. When the block size is set to 256 which is usually enough to fulfill the streaming multi-processor with adequate warps for the GPU device with CUDA capability 2.0, the highest branch efficiency (ratio of non-divergent branches to total branches [10]) of all executions with search range set to 1, 2, and 3 is 90.1%, 87.2%, and 85.9% respectively as collected by NVIDIA Visual Profiler. In theory, the less threads are put in one block, the less warp divergence occurrences will appear. Extremely, if there is only one thread in a block, then there will definitely not be warp divergence. However, the decrease of threads in each block implies the decrease of the CUDA cores usage associated to each streaming multi-processor. In order to analyze the tradeoff between performance and number of threads in a block, we have tested a set of different combinations of grid size and block size for the parallel SOM kernel. The configuration which makes the kernel run fastest is with block size of 8 with highest branch efficiency of 96.9%.

5.2   Comparative Results on GPU and CPU

During our experimental study, we have used the following platforms:

- *On the CPU side:* An Intel(R) Core(TM) 2 Duo CPU E8400 processor running at 2.67 GHz and endowed with four cores and 4 Gbytes memory. It is worth noting that only one single core executes the SOM process in our implementation.
- *On the GPU side:* A Nvidia GeForce GTX 570 Fermi graphics card endowed with 480 CUDA cores (15 streaming multi-processors with 32 CUDA cores each) and 1280 Mbytes memory.

Table 1. Experiment parameters

	α_{init}	α_{final}	σ_{init}	σ_{final}	iterations	δ	CRR[a]	SSR[b]	MRSR[c]
GPU[1]	1	0.01	12	1	100000	1	1	1	1000
CPU[1]	1	0.01	12	1	$100000 \times N$	–	100	1	–
GPU[2]	1	0.01	100	1	100000	1	1	3	1000
CPU[2]	1	0.01	100	1	$10000 \times N$	–	100	3	–

[1] Tests of small size instances. [2] Tests of large size instances.
[a] Cell refresh rate. [b] Spiral search range. [c] Memory reuse set rate.

We have done our tests with two groups of instances from either National TSPs (http://www.math.uwaterloo.ca/tsp/world/countries.html) and TSPLIB database [9]. One group consists of four small size instances from 124 cities to 980 cities, while the other consists of four large size instances from 8246 cities to 33708 cities. The parameter settings for the two groups are shown in Table

1. As discussed in Section 3.2, $T_{max} \times \lceil \sqrt{N \times \lambda} \rceil^2$ parallel SOM operations will be carried out as an extreme case by the GPU SOM program, with N the input instance size and λ set to 1.1. For the tests of small size instances, we set the total number of sequential iterations of the CPU version to $T_{max} \times N$, in order to make the total SOM operations approximately similar between GPU version and CPU version, and to reach similar quality results. Whereas for the tests with large size instances, we set it to $T_{max} \times N/10$, also to achieve similar quality results and because GPU operations depend on the cell activation probabilities and may be less than N at each GPU parallel iteration.

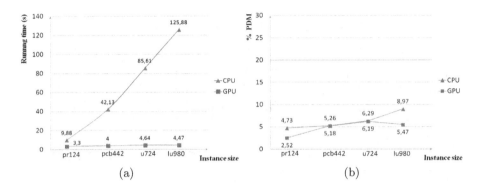

Fig. 4. Test results of small size instances

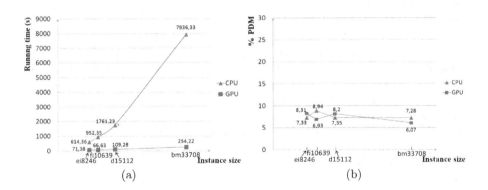

Fig. 5. Test results of large size instances

All the tests are done on a basis of 10 runs per instance. For each test case is reported the percentage deviation, called "%PDM", to the optimum tour length of the mean solution value obtained, i.e. %PDM = $(mean\ length - optimum) \times 100/optimum$. As well, is reported the percentage deviation from the optimum of the best solution value found over 10 runs, called "%PDB". Finally, is also reported the average computation time per run in seconds, called "Sec".

Table 2. Test results of small size instances

Problem	Optimal	GPU			CPU		
		%PDM	%PDB	Sec	%PDM	%PDB	Sec
pr124	59030	2.52	1.07	3.30	4.73	1.85	9.88
pcb442	50778	5.18	3.41	4.00	5.26	3.24	42.13
u724	41910	6.19	4.96	4.64	6.29	4.67	85.61
lu980	11340	5.47	3.40	4.47	8.97	4.58	125.88
Average		4.84	3.21	4.10	6.31	3.59	65.88

Table 3. Test results of large size instances

Problem	Optimal	GPU			CPU		
		%PDM	%PDB	Sec	%PDM	%PDB	Sec
ei8246	206171	8.31	7.12	71.38	7.33	6.88	614.36
fi10639	520527	6.93	6.49	66.63	8.94	8.10	952.35
d15112	1573084	8.20	7.66	109.28	7.35	7.14	1761.23
bm33708	959304	6.07	5.85	254.22	7.28	7.04	7936.33
Average		7.38	6.78	125.38	7.73	7.29	2816.07

As shown in Fig.4 and Fig.5, and in Table 2 and Table 3, respectively for the two instance groups, our GPU parallel SOM approach outperforms its counterpart CPU sequential version both on small size and large size instances, for similar tour length results. For small size instances, the ratio of CPU time by GPU time (called acceleration factor) varies from roughly factor 3 to factor 28, as the instance size grows. For large size instances, it varies from roughly factor 9 to factor 31 for the maximum size instance with up to 33708 cities. We think that the acceleration factor augmentation indicates a better streaming multi-processor occupancy as the instance size grows. We can note that the execution time of GPU version increases in a linear way with a very weak increasing coefficient, when compared to the CPU version execution time. We consider that such results are encouraging in that the parallel SOM model should really exploit the benefits of multi-processors, as the number of physical cores will augment in the future.

6   Conclusion

In this paper we propose a cellular-based parallel model for the self-organizing map and apply it to the large scale Euclidean traveling salesman problems. We did not find in the literature GPU implementations to such large size problems with up to 33708 cities. We think that this is because current GPU applications to the TSP concern memory consuming algorithms, such as ant colony, genetic algorithm or k-opt local search, which generally require $O(N^2)$ memory size. Whereas, our approach is dimension with $O(N)$ memory size. We implement our model on a GPU platform and compare the results with its counterpart CPU version. Test results shows that our GPU model has linear increasing execution time with a very weak increasing coefficient when compared to the CPU version, for both small size instances and large size instances.

Future work should deal with verification of effectiveness of the algorithm as the number of physical cores augments. More precisely, we should verify the possibility to design a weakly linear increasing, or ideally a near constant time algorithm, for bounded or uniform distributions, when the number of physical cores really increases as the instance size increases. It should be of interest also to study more CUDA programming techniques, for a better memory coalescing, or the use of shared memory. Moreover, implementations of the model to other parallel computing systems are also potential areas of research.

References

1. Papadimitriou, C.H.: The euclidean travelling salesman problem is np-complete. Theoretical Computer Science 4, 237–244 (1977)
2. Kohonen, T.: Self-organizing maps, vol. 30. Springer (2001)
3. Angeniol, B., de La Croix Vaubois, G., Le Texier, J.Y.: Self-organizing feature maps and the travelling salesman problem. Neural Networks 1, 289–293 (1988)
4. Cochrane, E., Beasley, J.: The co-adaptive neural network approach to the euclidean travelling salesman problem. Neural Networks 16, 1499–1525 (2003)
5. Créput, J.C., Koukam, A.: A memetic neural network for the euclidean traveling salesman problem. Neurocomputing 72, 1250–1264 (2009)
6. McConnell, S., Sturgeon, R., Henry, G., Mayne, A., Hurley, R.: Scalability of self-organizing maps on a gpu cluster using opencl and cuda. Journal of Physics: Conference Series 341, 012018 (2012)
7. Yoshimi, M., Kuhara, T., Nishimoto, K., Miki, M., Hiroyasu, T.: Visualization of pareto solutions by spherical self-organizing map and its acceleration on a gpu. Journal of Software Engineering and Applications 5 (2012)
8. Bentley, J.L., Weide, B.W., Yao, A.C.: Optimal expected-time algorithms for closest point problems. ACM Transactions on Mathematical Software (TOMS) 6, 563–580 (1980)
9. Reinelt, G.: Tsplib a traveling salesman problem library. ORSA Journal on Computing 3, 376–384 (1991)
10. NVIDIA: CUDA C Programming Guide 4.2, CURAND Library, Profiler User's Guide (2012), http://docs.nvidia.com/cuda
11. Sanders, J., Kandrot, E.: CUDA by example: an introduction to general-purpose GPU programming. Addison-Wesley Professional (2010)

Determination of Cardiac Ejection Fraction by Electrical Impedance Tomography Using an Artificial Neural Network

Rogerio G.N. Santos Filho, Luciana C.D. Campos,
Rodrigo Weber dos Santos, and Luis Paulo S. Barra

Federal University of Juiz de Fora
Juiz de Fora, Brazil
{rogerio.santos,luciana.campos,rodrigo.weber}@ice.ufjf.br,
luis.barra@ufjf.edu.br

Abstract. The cardiac ejection fraction (EF) is a clinical parameter that determines the amount of blood pumped by the heart in each cardiac cycle. An EF outside the normal range indicates the heart is contracting abnormally. Diverse non invasive methods can be applied to measure EF, like Computer Tomography, Magnetic Resonance. Nevertheless, these techniques cannot be used for the continuous monitoring of EF. On the other hand, Electrical Impedance Tomography (EIT) may be applied to obtain continuous estimations of cardiac EF. Low cost and high portability are also EITs features that justify its use. EIT consists in fixing a finite number of electrodes on the boundary of the tomography body, injecting low amplitude currents and recording the resulting potential differences. The problem we are interested is how to estimate the blood volume inside the ventricles by using the electric potentials obtained via the EIT technique. This problem is normally classified as a non-linear inverse problem. However, in this work we propose to face it as a classification problem. Because artificial neural networks (ANN) are nonlinear models simple to understand and to implement it was decided to use them in the context of EF estimation. The use of ANNs requires less computational resources than other methods. In addition, our ANN-based solution only requires as input the measurements of the electrical potentials obtained by the electrodes; and has as output only the scalar value that defines cardiac EF. In this work, ANNs were trained and tested with data from electrical potentials simulated computationally. Two-dimensional magnetic resonance images were used for the generation of synthetic EIT data set with various types of heart configurations, spanning from normal to pathological conditions. Our preliminary results indicate that the ANN-based method was very fast and was able to provide reliable estimations of cardiac EF. Therefore, we conclude that ANN is a promising technique that may support the continuous monitoring of patient's heart condition via EIT.

Keywords: Cardiac Mechanics, Medical Applications, Cardiac Ejection Fraction, Electrical Impedance Tomography, Artificial Neural Networks.

F. Castro, A. Gelbukh, and M. González (Eds.): MICAI 2013, Part II, LNAI 8266, pp. 130–138, 2013.
© Springer-Verlag Berlin Heidelberg 2013

1   Introduction

Cardiac Ejection Fraction is an important parameter to analyze the efficiency of the heart as a pump. It represents the amount of blood pumped out of each ventricle in each cardiac cycle. In other words, EF is a measure of blood fraction that the ventricle ejects. Clinically, it is more common to use only the ejection of the left ventricle to determine the ejection fraction. By definition, it is calculated as follows:

$$EF = \frac{PV}{EDV} = \frac{EDV - ESV}{EDV}, \tag{1}$$

where PV denotes the volume of blood pumped, given by the difference between the end-diastolic volume (EDV) and the end-systolic volume (ESV). Cardiac ejection fraction is a relevant parameter for its high correlation with the functional status of the heart. Diverse non-invasive techniques can be applied to determine EF, as echocardiography, cardiac magnetic resonance, and others. Although such techniques are able to produce high definition images for well-accurate diagnostics, they cannot be used for continuous monitoring, due specially to their high costs. In this work, a new method for continuous monitoring of cardiac ejection by Electrical Impedance Tomography (EIT) is presented based on its advantages in terms of lower costs and better portability, besides it does not use ionizing radiation.

Electrical Impedance Tomography produces an image of the conductivity distribution of part of the body using measures of current injection and potential protocols taken on the boundary of the domain. Usually, conducting electrodes are attached to the body of the patient and small currents are applied. Besides, this technique has been largely applied in different fields, as industrial monitoring [1], geophysics [2], and biomedical engineering [3–6]. In the context of the latest field, recent work [7] has discussed viability of EIT to continuous monitoring of cardiac ejection fraction, and other related works [8, 9] have shown preliminary results on the same subject. Some works use a method for generating an image of the ventricules and then the area is obtained for the estimate of EF, which is based on the partition of the body in small parts based on its resistivities.

In this work, the potential protocols taken by EIT are applied in an Artificial Neural Network (ANN) for calculation of EF. The measures of the potentials are used as ANN's input and the areas for both ventricles are obtained as ANN's output. Both areas are necessary to the EF's calculation. Thus, there is no need to generate an image of the body. Due to the lack of a real medical data base, for training and testing the ANN, a synthetically generated data set is used, containing various types of synthetic heart configuration (with anomalies or not). This synthetic data set was generated based on the work made by [10].

This paper is organized as follows. The second section describes the methods used for generating the data set. The third section presents our proposal: the Artificial Neural Network used to obtain the cardiac EF. The fourth section shows the simulation setup and his results obtained. In the last section, a conclusion is made with some ideas for future works.

2   Methods

2.1   Generation of Training Data Set

Parametrization. In [7] a parametrization is taken from an image of a human torso model provided by a magnetic resonance and the parameters that represent the regions of interest of the body are obtained. This image is segmented in five different regions: two for both lungs, one for the torso boundary and two for the heart ventricles. The shape of the regions are defined by a manual segmentation in two different image - one taken at the end of systole and another at the end of diastole. For simplicity matters, the shape of lungs and torso are considered constant during all heart cycle. The figure 1 illustrates the result of such manual segmentation.

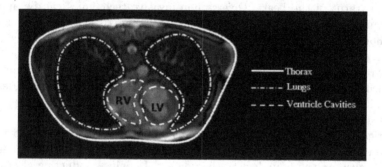

Fig. 1. Manual segmentation of a magnetic resonance image

To represent the boundary lines of the regions a extended x-spline curve is used with a minimum number of control points [11]. Since the lungs and torso are considered fixed, the control points critical for this work are the ones that represent the left and right ventricles. There are 7 control points for left ventricle and 8 for right ventricle. Each control point is represented by a coordinate with two axis. The coordinate of some control points is modified generating new splines curves that represents variations of the ventricles.

Also, a strategy is used to define the position of each control point in relation to the diastole and systole. Since the same amount of points is used for representation of diastole and systole, it is possible to represent the position of each control point i in a line, where $t_i = 0$ represents the point i at the end of the systole while $t_i = 1$ represents at diastole. As shown in figure 2.

Calculation of Electrical Potentials. As said before, this work uses an Artificial Neural Network that receives the electrical potentials synthetically calculated in function of the known resistivity and conductivity distribution of the body. As done in [7], the electrical potentials (ϕ) at each point of the regions must satisfy the Laplace's equation:

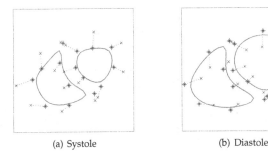

(a) Systole   (b) Diastole

Fig. 2. Position of each control point in relation to diastole and sytole

$$\nabla^2 \phi = 0, \tag{2}$$

subjected to the following conditions:

$$
\begin{aligned}
\sigma_L \nabla \phi . \eta &= \sigma_T \nabla \phi . \eta, & x \in \Gamma_1 \\
\sigma_B \nabla \phi . \eta &= \sigma_T \nabla \phi . \eta, & x \in \Gamma_2 \\
\sigma_T \nabla \phi . \eta &= J_i, & x \in \Gamma_3^{ie} \\
\nabla \phi . \eta &= 0, & x \in (\Gamma_3 - \Gamma_3^{ie})
\end{aligned}
$$

where Γ_1 represents the interface between lung and torso region; Γ_2 is the interface between the blood and torso region; Γ_3 is the external boundary of the body; Γ_3^{ie} is the portion of Γ_3 in which the ith electrode is placed on; J_i is the electric current injected through the ith electrode; and σ_T, σ_B and σ_L are, respectively, torso, blood and lung conductivities.

To solve this problem, an implementation of the Boundary Elements Method (BEM) [12] is used based on the method used by [13].

Generation of New Control Points for the Ventricles. In order to the ANN be capable to learn well, the training data set must be well representative with sufficient informations [14]. Since there is a lack of real data set, in this work, the data set used was synthetically generated. Aiming to cover all possible heart configuration, this data set was generated by pertubating some randomly chosen control points i as follows. The pertubation algorithm runs for each $t_i = 0, 0.1, 0.2...1$ alternating control points from right ventricle, left ventricle and both. Then, at each iteration of the algorithm half of total control points of left ventricle and of right ventricle are chosen. After that, some perturbations $x, t_i - 0.3 \leq x \leq t_i + 0.3$ are chosen and given to the control points predetermined. In this way, the areas for ventricles are well distributed with values between the systole and diastole. The figure 2.1 shows the histogram distribution for areas around the values from right and left ventricles from the generated synthetical data set.

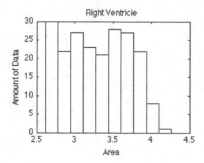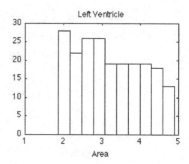

Fig. 3. Areas Histogram

2.2 Modelling the Artificial Neural Network

According to Haykin [14], ANNs are nonlinear computacional models, inspired by the structure of human brain, capable of learning, association, generalization and abstraction through experimental knowledge. ANNs are composed of structs called neurons and the connections between them. The connections are called synaptic weights and used to store the knowledge acquired. The adjustments of synaptic weights are provided by the learning algorithm, basically it consists in updates on the weights based on the error output. ANNs have been successfully applied to many problems in practical problems of prevision, classification and control. However, its performance is dependent on its configuration, such as weight initializations and number of neurons in the hidden layer.

In this work, a multilayer perceptron (MLP) neural network with one hidden layer was used. The implementation was provided by [15] which uses a Backpropagation Algorithm with the Levenberg-Marquardt optimization [16]. Different ANN configurations were trained changing the number of hidden neurons. For each configuration, some different weight inicializations was applied for training it. The comparison of all performance of trained configuration is based on the Mean Absolute Percentual Error(MAPE).

The data set has been divided in three different subsections: a training data set which is presented to the learning algorithm and is used to adjusts the synaptic weights; a validation set which secures that the ANN is generalizing well during the training phase; and finally, a test set which is used to measure the performance of the network after the training phase. In the training process, whenever the validation error begins to increase, an early stopping algorithm was applied for avoiding overfitting on the training set.

The data set division is made as following: the training set contains 63%, the validation contains 16% and the test contains 21% of the data set. All samples for each set are chosen randomly. Some ANN configurations have been trained with different numbers of hidden neurons and weights initializations. The best configuration is chosen by the smallest error(MAPE) among the others. In the following section, the results for the training phase is shown along with a test in a simulated case.

3   Results

For each ANN configuration trained - based on the number of hidden neurons, was obtained a minimum MAPE among all different weight inicializations. Also the mean of all weight inicializations MAPE was calculated. The Figure 4 shows the MAPE and the mean MAPE of all ANN configurations trained. In the lighter bars, the lowest MAPE achieved for that number of hidden neurons is represented and the darker bars represents the mean MAPE. The arrow sights the best trained configuration obtained.

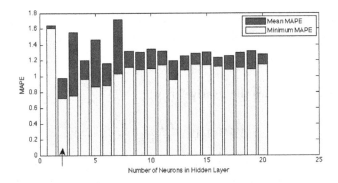

Fig. 4. Error based on Number of Hidden Neurons

In the present work, the areas that represents the ventricles are based in a transversal section of the heart cavities and is assumed to be proportional to their volumes. Assuming that, the EF can be calculated by

$$EF = \frac{EDA - ESA}{EDA}, \tag{3}$$

where EDA represents the area of the end of diastole, while ESA stands for the area of the ventricle at the end of the systole. Since the EF is calculated based on the area, the ANN gives as output the area corresponded to the electrical potentials, which is taken as inputs. Also a small error for the area corresponds to a small error on EF calculation.

The MAPE for the best ANN is 0.73% based on the test set. For the purpose of demonstration, an artificial cardiac dysfunction was generated to simulate a new heart cycle, in which EF of left ventricle is 33.02% and 17.25% for the right ventricle. In order o generate this target values, the end of systole is considered being greater than normal, while the disatole remains unaltered.

Applying the Equation 3, where the EDA remains the same, but ESA is the one used from the output of the ANN already trained, the result obtained was an EF of 33.37% of the left ventricle and 18.03% for the right ventricle, giving a relative error of 1.06% and 4.49%, respectively. In the methods used by [10] the results were 0.09% and 2.41%. These results are presented in the Table 1.

Table 1. Comparison between LM Method and ANN

Relative Errors (%)		
Method	RV	LV
LM	2.41	0.09
ANN	4.49	1.06

The equation 4 provides the relative error:

$$\Delta\% = 100 \times \frac{\tilde{EF} - EF}{EF},\tag{4}$$

where $\Delta\%$ is the relative error, $\tilde{EF}$ is the ejection fraction calculated from the values obtained using the ANN's output and EF is the target value for ejection fraction.

4   Conclusions

The main advantage of Electrical Impendance Tomography in relation to others tomography is its portability - the patient can stay in the hospital bedroom while making an EIT. Because of that, methods that gives low execution time is crucial for a continuous monitoring of the heart. As the results suggests, the Artificial Neural Network presents a low error and fast execution time, being capable to continuos monitoring the Ejection Fraction by EIT. Although its error was higher than the compared methods, the difference is not significant if you take in consideration that other errors was not included in the calculations, such as noise in electrical potentials due to irregularities in position of electrodes attached to the body

A problem for a neural network is its training phase, since a significant amount of data has to be provided. In this work, the data set was synthetically generated. But in a real world application, an image from a magnetic resonance of the patient would have to be taken in order to do the processes described here to train the network.

For further works, a three-dimension model can be used for better representation of the body. Besides, a data set provided from real EIT is interesting for the choose of the best method.

Acknowledgments. The first author would like to thank Departamento de Ciência da Computação of Universidade Federal de Juiz de Fora. All authors would like to thank the Programa de Pós-graduação em Modelagem Computacional of Universidade Federal de Juiz de Fora, FAPEMIG, CNPq, CAPES and FINEP.

References

1. Kim, M., Kim, K., Kim, S.: Phase boundary estimation in two-phase flows with electrical impedance tomography. Int. Comm. Heat Transfer 31, 1105–1114 (2004)
2. Trigo, F., Lima, R., Amato, M.: Electrical impedance tomography using extended kalman filter. I3ETBE 51, 72–81 (2004)
3. Polydorides, N., Lionheart, W.R.B., McCann, H.: Krylov subspace iterative techniques: On the brain activity with electrical impedance tomography. I3ETMI 21, 596–603 (2002)
4. Seo, J., Kwon, O., Ammari, H., Woo, E.: A mathematical model for breast cancer lesion estimation: Electrical impedance technique using ts2000 commercial system. I3ETBE 51, 1898–1906 (2004)
5. Moura, F.S., Lima, R.G., Aya, J.C.C., Fleury, A.T., Amato, M.B.P.: Dynamic imaging in electrical impedance tomography of the human chest with online transition matrix identification. IEEE Trans. Biomed. Engineering 57, 422–431 (2010)
6. Isaacson, D., Mueller, J.L., Newell, J.C., Siltanen, S.: Imaging cardiac activity by the d-bar method for electrical impedance tomography. Physiological Measurement 27, S43 (2006)
7. Peters, F.C., Barra, L.P.S., dos Santos, R.W.: Determination of cardiac ejection fraction by electrical impedance tomography - numerical experiments and viability analysis. In: Allen, G., Nabrzyski, J., Seidel, E., van Albada, G.D., Dongarra, J., Sloot, P.M.A. (eds.) ICCS 2009, Part I. LNCS, vol. 5544, pp. 819–828. Springer, Heidelberg (2009)
8. Barra, L.P.S., Peters, F.C., Martins, C.P., Barbosa, H.J.C.: Computational experiments in electrical impedance tomography. In: XXVII Iberian Latin American Congress on Computational Methods in Engineering, Belém, Brazil (2006)
9. Barra, L.P.S., Santos, R.W., Peters, F., Santos, E.P., Barbosa, H.: Parallel computational experiments in electrical impedance tomography. In: 18th Symposium on Computer Architecture and High Performance Computing, Ouro Preto, Brazil, Sociedade Brasileira de Computação, High Perfomance Computing in the Life Sciences, vol. 1, pp. 7–13 (2006)
10. Peters, F.C., Barra, L.P.S., Santos, R.W.: Determination of cardiac ejection fraction by electrical impedance tomography. In: Erondu, O.F. (ed.) Medical Imaging, pp. 253–270. InTech (2011)
11. Blanc, C., Schlick, C.: X-splines: a spline model designed for the end-user. In: Proceedings of the 22nd Annual Conference on Computer Graphics and Interactive Techniques, SIGGRAPH 1995, pp. 377–386. ACM, New York (1995)
12. Brebbia, C., Telles, J.C.F., Wrobel, L.C.: Boundary Elements Techniques: Theory and Applications in Engineering. Springer (1984)

13. Barra, L.P.S., Peters, F.C., Santos, R.W.: Numerical experiments for the viability analysis of the determination of the cardiac ejection fraction by the electrical impedance tomography. In: XXIX CILAMCE - Congresso Ibero Latino Americano de Métodos Computacionais em Engenharia, Maceió, Brasil (2008) (in Portuguese)
14. Haykin, S.: Neural Networks - A Comprehensive Foundation, 2nd edn. Person Education (2005)
15. MATLAB: Neural Network Toolbox. The MathWorks, Inc. (R2009b)
16. Hagan, M.T., Menhaj, M.: Training feed-forward networks with the marquardt algorithm. IEEE Transactions on Neural Networks 5, 989–993 (1999)

Bidirectional Recurrent Neural Networks
for Biological Sequences Prediction

Isis Bonet[1], Abdel Rodriguez[2], and Isel Grau[2]

[1] Escuela de Ingeniería de Antioquia, Envigado, Antioquia, Colombia
ibonetc@gmail.com
[2] Cetro de Estudios de Informática. Universidad Central "Marta Abreu" de Las Villas, Santa
Clara, Cuba
igrau@uclv.edu.cu

Abstract. The aim of this paper is to analyze the potentialities of Bidirectional
Recurrent Neural Networks in classification problems. Different functions are
proposed to merge the network outputs into one single classification decision.
In order to analyze when these networks could be useful; artificial datasets were
constructed to compare their performance against well-known classification
methods in different situations, such as complex and simple decision boundaries, and related and independent features. The advantage of this neural network
in classification problems with complicated decision boundaries and feature relations was proved statistically. Finally, better results using this network topology in the prediction of HIV drug resistance were also obtained.

Keywords: Bidirectional recurrent neural network, classification, feature relation, output combination, HIV drug resistance, bioinformatics.

1   Introduction

The classification task is based on assigning a new pattern to one class of a set of N
discrete classes. The pattern is represented by a vector $X = (x_1, x_2, ..., x_N)$ of N characteristics or features. Classification problems are just as common in bioinformatics as
they are in other areas. In this work we focused on the classification of biological
sequences, such as nucleotide and protein sequences.

Just like in any classification problem, the search for appropriate features is the
first step in building a knowledge database. The representation of biological sequences is particularly difficult; analyzing most biological sequences is easier if we
have the three-dimensional structure, but unfortunately it is very difficult and expensive to obtain. This is one of the motives to use primary or secondary structures as an
alternative to represent the sequences. These representations are linear and very
different to the three-dimensional structure. Complex relations between the amino
acids or between some parts of the sequence are hypothetically presumed in order to
relate these structures. To represent the sequences, some authors use biological properties such as: hydrophobicity, polarity, etc., in order to end the problem of the variable size of the sequences. However, sometimes it is common to keep the natural

F. Castro, A. Gelbukh, and M. González (Eds.): MICAI 2013, Part II, LNAI 8266, pp. 139–149, 2013

representation or replace the amino acids or nucleotides with any quantitative measure. This representation takes into account the complex relations that may exist between the elements; this representation can therefore be seen as a time sequence that induces the incentive to use dynamic structures to solve this problem.

Although we will use the primary structure to represent the biological sequences, the variable size is not the objective to use dynamic structures in this paper. In this paper we have supposed that the sequences are all the same sizes or an alignment method was applied. This assumption was done to compare the network against the classic classification methods. The motivation of this paper is to see the one specific structure's ability to deal with problems of complex relation between the features, that we suppose biological sequences have.

To solve classification problems there are some different models of machine learning. Recurrent Neural Network (RNN) has become an increasingly popular method in bioinformatics problems over recent years. Given its temporal connections, the RNN has the particularity of making possible a temporal memory, regardless of whether they are future or past times. Temporal problems are not the only ones that can be solved with this network. Just like a Multilayer Perceptron (MLP) or how a Support Vector Machine (SVM) does with nonlinear kernels, RNN makes an internal feature extraction, By separating the features in subsets associated with times, more complex feature extraction combinations can be achieved.

In particular Bidirectional Recurrent Neural Networks (BRNN) have been used for protein secondary structure prediction [1]. Currently this architecture is considered to be one of the best models for addressing this problem [2]. Some authors have used methods based on BRNN [3] or a combination with other methods [4].

Bidirectional Recurrent Neural Network is a type of Recurrent Neural Networks [5]. This structure has the advantage of not using fixed windows like MLP and can use information from both sides of the sequence, right and left.

The objective of this paper is to compare the behavior of BRNN and classical classification methods when dealing with problems of different dependencies of the features. The topology of BRNN used is the one proposed by Baldi [1], specifically the topology already described in [6]. The main difference between these topologies is the way they combine the outputs. In this paper some output combination functions are used to take into account that the network has one output for each time and in classification problems there is only one output.

Artificial databases with different dependences of the features were built in order to illustrate the potentiality of this type of network in datasets with complex relation between the features. In this paper, we selected a Multilayer Perceptron, as the classic neural network to classification problems as well as the Support Vector Machine and Bayes Network. With this comparison we don't pretend to generalize when the use of BRNN is appropriate. Our purpose is to justify that this method improves the prediction in some problems of biological sequences analysis in comparison to the classical classification methods.

To conclude this paper shows the results using the BRNN to solve the problem of prediction of HIV resistance, using the information of one protein: protease. Also, the results obtained by the BRNN are compared with the other methods.

2   Methods

2.1   Data Preparation

Artificial datasets were generated for this experiment. To build the datasets three factors were kept in mind: feature relation, direction of the relation and decision region of classes.

For each feature a further subset of features was randomly selected. A mathematical dependency was built between the feature and the selected subset. Dependencies were generated by linear, polynomial and piecewise polynomial functions $f(X)$ as can be seen in equations 1, 2 and 3 respectively. $X = (x_1, x_2, ..., x_N)$ represents the feature vector with dimension N.

$$f(X) = \frac{\sum_{i=1}^{N} a_i x_i + c}{\sum_{i=1}^{N} a_i + c} \quad (1)$$

In this linear function, a_i is the coefficient for each i, and c is an independent term. This function is finally normalized by the maximum possible value of the numerator, keeping in mind the features generated in the interval [0,1].

As was explain before each feature has a subset of features of which they are dependent upon, named as SDF_k. $SDF_k = (d_{k1}, d_{k2}, ..., d_{km})$, where d_{kj} represents the index of features and m is also generated randomly. The coefficient a_i is generated randomly if i is a member of SDF_k, or else the value will be 0.

In equation 2, the coefficients $b_i \in [1,10]$ are added, so the equation behaves polynomially.

$$f(X) = \frac{\sum_{i=1}^{N} a_i x_i^{b_i} + c}{\sum_{i=1}^{N} a_i + c} \quad (2)$$

On the other hand, piecewise generated by polynomial function $h(X)$ defines different behaviors for the last kind of functions: piecewise polynomial functions (equation 3).

$$f(X) = g_i(X), \qquad u_{i-1} \leq h(X) < u_i \quad (3)$$

Function g_i defines this behavior for each subdomain. A set of thresholds was generated at random: $U = (u_0, u_1, ..., u_R)$, where R represents the number of intervals (generated at random too in the [5,15] interval). A final consideration: $u_0=0$, $u_R=1$ and $\forall i \in [1,R]$: $u_{i-1} < u_i$.

At first, a subset without any feature relation was generated; and used as our reference for the comparison.

Dependencies between the features were analyzed in three ways: forward, backward and in both directions. To build dependencies forward, the selection of the subset of dependent features for a particular feature in the position i, a subset of indexes j were generated in the interval [0, i-1], to backward [i+1, N] and to both directions [1,N], $j \neq i$.

Additionally, the classes were generated with the same features described below.

In total, 285 datasets were generated, 95 datasets with the class generated from each function. Each dataset is described by 9 features and a dichotomy class.

2.2   Models Used

All models used in this paper were implemented in Weka (version 3.6; Waikato Environment for Knowledge Analysis), a software developed at the Waikato University, New Zealand, and available at: http://www.cs.waikato.ac.nz/ml/weka/index.html.

To compare the results, a Multilayer Perceptron, Support Vector Machine, Bayes Network (BayesNet) and C45 decision tree (named J48 in Weka) were selected.

Also BRNN mentioned before was implemented in Java using the Weka package and added to it.

2.3   Bidirectional Recurrent Network Topology

The use of these networks in dissimilar fields has increased in the last few years. These networks have the particularity of making a temporal memory given their temporal connections possible, no matter whether they are future or past times. There are many real problems with these characteristics.

In order to deal with biological sequences problems, a bidirectional model to establish recurrences in two directions was used. On the left in Figure 1 the proposed topology, with three-hidden-layers is shown. This makes the correlations independent of each time with the others. On the right, one can see the unfolded network to the time t. A size of window for the sequence is defined as a parameter of this model. The sequence is divided in sub-sequences according to the size of window (n) defined, where each one represents a time for the network. According to the size of windows it is also possible to define the number of neurons in the input layer. As is shown in figure 1, the topology has a recurrent to one step backward (time t-1) and one forward (time t+1), that is the unfolding is of T times, where T = Sequence Length / n. For example for a sequence divided into three parts (times), the unfolding of the network will be replicated exactly three times.

The network is trained with the Bakpropagation Through Times algorithm [7].

Once the basic algorithm steps for processing a problem have been defined, a procedure for combining the results was introduced.

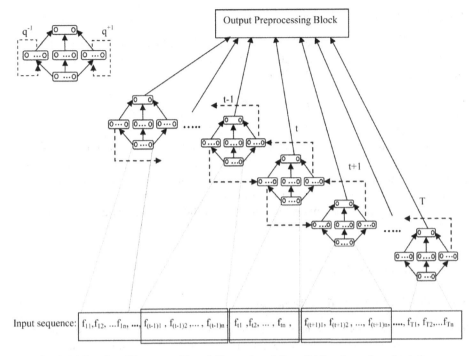

Fig. 1. Bidirectional Recurrent Neural Network and its unfolding in t, t-1 and t+1 times

Output Aggregation Functions

The outputs can be either labels or continuous values. Label outputs refer to the discrete value assigned to each class label. On the other hand, when continuous outputs are used, a c-dimensional vector $[d_1, d_2, ..., d_c]$ is provided, where d_j represents the support for the hypothesis that output vector comes from the jth class, and c is the total amount of classes.

The model can be compared with a multi-classifier, where each time is a classifier with its own output. Taking into account this idea, the model output can be represented as T vectors, one for each time.

In literature, several approaches for aggregating these values into a single output have been proposed and discussed. In this paper, we use the three following variants. Each function returns one vector of membership probabilities for each class, where the final result is the class associated to the index of value in the vector:

- Average function: Calculates the average of the probabilistic values associated with the class membership of the network outputs.
- Max Probability function: Calculates the highest value of class membership probability and returns the class with more probability.
- Mode function: Calculates the class with more probability for each network output and return the class that appears most often as result.

2.4   Performance Evaluation

As was mentioned before, the databases were built artificially with binary classes. The most commonly used parameter to assess the predictively of the classification models is the percent of well-classified cases (eq. 4).

$$Accuracy = \frac{TP + TN}{TP + FP + TN + FN} 100 \tag{4}$$

Where TP is the true positive rate (positives correctly classified/total positives), TN is the true negative rate (negatives correctly classified/total negatives), FP is the false positive rate (negatives incorrectly classified/total negatives) and FN is the false negative rate (positives incorrectly classified/total positives).

Here we used the accuracy and 10-fold cross-validation to show and compare the results.

3   Results and Discussion

3.1   Results from Artificial Databases

The training of the BRNN is based on the topology presented before. To simplify the experiment, three *times* and the same amounts of neurons for each hidden layer were selected: 4, 6, 8 and 10 neurons. Three output combination functions were tested: mode, max and average. Backpropagation Through Time algorithm was used with learning rate 0.01 and momentum 0.9.

We trained a J48, BayesNet, 10 SVMs with polynomial kernels (from 1 degree to 10 degrees), 10 MLPs with 2, 4, 6, 8, 10, 12, 14, 16, 18, and 20 neurons in the hidden layer. Then a 10-fold cross-validation was performed for each base, taking the accuracy as performance measures. Also statistical tests were applied.

The analysis of the results is focused on the three factors used to build the databases: feature relation, direction of this relation and the decision boundary, beginning with the last one.

When the class is obtained by a linear function the results of BRNN are not as good as the other methods. In this case, SVMs and MLPs provide better results than BRNNs. This could be due to their capability to find hyperplanes to separate the classes. They are also cheaper computationally speaking, so it is not advisable to use BRNNs in problems with linear separation.

On the other hand, when the class is obtained by polynomial or piecewise polynomial functions, BRNNs are superior to other classifiers depending on the output combination method used.

Figure 2 shows the results of accuracies in datasets with the features generated by a polynomial function. Vertical axes show results obtained by BRNNs with the proposed output combination functions (average, max and mode), and horizontal axes represent the highest accuracy values of the other classifiers: J48, BayesNet, SVM and MLP. The BRNN superiority can be seen, at first sight, in this unfair comparison.

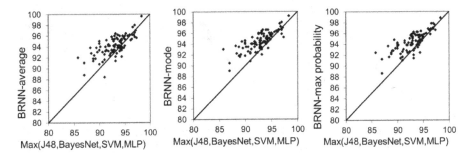

Fig. 2. BRNN accuracy using average, max and mode as combination functions against the J48, SVM, Bayes Net and MLP highest accuracy in datasets with class relation by polynomial function

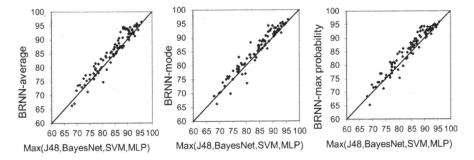

Fig. 3. BRNN accuracy using average, max and mode as combination functions against the J48, SVM, Bayes Net and MLP highest accuracy in datasets with class relation by piecewise polynomial function

The best results are obtained with the mode as output combination function.

Similar results are shown in figure 3, but in this case, the piecewise polynomial function to generate the features is being used. BRNNs are superior again. This suggests that when the decision boundary is complex the BRNN is an alternative method to solve the problem.

Taking into account the factor of feature relation, one could predict that, the results obtained by BRNN in datasets without relation between the features are not really better than others methods. BRNN is computationally expensive and complex. For this reason we suggest not using these networks when the problem has independent features. On the other hand, there are significant differences in datasets with feature relations, no matter the complexity of these relations. Fig 4 shows the comparison between the classical classification methods and the BRNN. Most of the time, BRNN achieve the higher result.

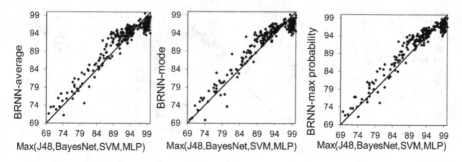

Fig. 4. BRNN accuracy using average, max and mode as combination functions against the J48, SVM, Bayes Net and MLP highest accuracy in datasets with feature relation by linear, polynomial and piecewise polynomial functions

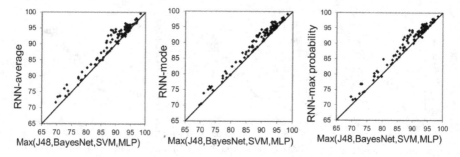

Fig. 5. BRNN accuracy using average, max and mode as combination functions against the J48, SVM, Bayes Net and MLP highest accuracy in datasets with feature and class relation by polynomial and piecewise polynomial function

In figure 5 only the database with relation between the features and a non-linear decision boundary is displayed. As can be seen, the results are now better for the BRNN, aiding towards a conclusion that the combination of a complex decision boundary and a dependency between features suggests that it is more suitable to use methods like BRNN for classification problems.

Additionally, the results obtained taking into account the directions of dependencies between features were analyzed. It is important to observe that BRNN achieves the best results again when the features have dependencies, in the three directions: forward, backward and in both directions. Although the BRNN achieves the best results for the three cases, the best are obtained when the data has dependence in both directions: forward and backward. The output combinations with best results are max probability and mode. As figure 6 illustrates, when features have both dependencies (forward + backward) and the output combinations are max probability or mode the BRNN is always superior or at least similar to the other methods.

To corroborate these conclusions statistic tests were used specifically nonparametric tests and more specifically the two-way Anova Friedman test. It was necessary to carry out a 2-related sample test to contrast the groups.

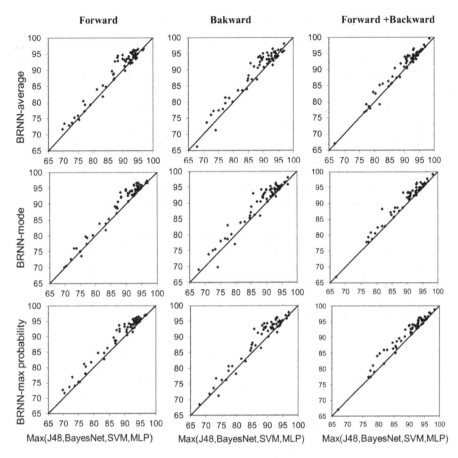

Fig. 6. BRNN accuracy using average, max and mode as combination functions against the J48, SVM, Bayes Net and MLP highest accuracy in datasets with different directions of dependencies between features

The Wilcoxon test shows highly significant differences between results obtained by BRNN and the other classifiers in those datasets where the class is obtained by polynomial and piecewise polynomial functions.

Furthermore, the comparison between the results related with features relation and with the dependencies between them reconfirms the superiority of the BRNN when the data has dependencies between the features in any direction.

Finally, output combinations were compared. Mode and max probability were best for accuracy, instead of the expected average function (the continuous central tendency measure).

3.2   Results Using the HIV Drug Resistance Database

The information to build the databases is from the "Stanford Database" [8]. There are 7 databases corresponding to drug resistance in the following protease inhibitors: Amprenavir (APV), Atazanavir (ATV), Indinavir (IDV), Lopinavir (LPV), Nelfinavir (NFV), Ritonavir (RTV) y Saquinavir (SQV).

In [6] the use of this BRNN topology is shown with mode as the output combination function, to solve this problem, but with another version of the database. Here more cases from the database were used. BRNN is compared with previous results with others methods. In [9] the results obtained by a lot of classification methods to predict the HIV drug resistance is shown.

Here the BRNN is trained with the three output combination functions used before. Also other classification models were trained: J48, SVM with different kernels: linear, polynomial and Gaussian; BayesNet, MLP.

In this work the amino acids are represented with their contact energies and the database is the last version of the Stanford Database. For these reason the obtained results are a slightly different to those obtained in [9] and [6].

Table 1 illustrates the results obtained by different models. BRNN achieves accurate similar or superior results in all cases. The best output combinations for this problem are mode and max probability.

Table 1. Results of accuracy for database of protease inhibitors

	J48	SVM linear	SVM Polynomial	SVM Gaussian	BayesNet	MLP	BRNN Average	BRNN Mode	BRNN Max Probability
APV	0.82	0.82	0.82	0.69	0.81	0.79	0.82	**0.83**	**0.83**
ATV	0.65	0.75	0.73	0.61	0.68	0.76	0.74	0.75	**0.77**
IDV	0.89	0.89	0.88	0.82	0.89	0.88	0.87	**0.90**	**0.90**
LPV	0.89	0.87	0.88	0.85	0.86	0.89	0.89	**0.91**	0.89
NFV	0.90	0.88	0.86	0.71	0.90	0.88	0.91	0.91	**0.92**
RTV	**0.93**	0.90	0.90	0.80	0.91	0.90	0.91	**0.93**	0.93
SQV	**0.76**	0.74	0.74	0.74	0.72	0.73	0.72	0.74	**0.76**
Average	0.83	0.84	0.83	0.74	0.83	0.83	0.84	**0.85**	**0.85**

In this biological sequence problem the BRNN also achieves the best or at least similar results in most of the databases, as is shown in table 1. Although the mode achieves better results with respect to the rest of methods, the max probability is now the aggregation function with best results.

4   Conclusions

BRNN is not the best classifier in linear decision boundary problems. In these problems, other simpler methods are in fact better, such as, SVM and MLP. However, in problems with complex decision boundaries, as soon as relations start emerging between features, BRNN becomes the best classifier. The best results of this model are when the features have dependencies in the sequences on both backward and forward. It is recommended to use the mode or the max probability as output combination.

In regards to the problem of HIV drug resistance the results of the topology of BRNN proposed has superior results or at least similar to the results obtained by the other techniques. These results and conclusions do not mean that the model described here is better than other methods for any type of biological problem, but it is a promising method to bear in mind.

Acknowledgements. The authors would like to thank Luke James for his help and proof reading.

References

1. Baldi, P., Brunak, S., Frasconi, P., Soda, G., Pollastri, G.: Exploiting the past and the future in protein secondary structure prediction. Bioinformatics 15, 937–946 (1999)
2. Agathocleous, M., Christodoulou, G., Promponas, V., Christodoulou, C., Vassiliades, V., Antoniou, A.: Protein Secondary Structure Prediction with Bidirectional Recurrent Neural Nets: Can Weight Updating for Each Residue Enhance Performance? In: Papadopoulos, H., Andreou, A.S., Bramer, M. (eds.) AIAI 2010. IFIP AICT, vol. 339, pp. 128–137. Springer, Heidelberg (2010)
3. Walsh, I., Martin, A.J.M., Di Domenico, T., Tosatto, S.C.E.: ESpritz: accurate and fast prediction of protein disorder. Bioinformatics 28, 503–509 (2012)
4. Ceroni, A., Frasconi, P., Passerini, A., Vullo, A.: A Combination of Support Vector Machines and Bidirectional Recurrent Neural Networks for Protein Secondary Structure Prediction. In: Cappelli, A., Turini, F. (eds.) AI*IA 2003. LNCS, vol. 2829, pp. 142–153. Springer, Heidelberg (2003)
5. Schuster, M., Paliwal, K.K.: Bidirectional recurrent neural networks. IEEE Transactions on Signal Processing 45, 2673–2681 (1997)
6. Bonet, I., García, M.M., Saeys, Y., Van de Peer, Y., Grau, R.: Predicting Human Immunodeficiency Virus (HIV) Drug Resistance Using Recurrent Neural Networks. In: Mira, J., Álvarez, J.R. (eds.) IWINAC 2007. LNCS, vol. 4527, pp. 234–243. Springer, Heidelberg (2007)
7. Werbos, P.J.: Backpropagation Through Time: What it does and How to do it, pp. 1550–1560 (1990)
8. HIV Drug Resistance Database, http://hivdb.stanford.edu//cgi-bin/GenoPhenoDS.cgi
9. Rhee, S.-Y., Taylor, J., Wadhera, G., Ben-Hur, A., Brutlag, D.L., Shafer, R.W.: Genotypic predictors of human immunodeficiency virus type 1 drug resistance. Proceedings of the National Academy of Sciences 103, 17355–17360 (2006)

Complete Diagnosis of Electrical Power Systems Using MDS and ANFIS

Juan Pablo Nieto González and Pedro Pérez Villanueva

Corporación Mexicana de Investigación en Materiales,
COMIMSA S.A. de C.V.
Ciencia y Tecnología No. 790, Fracc. Saltillo 400, C.P. 25290
Saltillo, Coahuila, México
juan.nieto@comimsa.com, pperez@comimsa.com

Abstract. The reasons because power systems monitoring is a challenging task are the complexity and high degree of interconnection present in electrical power networks, the presence of dynamic load changes in normal operation mode, the presence of both continuous and discrete variables, as well as noisy information and lack or excess of data. Therefore, in order to increase the efficiency of diagnosis, the need to develop more powerful approaches has been recognized, and hybrid techniques that combine several reasoning methods start to be used. This paper proposes a methodology based on the system's history data. It combines two techniques in order to give a complete diagnosis. The proposal is composed by two phases. The first phase is in charge of the fault detection by using Multidimensional Scaling (MDS). MDS acts like a first filter that gives the most probably state of each system's node. The second phase gives the final diagnosis using an Adaptive Neuro-Fuzzy Inference Systems (ANFIS) over the node(s) given by the first phase in order to look for the faulty line(s) and the time when the fault starts. This proposal can detect the presence of either symmetrical or asymmetrical faults. A set of simulations are carried out over an electrical power system proposed by the IEEE. To show the performance of the approach, a comparison is made against similar diagnostic systems.

Keywords: Fault Detection, Fault Diagnosis, Complex Systems, Electrical Power System, Dynamic Load Changes, Multidimensional Scaling, ANFIS.

1 Introduction

From the point of view of safety and reliability of electric power systems, it is necessary to have an early fault diagnosis scheme which can detect, isolate, diagnose the faults, and advise the system's operators to initiate corrective actions. During a disturbance, there is a great number of events related to the fault(s). Such events make the decision of the restoration actions to be carried out a difficult task to the power system's operator. Moreover, with advances in power system devices and communications, even more information will be presented to

F. Castro, A. Gelbukh, and M. González (Eds.): MICAI 2013, Part II, LNAI 8266, pp. 150–161, 2013.

operators, and alarm processing in large power systems calls for the treatment of a great bulk of information. The increase in information will enable a more complete view of the power systems state, but it will increase the need for fault diagnosis to effectively handle the system information. In this domain, the need to develop more powerful approaches has been recognized, and hybrid techniques that combine several reasoning methods start to be used.

An electrical power system fault detection and diagnosis methodology using a combination of the Multidimensional Scaling (MDS) and an Adaptive Neuro-Fuzzy Inference Systems (ANFIS) is proposed. The framework proposed is a process history based method. The organization of the paper is as follows. Section 2 reviews the state of the art. Section 3 gives the preliminaries and the background knowledge on MDS and ANFIS. Section 4 gives the approach general description. Section 5 shows how this framework works in a simulation example. Finally, conclusion ends this paper in section 6.

2   State of the Art

The reasons behind the increased interest in fault diagnosis in power networks are the complexity and high degree of interconnection present in electrical power networks, that can lead to an overwhelming array of alarms and status messages being generated as a result of a disturbance. This can have a negative impact on the speed with which operators can respond to a contingency. Therefore, in order to increase the efficiency of diagnosis, it is necessary to use automated tools, which could help the operator to speed up the process.

[8] presents a methodology that uses artificial neural networks integrated with other several statistical techniques. Among the numerical and statistical tools used in the approach is the Fourier parameters, the RMS values (RMS), the constant of false alarm rates (CFAR), the skewness values (SV), the Kurtosis measures (KM), the ratio of power (ROP), symmetrical components (SC), which seek to identify in a integrated way between a normal operation situation and a transient occurrence situation. When there is a fault, an artificial neural network of multilayer perceptron type classifies it. In [9] there are multiple ANFIS units which are Fault Detection, Fault Classification and Fault Location units to carry out the diagnosis of a long transamission line. They are instituted by training different data that are carried out at various situations of fault and no fault conditions. The input data ANFIS detection units are firstly derived from the fundamental values of the voltage and current measurements using digital signal processing via Fourier transform. [6] uses readings of the phase current only during the first one-forth of a cycle in an integrated method that combines symmetrical components technique with the principal component analysis (PCA) to declare, identify, and classify a fault. This approach also distinguishes a real fault from a transient one and can be used in either a transmission or a distribution system. [4] presents a framework that uses a probabilistic neural network to classify the most probably node's state based on the eigenvalues of the line's voltages correlation matrix. Then a comparison against a fault signature is made to diagnose the type of fault. [7] proposes an Augmented Naive

Bayesian power network fault diagnosis method based on data mining to diagnose faults in power network. The status information of protections and circuit breakers are taken as conditional attributes and faulty region as decision-making attribute. [2] can analyze faults occurring between two buses that are equipped with measurement units. The first step of the framework is to detect the presence of a fault in the power system in real time. Then, the method of symmetrical components is used to convert the three-phase power signals to three sets of independent components, which are positive, negative, and zero sequences. [5] proposes a two phase methodology. First phase uses a probabilistic neural network to obtain the most probably operation mode of the nodes, then a second phase performs an ANFIS to determine the real state of each node's lines. The present work proposes a variant of the approaches shown on [4] and [5].

The methodology presented in the present paper, carries out a complete diagnosis in two phases. The main difference is the way the detection process is done. A set of simulations are carried out over an electrical power system proposed by the IEEE. To show the performance of the approach, a comparison is made against similar diagnostic systems. The results have shown promising results for this new proposal.

3   Preliminars

3.1   Multidimensional Scaling

Multidimensional Scaling (MDS) techniques are applied when for a set of observed similarities (or distances) between every pair of N items, it is wanted to find a representation of the items in fewer dimensions such that the inter-item proximities nearly match the original similarities (or distances). It may not be possible to match exactly the ordering of the original similarities (distances). Consequently, scaling techniques attempt to find configurations in $q \leq N - 1$ dimensions such that the match is as close as possible. The numerical measure of closeness is called the *stress*. [3] summarizes the MDS algorithm as follows:

- For N items, obtain

$$M = \frac{N(N - 1)}{2} \tag{1}$$

  similarities (distances) between distinct pairs of items.
- Order the similarities as

$$s_{i_1 k_1} < s_{i_2 k_2} < ... < s_{i_M k_M} \tag{2}$$

  where $s_{i_1 k_1}$ is the smallest of the M similarities.
- Using a trial configuration in q dimensions, determine the inter-item distances

$$d_{i_1 k_1}^{(q)} > d_{i_2 k_2}^{(q)} > ... > d_{i_M k_M}^{(q)} \tag{3}$$

– Minimize the *stress*

$$Stress = \left[\frac{\sum_{i<k} \sum (d_{ik}^{(q)} - \hat{d}_{ik}^{(q)})^2}{\sum_{i<k} \sum (d_{ik}^{(q)})^2} \right]^{\frac{1}{2}} \tag{4}$$

– Using the $\hat{d}_{ik}^{(q)}$'s, move the points around to obtain an improved configuration. A new configuration will have new $d_{ik}^{(q)}$'s new $\hat{d}_{ik}^{(q)}$'s and smaller stress. The process is repeated until the best (minimum stress) representation is obtained.

Thus, MDS allows to visualize how near points are to each other for many kinds of distance or dissimilarity measures and can produce a representation of data in a small number of dimensions. MDS does not require raw data, but only a matrix of pairwise distances or dissimilarities. A matrix is a similarity matrix if larger numbers indicate more similarity between items, rather than fewer. A matrix is a dissimilarity matrix if larger numbers indicate less similarity.

3.2 Adaptive Neuro-Fuzzy Inference Systems

Adaptive Neuro-Fuzzy Inference Systems (ANFIS) are a class of adaptive networks that are functionally equivalent to fuzzy inference systems. For simplicity, assume that the fuzzy inference system under consideration has two inputs x and y and one output z. For a first order Sugeno fuzzy model (shown in Fig. 1) a common rule set with two fuzzy if-then rules is of the form

– Rule 1: If x is A_1 and y is B_1, then $f_1 = p_1x + q_1y + r_1$
– Rule 2: If x is A_2 and y is B_2, then $f_2 = p_2x + q_2y + r_2$

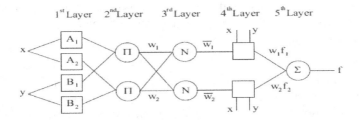

Fig. 1. ANFIS architecture

Every node i in layer 1 has a node function

$$O_{1,i} = \mu_{A_i}(x) \quad for \ i = 1, 2, \tag{5}$$

where $O_{1,i}$ is the membership grade of a fuzzy set A ($A = A_1, A_2, B_1$ or B_2) and it specifies the degree in which the given input x satisfies the quantifier A.

These are the premise parameters. In layer 2 every node is a fixed node labeled Π, whose output is the product of all the incoming signals

$$O_{2,i} = w_i = \mu A_i(x)\mu B_i(y) \quad i = 1, 2 \tag{6}$$

each node output represents the firing strength of a rule. Every node in layer 3 is a fixed node labeled N. The ith node calculates the ratio of the ith rule's firing strength to the sum of all rules' firing strengths

$$O_{3,i} = \bar{w}_i = \frac{w_i}{w_1 + w_2} \quad i = 1, 2 \tag{7}$$

In layer 4 every node i is an adaptive node with a node function

$$O_{4,i} = \bar{w}_i f_i = \bar{w}_i(p_i x + q_i y + r_i) \tag{8}$$

these are the consequent parameters. The single node in layer 5 is a fixed node labeled $\sum$, which computes the overall output as the summation of all incoming signals

$$overall \;\; output = O_{5,i} = \sum_i \bar{w}_i f_i = \frac{\sum_i w_i f_i}{\sum_i w_i} \tag{9}$$

4   Framework Description

This is a variant of the proposals shown in [4] and [5]. The general fault detection and diagnosis framework proposed in the present work is shown in Fig. 2. According to [10] this proposal is a process history-based method because of the need of a data set when the system runs under normal operating conditions. The framework only requires a big quantity of historical data, containing normal operation data in the system. The approach is composed by two phases. First phase is the detection process and the second phase gives the final diagnosis.

The two phases of the complete fault detection and diagnosis system performs their functions as follows:

1. As depicted in figure 2, the very first step is to take data sets of normal operation and split them in windows of n samples. Then a multidimensional scaling (MDS) procedure is carried out. The output of this MDS will be a set of vectors in p dimensional space such that the matrix of Euclidean distances among them corresponds as closely as possible to some function of the input matrix according to a criterion function called *stress*. These distances could be plotted and will give an idea of how the samples group in a two dimensional space. MDS is used as a feature extraction step to learn the normal operation dynamics of the system. Feature extraction could include several different methods to extract relevant aspects that will serve as a-priori knowledge of the normal behavior of the system. In this paper the feature extraction is carried out only by the MDS. MDS gives the distances between the lines of each system's nodes. Then from these distances, the

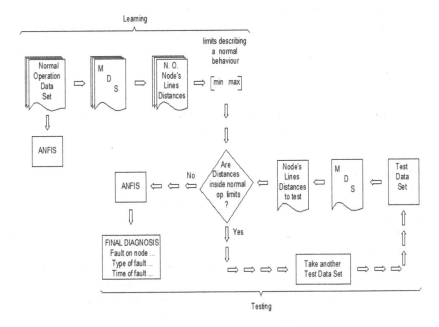

Fig. 2. General fault detection and diagnosis framework

minimum and maximum limits are obtained describing in this way the normal operation mode. When monitoring the system, MDS is performed over the test data set to extract the distances between the lines of each system's node and then they are compared against the minimum and maximum limits that describe the normal operation. When faulty data is present the output of this phase will give which node is on a faulty condition based on the fact that at least one of the distances between its lines must be out of their normal operation limits. The use of MDS is to quickly locate the suspicious nodes instead of performing the second phase of the methodology over the entire original system. Thus the search space for a fault presence is reduced to only for those nodes whose distances between their lines lay outside the normal operation limits providing the advantage of speeding up the fault detection process. If the features extracted are inside the normal operation limits then the monitoring system continues its process by taking another data set to test.

2. If the features extracted lay outside the normal operation limits the second phase of the methodology starts. Here an ANFIS is used to look for the type of fault present and to give the final diagnosis. In this second phase an ANFIS is built as shown in section 3.2 using for this task according with the most probably state of the system the corresponding variables (electrical node's lines) that are found in normal operation as the predictor variables for each one of the rest of variables. Thus, the ANFIS for a specific variable will predict the value of the variable monitored being this output, its normal

operation value. With this value it is obtained a normal operation interval with respect to the normal operation predicted value. Finally a comparison against the normal operation limits is carried out in order to detect which of the variables has a fault present. This comparison serves as a classifier that gives the real variables' state and can be used to locate the period of time or sample number where the fault occurs.

The algorithm for this approach could be summarized as follows:

Learning steps of the monitoring system

1. *Take a normal operation data set*
2. *Carry out the feature extraction for learning. In this work this is as follows:*
   (a) *Split the original data set in smaller windows*
   (b) *Apply MDS*
   (c) *Obtain the minimum and maximum distances between the electrical lines of each node*
   (d) *Stablish the normal operation distances limits for the electrical lines*
3. *Form and train an ANFIS using the corresponding variables (electrical node's lines) that are found in normal operation as the predictor variables for each one of the rest of variables.*

When monitoring a data set the system performs as follows:

4. *Take a test data set. This is a window of n samples as depicted in step 2(a).*
5. *Carry out the feature extraction for testing. Do the same as in step 2 (b) and 2 (c).*
6. *Compare the distances between the electrical lines of a suspicious faulty node against the limits of normal operation data distances. Verify if these distances are inside the limits obtained in step 2 (d).*
7. *If all of the distances are between the normal operation limits return to step 4 else go to step 8*
8. *Perform an ANFIS for the suspicious node*
9. *Look for the variables that have actual different values from those predicted by the ANFIS*
10. *Look for the position of the samples that differ from the right predicted value given by the ANFIS obtained in step 3*
11. *Give the final diagnosis. Show the variable that is in faulty mode as well as its location*

5 Case Study

The present section shows the performance of the framework proposed for multiple-fault diagnosis over the IEEE network shown in Fig. 3. This figure depicts an electrical power system having dynamic load changes. The performance of the methodology proposed for multiple-fault diagnosis was observed within

50 simulation databases of the IEEE network. In order to make the comparison, it has been used those 50 databases containing symmetrical and asymmetrical faults at random nodes, taking into account multiple simultaneous faults scenarios with up to five different faults at a time, and combining faults such as: one line to ground, two lines to ground, three lines to ground, fault between two lines and the no fault mode.

The diagnosis system proposed was tailored according to the steps described on section 4 as follows:

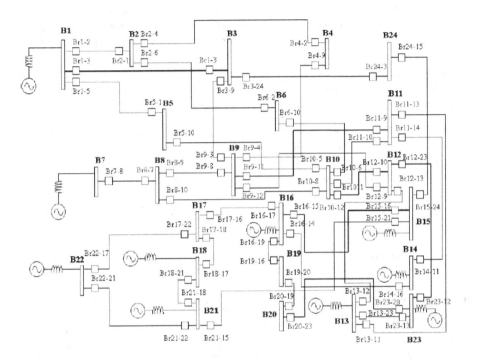

Fig. 3. IEEE reliability test system single line diagram

1. *Obtain windows of 100 samples from normal operation history data process (electrical voltage in each node's lines).*
2. *Obtain MDS minimum and maximum distances between the electrical lines of each of the 24 nodes of the system.*
3. *Stablish the normal operation distances limits for each of the 24 nodes.*
4. *Train an ANFIS with voltage's amplitude of normal operation mode.*
5. *Take a test data set of 100 samples from the electrical power system being monitored.*
6. *First Phase: Use MDS to obtain the distances between the electrical lines of each of the 24 nodes of the system.*
7. *Identify which nodes have their distances out of the normal operation limits.*

8. *Second Phase: Carry out and ANFIS for each of the lines involved on the most probably faulty node given by the first phase output (see step 7). Then compare the suspicious samples with the output of the ANFIS in order to determine the real state of the system and if there is a fault present, classify and locate it.*
9. *Give the final diagnosis of each node being monitored. If a fault is present in a specific node give the node's number, the type of fault present and the time when it appears, else print NO FAULT.*

We have considered on the simulations that voltages from the three lines of each of the 24 nodes from the electrical network are measured and registered on a database. The methodology has been applied under the consideration that voltage's information is known, nevertheless on electrical power systems the only available information could be the electrical network's breakers state instead of voltages or electrical current's values. The proposal takes sample windows of 100 data and takes into account three possible cases.

– **Case 1:** System is working properly during the first 25 samples from a total of 100, that means 25 samples are ok and 75 samples correspond to fault present on system.
– **Case 2:** Takes 50 samples of normal operation data and 50 samples with fault present.
– **Case 3:** Takes 75 samples of normal operation and 25 with fault present.

Table 1. Comparison of the diagnosis systems general performance's percentages of detection by fault type for each proposal after 50 simulations

Component State	Probabilistic Logic [1]	PNN + EIG [4]	MDS + ANFIS
A-B-C GND	100	100	100
A-B GND	100	100	100
A GND	86	93	100
A-B	83	78	88
B-C	100	79	88
NO FAULT	71	64	88

Table 2. Comparison of the diagnosis systems general performances percentages for each of the proposals for case 1 after 50 simulations of different fault scenarios

Proposal [Reference]	Detection	Identification	Location
Probabilistic Logic [1]	88	88	70
PNN + EIG [4]	85	85	60
MDS + ANFIS	85	90	90

Table 3. Comparison of the diagnosis systems general performances percentages for each of the proposals for case 2 after 50 simulations of different fault scenarios

Proposal [Reference]	Detection	Identification	Location
Probabilistic Logic [1]	85	83	65
PNN + EIG [4]	79	79	50
MDS + ANFIS	80	85	85

Table 4. Comparison of the diagnosis systems general performances percentages for each of the proposals for case 3 after 50 simulations of different fault scenarios

Proposal [Reference]	Detection	Identification	Location
Probabilistic Logic [1]	80	79	50
PNN + EIG [4]	75	75	45
MDS + ANFIS	75	80	80

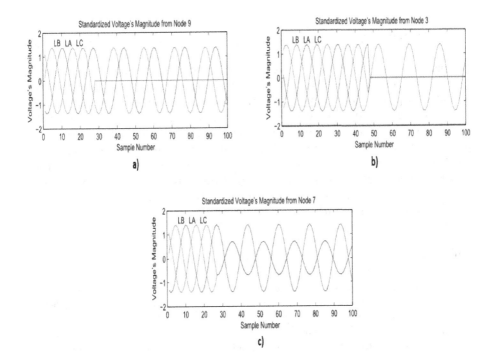

Fig. 4. Different fault scenarios. a)Case 1 for node 9, one line to ground. b)Case 2 for node 3, two lines to ground, c)Case 1 for node 7, fault between two lines.

Fig. 4 shows the voltages' magnitud for different scenarios. Those scenarios are the following: Fig.4a) represents a fault present on node 9 for case 1 and the type of fault is one line to ground. Fig.4b) shows a two lines to ground fault on node 3 for case two and Fig.4c) depicts case 1 fault between two lines for node 7.

To observe the performance of the new proposal, a comparison against a diagnostic system based on probabilistic logic taken from [1] and the framework proposed on [4] has been carried out. Table 1 shows the comparison of the performance's percentages of detection by fault type for each proposal. It clearly shows that the new approach has the best performance of the three diagnostic systems being compared.

Tables 2, 3 and 4 show the comparison of the present fault diagnosis system against those used in [4] and in [1]. The comparison was made for Case 1, Case 2 and Case 3 respectively. The percentages were obtained after carry out 50 simulations for each case and combining different fault scenarios. First column shows the methods used on each proposal. Second column gives the general percentage of fault detection, that is the percentage of correct detection of a fault present for the 50 simulations. Third column is the general percentage of the correct identification of type of fault present on the system. Fourth column shows the general percentage of the correct sample location when the fault occurs.

6   Conclusion

This paper has presented a new proposal to carry out a complete fault detection and diagnosis of electrical power systems with dynamic load changes. The methodology proposed is composed by two phases. First phase is the fault detection process. This is done by using MDS technique in order to obtain the limits of the distances between the voltage samples of each node that define the normal operation of the system. The output of the second phase is the final diagnosis. This is carried out by a comparison between the observed variables and those predicted by an ANFIS. This allows to give which line(s) are in faulty mode. The simulations carried out has shown the promising results obtained with this approach in comparison with similar frameworks.

References

1. Garza, L.: Hybrid Systems Fault Diagnosis with a Probabilistic Logic Reasoning Framework. PhD thesis, Instituto Tecnológico y de Estudios Superiores de Monterrey, Campus Monterrey (2001)
2. Wang, Y.C., Hung, C.H., Wang, J.Y., Lee, C.H., Jiang, J.A., Chuang, C.L., Hsiao, Y.T.: A hybrid framework for fault detection, classification, and locationpart i: Concept, structure, and methodology. IEEE Transactions on Power Delivery 26(3), 1988–1998 (2011)
3. Johnson, R., Wichern, D.: Applied Multivariate Statistical Analysis. Prentice Hall (2004)

4. Garza, L.E., Nieto, J.P., Morales, R.: Multiple fault diagnosis in electrical power systems with dynamic load changes using probabilistic neural networks. Computación y Sistemas Magazine 14(1), 17–30 (2010)
5. González, J.P.N.: Multiple fault diagnosis in electrical power systems with dynamic load changes using soft computing. In: Batyrshin, I., Mendoza, M.G. (eds.) MICAI 2012, Part II. LNCS, vol. 7630, pp. 317–328. Springer, Heidelberg (2013)
6. Abdel-Qader, I., Alsafasfeh, Q., Harb, A.: Symmetrical pattern and pca based framework for fault detection and classification in power systems. In: IEEE International Conference on Electro Information Technology, pp. 1–5 (2010)
7. Qianwen, N., Youyuan, W.: An augmented naive bayesian power network fault diagnosis method based on data mining. In: Asia-Pacific Power and Energy Engineering Conference (APEEC), pp. 1–4 (2011)
8. da Silva, I.N., Flauzino, R.A., Ziolkowski, V., de Souza, D.M.B.S.: Hybrid intelligent architecture for fault identification in power distribution systems. In: IEEE Power & Energy Society General Meeting, PES 2009, pp. 1–6 (2009)
9. Moustafa Hassan, M.A., Kamel, T.S., El-Morshedy, A.: Advanced distance protection scheme for long transmission lines in electric power systems using multiple classified anfis networks. In: Fifth International Conference on Soft Computing with Words and Perceptions in System Analysis, Decision and Control, pp. 1–5 (2009)
10. Yin, K., Venkatasubramanian, V., Rengaswamy, R., Kavuri, S.N.: A review of process fault detection and diagnosis part i: Quantitative model-based methods. Computers and Chemical Engineering 27(3), 293–311 (2003)

Intelligent Rotor Time Constant Identification Approach in Indirect Field Oriented Induction Motor Drive

Moulay Rachid Douiri and Mohamed Cherkaoui

Mohammadia Engineering School, Department of Electrical Engineering,
Ibn Sina Avenue, 765, Agdal-Rabat, Morocco
douirirachid@hotmail.com

Abstract. This paper proposes a novel control scheme for rotor time constant identification using artificial neural networks. This approach, based on estimation of the rotor time constant from motor terminal variables (stator voltage, stator current and rotor speed), can be applied to indirect field oriented control and used to tune the actual rotor time constant of the induction motor to its set value programmed in the decoupling controller. The neural estimators use the backpropagation learning process to update their weights. The performance of the proposed scheme is carried out by extensive simulations confirming the feasibility of the proposed control strategy.

Keywords: artificial neural networks, indirect field oriented control, induction motor drives, rotor time constant.

Nomenclature

ANNs	Artificial Neural Networks
d, q	direct and quadrature components
R_s, R_r	stator and rotor resistance [Ω]
i_{ds}, i_{qs}	stator current dq –axis [A]
i_{dr}, i_{qr}	rotor current dq –axis [A]
v_{ds}, v_{qs}	stator voltage dq-axis [V]
v_{dr}, v_{qr}	rotor voltage dq-axis [V]
L_s, L_r, L_m	stator, rotor and mutual inductance [H]
λ_{ds}, λ_{qs}	dq stator fluxes [Wb]
λ_{dr}, λ_{qr}	dq rotor fluxes [Wb]
T_{em}	electromagnetic torque [N.m]
ω_r, ω_e, ω_{sl}	rotor, synchronous and slip frequency [rad/s]
τ_r	rotor time constant
J	inertia moment [Kg.m^2]
n_p	motor pole number
σ	leakage coefficient

F. Castro, A. Gelbukh, and M. González (Eds.): MICAI 2013, Part II, LNAI 8266, pp. 162–171, 2013.

1   Introduction

Development of vector control techniques applied to induction motors, power converters and digital controllers has initiated the decline of the supremacy of DC machines in high performance adjustable speed drives. The vector control can be realized in a direct or indirect fashion [1]. The latter arouses more interest since it does not imply any modification to the structure of the machine. The method of indirect orientation of the rotor flux is widely used due to its simplicity and because it lends itself well to a generalized implementation for general-purpose induction motors. The principal drawback of the indirect method is its sensitivity to parameters variation [2]. The differences between the parameter programmed in the regulators and the real parameters of the machine deteriorate the performances of the drive not only in transients, but also in steady state [3]. The estimation of the rotor time constant is thus necessary for the implementation of high performance vector control schemes based on indirect method of rotor flux orientation. Various techniques are explored nowadays by research team's all around the world. All have the aim of obtaining correct values of the motor parameters, required in the implementation of indirect vector controls insensitive to parameters variation [4]-[5]-[6]-[7]-[8]-[9]-[10]-[11].

The contribution of this paper lies in the use of artificial neural networks (ANNs) for the implementation of vector controlled induction motor. The advantages of ANNs have been highlighted in several fields of application and they arouse, currently, much interest in the fields of power electronics and electrical machines control [12]. The main objective of this research is to estimate the rotor time constant of an induction motor drive, in order to realize an indirect field oriented control insensitive to the variation of this parameter. The originality of this work lies in the approaches used. Indeed, three new estimation strategies have been developed. These techniques use either ANNs or the motor model equations under dynamic conditions in the stationary reference frame. To achieve this goal, several sub-objectives are to consider in particular, the development of a simulation library of induction motor, the development of learning methods ANNs, and finding appropriate architectures.

2   Indirect Field Orientated Control

The indirect field orientation uses the slip relation to estimate the flux position to the rotor. There are no sensing devices placed inside the motor, meaning there is no direct measurement of the magnetic field. Instead, the rotor speed (i.e. rotor frequency) is measured and slip frequency is calculated. Addition of these frequencies yields an optimal stator frequency for motor control. A sensor on the motor shaft measures the rotor angle θ_r (or measures the rotor speed ω_r, followed by an integrator for calculation of the angle). The input signals for current control are used for calculation of the desired slip frequency, ω_{sl}, which is integrated, giving a slip angle, θ_{sl}, which is added to the rotor angle. (The slip angle is required to adjust the inclination of the d-axis so that the magnetization of the motor is along this axis). The sum of the two angles gives the instantaneous rotor flux position angle.

The decoupling conditions may be written:

$$\lambda_r = \lambda_{dr} + j\lambda_{qr} = \lambda_{dr}, \quad \lambda_{qr} = 0, \quad \text{and} \quad i_{qs} = \left(-\frac{L_r}{L_m}\right)i_{qr} \tag{1}$$

Then, the torque equation becomes:

$$T_{em} = \frac{3n_p L_m}{2L_r}\lambda_r i_{qs} \tag{2}$$

And the rotor flux equation becomes:

$$\lambda_r = \left(\frac{L_m}{1+s\tau_r}\right)i_{ds} \tag{3}$$

The slip equations for an induction motor in an arbitrary synchronously rotating reference frame are given by:

$$\omega_e - \omega_r = \omega_{sl} = -\frac{R_r i_{qr}}{\lambda_{dr}} = \frac{R_r L_m}{\lambda_{dr} L_r}i_{qs} = \left[\left(1+s\frac{L_r}{R_r}\right)\frac{1}{i_{ds}}\right]\frac{R_r}{L_r}i_{qs} \tag{4}$$

when i_{ds} and i_{qs} are decided by ω_{sl}, rotor flux position θ_e is given by:

$$\theta_e = \int_0^t \omega_e dt = \int_0^t (\omega_r + \omega_{sl})dt \tag{5}$$

Indirect field orientation does not have inherent low speed problems (unlike direct field oriented control), and is thus preferred in most systems that must operate near zero speed. As well, flux can be obtained even down to zero frequency, making it suitable for position control. A major drawback, however, is that calculation of the rotor flux depends on the rotor the constant τ_r, where $\tau_r = L_r/R_r$. This time constant is dependent on rotor resistance, which is a function of rotor temperature and therefore tends to vary significantly due to temperature variations and the skin effect. This affects the accuracy of the flux magnitude and angle estimation, leading to degradation in system performance and quality of control.

3   Mathematical Development of Rotor Time Constant Estimator and Rotor Flux

Consider the stator voltages equations and calculate the term: $(v_{ds}i_{qs} - v_{qs}i_{ds})$,

$$v_{ds}i_{qs} - v_{qs}i_{ds} = \frac{d\lambda_{ds}}{dt}i_{qs} - \frac{d\lambda_{qs}}{dt}i_{ds} \tag{6}$$

Let us know that:

$$\lambda_{ds} = \frac{L_m}{L_r}\lambda_{dr} + \sigma L_s i_{ds} \tag{7}$$

$$\lambda_{qs} = \frac{L_m}{L_r}\lambda_{qr} + \sigma L_s i_{qs} \tag{8}$$

$$\frac{d\lambda_{dr}}{dt} = \frac{R_r}{L_r}\left(L_m i_{ds} - \lambda_{dr}\right) - \omega_r \lambda_{qr} \tag{9}$$

$$\frac{d\lambda_{qr}}{dt} = \frac{R_r}{L_r}\left(L_m i_{qs} - \lambda_{qr}\right) - \omega_r \lambda_{dr} \tag{10}$$

We replace (λ_{ds} and λ_{qs}) by their values given by (7) and (8), we find:

$$v_{ds}i_{qs} - v_{qs}i_{ds} = \left(\frac{L_m}{L_r}\frac{d\lambda_{dr}}{dt} + \sigma L_s \frac{di_{ds}}{dt}\right)i_{qs} - \left(\frac{L_m}{L_r}\frac{d\lambda_{qr}}{dt} + \sigma L_s \frac{di_{qs}}{dt}\right)i_{ds} \tag{11}$$

We replace ($d\lambda_{ds}/dt$ and $d\lambda_{qs}/dt$) by their values given by (9) and (10), we find:

$$v_{ds}i_{qs} - v_{qs}i_{ds} = \frac{L_m}{L_r}\left(-\frac{R_r}{L_r}\left(\lambda_{dr}i_{qs} - \lambda_{qr}i_{ds}\right) - \omega_r\left(\lambda_{qr}i_{qs} - \lambda_{dr}i_{ds}\right)\right)$$
$$+\sigma L_s\left(\frac{di_{ds}}{dt}i_{qs} - \frac{di_{qs}}{dt}i_{ds}\right) \tag{12}$$

Hence, we can derive the expression of the rotor time-constant ($\tau_r = L_r/R_r$):

$$\tau_r = \frac{\left(\lambda_{qr}i_{ds} - \lambda_{dr}i_{qs}\right)}{\frac{L_r}{L_m}\left(\left(\lambda_{ds}i_{qs} - \lambda_{qr}i_{ds}\right) - \sigma L_s\left(\frac{di_{ds}}{dt}i_{qs} - \frac{di_{qs}}{dt}i_{ds}\right)\right) + \omega_r\left(\lambda_{qr}i_{qs} + \lambda_{dr}i_{ds}\right)} \tag{13}$$

Due to the mathematical complexity and quantity calculations of rotor time constant estimators, an implantation using ANNs seems interesting.

4   Neural Rotor Time Constant Estimator

Among the various neural networks and their associated algorithms, our choice fell on the study of continuous multilayer neural networks. This type of network has excellent characteristics in the estimation and signal processing. In our application, we developed three ANNs that can be used in achieving a high performance control of induction motors controlled by indirect method of rotor flux orientation. ANNs we used are multi-layer networks, simple (the neurons of a layer are connected only to neurons of the next layer) and each neuron is connected to all neurons of the next layer. The network consists of an input layer, a hidden layer and an output layer. We also tried two hidden layers networks, but the results and the learning curve is very comparable, for the same number of neurons, to those obtained from a hidden layer. Neurons used in ANNs developed are continuous neurons (sigmoid and linear). The methodology used consisted in preparing a databank fairly representative. This bank should take into account the maximum information on the different modes of training, enrolling in range where it is required to operate. Once this databank prepared and normalized, a part representing 20% is chosen to test the network generalization for data never learned. The remaining 80% is used as databank learning will be used to adapt the weights and biases of the ANN. As we mentioned goal is to realize ANNs capable of well generalize, the structure of ANNs has been developed following the cross-validation procedure proposed by [13]. Once the databank learning and the structure of ANNs determined, the learning phase is started using the toolbox neural network MATLAB. During this learning phase, we proceed regularly to verify the network generalization. At the beginning of this phase, the training error and those generalization decrease progressively as the number of iterations increases. However, from a number of iterations, the generalization error starts to grow while the learning continues to decline. This is due to the fact that ANNs begins to learn by heart the training data (memorization).

As the goal is to develop ANNs that generalize, it is necessary that the learning phase to be stopped as soon as the generalization error starts to grow. If both errors are far from the desired error, we add some neurons and restart the learning phase until obtaining a good compromise between the desired errors, learning and generalization.

Once the ANN has converged to an acceptable error, the optimal weights and biases are saved.

Development of the Neural Network

A neural network has been trained for estimating the rotor time constant variation in line using speed measurements, voltage and stator current (v_{ds}, v_{qs}, i_{ds}, i_{qs}, ω_r).

Signals networks learning were prepared from the machine phase model in which we programmed the rotor resistance variations. In addition, survey data from the machine experimental magnetization characteristic were used to develop a model that takes into account the saturation. For each rotor resistance variation, the rotor time constant is calculated and stored. A databank has been constructed from the input signals (v_{ds}, v_{qs}, i_{ds}, i_{qs}, ω_r), and network output τ_r. In preparing this databank, different operating conditions (torque and flux variables) were simulated. For the couple, the operations in the two rotation directions and even stoppage were simulated. It should be noted that learning could also be done with real signals captured in the laboratory, if we can by one means or another to vary the rotor time constant value. This is simpler in the case of a wound rotor machine, which can easily apply variations in rotor resistance. Each time constant value corresponds to a very precise combination of input signals. The artificial neural network role is therefore able to detect in the modifications imposed on the input signals, due to the rotor resistance variation, the time constant value at machine level. Once this databank prepared, it was subdivided at random into two subsets, one for training whose size represents 80% of this databank and another representing approximately 20% was reserved for testing the network generalization for data never learned. The databank contains prepared 5000 combinations of input signals - rotor time constant, which represents a reasonable size for bank learning ANNs.

$$I_s^2 = i_{ds}^2 + i_{qs}^2 \tag{14}$$

$$i_{qs} = \sqrt{I_s^2 - \left(\frac{\lambda_r}{L_m}\right)} \tag{15}$$

$$\lambda_r = \frac{L_m I_s}{\left(1 + s\tau_r^*\right)\sqrt{\left(\frac{1}{1 + s\tau_r^*}\right)^2 + \tau_r^2 \left(\frac{L_m i_{qs}^*}{\tau_r^* \lambda_r^*}\right)^2}} \tag{16}$$

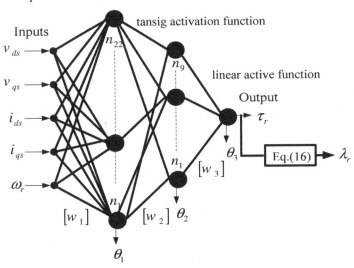

Fig. 1. Neural network for rotor time constant calculation

A three-layer network with a total of 37 hard limit neurons is employed to implement the rotor time constant estimator as shown in Fig.1. The first hidden layer has 22 neurons (square activation function neuron with the w_1 and bias θ_1), 8 neurons in the second hidden layer (tansig activation function neuron with the weight w_2 and bias θ_2), and the output layer has one neuron (linear active function neuron with the weight w_3 and bias θ_3). The network is trained by a supervised method. After 435 training epochs, the sum squared error arrives at zero.

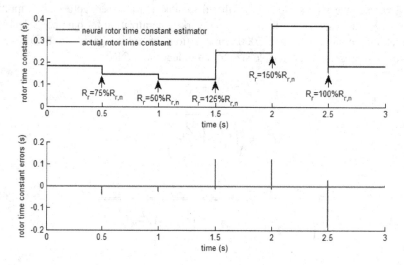

Fig. 2. Estimation results of the neural rotor time constant and estimation errors

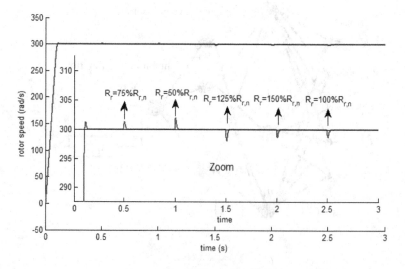

Fig. 3. Rotor speed

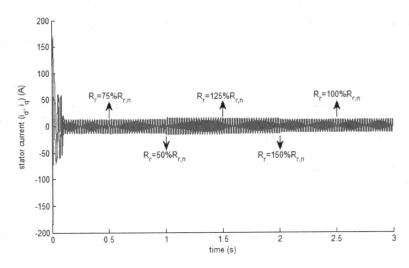

Fig. 4. Stator current (i_d, i_q)

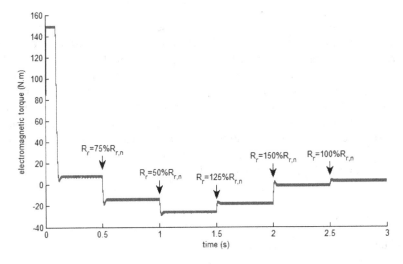

Fig. 5. Electromagnetic torque

Fig.2 shows the results of neural rotor time constant estimating. This result is presented for rotor flux oriented drive operating at nominal set-points flux and torque, in which we have programmed a rotor resistance which varies between 100%, 75%, 50%, 125%, 150% and 100% at $t = 0.5s$, $t = 1s$, $t = 1.5s$, $t = 2s$ and $t = 2.5s$ respectively. The neural network was also used to adjust a rotor flux oriented drive with respect to the rotor resistance variation. The rotor time constant estimated by this ANNs is used to correct the set-point slip at vector controller level.

You can see in this figure the transient behavior of rotor time constant estimator based ANNs. We can also see that it responds precisely and variation index instantly applied to the rotor time constant. Indexical variations were used here in order to verify the dynamic performance estimation scheme. However, in practice the rotor time constant varies exponentially with the heating of the machine.

The rotor speed response shows that the drive can follow the low command speed very quickly and rapid rejection of disturbances, with a low dropout speed (Fig. 3).

The current responses are sinusoidal and balanced, and its distortion is small (Fig. 4).

The current and electromagnetic torque (Figs. 4 and 5) curves remain at their respective set-points despite the variation applied to the rotor resistance. This proves that the adaptation process of this parameter is actually performed and that decoupling is maintained, seen that electromagnetic torque and current in the machine remain at their respective set-points.

Induction motor parameters:

P_n = 2.2kW, V_n = 220/380V, f = 60Hz, R_s = 0.84Ω, R_r = 0.3858Ω, L_s = 0.0706H, L_r = 0.0706H, L_m = 0.0672H, J = 0.008kg·m², n_p = 2.

5   Conclusions

In this paper we presented the analysis and the discussion of the effect of the rotor time constant variations on the dynamic performance of rotor flux indirect field orientation drives. We proposed a novel method for the adaptation of this quantity based on artificial neural networks. The computer simulations have shown the validity and the feasibility of the proposed method that possesses the advantages of neural network implementation: the high speed of processing. In addition this method is more adapted for practical implementation because it uses only stator terminal quantities (voltage, current and frequency) in the estimation of the rotor time constant. This approach should be useful in various applications where rotor time constant changes can seriously deteriorate the performance of the drive.

References

1. Novotny, D.W., Lipo, T.A.: Vector Control and Dynamics of AC Drives. Oxford University Press (1996)
2. De Wit, P.A.S., Ortega, R., Mareels, I.: Indirect field-oriented control of induction motors is robustly globally stable. Automatica 32(10), 1393–1402 (1996)
3. Krishnan, R., Bharadwaj, A.S.: A review of parameter sensitivity and adaptation in indirect vector controlled induction motor drive systems. IEEE Transactions on Power Electronics 6(4), 695–703
4. Wang, G., Yang, R., Zhang, J., Yu, Y., Ma, J., Cai, L., Xu, D.: Rotor time constant on-line estimation of induction motors based on MRAS. Diangong Jishu Xuebao/Transactions of China Electrotechnical Society 27(4), 48–53 (2012)

5. Dong, K., Diao, L., Sun, D., Ruan, B., Liu, Z.: MRAS-based rotor time constant estimation for indirect vector controlled induction motor drive. Advanced Materials Research 433-440, 6812–6818 (2012)
6. Bianchunyuan, Caoruixia, Manyongkui, Songchonghui: A rotor time constant identification method with compensation algorithm. Applied Mechanics and Materials 127, 12–18 (2012)
7. Li, Q., Yang, T.: A novel identification method of rotor time constant of induction motor. Applied Mechanics and Materials 87, 249–254 (2011)
8. Aydeniz, M.G., Şenol, I.: A Luenberger-sliding mode observer with rotor time constant parameter estimation in induction motor drives. Turkish Journal of Electrical Engineering and Computer Sciences 19(6), 901–912 (2011)
9. Yu, S.-Y., Zhang, Y.-C., Gao, J.-S., Gui, W.-H.: Identification of rotor time constant based on reactive power model in vector control system of induction motor. Zhongnan Daxue Xuebao (Ziran Kexue Ban)/Journal of Central South University (Science and Technology) 40(5), 1318–1322 (2009)
10. Zidani, F., Naït Saïd, M.S., Abdessemed, R., Benbouzid, M.E.H.: A fuzzy method for rotor time constant estimation for high-performance induction motor vector control. Electric Power Components and Systems 31(10), 1007–1019 (2003)
11. Zai, L.-C., DeMarco, C.L., Lipo, T.A.: An extended Kalman filter approach to rotor time constant measurement in PWM induction motor drives. IEEE Transactions on Industry Applications 28(1), 96–104 (1992)
12. Soulié, F.F., Gallinari, P.: Industrial Applications of Neural Networks. World Scientific Publishing Co. Pte. Ltd. (1998)
13. Haykin, S.: Neural Networks and Learning Machines, 3rd edn. Prentice Hall (2009)

Flame Classification
through the Use of an Artificial Neural Network
Trained with a Genetic Algorithm

Juan Carlos Gómez[1], Fernando Hernández[1], Carlos A. Coello Coello[2],
Guillermo Ronquillo[1], and Antonio Trejo[1]

[1] Applied Research Management, CIDESI, Queretaro, Mexico
[2] Computer Science Department, CINVESTAV-IPN, Mexico

Abstract. This paper introduces a Genetic Algorithm (GA) for training
Artificial Neural Networks (ANNs) using the electromagnetic spectrum
signal of a combustion process for flame pattern classification. Combustion requires identification systems that provide information about the
state of the process in order to make combustion more efficient and clean.
Combustion is complex to model using conventional deterministic methods thus motivate the use of heuristics in this domain. ANNs have been
successfully applied to combustion classification systems; however, traditional ANN training methods get often trapped in local minima of the
error function and are inefficient in multimodal and non-differentiable
functions. A GA is used here to overcome these problems. The proposed
GA finds the weights of an ANN than best fits the training pattern with
the highest classification rate.

Keywords: Genetic Algorithms, Artificial Neural Networks, Flame
Classification, Electromagnetic Spectrum.

1 Introduction

Currently Combustion is the most important source of energy for power generation, heating, and transportation in the world and this trend is expected to
continue in the foreseeable future [1]. Control systems that provide information about combustion are of great importance for the energy saving. However,
combustion is a dynamic, highly nonlinear and multivariable process, which is
particularly complex to model using conventional deterministic methods.

Diagnostic methods based on flame monitoring have been implemented as
strategies to provide a status in combustion process with which can implement
control and optimization systems to make more efficient combustion process,
optimizing fuel consumption and reducing emissions. Several monitoring flame
techniques have been developed for combustion processes using Fuzzy Logic [2],
Expert systems [1], Support Vector Machines [3], Artificial Neural Networks
(ANNs) [4] and Genetic Algorithms (GAs) [5, 6], focussing mainly on combustion
gases analysis and prediction.

F. Castro, A. Gelbukh, and M. González (Eds.): MICAI 2013, Part II, LNAI 8266, pp. 172–184, 2013.
© Springer-Verlag Berlin Heidelberg 2013

Monitoring flames through spectral analysis approaches arises as an alternative to monitoring techniques such as image analysis, which are difficult to implement in combustion systems and require more computer processing. Combustion processes such as those occurring in power generation industry frequently make use of optical sensors as a safety measure indicating the presence or absence of the flame inside the furnace. However these sensors could provide more information about the flame state that can be used for combustion optimization.

GAs are heuristic search methods based on the mechanism of genetics and natural selection. GAs require minimum specific domain knowledge about the search space, which makes their use very general. GAs are also easy to use and can be particularly useful when dealing with optimization problems having a very large, complex and little known search space, in which traditional mathematical programming techniques tend to fail [7].

Performance of ANNs is largely influenced by the architecture as well as by the weights used for its connections. The training stage in an ANN is the process of adjusting the weights such that the training patterns fit with the lowest error while having a profitable generalization ability to recognize new patterns. Traditional training methods for ANNs are based on gradient descent and get often trapped in local minima of the error function. Therefore, such methods are very inefficient in multimodal and non-differentiable functions [8]. In such cases, the use of metaheuristics such as a GA is more appropriate. The GA proposed here aims to adapt the weights of the connections of an ANN[9], different approaches include the evolution of architecture [10–12] and the evolution of learning rules and transfer functions [13].

The study reported here focuses on the electromagnetic spectrum signal analysis and GAs to train an ANN for the classification of pattern flames of a combustion process. The remainder of this paper is organized as follows. In Section 2, we describe the methodology adopted for our study, including a description of the data acquisition and the features extraction processes of the electromagnetic spectrum. In Section 3, we describe the main features of the GA that is used to train an ANN and we also provide a description of the experimental design adopted.Our results are shown in Section 4 and our conclusions and some possible paths for future research are provided in Section 5.

2   Methodology

This section provides a description of the methodologies that have been used for flame classification. In Figure 1, we show a general diagram of the system adopted in our study, which includes three main stages: 1) data acquisition, 2) features extraction and 3) the use of an ANN trained by a GA.

2.1   Data Acquisition

In our study, the electromagnetic spectrum of a combustion process was measured using a flame scanning system with a solid-state optical sensor that operates between the ultraviolet peak at 350 nm and the infrared peak at 700

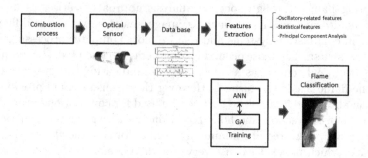

Fig. 1. Diagram of the system adopted in our study

nm. The scanning system output is 450 hexadecimal data, containing the sensor configuration and the flame signal in both the time and frequency domains.

In combustion process optimization one of the most important condition is the air/fuel ratio. Particularly there are tree conditions related to this ratio balance: fuel rich, fuel lean and air/fuel balance. In Figure 2, we show the signals associated to the following flame states:

1. No flame (background radiation)
2. Stable flame(air fuel balance)
3. Flame with air excess (fuel lean)
4. Flame with fuel excess (fuel rich)

A database was created using signals of the four flames states using a program written in Visual Basic for data acquisition. The database is composed of 480 signals (we stored 120 for each flame pattern). Each signal contains 256 values corresponding to the voltage equivalent to the flame intensity in 500 ms.

The database was divided in three subsets:

1. *Data Training:* Data used for training our ANN (see Section 3). The quadratic error is minimized in the fitness function of the GA adopted to train the ANN. This data corresponds to 50% of the total data set.
2. *Data Validation:* Data for computing the percentage of generalization. This data corresponds to 20% of the total data set.
3. *Data Test:* New data to test the ANN. This data corresponds to 30% of the total data set.

2.2   Features Extraction

Flame signals were preprocessed to extract features that capture the whole possible information (e.g., trends, periodicity, signatures of chaos) required to describe the flame patterns. We provide next a description of the formulation of these features.

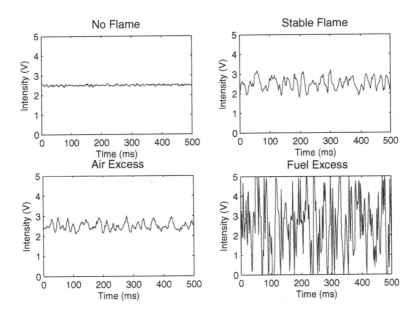

Fig. 2. Signal of the four flame patterns considered in our study

2.3   Statistical Features

Statistical Moments. Statistical moment analysis is a technique that can be used for data series characterization, since it gives a set of parameters that describe and provide information of a probability distribution function. The second, third, and fourth normalized central moments of the distribution of the flame signal intensity were calculated in order to provide information derived from the comparison of the shape of the electromagnetic spectra.

The formal definition of a statistical moment is:

$$M_k = E[x - E(x)]^k \tag{1}$$

Where:
M_k= k order statistical moment
$E[\ ]$=Expected value
x= Data signal

Autocorrelation Sum (Box-Pierce). Autocorrelation measures the linear correlation in a time series. The autocorrelation sum is calculated as:

$$Q(\tau_{max}) = n\Sigma_{\tau=1}^{\tau_{max}} r(\tau)^2 \tag{2}$$

where:

$$r(\tau) = \frac{\sum_{t=\tau+1}^{n} (x_t x_{t-\tau} - \bar{x}^2)}{\sum_{t=\tau+1}^{n} x_t^2 - \bar{x}^2} \tag{3}$$

2.4 Oscillation-Related Features

Oscillation-related features have been applied considering an oscillating behavior in the flame signal (although this is not always true) and are calculated as in [14]. The signal is spanned with a data window of length k, and we checked if the center is either a minimum or a maximum. The oscillation period is defined as the time between successive peaks. The Oscillation-related features calculated are the mean, and standard deviation of the period and peak, which are defined as:

Period average:

$$\bar{T} = \frac{1}{n} \Sigma_{i=1}^{n} T_i \tag{4}$$

where:
$T_i =$ Period of the ith oscillation.

Peak average:

$$\bar{z} = \frac{1}{n} \Sigma_{i=1}^{n} z_i \tag{5}$$

where:
$z_i =$ Peak of the ith oscillation.

Period standard deviation

$$S_T = \sqrt{\frac{1}{n-1} \Sigma_{i=1}^{n} (T_i^2 - \bar{T}^2)} \tag{6}$$

Peak standard deviation

$$S_z = \frac{1}{n-1} \Sigma_{i=1}^{n} (z_i - \bar{z}^2) \tag{7}$$

2.5 Principal Components Analysis

Principal Components Analysis (PCA) is a data transformation technique that can be useful to reveal simple structures, patterns or tendencies underlying in complex data sets using analytical solutions. This technique provides a measure to quantify the relative importance of each dimension allowing the characterization of large data sets with a reduced number of components.

Let X be a $(m \times n)$ matrix and $X^t X$ a quadratic matrix of range q. Then, X could be expressed as:

$$X = U \Sigma V^t \tag{8}$$

where U and V are m order matrices containing the eigenvector of $X^t X$ and Σ is a diagonal matrix that contains the square roots of the eigenvalues of $X^t X$: $(\sigma_1, \sigma_2, \sigma_3, ..., \sigma_q)$, with $\sigma_1 \geq \sigma_2 \geq \sigma_3 \geq, ..., \sigma_q > 0$.

In this study, we first compute the distance matrix of the data of a flame signal and then, PCA is applied.

Principal Components Selection. It is expected that keeping $n \ll m$ components produces a high variance of the original data set. Then, the number of components to retain is based on the cumulative contribution of the variance of the first several components, which can be expressed as:

$$CV_k = \sum_{i=1}^{k} \frac{100 \lambda_i}{\sum_{j=1}^{m} \lambda_j} \tag{9}$$

where:
$CV_k =$ cumulative variance of the component k
$m =$ Total number of components

In Figure 3 we show the cumulative variance of the first 20 principal components of a flame signal. As we can see, the first five components explain the 92.7% variability percentage and the 6th component increases it by only 1.28%. Therefore, since the first five components have a high percentage of variability, only these are retained.

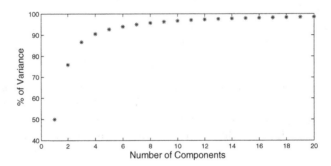

Fig. 3. Cumulative variance of the first 20 principal components

3 Genetic Algorithm Parameters

A real-coded GA was implemented, together with a two-layer feedforward neural network using a hyperbolic tangent transfer function in both the hidden and output layers. Figure 4 highlights the architecture of the ANN and in Figure 5 we show the weights encoding scheme adopted.

The inputs vector of the ANN is formed by the 13 features described in the previous section, while the outputs correspond to the four different flame patterns being considered. In Figure 6, we show the targets for the flame states.

Algorithm 1. Pseudocode of the GA used to train our ANNs

Require: Population size N, Maximum number of generations G
Ensure: Trained artificial neural network
 1: Load features extracted from flame signals.
 2: Normalize features.
 3: Perform data training, data validation and data testing.
 4: Initialize the population P_i of N individuals:
 5: $k = 1$
 6: **repeat**
 7:     Generate random weights for the adjacency matrix of ANN_k .
 8:     Define the first chromosome with a concatenation of the weights of the hidden layer of the adjacency matrix.
 9:     Define the second chromosome with a concatenation of the the weights of the output layer of the adjacency matrix.
10:     Perform an elimination of the connection weights using the connection elimination operator with a probability of 0.35.
11:     $k = k + 1$
12: **until** $k = N$
13: $i \leftarrow 0$
14: **repeat**
15:     Evaluate fitness of population P_i.
16:     Perform roulette wheel selection
17:     Generate offspring P'_i.
18:     Apply mutation operator to P'_i.
19:     Apply the elimination connection operator to P'_i with a probability of $\frac{P_{mut}}{2}$.
20:     Apply elitism$P_{i+1} \leftarrow P'_i$.
21:     $i \leftarrow i + 1$
22: **until** Termination condition is reached

The pseudocode of the GA that we implemented is depicted in Algorithm 1.

Our GA uses elitism (the best individual from each generation passes intact to the next one), as well as roulette wheel selection, arithmetic crossover [15] and uniform mutation. Each of the main elements of our GA are briefly described next.

3.1   Initial Population

The initial population is created with randomly generated real values in the range $[-50, 50]$ for both chromosomes. Then, a connection elimination operator in applied. This operator sets the weights equal to zero with a probability of 0.35.

3.2   Fitness Function

The objective function commonly used to adjust the weights of an ANN is the mean squared error (MSE). However, this is not necessarily the best choice when

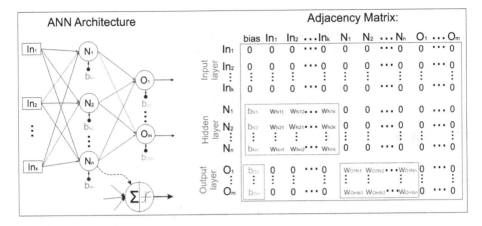

Fig. 4. Architecture of the ANN adopted and the representation as a adjacency matrix

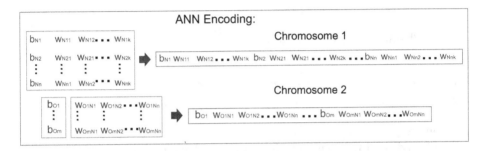

Fig. 5. Adjacency matrix encoding in our GA

No flame	Stable	Oxigen excess	Fuel excess
$\begin{bmatrix} 1 \\ -1 \\ -1 \\ -1 \end{bmatrix}$	$\begin{bmatrix} -1 \\ 1 \\ -1 \\ -1 \end{bmatrix}$	$\begin{bmatrix} -1 \\ -1 \\ 1 \\ -1 \end{bmatrix}$	$\begin{bmatrix} -1 \\ -1 \\ -1 \\ 1 \end{bmatrix}$

Fig. 6. Targets for the four flame classes during the ANN training

using a GA. In our study, we adopted a different scheme in which we aim to find the weights of an ANN that provide a good generalization performance while also providing the best matching with respect to the training set.

Thus, the fitness function adopted by our GA is:

$$Fitness = \| \prod_{i=1}^{n} (1 + e_i^2), \sum_{i=1}^{n} e_i^2, E_{test} \| \qquad (10)$$

where:

e_i=Error associated to the training data set i

E_{test}=Percentage of misclassifications in the test data set

n=Size of the training data set

From now on, this fitness function will be referred to as the *error norm*.

3.3   Genetic Operators

As indicated before, we adopted roulette wheel selection with a probability of 0.9.

We also incorporated uniform crossover, which is defined as follows:

Let's consider the following two parents F_1 and F_2:

$$F_1 = \langle v_1, \ldots, v_k, \ldots, v_m \rangle \tag{11}$$

$$F_2 = \langle w_1, \ldots, w_k, \ldots, w_m \rangle \tag{12}$$

Their offspring are generated, using:

$$O_1 = \langle av_1 + (1-a)w1, \ldots, a \times w_k + (1-a)w_k, \ldots, a \times v_m + (1-a)w_m \rangle \tag{13}$$

$$O_2 = \langle aw_1 + (1-a)v1, \ldots a \times w_k + (1-a)v_k, \ldots, a \times w_m + (1-a)v_m \rangle \tag{14}$$

In our case, we adopted $a = 0.6$.

We also adopted uniform mutation with a probability $P_{mut} = 0.05$.

Given an individual P, the mutated version is:

$$P' = \langle v_1, \ldots, v'_k, \ldots, v_m \rangle \tag{15}$$

where

$$v'_k = \begin{cases} v_k + m_k & \text{if } LB \leq v_k + m_k \leq UB, \\ v_k - m_k & \text{other case.} \end{cases} \tag{16}$$

and:

$m_k = rand(LB, UB)$ and $[LB, UB]$ are the lower bound (LB) and upper bound (UB) of v_k, which is the original position of the individual to be mutated.

Finally, we also adopted the elimination connection operator, in order to allow the remotion of connections during the evolutionary search. This operator was applied with a probability of $\frac{P_{mut}}{2}$ (except for the initial generation in which a higher probability was used, as indicated before).

3.4   Experimental Design

The 13 features extracted from the database of the four experimental flames patterns were linearly normalized and were used as the inputs of our ANN. The

GA was tested with a population of 30 ANNs having 10 neurons in the hidden layer. First, MSE was used as our fitness function and then we adopted the fitness function defined in equation (10).

The stopping criterion for all the runs of the GA was to reach the best possible fitness value (i.e., $Fitness = 1$ for equation (10) and $Fitness = 0$ for MSE), or when reaching 2000 generations (whatever happened first).

The results obtained from the GA when using equation (10) were compared with respect to those produced by the scaled conjugate gradient method (SCG) [16], which is a traditional approach for training ANNs. Our result are presented next.

4   Discussion of Results

In Figure 7, we plot the fitness values versus the generation number. We show there the results corresponding to the best individual found in a run of the GA using equation (10). This plot shows how, in a few generations, an individual with a fitness value of one (i.e., the best possible value) was found.

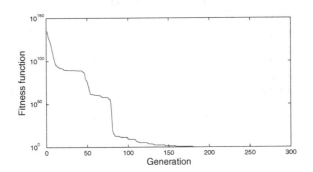

Fig. 7. Fitness function of the best individual as defined in equation (10)

Table 1. ANN training with GA. Average of 10 runs

	average % correct classification	average generations
MSE	98.1712963	2000
Norm	99.5138889	913.333333

In Table 1, we provide the results of the ANN training when using MSE as the fitness function. In Figure 8, we show a comparison of the MSE of the best individual using both fitness functions. As we can see, the use of MSE needs more generations to reach an acceptable fitness value, whereas the use of equation (10) provides good results with a lower number of generations.

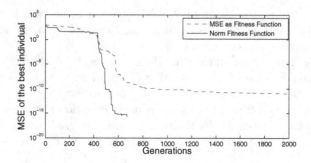

Fig. 8. Comparison of the MSE with the two different fitness functions adopted in our study

Table 2. Average of 30 independent runs of ANN training using a GA

	Average MSE	Total misclassified signals	Average % Correct Classification	Average of misclassified signals
Class 1	5.7628E-17	2	99.9444444	0.06666667
Class 2	6.8257E-15	52	98.5555556	1.73333333
Class 3	1.421E-13	13	99.6388889	0.43333333
Class 4	1.0938E-17	0	100	0
Total data set	2.3157E-15	67	99.5347222	2.23333333

Table 3. ANN training using SCG. Average of 30 independent runs

	Total misclassification	Average % Correct Classification	Average of misclassified signals
Class 1	120	96.66666667	4
Class 2	121	96.63888889	4.03333333
Class 3	1	99.97222222	0.03333333
Class 4	246	93.16666667	8.2
Total data set	488	96.61111111	4.06666667

The results of 30 runs of the GA with the fitness function defined in equation (10) are given in Table 2. A fitness value equal to 1 was reached, on average, after 881.4 generations. Having a low average MSE implies a good fit with the data training set, and having a high percentage of correct classification corresponds with a good generalization ability. As Table 3 indicates, our results are better than those obtained using SCG (this approach produced higher MSE values than our GA using the fitness function defined in equation (10)).

Table 4. MSE results with Scaled Conjugate Gradient method

	Average MSE	Average %error
training	0.0084154	3.26385333
validation	0.0088272	3.33308833
test	0.00959884	3.63403133

In Table 5, we compare the best and worst results of both training algorithms. The best results obtained by our proposed GA significantly outperform the results obtained by SCG.

Table 5. Comparison of the best and worst results obtained with a GA and with the Scaled Conjugate Gradient method

	MSE training	MSE Validation	MSE Test	% Correct Classification
AG best result	6.77E-18	7.62E-18	9.01E-16	100
AG worst result	2.77E-13	1.66E-09	9.66E-01	98.95833
SCG best result	9.25E-08	8.81E-08	3.30E-04	100
SCG worst result	6.73E-02	6.10E-02	6.10E-02	74.8

5   Conclusions and Future Work

A Genetic Algorithm was developed to train Artificial Neural Networks for flames classification using the electromagnetic spectrum. The proposed GA was compared with respect to the use of the Scaled Conjugate Gradient method in the training of artificial neural networks. Our preliminary results indicate our proposed approach is able to produce better performance, since it generates solutions with less error and an improved generalization ability. Additionally, our results show that the features extracted from signal spectra could provide information about the combustion state and could be used for flame characterization and combustion monitoring. All flame classes were classified with a high percentage while using ANNs trained with our proposed GA.

As part of our future work, we are considering the use of ANNs for the classification of signals of a combustion process in power generation systems, in which there is a more complicated dynamics. We are also interested in evolving weights connections of different ANN architectures, such as recurrent ANNs and generalized multilayer perceptrons, using Genetic Algorithms.

Acknowledgments. The third author gratefully acknowledges support from CONACyT project no. 103570.

References

1. Mahajan, A., Mahajan, R.: Expert system for flame analysis. In: 2004 IEEE Conference on Cybernetics and Intelligent Systems, vol. 2, pp. 1160–1165. IEEE (2004)
2. Xu, L., Yan, Y., Cornwell, S., Riley, G.: On-line fuel identification using digital signal processing and fuzzy inference techniques. IEEE Transactions on Instrumentation and Measurement 53(4), 1316–1320 (2004)
3. Torres, C.I., Hernández, F., Trejo, A., Ronquillo, G.: Support vector machines applied to a combustion process
4. Li, X., Sun, D., Lu, G., Krabicka, J., Yan, Y.: Prediction of nox emissions through-flame radical imaging and neural network based soft computing. In: 2012 IEEE International Conference on Imaging Systems and Techniques (IST), pp. 502–505. IEEE (2012)
5. Hao, Z., Qian, X., Cen, K., Jianren, F.: Optimizing pulverized coal combustion performance based on ann and ga. Fuel Processing Technology 85(2), 113–124 (2004)
6. Kesgin, U.: Genetic algorithm and artificial neural network for engine optimisation of efficiency and nox emission. Fuel 83(7), 885–895 (2004)
7. Palmes, P.P., Hayasaka, T., Usui, S.: Mutation-based genetic neural network. IEEE Transactions on Neural Networks 16(3), 587–600 (2005)
8. Yao, X.: Evolving artificial neural networks. Proceedings of the IEEE 87(9), 1423–1447 (1999)
9. Sexton, R.S., Dorsey, R.E., Johnson, J.D.: Toward global optimization of neural networks: a comparison of the genetic algorithm and backpropagation. Decision Support Systems 22(2), 171–185 (1998)
10. Rivero, D., Dorado, J., Fernández-Blanco, E., Pazos, A.: A genetic algorithm for ANN design, training and simplification. In: Cabestany, J., Sandoval, F., Prieto, A., Corchado, J.M. (eds.) IWANN 2009, Part I. LNCS, vol. 5517, pp. 391–398. Springer, Heidelberg (2009)
11. Yao, X., Islam, M.M.: Evolving artificial neural network ensembles. IEEE Computational Intelligence Magazine 3(1), 31–42 (2008)
12. Ballabio, D., Vasighi, M., Consonni, V., Kompany-Zareh, M.: Genetic algorithms for architecture optimisation of counter-propagation artificial neural networks. Chemometrics and Intelligent Laboratory Systems 105(1), 56–64 (2011)
13. Annunziato, M., Bertini, I., Lucchetti, M., Pizzuti, S.: Evolving weights and transfer functions in feed forward neural networks. In: Proc. EUNITE 2003, Oulu, Finland (2003)
14. Tsimpiris, A., Kugiumtzis, D.: Feature selection for classification of oscillating time series. Expert Systems 29(5), 456–477 (2012)
15. Michalewicz, Z.: Genetic algorithms + data structures = evolution programs. Springer (1996)
16. Møller, M.F.: A scaled conjugate gradient algorithm for fast supervised learning. Neural Networks 6(4), 525–533 (1993)

Traffic Sign Recognition
Based on Linear Discriminant Analysis

Sheila Esmeralda Gonzalez-Reyna*, Juan Gabriel Avina-Cervantes,
Sergio Eduardo Ledesma-Orozco,
Ivan Cruz-Aceves, and M. de Guadalupe Garcia-Hernandez

Universidad de Guanajuato, Division de Ingenierias Campus Irapuato-Salamanca
Carretera Salamanca-Valle de Santiago km 3.5 + 1.8 km. Comunidad de Palo Blanco,
C.P. 36885. Salamanca, Gto., Mexico
{se.gonzalezreyna,avina,selo,i.cruzaceves,garciag}@ugto.mx

Abstract. Traffic Signs provide visual information to drivers, in order
to warn them from possible danger on the road, set rules for pedes-
trian protection and inform people about their environment, to name
a few. Therefore, Traffic Sign Detection and Recognition Systems have
increased their interest in the scientific community. Applications include
autonomous driving systems, road sign inventory and driver support assistance systems. This paper presents a traffic sign recognition algorithm
for velocity signs, based on Linear Discriminant Analysis that performs
dimensionality reduction and it improves class separability. The tests
were performed on the German Traffic Sign Recognition Benchmark, using a Multi-Layer Perceptron as a classification tool. LDA classification
and k-Nearest Neighbors were also used for comparison. Experimental results demonstrate the validity of the proposed approach, having a 99.1%
of attributes reduction and a 96.5% of classification accuracy.

Keywords: Traffic Sign Recognition, Linear Discriminant Analysis, Artificial Neural Networks, Pattern Recognition.

1 Introduction

Driving a car is almost a purely visual task. Therefore, traffic signs are some
kind of visual language for drivers, with the main purpose of describing the
road, restrict or allow certain actions (parking, speed limits, etc.), warn from
possible risks, among others.

Traffic Sign Detection and Recognition is a computer vision field which automatically localizes and identifies road signs immerse in images, taken from a
moving car. It is also an important part of Driver Assistance Systems (DAS),
that provides information to the driver for incident avoidance.

Road sign detection and recognition is a hard task due to several factors (see
Fig. 1 for some examples):

---

* Corresponding author.

F. Castro, A. Gelbukh, and M. González (Eds.): MICAI 2013, Part II, LNAI 8266, pp. 185–193, 2013.
© Springer-Verlag Berlin Heidelberg 2013

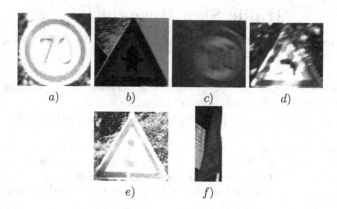

Fig. 1. Factors that affect automatic traffic sign recognition. a) Bright images, b) dark images, c) blurring, d) shadows, e) lackluster color and f) perspective.

- color appreciation changes depending on the time of the day,
- weather conditions like rain, clouds, sun or fog affect visibility,
- road signs might be disoriented or rotated,
- lackluster color due to sunlight exposure, and
- blurring caused by camera moving velocity, among others.

In the Traffic Sign Recognition field, there have been a lot of different approaches. Original traffic sign images are commonly taken on RGB color space. However, sometimes it can be convenient to work on a different color space due to its relative illumination invariance, such spaces include CIELab [1], HSI [2], HSV [3,4], and CIECAM97 [5]. However, there are some previous works that offer good results using RGB color space [6].

Some authors have proposed to apply different image processing algorithms, in order to improve sign color, contrast and appreciation. There is a wide variety of image processing algorithms used for traffic sign recongition: color segmentation [2,3,6], Scale Invariant Feature Transform (SIFT) [1], Histograms of Orientations [4,5] and Principal Component Analysis (PCA) [3].

There are several methods to classify the signs: Artificial Neural Networks [6], Support Vector Machines (SVM) [2,4], k-Nearest Neighbors with different similarity measures [3,5].

In the present study, a method for velocity Traffic Sign Recognition (TSR) is proposed. The original images were taken from the German Traffic Sign Recognition Benchmark (GTSRB) [7]. However, images contain a huge amount of information, making a dimensionality reduction algorithm necessary. Therefore, Linear Discriminant Analysis (LDA) has been chosen, given its ability to project data taking into account the largest between-class separability. Classification will be performed by the use of a Multi-Layer Perceptron (MLP), the simplest type of Artificial Neural Networks, due to its noise robustness and generalization abilities. LDA classification and Nearest Neighbors (k-NN) were also used for comparison.

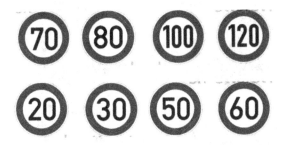

Fig. 2. Eight different classes of speed traffic signs

The rest of this document is organized as follows. Section 2 describes preprocessing steps and the Multivariate Linear Discriminate Analysis. Experimental results are detailly described on Sect. 3. Finally, Sect. 4 presents some conclusions and directions for future work.

2   Methodology

2.1   Image Preprocessing Stage

The GTSRB, contains over 50000 images, ordered in 43 different classes. Images are taken under different illumination, movement, rotation, scaling, and weather conditions. In this study, only speed signals on the GTSRB were used, due to their importance in safe and legal driving, which correspond to eight classes, this specific database is already divided into 12780 images for training, and 4170 for validation (see Fig. 2).

The original images present varying illumination conditions, making recognition task unreliable when the contrast is low or when the brightness is extremely high. Therefore, it is convenient to apply a preprocessing stage, in order to create a semi-uniform data set in what it refers to luminance.

A gamma correction algorithm was applied only dark and bright images. For that purpose, two thresholds were found by tuning, based on the average luminance value (gray scale images). All dark images (mean below 65, for $[0, 255]$ gray scale) were transformed with a gamma factor of 0.4545. While all bright images (mean above 180) were transformed used a gamma factor of 2.2. The remaining images were not modified. The first row in Fig. 3 shows an example of the three possibilities: dark, bright and ideal images. The second row of the same figure shows the same images after the gamma correction was applied.

2.2   Multivariate Linear Discriminant Analysis

In pattern recognition, preprocessing stages might simplify data representation if feature extraction is used, and therefore improve class separability. Linear Discriminant Analysis (LDA) may find the best set of features to discriminate existing classes.

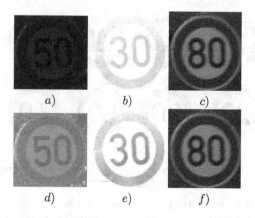

Fig. 3. Adaptive gamma correction. a), b) and c) are original dark, bright and ideal images. d), e) and f) are corrected with gamma values of 0.4545, 2.2 and 1.0, respectively.

For the multivariate LDA, we used the method proposed by Croux, Filzmoser and Joossens [8]. The algorithm is described below.

Let $\overrightarrow{X}$ be an N^2-dimensional vector, corresponding to an $N \times N$ image. The data set would be fully contained on an $N^2 \times M$ matrix $\mathbf{A}$, where M is the total number of samples. Now consider the existence of C different classes to be discriminated, each with their correspondent mean vectors $\overrightarrow{\mu_i}$ and covariance matrices $\mathbf{S}_i$, $i = 1, \ldots, C$. The probability that a given sample test belongs to class i is given by π_i, and can be estimated by the frequency of observations in the training set.

The *Between-Class* covariance matrix is defined as,

$$\mathbf{B} = \sum_{i=1}^{C} \pi_i \left(\overrightarrow{\mu_i} - \overrightarrow{m} \right) \left(\overrightarrow{\mu_i} - \overrightarrow{m} \right)^T \tag{1}$$

where,

$$\overrightarrow{m} = \sum_{i=1}^{C} \pi_i \overrightarrow{\mu_i}. \tag{2}$$

Additionally, a *Within-Class* covariance matrix is defined as,

$$\mathbf{W} = \sum_{i=1}^{C} \pi_i \mathbf{S}_i. \tag{3}$$

In order to find the projection space, eigenvalues λ_i and eigenvectors $\overrightarrow{V}_i$ of the product $\mathbf{W}^{-1}\mathbf{B}$ shall be found. Furthermore, if dimensionality reduction is required, only the first k eigenvectors which correspond to the highest k eigenvalues should be considered. Finally, the new data is a projection from the original data set by the means of the k-eigenvectors set, as it can be seen in (4).

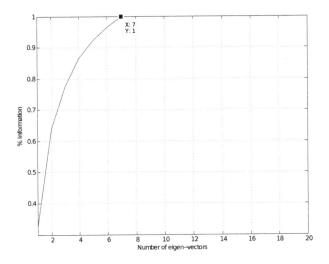

Fig. 4. LDA amount of information for dimensionality reduction

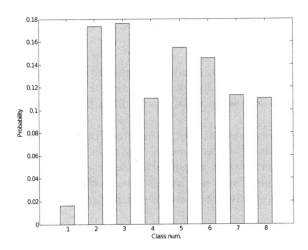

Fig. 5. Training set per class probability (Frequency of observations divided by the total number of samples)

$$\mathbf{Y} = \mathbf{V}^T \left(\mathbf{A} - \overrightarrow{m} \right), \tag{4}$$

where $\mathbf{V} = \{ \overrightarrow{V}_1, \ldots, \overrightarrow{V}_q \}$ is the set of eigenvectors, with $q = N^2$ for classical projection and $q = k$ for dimensionality reduction.

The first question in the described LDA methodology would be, how to know the optimal number of eigenvectors for dimensionality reduction. The answer is simple: taking the $\sum_{i=1}^{N^2} \lambda_i$ as a total amount of information, $\sum_{i=1}^{q} \lambda_i$, $q =$

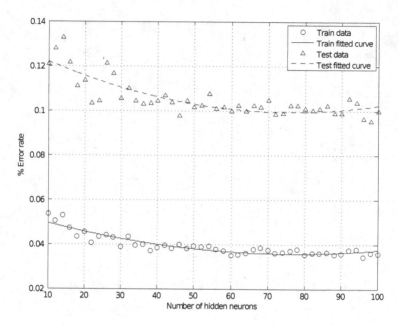

Fig. 6. Training and Testing stages error rates with varying number of hidden neurons

$1, \ldots, N^2$ will represent the information taking the first q eigenvalues. Choose q that represents the minimal loss of information. Figure 4 shows the result of these process. With only seven eigenvectors, LDA has a loss of information of $4.58 \times 10^{-11}\%$.

Figure 5 shows the actual training set per class probabilities. If data sets are not balanced (the number of elements per class is different), classes that contain more samples will have larger classification accuracies than those with fewer number of observations. However, when the class probability is considered in the algorithm, all classes will tend to have similar recognition accuracies.

3   Results

A MLP is a feed-forward neural network capable of discriminate nonlinear patterns. Some of its greatest advantages are noise robustness, and generalization capabilities. A MLP is characterized by simple units of processing named neurons, which are organized in layers.

For the experiments presented here, the number of input neurons is equal to the number of final attributes, and the number of outputs must be equal to the number of classes (in this case, eight). The real problem is to find the optimal number of neurons in the hidden layer of the network. In order find this number, a performance test was implemented, by successively incrementing the number of neurons in the hidden layer. Figure 6 shows that after sixty neurons, the

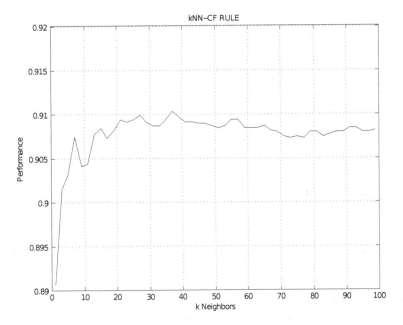

Fig. 7. Classification accuracy with varying the number of Neighbors in kNN-CF algorithm

classification error rate does not decrease significatively for training, neither for testing (validation).

LDA classification can be achieved by comparing the similitude of the desired sample with the ones existing in the training set. This process can also be known as the Nearest Neighbor process. Another version of this algoritm, uses the comparison of the current sample against a larger number of Neighbors, generating the k-Nearest Neighbors algorithm for classification. In this study, a variant to this process, the kNN-CF is used, a detailed description can be found in [9], due to its ability to manage unbalanced datasets. Another tuning process was performed in order to find the number of neighbors which best classify the data, the results of this experiment are shown in Fig. 7, where it is observed that the highest accuracy is obtained for $k = 37$.

Table 1 lists the performance per class obtained when these classification methods were applied to the same data set. For MLP both training and testing performances are presented. In LDA and kNN-CF, euclidean distance was used.

For the MLP classification, it can be observed that for training, class 1 reached the highest identification accuracy, however, it is also the worst recognition rate for testing. This might be related to the fact that this is the class with lower frequency of observations. The average performance for MLP and kNN-CF classification are above 90%.

Table 1. Per Class performance accuracy and average performance for training and testing sets

Class number	MLP Training	MLP Test	LDA	kNN-CF
1	99.5%	82.3%	89.7%	95.0%
2	96.8%	87.7%	87.0%	90.3%
3	96.1%	88.7%	88.6%	93.7%
4	95.8%	88.1%	83.8%	94.4%
5	97.8%	95.5%	96.0%	91.4%
6	94.9%	88.2%	85.9%	86.0%
7	97.2%	95.8%	92.7%	87.8%
8	96.9%	91.2%	90.5%	93.6%
average performance	**96.5%**	**90.3%**	**89.06%**	**91.0%**

In 2011, Fleyeh and Davami [3] proposed the "Eigen-based" traffic sign recognition. The essential differences between their work and ours are enumerated in Table 2. In the present study, segmentation step is not required. Furthermore, since a known, free database is used, experiments can be easily reproduced and compared to the proposed approach. The number of images is also an important factor, because the classification tool presents better generalization capabilities depending on the number of samples in the training step. Attributes reduction is larger for this work, which is always a desirable characteristic in pattern recognition. Although when recognition accuracy is a bit lower, good results were obtained using a more complex database. However, direct comparison of performances might be difficult due to the different amount of images used for both experiments, and it is not known if the dataset used by Fleyeh and Davami is balanced.

Table 2. Comparative results between the proposed method and [3]

	Our work	Fleyeh and Davami, 2011
Image preprocessing	Gamma correction	HSV color space segmentation
Feature extraction algorithm	LDA	PCA
Classification tool	MLP	SVM
Train and test images	12780, 4170	648
Image dataset	GTSRB	Private
Number of Final Attributes	7	20
Recognition accuracy	96.5%	97.9%

4   Conclusions

In this paper, a Traffic Sign Recognition system based on LDA is presented. We conclude that speed traffic signs can be accurately classified by applying a gamma correction algorithm to decrease luminance variations and LDA for attributes optimization and reduction. A factor that could increase identification performance is the inclusion of more rotated signs in the training dataset. Consequently, the final system will have a stronger rotation robustness.

This method can be applied for TSR with more than eight classes, having a pre-classification step for Traffic Signs subgroups (e.g. prohibition, speed limits, warnings).

Aknowledgements. This work has been supported by the National Council of Science and Technology of Mexico (**CONACYT**) under Grant number 329483/229696, and for Universidad de Guanajuato through PIFI-2012.

References

[1] Guo, H.R., Wang, X.J., Zhong, Y.X., Lu, P.: Traffic signs recognition based on visual attention mechanism. The Journal of China Universities of Posts and Telecommunications 18, 12–16 (2011)

[2] Maldonado-Bascon, S., Lafuente-Arroyo, S., Gil-Jimenez, P., Gomez-Moreno, H., Lopez-Ferreras, F.: Road-sign detection and recognition based on support vector machines. IEEE Transactions on Intelligent Transportation Systems 8, 264–278 (2007)

[3] Fleyeh, H., Davami, E.: Eigen-based traffic sign recognition. IET Intelligent Transport Systems 5, 190–196 (2011)

[4] Boi, F., Gagliardini, L.: A support vector machines network for traffic sign recognition. In: The 2011 International Joint Conference on Neural Networks (IJCNN), pp. 2210–2216 (2011)

[5] Gao, X.W., Podladchikova, L., Shaposhnikov, D., Hong, K., Shevtsova, N.: Recognition of traffic signs based on their colour and shape features extracted using human vision models. Journal of Visual Communication & Image Representation 17, 675–685 (2006)

[6] de la Escalera, A., Armingol, J.M., Mata, M.: Traffic sign recognition and analysis for intelligent vehicles. Image and Vision Computing 11, 247–258 (2003)

[7] Stallkamp, J., Schlipsing, M., Salmen, J., Igel, C.: Man vs. computer: Benchmarking machine learning algorithms for traffic sign recognition. Neural Networks 32, 323–332 (2012)

[8] Croux, C., Filzmoser, P., Joossens, K.: Classification efficiencies for robust linear discriminant analysis. Statistica Sinica 18, 581–599 (2008)

[9] Zhang, S.: KNN-CF Approach: Incorporating certainty factor to kNN classification. IEEE Intelligent Informatics Bulletin 11, 24–33 (2010)

Association Measures and Aggregation Functions

Ildar Batyrshin

Research Program of Applied Mathematics and Computations
Mexican Petroleum Institute
batyr1@gmail.com

Abstract. The concept of association measure generalizing the Pearson correlation coefficient is introduced. The methods of generation of association measures by means of pseudo-difference associated to some t-conorm and by similarity measures are proposed. The association measure can be introduced on any set with involutive reflection operation and suitably defined similarity measure. The methods of construction of association measures by Minkowski metric and data standardization using the aggregation functions are considered. The cosine similarity and the Pearson's correlation coefficient are obtained as partial cases of the proposed general methods.

Keywords: association measure, t-conorm, pseudo-difference, similarity measure, Minkowski distance, correlation coefficient, cosine similarity, involutivity, reflection, idempotence, data standardization.

1   Introduction

The Pearson correlation coefficient plays an important role in data analysis giving possibility to measure possible direct and inverse relationships between variables. It is considered as a measure of the strength of linear relationship between variables but it is not always suitable for measuring possible associations between variables in general case [1] and for measuring associations between time series shapes [2]. It arises the problem of creation of association measures suitable for different applications. An axiomatic definition of time series shape association measures generalizing the properties of correlation coefficient has been considered in [4]. In [3], the general methods of construction of association measures satisfying to the axioms of time series shape association measure have been proposed. In the present work the results of [3] are extended in several directions. First, the problem of definition and construction of association measures is considered here from the more general point of view of the theory of aggregation functions [6]. It gives possibility to extend the methods of generation of association measures using the concept of pseudo difference associated with some *t*-conorm. Second, the concept of association measure is extended from the set of time series on a general domain where some involutive mapping together with a similarity measure related with this mapping can be introduced. It gives possibility to extend the class of association measures that can be considered and generated

F. Castro, A. Gelbukh, and M. González (Eds.): MICAI 2013, Part II, LNAI 8266, pp. 194–203, 2013.
© Springer-Verlag Berlin Heidelberg 2013

on wide class of objects different from time series. The cosine similarity and the Pearson correlation coefficient are obtained as particular cases of the proposed approach.

The paper has the following structure. Section 2 gives definitions of t-conorms and pseudo-differences. Section 3 introduces the concept of the association measure and proposes the methods of construction of these measures on the sets with involutive reflection operation and suitably defined similarity measures. Section 4 considers a set of n-tuples of real values (vectors, time series or samples) where association measures can be defined and discusses the methods of standardization of n-tuples. Section 5 shows how dissimilarity measures and the Minkowski distance together with standardizations can be used for constructing association measures considered in Section 3. The cosine similarity and the Pearson's correlation coefficient are obtained from the general methods of construction of association measures using standardization transformation and Minkowski distance. Conclusions are given in Section 6.

2   Basic Definitions

Consider some definitions from [5-7].

A t-**conorm** is a function $S:[0,1]^2 \to [0,1]$ such that for all $a,b,c \in [0,1]$ the following axioms are satisfied:

$$S(a,b) = S(b,a), \qquad \text{(commutativity)}$$

$$S(a,S(b,c)) = S(S(a,b),c), \qquad \text{(associativity)}$$

$$S(a,b) \leq S(a,c), \text{ whenever } b \leq c, \qquad \text{(monotonicity)}$$

$$S(a,0) = a. \qquad \text{(boundary condition)}$$

From the definition of t-conorms it follows for all $a \in [0,1]$:

$$S(1,a) = S(a,1) = 1, \qquad S(0,a) = a.$$

An element $a \in]0,1[$ will be referred to as **a nilpotent element** [5] of S if there exists some $b \in]0,1[$ such that $S(a,b) = 1$. A t-conorm S has no nilpotent elements if and only if on $[0,1]$ it is fulfilled:

$$\text{from } S(a,b) = 1 \text{ it follows } a = 1 \text{ or } b = 1.$$

Consider simplest t-conorms:

$$S_M(a,b) = max\{a,b\}, \qquad \text{(maximum)}$$

$$S_L(a,b) = min\{a+b, 1\}, \qquad \text{(Lukasiewicz } t\text{-conorm)}$$

$$S_P(a,b) = a+b-ab. \qquad \text{(probabilistic sum)}$$

It is clear that the maximum and the probabilistic sum have no nilpotent elements but the Lukasiewicz t-conorm has.

Let S be a t-conorm. The **S-difference** is defined by [6]:

$$a \overset{S}{-} b = inf\{c \in [0,1] | S(b,c) \geq a\}$$

for any a,b in $[0,1]$.

From the properties of t-conorms it follows:

$$1 \overset{S}{-} 0 = 1,$$

$$1 \overset{S}{-} b = 1, \text{ if } b < 1 \text{ and } t\text{-conorm } S \text{ has no nilpotent elements.}$$

Let S be a t-conorm. The **pseudo-difference** associated to S is defined by [6]:

$$a(-)_S b = \begin{cases} a \overset{S}{-} b, & if \ a > b \\ -\left(b \overset{S}{-} a\right), & if \ a < b \\ 0, & if \ a = b \end{cases}$$

for any a,b in $[0,1]^2$. Equivalently

$$a(-)_S b = sign(a - b)(max \ (a,b) \overset{S}{-} min \ (a,b)).$$

The following pseudo-differences are associated with t-conorms S_M, S_L and S_P respectively:

$$a(-)_M b = \begin{cases} a, & if \ a > b \\ -b, & if \ a < b \\ 0, & if \ a = b \end{cases},$$

$$a(-)_L b = a - b,$$

$$a(-)_P b = (a - b)/(1 - min \ (a,b)).$$

3   Association Measures

Suppose X is a set with a mapping $N{:}X \to X$ satisfying for all elements x from X the property:

$$N(N(x)) = x. \hspace{3cm} \text{(involutivity)}$$

This mapping will be called **a reflection operation**.

As an example of a set with a reflection operation one can consider the set $X = [0,1]$ with an involutive negation N, defined, e.g. by [7]: $N(x) = 1\text{-}x$, the set of fuzzy sets X with an involutive negation of fuzzy sets, the set of vectors or time series of the length n with real valued elements $x = (x_1,...,x_n)$ and reflection operation $N(x)=(-x_1, ..., -x_n)$ etc.

Suppose A is a function $A:X{\times}X \to [-1,1]$ satisfying for all x and y from X the properties:

$$A(x,y) = A(y,x), \qquad \text{(symmetry)}$$

$$A(x,x) = 1, \qquad \text{(reflexivity)}$$

and N is a reflection operation on X. The function A will be called an **association measure** (with respect to N) if for all x from X such that $A(N(x),x) \neq 1$, it is fulfilled:

$$A(N(x),x) = -1, \qquad \text{(inverse reflexivity)}$$

$$A(N(x),y) = -A(x,y). \qquad \text{(inverse relationship)}$$

Generally, a function $SIM:X{\times}X \to [0,1]$ satisfying for all x and y from X the properties:

$$SIM(x,y) = SIM(y,x), \qquad \text{(symmetry)}$$

$$SIM(x,x) = 1, \qquad \text{(reflexivity)}$$

will be referred to as a **similarity measure**.

Suppose SIM for all x, y satisfies some of the following properties:

$$SIM(N(x),y) = SIM(x,N(y)), \qquad \text{(permutation of reflections)}$$

$$SIM(N(x),x) < 1, \qquad \text{(weak similarity of reflections)}$$

$$SIM(N(x),x) = 0. \qquad \text{(non-similarity of reflections)}$$

It is clear that from the non-similarity of reflections it follows the weak similarity of reflections. Below it is a generalization of the result from [3] on pseudo-differences and reflection operation N.

Theorem 1. Suppose SIM is a similarity measure satisfying the property of permutation of reflections and S is a t-conorm. Then the function:

$$A_{SIM}(x,y) = SIM(x,y)(-)_S SIM(x,N(y))$$

defined for all y such that $SIM(N(y),y) \neq 1$ is an association measure if one of the following is fulfilled:

1. SIM satisfies the non-similarity of reflections;
2. SIM satisfies the weak similarity of reflections and t-conorm S has no nilpotent elements.

Since maximum S_M and probabilistic S_P t-conorms has no nilpotent elements but Lukasiewicz t-conorm S_L has, from the Theorem 1 the following specific methods for construction of association measures can be obtained.

Corollary 2. Suppose *SIM* is a similarity measure satisfying the property of permutation of reflections. For all y such that $SIM(N(y),y) \neq 1$ the association measure can be defined as follows. If *SIM* satisfies the non-similarity of reflections then the function:

$$A_{SIM,L}(x,y) = SIM(x,y) - SIM(x,N(y))$$

is an association measure. If *SIM* satisfies the weak similarity of reflections then the following functions are association measures:

$$A_{SIM,M}(x,y) = \begin{cases} SIM(x,y), & if\ SIM(x,y) > SIM(x,N(y)) \\ -SIM(x,N(y)), & if\ SIM(x,y) < SIM(x,N(y)) \\ 0, & if\ SIM(x,y) = SIM(x,N(y)) \end{cases},$$

$$A_{SIM,P}(x,y) = (SIM(x,y) - SIM(x,N(y)))/(1 - \min(SIM(x,y), SIM(x,N(y)))).$$

In the following section, we will consider the set X of n-tuples of real values $x = (x_1,\dots,x_n)$ of the length n with the reflection operation $N(x) = -x = (-x_1,\dots,-x_n)$. In this case a symmetric and reflexive function A will be an association measure if for all x from X such that $A(-x,x) \neq 1$, it is fulfilled:

$$A(-x,x) = -1, \qquad\qquad \text{(inverse reflexivity)}$$

$$A(-x,y) = -A(x,y). \qquad\qquad \text{(inverse relationship)}$$

The corresponding properties of similarity measures related with reflection operation will have the following notations:

$$SIM(-x,y) = SIM(x,-y), \qquad \text{(permutation of reflections)}$$

$$SIM(-x,x) < 1, \qquad \text{(weak similarity of reflections)}$$

$$SIM(-x,x) = 0. \qquad \text{(non-similarity of reflections)}$$

Generally we do not require as in [3] that association measure satisfies for any real value q the following property:

$$A(x+q,y) = A(x,y). \qquad\qquad \text{(translation invariance)}$$

But this property will be considered as necessary if X is a set of time series $x = (x_1,\dots,x_n)$ [3]. The association measure will be referred to as scale invariant if for all positive real values p it is fulfilled [3]:

$$A(px,y) = A(x,y). \qquad\qquad \text{(scale invariance)}$$

It is clear that A_{SIM} is translation or scale invariant if *SIM* satisfies the corresponding properties.

4   Standardization

For any n-tuples x, y and real values p,q define $x+y = (x_1+y_1, ..., x_n+y_n)$, $px+q= (px_1+q, ...,px_n+q)$. Denote $q_{(n)}$ a constant n-tuple with all elements equal to q. We will write $x= const$ if $x = q_{(n)}$ for some q, and $x \neq const$ if $x_i \neq x_j$ for some $i \neq j$ from $\{1,...,n\}$. From definitions above it follows: $px+q = px+q_{(n)}$.

A transformation $F:R^n \rightarrow R^n$ is said to be a **standardization** if for all $x \in R^n$ it is fulfilled $F(x) \neq const$ if $x \neq const$:

$$F(F(x)) = F(x), \qquad\qquad \text{(idempotence)}$$

$$F(q_{(n)}) = 0_{(n)}, \quad \text{for any real value } q.$$

A n-tuple x is said to be in a **standard form wrt a standardization F** if $F(x) = x$.

As it follows from the definition, a standardization F transforms any x into a standard form $F(x)$. We will say that $F(x)$ satisfies r-**normality** for some $r = 1,2,....$ if:

$$\sum_{i=1}^{n} |F(x)_i|^r = 1 .$$

A transformation $E:R^n \rightarrow R$ is said to be an **estimate** if $E(q_{(n)})=q$ for any real value q.

It is clear that any aggregation function [6] is an estimate.

We will use the following terminology, if for all n-tuples x,y, for any real value q and for any positive value $p > 0$, F satisfies the properties:

$$F(x+q) = F(x)+q, \qquad\qquad \text{(translation additivity)}$$

$$F(x+q) = F(x), \qquad\qquad \text{(translation invariance)}$$

$$F(x+y) = F(x)+F(y), \qquad\qquad \text{(additivity)}$$

$$F(px) = pF(x), \quad p > 0, \qquad\qquad \text{(scale proportionality)}$$

$$F(px) = F(x). \qquad\qquad \text{(scale invariance)}$$

Note that in literature the translation additivity is often referred to as shift invariance or translation invariance, the scale proportionality is referred to as scale invariance or homogeneity of degree 1. It is clear that from the additivity of F it follows its translation additivity. The same terminology will be used for E.

Proposition 3. The following transformations are standardizations:

1. $F_1(x)= x-E_1(x)$, if E_1 is a translation additive estimate.
   F_1 is translation invariant and $E_1(F_1(x))= 0$.

2. $F_2(x)= x/E_2(x)$, for $x \neq const$, if E_2 is a scale proportional estimate and $E_2(x) > 0$ for all x.
   F_2 is scale invariant and $E_2(F_2(x))= 1$.

If $E_2(x) = \sqrt[r]{\sum_{i=1}^{n}|x_i|^r}$, then $F_2(x)$ satisfies the r-normality property.

If $E_2(x) = \sum_{i=1}^{n} x_i$, then $F_2(x)$ satisfies the normality property: $\sum_{i=1}^{n} F(x)_i = 1$.

3. $F_3(x) = (x - E_{13}(x))/E_{23}(x)$, if E_{13} is a translation additive and scale proportional estimate, E_{23} is a translation invariant and a scale proportional estimate, and $E_{23}(x) > 0$, for all x.

F_3 is translation and scale invariant, $E_{13}(F_3(x)) = 0$.

If $E_{23}(x) = (\sum_{i=1}^{n}|x_i - E_{13}(x)_i|^r)^{1/r}$ then $F_3(x)$ satisfies the r-normality property.

An estimate E is said to be a **mean** if it satisfies the condition [6]:

$$\min\{x_1,\dots, x_n\} \le E(x) \le \max\{x_1,\dots, x_n\}.$$

Most of the means [6] are translation additive and scale proportional estimates and they can be used for generation standardizations considered above. Below are examples of standardizations $F(x) = f(x)$, where the arithmetic mean is denoted by $\bar{x} = \dfrac{1}{n}\sum_{j=1}^{n} x_j$:

$$f_1(x)_i = x_i - \bar{x},$$

$$f_2(x)_i = x_i - MIN(x),$$

$$f_3(x)_i = \frac{x_i - \bar{x}}{\sqrt{\sum_{j=1}^{n}(x_j - \bar{x})^2}}.$$

5   Dissimilarity Measures

A **dissimilarity measure** $D(x,y)$ is a real valued function satisfying for all n-tuples x and y the properties:

$$D(x,y) = D(y,x),$$

$$D(x,y) \ge D(x,x) = 0.$$

D will be called **normalized** if it takes values in $[0,1]$.

Define dissimilarity measure by Minkowski metric and a standardization F:

$$D_{r,F}(x, y) = (\sum_{i=1}^{n}|F(x)_i - F(y)_i|^r)^{1/r}.$$

$D_{r,F}$ satisfies permutation of reflections property $D_{r,F}(-x,y) = D_{r,F}(x,-y)$ if standardization F used in Minkowski distance is an **odd function,** i.e. it satisfies: $F(-x) = -F(x)$. Standardization F_2 defined in Proposition 3 is an odd function. Standardizations F_1 and F_3 from Proposition 3 will be odd functions if the estimates E_1 and E_{13} are odd functions [3].

If U is a strictly decreasing nonnegative function such that $U(0) = 1$ then the function $SIM_D(x,y) = U(D_{r,F}(x,y))$ with odd standardizations F will be a similarity measure satisfying permutation of reflections property. The property of a weak similarity of reflections $SIM_D(-x,x) < 1$, will be fulfilled because $D_{r,F}(x,-x) > 0$ for odd standardizations F. Such $SIM_D(x,y) = U(D_{r,F}(x,y))$ can be used for generating association measures $A_{SIM,M}$ and $A_{SIM,P}$ considered in Corollary 2 and generally for A_{SIM} from Theorem 1 when t-conorm S has no nilpotent elements. For example, we can use one of the following definitions of SIM, where $D = D_{r,F}$ and C is a positive constant:

$$SIM_D(x,y) = \frac{c}{D(x,y)+c},$$

$$SIM_D(x,y) = \frac{1}{e^{D(x,y)}}.$$

Consider the method of construction of association measure $A_{SIM,L}$ from Corollary 2 by means of standardizations F_2 or F_3 from Proposition 3. If it exists some positive constant H such that $H \geq D(x,y)$ for all x,y, and W is a strictly increasing function such that $W(0) = 0$, $W(H) \leq 1$, then a similarity measure can be defined as follows:

$$SIM_D(x,y) = 1 - W(D(x,y)).$$

Such similarity measure will satisfy non-similarity of reflections property if for all n-tuples x,y the following will be fulfilled: $D(-x,x) = H \geq D(x,y)$, $H > 0$, and $W(H) = 1$. If D is normalized then one can define similarity measure by:

$$SIM_D(x,y) = 1 - D(x,y).$$

Such similarity measure satisfies non-similarity of reflections property if $D(-x,x) = 1$.

Proposition 4. Suppose $D_{r,F}(x,y)$ is a dissimilarity measure defined by Minkowski distance, F is an odd standardization satisfying r-normality and W is a strictly increasing function such that $W(0) = 0$, $W(2) = 1$, then the function:

$$A_{SIM,L}(x,y) = W(D_{r,F}(x,-y)) - W(D_{r,F}(x,y)), \tag{1}$$

defined for all $x,y \neq const$, is an association measure.

The simplest functions $W(D_{r,F}(x,y))$ considered in Proposition 4 have the form:

$$W(D_{r,F}(x,y)) = \left(\frac{D_{r,F}(x,y)}{2}\right)^p, \tag{2}$$

where p is a positive constant. For $p = 1$ we have:

$$A_{SIM,L}(x,y) = 0.5(D_{r,F}(x,-y)-D_{r,F}(x,y)).$$

For $p = r$ the association measure defined by (1), (2) has the form:

$$A_{SIM,L}(x, y) = \frac{1}{2^r}\left(\sum_{i=1}^{n}\left(|F(x)_i + F(y)_i|^r - |F(x)_i - F(y)_i|^r\right)\right).$$

Corollary 5. A shape association measure defined by (1), (2) with parameters $p=r=2$ coincides with a cosine similarity measure:

$$A_{cos,F}(x,y) = cos(F(x),F(y)).$$

Corollary 6. The shape association measure $A_{cos,F}(x,y) = cos(F(x),F(y))$ with standardization

$$f_3(x)_i = \frac{x_i - \bar{x}}{\sqrt{\sum_{j=1}^{n}\left(x_j - \bar{x}\right)^2}}$$

coincides with the sample Pearson's correlation coefficient:

$$A(x, y) = \frac{\sum_{i=1}^{n}(x_i - \bar{x})(y_i - \bar{y})}{\sqrt{\sum_{i=1}^{n}(x_i - \bar{x})^2 \cdot \sum_{i=1}^{n}(y_i - \bar{y})^2}}.$$

6   Conclusions

The paper introduces the concept of association measure in the rapidly developed area of aggregation functions. The operation of pseudo-difference associated to t-conorm S considered in the theory of aggregation functions [6] gives possibility to generalize the methods of construction of association measures considered in [3] and to propose new methods of construction of such measures. The pseudo-differences associated to t-conorms without nilpotent elements play an important part in these methods. Such t-conorms are dual to t-norms without zero devisors have been considered in the theory of t-norms [5,7]. The main results are given for a wide class of sets with a reflection operation and a suitably defined similarity measure. It gives possibility to introduce association measures on feature spaces, in fuzzy logic, on the set of fuzzy sets, etc. The obtained results can be used for generation of association measures in various application areas, for example, is time series data mining [3]. Possible extensions of considered results can be based on the methods of definition of similarity measures used for generation of association measures. These similarity measures can be given by indistinguishability operators [9], by metrics related with the Archimedian norms [10], by some shape function [8] or kernel function etc.

Acknowledgements. The work presented in the paper has been partially supported by the projects D.00507 of IMP and by PIMAyC research Program of IMP. The author is thankful to reviewers of WCSC 2013 for their comments where the first version of this paper has been accepted.

References

1. Anscombe, F.J.: Graphs in Statistical Analysis. American Statistician 27, 17–21 (1973)
2. Batyrshin, I.: Up and Down Trend Associations in Analysis of Time Series Shape Association Patterns. In: Carrasco-Ochoa, J.A., Martínez-Trinidad, J.F., Olvera López, J.A., Boyer, K.L. (eds.) MCPR 2012. LNCS, vol. 7329, pp. 246–254. Springer, Heidelberg (2012)
3. Batyrshin, I.: Constructing Time Series Shape Association Measures: Minkowski Distance and Data Standardization. In: BRICS CCI 2013, Brasil, Porto de Galhinas. IEEE Computer Society, Conference Publishing Services (CPS) (in print, 2013)
4. Batyrshin, I., Sheremetov, L., Velasco-Hernandez, J.X.: On Axiomatic Definition of Time Series Shape Association Measures. In: ORADM 2012, Workshop on Operations Research and Data Mining, Cancun, pp. 117–127 (2012)
5. Fodor, J., Roubens, M.: Fuzzy Preference Modelling and Multi-Criteria Decision Support. Kluwer, Dordrecht (1994)
6. Grabisch, M., Marichal, J.-L., Mesiar, R., Pap, E.: Aggregation Functions. Cambridge University Press, Cambridge (2009)
7. Klement, E.P., Mesiar, R., Pap, E.: Triangular Norms. Kluwer, Dordrecht (2000)
8. Mesiar, R., Spirková, J., Vavríková, L.: Weighted aggregation operators based on minimization. Information Sciences 178, 1133–1140 (2008)
9. Recasens, J.: Indistinguishability Operators. In: Recasens, J. (ed.) Indistinguishability Operators. STUDFUZZ, vol. 260, pp. 189–199. Springer, Heidelberg (2010)
10. Wagenknecht, M.: On some Relations Between Fuzzy Similarities and Metrics under Archimedian t-norms. The Journal of Fuzzy Mathematics 3, 563–572 (1995)

JT2FIS
A Java Type-2 Fuzzy Inference Systems Class Library for Building Object-Oriented Intelligent Applications

Manuel Castañón–Puga, Juan Ramón Castro,
Josué Miguel Flores–Parra, Carelia Guadalupe Gaxiola–Pacheco,
Luis-Guillermo Martínez–Méndez, and Luis Enrique Palafox–Maestre

Universidad Autónoma de Baja California,
Calzada Universidad 14418, Tijuana, BC, México. 22390
{puga,jrcastror,flores31,cgaxiola,
luisgmo,lepalafox}@uabc.edu.mx
http://www.uabc.edu.mx

Abstract. This paper introduces JT2FIS, a Java Class Library for Interval Type-2 Fuzzy Inference Systems that can be used to build intelligent object-oriented applications. The architecture of the system is presented and its object-oriented design is described. We used the water temperature and flow control as a classic example to show how to use it on engineering applications. We compared the developed library with an existing Matlab® Interval Type-2 Fuzzy Toolbox and Juzzy Toolkit in order to show the advantages of the proposed application programming interface (API) features.

Keywords: Interval Type-2 Fuzzy Inference Systems, Java Class Library, Object-Oriented Intelligent Applications.

1 Introduction

Fuzzy inference systems (FIS) have been broadly used for a wide range of engineering applications. FIS's have been applied successfully in control [1] and classification systems [2], which have been under constant improving. Their main advantage is the way they deal with imprecise information of some system variables and it allows to work with it.

Most of the FIS's models used until now are based on a Type-1 model [3], but lately, a Type-2 models have been developed and others applications have been extended with it [4]. The fuzzy system state of the art leads us to Type-2 General Fuzzy Inference Models [5] that have been developed as the next step on the way to have FIS's with more capabilities to model real-world things [6].

The purpose of this paper is to present a Java Class Library for fuzzy systems that can be used to build an Interval Type-2 Fuzzy Inference System.

F. Castro, A. Gelbukh, and M. González (Eds.): MICAI 2013, Part II, LNAI 8266, pp. 204–215, 2013.
© Springer-Verlag Berlin Heidelberg 2013

1.1   Type-2 Fuzzy Inference System

A fuzzy inference system (FIS) is based on logical rules that can work with numeric values or fuzzy inputs, these rules and individual results are evaluated together to form a fuzzy output, then, a numerical value must be passed through a process of defuzzification if necessary. Figure 1 shows a block diagram of the classic structure of a FIS.

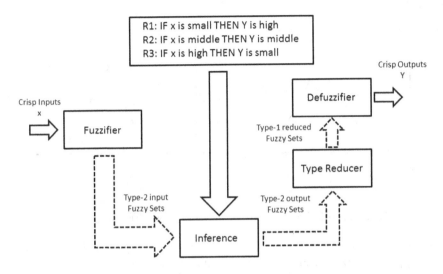

Fig. 1. Type-2 Fuzzy Inference System block diagram

The concept of a Type-2 fuzzy set was introduced by Zadeh [7] as an extension of the concept of usually type-1 fuzzy sets. A Type-2 fuzzy set is characterized by a membership function whose membership value for each element of the universe is a membership function within the range [0, 1], unlike the type-1 fuzzy sets where the value of membership is a numeric value in the range [0, 1]. The creation of a fuzzy set depends on two aspects: the identification of a universe of appropriate values and specifying a membership function properly. The choice of membership function is a subjective process, meaning that different people can reach different conclusions on the same concept. This subjectivity derives from individual differences in the perception and expression of abstract concepts and it has very little to do with randomness. Therefore, subjectivity and randomness of a fuzzy set are the main difference between the study of fuzzy sets and probability theory [8].

In type-1 fuzzy sets, once the membership function is defined for a concept, this is based on the subjective opinion of one or more individuals and shows no more than one value for each element of the universe. In doing so, it loses some of the ambiguity of the discussed concepts, especially where people may have a slightly different opinion, but they are considered valid. The Type-2 fuzzy sets allow handling linguistic and numerical uncertainties. Figure 2 depicts two graphics of fuzzy sets: a) with type-1 fuzzy logic, and b) with Type-2 fuzzy logic.

In a) the values set shown are $A = \{(x, \mu_A(x)) | x \in X\}$ where $A \subseteq X$, X $A \subseteq X$, X is the universe of valid values and $\mu_A(x)$ is the membership function (MF) that contains a map of each value of X with its membership value corresponding to a value between $[0, 1]$. For b) the values set are $\tilde{A} = \{((x, u), \mu_{\tilde{A}}(x, u))\}$, where MF $\mu_{\tilde{A}}(x, u)$ has a membership value for each element of the universe as a function of membership in the range $[0, 1]$, so the footprint can be seen around the curve of a).

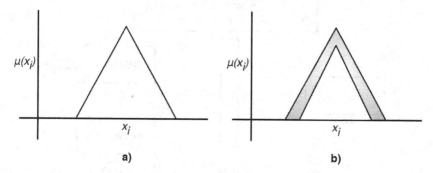

a)   b)

Fig. 2. Type-1 fuzzy set and Type-2 fuzzy set with uncertainty

1.2   Type-2 Fuzzy Inference System Applications

Concepts such as large/small or fast/slow can be represented as fuzzy sets, thus allowing slight variations in the definition of common concepts, an example of this is presented in [9]. When dealing with a fixed set of actions but with a different criteria to decide what action to take, you can use fuzzy logic as a viable option to define behavior profiles. There are many applications where fuzzy logic has been used, for example: a simulation of bird age-structured population growth based on an interval Type-2 fuzzy cellular structure [10], optimization of interval Type-2 fuzzy logic controllers using evolutionary algorithms [11], a hybrid learning algorithm for a class of interval Type-2 fuzzy neural networks [12], Type-1 and Type-2 fuzzy inference systems as integration methods in modular neural networks for multimodal biometry and its optimization with genetic algorithms [13] and face recognition with an improved interval Type-2 fuzzy logic sugeno integral and modular neural networks [14].

1.3   Object-Oriented Fuzzy Inference Systems

There are available code libraries and tool-kits to build Fuzzy Inference Systems [15]. Some of these packages are object-oriented class libraries that are developed mainly to build Type-1 Fuzzy Logic with object-oriented programming language [16]. jFuzzyLogic [17] and Juzzy [18] are examples of a class library written in Java. The advantage of a Fuzzy Inference System in Java is that we can build intelligent systems with Type-2 Fuzzy Logic capabilities using an object-oriented programming language. Java is a robust general use object-oriented programming language used in a wide range of applications.

There are already discussions about the advantages and disadvantages of using Java in scientific research [19], but the Java library becomes very important due to the convenience of reuse, legibility of coding and system portability from an engineering point of view and compared with other industrial used programming languages [20].

2   The JT2FIS Class Library

JT2FIS is a class library developed for Java. The main purpose is to deploy a library to building Type-2 fuzzy inference systems with an object-oriented programming language.

2.1   JT2FIS Design

JT2FIS is integrated by a package structure that contains all class collection. The package containment is organized and depicted in Table 1.

The library takes advantage of heritage capability of the object-oriented paradigm to integrate new membership features. Figure 3 depicts JT2FIS expressed in Unified Modeling Language (UML) and class structure JT2FIS is shown.

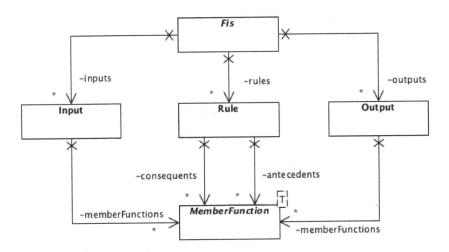

Fig. 3. JT2FIS core class structure

In JT2FIS we have a set of core Type-1 and Type-2 member functions(Gauss, Triangular, Trapezoidal). Table 2 list Type-2 member function available in the library.

Table 1. JT2FIS library packages content

fis package	FIS class		
	Mamdani class		
	Sugeno class		
defuzzifier package	Defuzzifier class		
	TypeReducer class		
fuzzifier package	Fussify class		
	PointFuzzy class		
mf package	MemberFunction class		
	type1 package	BellMemberFunction class	
		GaussMemberFunction class	
		TrapezoidalMemberFunction class	
		TriangulerMemberFunction class	
	type2 package	GaussCutMemberFunction class	
		GaussUncertaintyMeanMemberFunction class	
		GaussUncertaintyStandardDesviationMemberFunction class	
		TrapaUncertaintyMemberFunction class	
		TrapezoidalUncertaintyMemberFunction class	
		TriangulerUncertaintyMemberFunction class	
		TriUncertaintyMemberFunction class	
structure package	Input class		
	Output class		
	Rule class		
util package	LinSpace class		
	Sorter class		
	Utilities class		

Table 2. JIT2FIS Type-2 Member Functions

PackageType-2 Member Functions	Description
GaussCutMemberFunction	Params=[sigma mean alfa]
GaussUncertaintyMeanMemberFunction	Params=[sigma mean1 mean2]
GaussUncertaintyStandardDesviationMemberFunction	Params=[sigma1 sigma2 mean]
TrapaUncertaintyMemberFunction	Params=[a1 b1 c1 d1 a2 b2 c2 d2 alfa]
TrapezoidalUncertaintyMemberFunction	Params=[a d sa sd sn alfa]
TriangulerUncertaintyMemberFunction	Params=[a c sa sc]
TriUncertaintyMemberFunction	Params=[a1 b1 c1 a2 b2 c2]

The Fis class instances are composed by a set of inputs (Input class), outputs (Output class) and rules (Rule class). Each input and output contain a set of member functions (MemberFunction class) and each one could be a specific type of member function. The Fis class provides the main features of an Interval Type-2 Fuzzy Inference System. It is an abstract class that establishes the core functionality and extends to Mamdani and Sugeno concrete classes which implements different approaches.

We can start a FIS extending the `Mamdani` or `Sugeno` class. This core classes are extensions of the basic `Fis` class and `Mamdani` and `Sugeno` subclasses implements all functionality of each model respectively, but share the same interface with structural `Input`, `Output` and `Rule` classes.

Creating a new FIS Instance To build an Interval Type-2 Fuzzy Inference System with JT2FIS, first we must create an instance of `Mamdani` or `Sugeno` classes, depending of the selected model to implement. Then, we must add inputs, outputs and rules creating the corresponding objects to classes. For each input and output instances, we must add a member function that will represents a linguistic variable within the system. Member functions could be from different type, depending on the application.

Listing 1.1 shows an example of how to code a FIS with JT2FIS class library.

Listing 1.1. Object-oriented coding example

```
//Creating a new FIS instance
Mamdani fis = new Mamdani("FIS");
//Creating a new Input instance
Input input = new Input("Input");
//Creating a input member function
GaussUncertaintyMeanMemberFunction inputMF = new
    GaussUncertaintyMeanMemberFunction("InputMF");
//Adding member function to Input instance
input.getMemberFunctions().add(inputMF);
//Adding input to FIS instance
fis.getInputs().add(input);
//Etc.
...
```

The written code is full object-oriented programming style, and could be offered a better coding experience for object-oriented programmers.

3   Test Cases and Results

In order to show JT2FIS features and capabilities, on this paper we are showing three different test cases to compare JT2FIS with other Type-2 Fuzzy Logic libraries. First we going to compare JT2FIS with Matlab® Interval Type-2 Fuzzy Toolbox using Water Temperature and Flow Control Test Case. Second, we going to compate JT2FIS with Matlab® Interval Type-2 Fuzzy Toolbox and Juzzy Toolkit using Water Temperature and Flow Control Test Case Variation. Finally, we going to compare JT2FIS with Matlab® Interval Type-2 Fuzzy Toolbox and Juzzy Toolkit using Rule Sets Test Case.

3.1   Test Case 1: Comparing JT2FIS with Matlab® Interval Type-2 Fuzzy Toolbox Using Water Temperature and Flow Control Test Case

Water Temperature and Flow Controller is a proposed problem provided by Matlab® as an example to show how to use the Fuzzy Logic Toolbox. In [15] extends Matlab® Toolbox to Type-2 Fuzzy Logic, so we used this toolbox to compare our approach to it. The system implements the following set of rules (see Table 3):

Table 3. Rules example "ISHOWER"

Antecedent (IF)	Consequent (THEN)
(Temp is Cold) and (Flow is Soft)	(Cold is openSlow)(Hot is openFast)
(Temp is Cold) and (Flow is Good)	(Cold is closeSlow)(Hot is openSlow)
(Temp is Cold) and (Flow is Hard)	(Cold is closeFast)(Hot is closeSlow)
(Temp is Good) and (Flow is Soft)	(Cold is openSlow)(Hot is openSlow)
(Temp is Good) and (Flow is Good)	(Cold is Steady)(Hot is Steady)
(Temp is Good) and (Flow is Hard)	(Cold is closeSlow)(Hot is closeSlow)
(Temp is Hot) and (Flow is Soft)	(Cold is openFast)(Hot is openSlow)
(Temp is Hot) and (Flow is Good)	(Cold is openSlow)(Hot is closeSlow)
(Temp is Hot) and (Flow is Hard)	(Cold is closeSlow)(Hot is closeFast)

For Test Case 1 we configured Type-2 FISs in JT2FIS and Matlab® Interval Type-2 Fuzzy Toolbox implementations using the same parameters showed in Table 4.

Using 101 points and Centroid reduction type, we evaluate both systems implementations with the same set of input data. Table 5 shows that there's no difference between tools by obtaining the same response.

We evaluated performance by increasing the number of discretizations points in order to increment complexity of processing inputs and outputs (fuzzing and de-fuzzing).

Table 6 showed that JT2FIS is faster than Matlab® Interval Type-2 Fuzzy Logic Toolbox.

3.2   Test Case 2: Comparing JT2FIS with Matlab® Interval Type-2 Fuzzy Toolbox and Juzzy Toolkit using Water Temperature and Flow Control Test Case Variation

[18] introduced Juzzy, a Java based Toolkit for Type-2 Fuzzy Logic. To compare the JT2FIS with Juzzy Toolkit we used a Water Temperature and Flow Controller test variation. The use of this Toolkit is to compare Matlab® Interval Type-2 Fuzzy Toolbox and our approach to it. For Test Case 2 we configured Type-2 Fuzzy Inference Systems in JT2FIS, Matlab® Interval Type-2 Fuzzy

Table 4. Inputs, Outputs example "ISHOWER"

Type	MemberFunction	Params
Input1	TrapaUncertaintyMemberFunction	a1=-31,b1=-31,c1=-16,d1=-1, a2=-29,b2=-29,c2=-14,d2=1.0,alfa=0.98
Input1	TriUncertaintyMemberFunction	a1=-11,b1=-1,c1=9,a2=-9,b2=1,c2=11
Input1	TrapaUncertaintyMemberFunction	a1=-1,b1=14,c1=29,d1=29, a2=1,b2=16,c2=31,d2=31,alfa=0.98
Input2	TrapaUncertaintyMemberFunction	a1=-3.1,b1=-3.1,c1=-0.9,d1=-0.1, a2=-2.9,b2=-2.9,c2=-0.7,d2=0.1,alfa=0.98
Input2	TriUncertaintyMemberFunction	a1=-0.45,b1=-0.05,c1=0.35,a2=-0.35,b2=0.05,c2=0.45
Input2	TrapaUncertaintyMemberFunction	a1=-0.1,b1=0.7,c1=2.9,d1=0.1, a2=0.9,b2=3.1,c2=3.1,d2=0.1,alfa=0.98
Output1	TriUncertaintyMemberFunction	a1=-1.05,b1=-0.65,c1=-0.35,a2=-0.95,b2=-0.55,c2=-0.25
Output1	TriUncertaintyMemberFunction	a1=-0.65,b1=-0.35,c1=-0.05,a2=-0.55,b2=-0.25,c2=0.05
Output1	TriUncertaintyMemberFunction	a1=-0.35,b1=-0.05,c1=0.25,a2=-0.25,b2=0.05,c2=0.35
Output1	TriUncertaintyMemberFunction	a1=-0.05,b1=0.25,c1=0.55,a2=0.05,b2=0.35,c2=0.65
Output1	TriUncertaintyMemberFunction	a1=0.25,b1=0.55,c1=0.95,a2=0.35,b2=0.65,c2=1.05
Output2	TriUncertaintyMemberFunction	a1=-1.05,b1=-0.65,c1=-0.35,a2=-0.95,b2=-0.55,c2=-0.25
Output2	TriUncertaintyMemberFunction	a1=-0.65,b1=-0.35,c1=-0.05,a2=-0.55,b2=-0.25,c2=0.05
Output2	TriUncertaintyMemberFunction	a1=-0.35,b1=-0.05,c1=0.25,a2=-0.25,b2=0.05,c2=0.35
Output2	TriUncertaintyMemberFunction	a1=-0.05,b1=0.25,c1=0.55,a2=0.05,b2=0.35,c2=0.65
Output2	TriUncertaintyMemberFunction	a1=0.25,b1=0.55,c1=0.95,a2=0.35,b2=0.65,c2=1.05

Table 5. Comparing JT2FIS outputs versus Matlab$^{\circledR}$ Interval Type-2 Fuzzy Logic Toolbox outputs

Inputs		JT2FIS			Interval Type-2 Fuzzy Logic Toolbox		
x1	x2	Output 1	Output 2	Time(ms)	Output 1	Output 2	Time(ms)
-16	-0.8	0.3	0.6328	1.24	0.3	0.6328	8.6
-12	-0.6	0.3	0.6342	1.24	0.3	0.6342	8.6
-8	-0.4	0.2211	0.5184	1.24	0.2211	0.5184	8.6
-4	-0.2	-0.0098	0.2545	1.24	-0.0098	0.2545	8.6
0	0	0	0	1.24	0	0	8.6
4	0.2	0.0098	-0.2545	1.24	0.0098	-0.2545	8.6
8	0.4	-0.22113	-0.5184	1.24	-0.22113	-0.5184	8.6
12	0.6	-0.2999	-0.6342	1.24	-0.2999	-0.6342	8.6
16	0.8	-0.3	-0.6328	1.24	-0.3	-0.6328	8.6
20	1	-0.3	-0.6328	1.24	-0.3	-0.6328	8.6

Toolbox and Juzzy Toolkit implementations using the same parameters showed in Table 7. The Juzzy Toolkit does not have an available Gaussian type member function for the Type-2 systems, so we used the new configuration for all systems using "Triangular with Uncertainty" member functions.

Table 6. Comparing JT2FIS times(ms) versus Matlab® Interval Type-2 Fuzzy Logic Toolbox times(ms) with different discretizations points for input1=20 and input2=1

Number Points	JT2FIS Time(ms)	Interval Type-2 Fuzzy Logic Toolbox Time(ms)
101	1.24	8.6
1001	4.96	13.7
10001	45.42	71.2

Table 7. Inputs, Outputs example "ISHOWER" Trianguler

Type	MemberFunction	Params
Input1	TriUncertaintyMemberFunctionn	a1=-20.0,b1=-20.0,c1=1.06,a2=-20.0,b2=-20.0,c2=-1.0
Input1	TriUncertaintyMemberFunction	a1=-11.0,b1=0.0,c1=11.0,a2=-9.0,b2=0.0,c2=9.0
Input1	TriUncertaintyMemberFunction	a1=-1.0,b1=20.0,c1=20.0,a2=1.0,b2=20.0,c2=20.0
Input2	TriUncertaintyMemberFunction	a1=-1.0,b1=-1.0,c1=0.1,a2=-1.0,b2=-1.0,c2=-0.1
Input2	TriUncertaintyMemberFunction	a1=-0.5,b1=-0.0,c1=0.5,a2=-0.3,b2=0.0,c2=0.3
Input2	TriUncertaintyMemberFunction	a1=-0.1,b1=1.0,c1=1.0,a2=0.1,b2=1.0,c2=1.0
Output1	TriUncertaintyMemberFunction	a1=-1.05,b1=-0.6,c1=-0.25,a2=-0.95,b2=-0.6,c2=-0.35
Output1	TriUncertaintyMemberFunction	a1=-0.65,b1=-0.3,c1=0.05,a2=-0.55,b2=-0.3,c2=-0.05
Output1	TriUncertaintyMemberFunction	a1=-0.35,b1=0.0,c1=0.35,a2=-0.25,b2=0.0,c2=0.25
Output1	TriUncertaintyMemberFunction	a1=-0.05,b1=0.3,c1=0.65,a2=0.05,b2=0.3,c2=0.55
Output1	TriUncertaintyMemberFunction	a1=0.25,b1=0.6,c1=1.05,a2=0.35,b2=0.6,c2=0.95
Output2	TriUncertaintyMemberFunction	a1=-1.05,b1=-0.6,c1=-0.25,a2=-0.95,b2=-0.6,c2=-0.35
Output2	TriUncertaintyMemberFunction	a1=-0.65,b1=-0.35,c1=-0.05,a2=-0.55,b2=-0.25,c2=0.05
Output2	TriUncertaintyMemberFunction	a1=-0.35,b1=0.0,c1=0.35,a2=-0.25,b2=0.0,c2=0.25
Output2	TriUncertaintyMemberFunction	a1=-0.05,b1=0.3,c1=0.65,a2=0.05,b2=0.3,c2=0.55
Output2	TriUncertaintyMemberFunction	a1=0.25,b1=0.6,c1=1.05,a2=0.35,b2=0.6,c2=0.95

Using 101 points and Centroid reduction type, we evaluate all system implementations with the same set of input data. Table 8 shows no difference between JT2FIS and Matlab® Interval Type-2 Fuzzy Toolbox tools, obtaining the same response, but we noticed little differences between JT2FIS and Juzzy Toolkit.

We evaluated performance by increasing the number of discretizations points in order to increase complexity of processing inputs and outputs (fuzzing and defuzzing). Table 9 shows that Juzzy Toolkit is faster than JT2FIS and Matlab® Interval Type-2 Fuzzy Logic Toolbox.

3.3   Test Case 3: Comparing JT2FIS with Matlab® Interval Type-2 Fuzzy Toolbox and Juzzy Toolkit Using Rule Sets Test Case

Alternatively, to compare performance between JT2FIS, Matlab® Interval Type-2 Fuzzy Toolbox and Juzzy Toolkit we used the rule set to configure and test inference systems, increasing the number of rules on each test in order to increment complexity on processing rules.

Table 8. Comparing JT2FIS outputs versus Matlab® Interval Type-2 Fuzzy Logic Toolbox outputs y Juzzy Toolkit

Inputs		JT2FIS			Interval Type-2 Fuzzy Logic Toolbox			Juzzy Toolkit		
x1	x2	Output 1	Output 2	Time(ms)	Output 1	Output 2	Time(ms)	Output 1	Output 2	Time(ms)
-16	-0.8	0.3	0.6336	1.24	0.3	0.6336	8.6	0.2999	0.6346	0.67
-12	-0.6	0.3	0.6363	1.24	0.3	0.6363	8.6	0.2999	0.6374	0.67
-8	-0.4	0.1822	0.4890	1.24	0.1822	0.4890	8.6	0.1824	0.4905	0.67
-4	-0.2	-0.0052	0.2337	1.24	-0.0052	0.2337	8.6	-0.0053	0.2356	0.67
0	0	-3.4694E-17	-3.4694E-17	1.24	-3.4694E-17	-3.4694E-17	8.6	-5.5511E-17	-5.5511E-17	0.67
4	0.2	0.0052	-0.2337	1.24	0.0052	-0.2337	8.6	0.0053	-0.2356	0.67
8	0.4	-0.1822	-0.4890	1.24	-0.1822	-0.4890	8.6	-0.1824	-0.4905	0.67
12	0.6	-0.2999	-0.6363	1.24	-0.2999	-0.6363	8.6	-0.2999	-0.6374	0.67
16	0.8	-0.3	-0.6336	1.24	-0.3	-0.6336	8.6	-0.2999	-0.6346	0.67
20	1	-0.3	-0.6324	1.24	-0.3	-0.6324	8.6	-0.2999	-0.6334	0.67

Table 9. Comparing JT2FIS times(ms) versus Matlab® Interval Type-2 Fuzzy Logic Toolbox times(ms) and Juzzy Toolkit times(ms) with different discretizations points for input1=20 and input2=1

Number Points	JT2FIS Time(ms)	Interval Type-2 Fuzzy Logic Toolbox Time(ms)	Juzzy Toolkit Time(ms)
101	1.24	8.6	0.67
1001	4.96	13.7	1.23
10001	45.42	71.2	8.48

Table 10. Inputs, Outputs example "ISHOWER" Trianguler

Type	MemberFunction	Params
Input1	GaussUncertaintyStandardDesviationMemberFunction	deviation1=0.1623, deviation2=0.2623 mean=0.0
Input1	GaussUncertaintyStandardDesviationMemberFunction	deviation1=0.1623, deviation2=0.2623 mean=0.5
Input1	GaussUncertaintyStandardDesviationMemberFunction	deviation1=0.1623, deviation2=0.2623 mean=1.0
Output1	TriUncertaintyMemberFunction	a1=-0.5833,b1=-0.08333,c1=0.4167,a2=-0.4167,b2=-0.08333,c2=0.5833
Output1	TriUncertaintyMemberFunction	a1=-0.08333,b1=0.4167,c1=0.9167,a2=0.08333,b2=0.4167,c2=1.083
Output1	TriUncertaintyMemberFunction	a1=0.4167,b1=0.9167,c1=1.417,a2=0.5833,b2=0.9167,c2=1.583

Using 101 points and Centroid reduction type, we evaluate all system implementations with different rule sets.

Table 11 shows significant differences between JT2FIS, Matlab® Interval Type-2 Fuzzy Toolbox and Juzzy Toolkit. JT2FIS showed better performance when the rule set was increased.

Table 11. Comparing JT2FIS times(ms) versus Matlab® Interval Type-2 Fuzzy Logic Toolbox times(ms) and Juzzy Toolkit times(ms) with different number of rules for input1=20 and input2=1

Number Inputs	Number Rules	JT2FIS Time(ms)	Interval Type-2 Fuzzy Logic Toolbox Time(ms)	Juzzy Toolkit Time(ms)
2	9	0.72	4	0.74
3	27	1.09	5.5	2.03
4	81	1.95	10	10.77
5	243	5.807	30	148.19
6	729	16.44	70	3621.2

4   Conclusions and Future Work

JT2FIS is an object-oriented class library that can be used to build intelligent applications based on type-2 fuzzy systems. We presented an architecture of an object oriented design. We compared outputs response between JT2FIS, Matlab® Interval Type-2 Fuzzy Toolbox and Juzzy Toolkit in order to validate robustness and performance.

The proposed class library are prospected to cover the need of a type-2 fuzzy system library in Java. Matlab® Interval Type-2 Fuzzy Logic Toolbox have been traditionally used in research, but has been difficult to transfer some designs and implementations from Matlab® to commercial applications. In other hand, Java is a very used programming language by academics and professionals, and are fully accepted by software industry due the convenience of reuse, legibility of coding and system portability.

As a future work, first, we will continue adding features to the library and re-factoring the code in order to improve performance and usability. Finally, we are planning to extend the JT2FIS capabilities to Generalized Type-2 Fuzzy Inference Systems.

Acknowledgment. The work was partially supported by the Internal Fund for Research Projects (Grant No. 300.6.C.62.15 and 300.6.C.135.17) of the Autonomous University of Baja California, México.

References

1. Castillo, O., Melin, P.: A review on the design and optimization of interval type-2 fuzzy controllers. Appl. Soft Comput. 12(4), 1267–1278 (2012)
2. Melin, P., Olivas, F., Castillo, O., Valdez, F., Soria, J., García-Valdez, J.: Optimal design of fuzzy classification systems using pso with dynamic parameter adaptation through fuzzy logic. Expert Syst. Appl. 40(8), 3196–3206 (2013)
3. Zadeh, L.: The concept of a linguistic variable and its application to approximate reasoning. Information Science 8(3), 199–249 (1975)

4. Zadeh, L.: Outline of a new approach to the analysis of complex systems and decision processes. IEEE Transactions on Systems, Man, and Cybernetics 3(1), 28–44 (1973)
5. Lucas, L., Centeno, T., Delgado, M.: General type-2 fuzzy inference systems: Analysis, design and computational aspects. In: Fuzzy Systems Conference, pp. 1–6. IEEE Press (2007)
6. Castillo, O., Melin, P., Castro, J.: Computational intelligence software for interval type2 fuzzy logic. Journal Computer Applications in Engineering Education, 1–7 (2010)
7. Zadeh, L.: Fuzzy Sets. Information and Control 8, 338–353 (1965)
8. Jang, J., Sun, C., Mizutani, E.: Neuro-Fuzzy and Soft Computing: A Computational Approach to Learning and Machine Intelligence. MATLAB Curriculum Series. Prentice Hall (1997)
9. Wagner, C., Hagras, H.: Fuzzy composite concepts based on human reasoning. In: IEEE International Conference on Information Reuse and Integration. IEEE Press, Las Vegas (2010)
10. Leal-Ramírez, C., Castillo, O., Melin, P., Rodríguez-Díaz, A.: Simulation of the bird age-structured population growth based on an interval type-2 fuzzy cellular structure. Information Sciences 181(3), 519–535 (2011)
11. Castillo, O., Melin, P., Alanis, A., Montiel, O., Sepulveda, R.: Optimization of interval type-2 fuzzy logic controllers using evolutionary algorithms. Soft Computing 15(6), 1145–1160 (2011)
12. Castro, J., Castillo, O., Melin, P., Rodríguez-Díaz, A.: A hybrid learning algorithm for a class of interval type-2 fuzzy neural networks. Information Sciences 179(13), 2175–2193 (2009)
13. Hidalgo, D., Castillo, O., Melin, P.: Type-1 and type-2 fuzzy inference systems as integration methods in modular neural networks for multimodal biometry and its optimization with genetic algorithms. Information Sciences 179(13), 2123–2145 (2009)
14. Melin, P., Mendoza, O., Castillo, O.: Face recognition with an improved interval type-2 fuzzy logic sugeno integral and modular neural networks. IEEE Transactions on Systems, Man, and Cybernetics 41(5), 1001–1012 (2011)
15. Castro, J., Castillo, O., Martínez, L.: Interval type-2 fuzzy logic toolbox. Engineering Letters 1 (2007)
16. García-Valdez, M., Licea-Sandoval, G., Alaníz-Garza, A., Castillo, O.: Object oriented design and implementation of an inference engine for fuzzy systems. Engineering Notes 15(1) (2007)
17. Cingolani, P., Alcala-Fdez, J.: jfuzzylogic: a robust and flexible fuzzy-logic inference system language implementation. In: 2012 IEEE International Conference on Fuzzy Systems, pp. 1–8 (2012)
18. Wagner, C.: Juzzy a java based toolkit for type-2 fuzzy logic. In: Proceedings of the IEEE Symposium Series on Computational Intelligence, Singapore (2013)
19. Gudenberg, J.: Java for scientific computing, pros and cons. Journal of Universal Computer Science 4(1), 11–15 (1998)
20. Stein, M., Geyer-Schulz, A.: A comparison of five programming languages in a graph clustering scenario. Journal of Universal Computer Science 19(3), 428–456 (2013)

Fault Detection and Diagnosis of Electrical Networks Using a Fuzzy System and Euclidian Distance

César Octavio Hernández Morales[*] and Juan Pablo Nieto González

Corporación Mexicana de Investigación en Materiales S.A. de C.V. (COMIMSA),
Ciencia y Tecnología No. 790, Fracc. Saltillo 400, C.P. 25290
Saltillo, Coahuila, México
{cesarhdz,juan.nieto}@comimsa.com

Abstract. In this work a diagnosis system for an electrical network is proposed. The approach carries out the monitoring of an electrical system with dynamical load changes proposed by the IEEE. The framework is composed by two phases. The detection phase which uses a fuzzy system, and the diagnosis phase that computes the Euclidean distances between samples in order to identify a pattern on the system's elements. The proposal is able to diagnose asymmetrical electrical faults. Promissory results of the proposal are shown.

Keywords: Fault Detection, Diagnosis, Electrical Networks, Fuzzy System and Euclidian Distance.

1   Introduction

The fault detection and diagnosis field is taking an important role in many industrial areas in which engineering is involved. This is due to the complex systems that industries have today working on their processes. This complexity is given by the presence of a lot of variables taking part of a process or system being monitored. Thus, the identification of abnormal operation conditions in a system or a process is needed. An alternative solution to the monitoring task of a lot of variables, is that the implementation of intelligent models are used to make faster diagnosis when a fault is present and to make more precise systems that diminish the presence of false alarms. Avoiding in this way the economic losses and preventing the risk to the operators working on dangerous processes. Thus, the aim of this paper is to generate a system for fault detection and diagnosis of a complex system that helps the operators to quickly identify a fault presence and the location of it. In this paper a methodology has been proposed to diagnose an electrical power system with dynamical load changes that uses historical data of the process to carry out a fault detection and diagnosis. The framework proposed is composed by two steps. The first step uses a fuzzy logic system to do the fault detection and the second step gives the final diagnosis measuring the Euclidean distance between the voltages of the lines for each node. These steps are done to

---

[*] Corresponding author.

F. Castro, A. Gelbukh, and M. González (Eds.): MICAI 2013, Part II, LNAI 8266, pp. 216–224, 2013.
© Springer-Verlag Berlin Heidelberg 2013

obtain a more robust and accurate monitoring system diminishing the presence of false alarms in the final diagnosis.

2   State of the Art

Since the beginning of the use of the machines, the need to monitor if they are working properly has been a common task. In this way some important concepts related to this field have been appeared. For instance, a fault is defined as a not allowed deviation by at least one property, characteristic or parameter to acceptable conditions, usual or normal operation of a system. Fault detection is to determine when a fault is present on a system. Fault isolation is to determine the type and location of a fault. Fault identification is to determine the size and variation in time of a fault. Finally, fault diagnosis is to determine the type, size, location and time of detection. Finally, the system is intervened to recover its normal operation[1]. According to [2], figure 1 shows the detection and diagnosis general methodology employed.

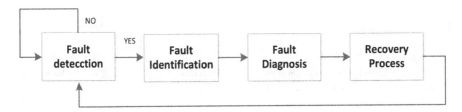

Fig. 1. Process monitoring system (Adapted from [2])

Once exposed the basic concepts in the field of fault detection and diagnosis, the classification of the general methods is presented. Until now, researchers have addressed the problem of faults detection in different ways. [3] and [4] classifies the detection methods in three different categories. Quantitative models that make use of mathematical models, qualitative models which perform detection using graph theory and partially mathematical models of the system and finally models that make use of historical data to carry out a complete monitoring system. Another point of view are the models described by [2], which describes the processes as invasive. For instance those taking into account large linear systems that are often incorporated into the system or process and as non-invasive such as those requiring data drive to detect if the system is in faulty mode. In this same way, it characterizes as rigid models those which depend directly on a mathematical model and the flexible models those that make use of historical data. The use of these flexible models sometimes is more feasible because there are applications where it is not possible to mathematically model the dynamics of the system. This could happen even when the monitoring system designer has much experience or know very well the process. Additionally it has been shown that flexible models can work complementing mathematical models [5] since most of today's systems try to emulate the human behavior.

The methods based on historical data of the process, are widely used nowadays in most of the processes or systems due to its simplicity and efficiency [5]. In the particular case of electrical systems, the soft computing techniques such as: fuzzy logic, artificial neural networks, probabilistic reasoning and evolutionary algorithms are employed as classifiers. [6] uses fuzzy logic to do the fault detection process in real time on a fuel injection system in a diesel engine. [7] proposes a control level system of three tanks with the use of signals from various sensors. The main objective of this system is to detect abnormal signals from these sensors, using fuzzy logic to carry out fault detection and the diagnosis phase evaluates the data measurement provided. This evaluation is done with the purpose of provide a robust system. Euclidean distances are used as in [8] and [9]. The former applies decision rules at the photolithography stage in the manufacturing process of an integrated circuit. The second calculates the distances in a study case related with semiconductors in order to give the fault diagnosis.

3　Preliminaries

3.1　Fuzzy Logic

Fuzzy logic systems are based on if-then rules that capture the experts' knowledge. Each rule is an instruction represented in mathematical language. On it, the words are characterized by membership functions such as those described below.

- Membership Functions

The membership functions fuzzify data. That is to defined a fuzzy set A on a universe of discourse X of the form $\mu_A: X \rightarrow [0,1]$, Taking the máximum value of $\mu_A(x)=1$ and mínimum value $\mu_A(x)=0$. A membership function allows to represent graphically a fuzzy set.

$$\mu_{A(x)} = \begin{cases} 0 & \text{si } x < a \\ \dfrac{x-a}{m-a} & \text{si } a < x \leq m \\ \dfrac{b-a}{b-m} & \text{si } a < x < m \\ 0 & \text{si } x \geq b \end{cases} \tag{1}$$

Where a is defined as the lorwer value, b is the higher value and m is mean value, x is any input value in the membership functions.

- Fuzzy Operators

Fuzzy operators are applied to do basic operations with fuzzy sets. The basic operators for complement, union, and intersection are defined as:
The complement:

$$\mu_{\bar{A}(x)} = 1 - \mu_{A(x)} \tag{2}$$

The union or t-norm:

$$\mu_{A \cup B_{(x)}} = \max \left[\mu_{A(x)}, \mu_{B(x)} \right] \tag{3}$$

The intersection or s-norm:

$$\mu_{A \cap B_{(x)}} = \min \left[\mu_{A(x)}, \mu_{B(x)} \right] \tag{4}$$

- Fuzzy Implications

The output of fuzzy the system is represented by a membership value which needs to be transformed onto a crisp number. To perform this transformation is required a fuzzifier such as: centroid defuzzfier.

$$\mu_{MM}(x, y) = \min \left[\mu_{FP_1}(x), \mu_{FP_2}(y) \right] \tag{5}$$

or

$$\mu_{MP}(x, y) = \mu_{FP_1}(x) * \mu_{FP_2}(y) \tag{6}$$

- Defuzzification

To get a solution to a decision problem, the obtention of a crisp number is required in order to no use a fuzzy output. Therefore, this fuzzy output is transformed using the centroid method [10].

$$g = \frac{\sum_{1=1}^{n} x_i . u(x_i)}{\sum_{1=1}^{n} u(x_i)} \tag{7}$$

3.2   Euclidean Distance

Euclidean distance is defined as the ordinary distance between two points that is deduced with the Pythagorean Theorem. This is using a bidimentional space, to obtain the distance between two points P1 y P2, in coordinates (x_1, y_1) and (x_2, y_2) respectively, is [11]:

$$d_e(P_1, P_2) = \sqrt{(x_2 - x_1)^2 + (y_2 - y_1)^2} \tag{8}$$

4   Framework Description

In this paper it is proposed the implementation of a new methodology described in Figure 2 in order to perform the detection and diagnosis of an electrical power system proposed by the IEEE. The methodology consists of two steps. The first step is the detection process in which it is used fuzzy logic to perform the task of evaluating the operating conditions of the system. The second step gives the final diagnosis measuring the Euclidean distances in order to obtain a normal operation pattern between the voltages of each of the 24 nodes of the system. Thus, when a fault is present it determines which of the lines have the problem.

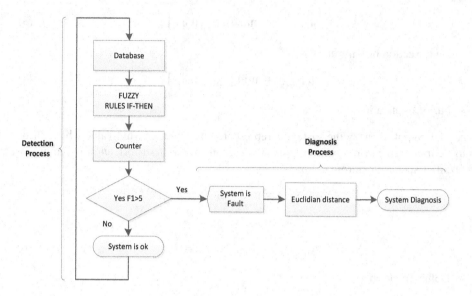

Fig. 2. General fault detection and diagnosis framework of the proposal

The steps of the proposal are summarized as follows:

1. To obtain the system's databases in normal operation and faulty mode.
2. To generate a fuzzy system that evaluates each system's nodes whose output will be a zero for a node of the monitored system when it is found in faulty mode otherwise it will give a nonzero value.
3. To count the number of consecutives zero's output of the fuzzy system for a specific node to determine whether the system is faulty or not.
4. If the system has a faulty node(s) then measure the Euclidean distances between the voltages of the lines of each suspicious node(s) of the system.
5. To perform a comparison of the distances obtained on step 4 against those of the normal operation voltages' distances magnitudes in order to give the final diagnosis showing which line(s) is in faulty mode.

5   Case Study

This work is addressed to analyze an electrical power system with dynamic load changes proposed by the IEEE. This system consists of 24 nodes with 3 lines each. Given in this way a total of 72 variables to monitor. The electrical system is depicted in Figure 3.

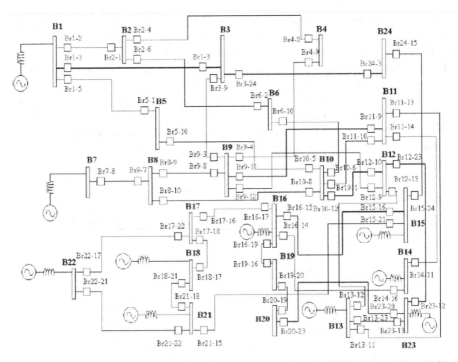

Fig. 3. Reliability test system single line diagram proposed by the IEEE (Adapted from [12])

The fuzzy system model was trained with the samples of only one of the nodes of the original system. This represents a great advantage because it was not needed to design and to train 24 different fuzzy systems in order to monitor each bus of the original electrical power system. For the simulations it was considered two fault types. Symmetrical faults that occurs between two lines and asymmetrical faults occurring   when one or more lines fall to ground.

The proposed methodology was applied in the following manner.

The first step is the detection process and is composed by the blocks shown in Figure 4. Each block performs as follows:

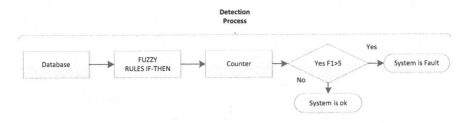

Fig. 4. Fault Detection step

1. The Database block indicates that it is needed the acquisition and analysis of historical data from the electrical power system described above. This analysis was

performed evaluating the amplitudes of the voltages of each node's lines taking data windows of 100 samples using normal operation and faulty databases.

2. In the Fuzzy Rules block are contained the steps 2 to 6

3. In this block the selection of a membership function is needed. In this case it was selected triangular functions due to their simplicity.

4. Additionally with the databases taken on step 1, the fuzzy rules describing the system's behavior were generated. These rules are shown on table 1.

5. The fuzzy operators and fuzzy implication were selected as those depicted on equations 2 to 6. This selection was made because the use of these operators and implications were enough to explain relatively well the behavior of the system.

Table 1. Fuzzy rules

Rule	Line 1	Line 2	Line 3	Fault
1	More	Less	More	No
2	More	Less	Less	No
3	More	More	Less	No
4	Less	More	More	No
5	Less	Less	More	No
6	Less	More	Less	No
7	More	More	More	Yes
8	Less	Less	Less	Yes
9	Zero	Zero	Zero	Yes

The range considered for the amplitudes of the voltages observed in each line was from -200 to 200 volts.

6. It has been selected the centroid method to carry out the defuzzification step described in Eq. 7. because this is the most commonly method used.

7. The output of the fuzzy system will be a zero if the system is found on a faulty mode and otherwise it will give a nonzero output.

8. The counter block contains a counter that is adjusted by the user in order to give sensibility to the detection process. The counter increments in one its counting when there exist consecutive zeroes given by the fuzzy system.

9. Several tests have been carried out and there were found the results showing on table 2. This table shows the percentage of detection obtained for different preset values of the counter.

Table 2. Percentage of detection for different counter preset values

Counter	F1=3	F1=4	F1=5
Porcentage	80%	100%	100%

For the second step the diagnosis process is carried out as described below and this process is shown in Figure 5.

After analyzed the operating conditions of the system for the possible different faults that could be present, the relationship founded for the Euclidean distances measured gives the different possible faults signature. These relationships are described below.

One line to ground fault.

If when comparing the distances between L1-L2-L3, those of L2-L3 are equal values, then the fault is present on line L1. If those of L1-L3 are equal values, then the fault is present on line L2. And in the same way if the distances between L1-L2 are equal values then the fault is present on line L3.

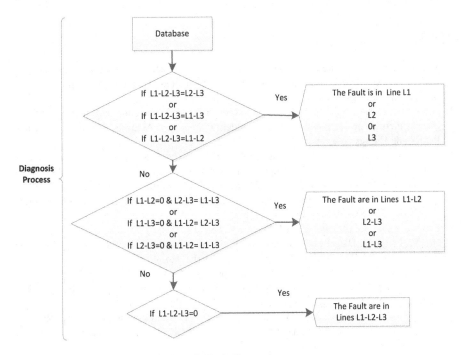

Fig. 5. Fault diagnosis step

Two lines to ground fault.

If the distances between L1-L2 are equal to zero, and L2-L3, L1-L3 are equal, the fault is present in the lines L1 and L2. If the distances between L1-L3 are equal to zero, and L1-L2, L2-L3 are equal, the fault is present in the lines L1 and L3. Or, If the distances between L2-L3 are equal to zero, and L1-L2, L1-L3 are equal, the fault is present in the lines L2 and L3.

Three lines to ground fault.

If the distances between the three lines L1-L2-L3 are zero then the type of fault present is a three lines to ground fault.

Thus, as it can be seen the comparison carried out in the second step of the proposal, determines which line has the asymmetrical fault present on it.

6   Conclusion

This paper has proposed a fault detection and diagnosis system that uses a fuzzy logic system for the detection process and a comparison of the measured Euclidean distances between the voltages magnitude of an electrical power system to give the final diagnosis. The proposal is a process history data based method. This approach was validated in an electrical power system of 24 nodes having dynamic load changes proposed by the IEEE. This work was done with the purpose to give a robust methodology using these two techniques for a safer detection and diagnosis.

References

1. Valenzuela, J.C.R.: Diagnóstico de fallos en sistemas industriales basado en razonamiento borroso y posibilístico, Universidad politécnica de valencia Departamento de Ingeniería de Sistemas y Automática (2007)
2. Ajami, A., Daneshvar, M.: Data driven approach for fault detection and diagnosis of turbine in thermal power plant using Independent Component Analysis (ICA). In: Electrical Power and Energy Systems, pp. 728–735 (2012)
3. Venkatasubramanian, V., Rengaswamy, R., Yin, K., Kavuri, S.: A review of process fault detection and diagnosis Part I. Computers and Chemical Engineering 27, 293–311 (2003)
4. Nieto González, J.P., Castañón, L.G., Menéndez, R.M.: Multiple Fault Diagnosis in Electrical Power Systems with Dynamic Load Changes Using Probabilistic Neural Networks. Computación y Sistemas 14(1), 17–30 (2010)
5. Cox, E.: Fuzzy fundlmentals. IEEE Spectrum, 58–61 (2002)
6. He, Y., Feng, L.: Diesel Fuel Injection System Faults Diagnosis Based on Fuzzy Injection Pressure Pattern Recognition. In: Proceedings of the 5th World Congress on Intelligent Control and Automation, June 15-19. Hangzhou, P.R., China, pp. 1654–1657 (2004)
7. Lu, S.P.: Signal Processing and Fuzzy Cluster Based Online Fault Diagnosis. In: IEEE Eurocon 2009. IEEE Conference Publications, pp. 1454–1459 (2009)
8. Verdier, G., Ferreira, A.: Adaptive Mahalanobis Distance and k-Nearest Neighbor Rule for Fault Detection in Semiconductor Manufacturing. IEEE Transactions on Semiconductor Manufacturing 24(1), 59–67 (2011)
9. Luo, M., Zheng, Y., Liu, S.: Data-based Fault-tolerant Control of the Semiconductor Manufacturing Process based on K-Nearest Neighbor Nonparametric Regression. In: Proceedings of the 10th World Congress on Intelligent Control and Automation, pp. 3008–3012 (2012)
10. Wang, L.-X.: A course in fuzzy systems and control, 2nd edn. Prentice-Hall International Inc. (1997) ISBN 0-13-540882-2
11. Deza, E., Deza, M.M.: Encyclopedia of Distances, p. 94. Springer (2009)
12. Nieto González, J.P.: Complex Systems Fault Diagnosis Using Soft Computing and Statistical Methods. In: Instituto Tecnológico y de Estudios Superiores de Moterrey Campus Monterrey, Escuela de Ingeniería y Tecnologías de Información (2012)

An Embedded Fuzzy Agent for Online Tuning of a PID Controller for Position Control of a DC Motor

Luis A. Alvarado-Yañez, Luis M. Torres-Treviño, and Angel Rodríguez-Liñán

Universidad Autónoma de Nuevo León, FIME Avenida Universidad S/N Ciudad Universitaria, 66451, San Nicolás de los Garza, Nuevo León, México

Abstract. The aim of the presented work is to illustrate the performance of embedded fuzzy agent for online tuning of a PID controller. A DC motor is used for illustration of its position control. An agent is built using an embedded fuzzy system type 1. Performance of the PID controller is evaluated on line and this performance is improved in low cycles of tuning by the agent.

1 Introduction

1.1 Pid Control Systems

Nowadays, there is an existing problem generalized with the tuning of PID control systems, which generally are set through the developer's experience, which means, that the gains are set in an heuristic way.

The PID schemes, based in the classic control theory, have been widely used in the control industry for a long time. So, in order to improve the control quality, developers use the nonlinear characteristics to modify the traditional PID control[3,4].

The integral square error, is more effective for considerable error than with minimum errors, it tends to eliminate them in a prompt way, even though the initial response overshoots, this one decays rapidly. Basically, various small peaks are tolerated for reducing the magnitude of the principal peak. This type of behavior is usually non desire in the process, whereby a gains optimization is a desired process in the controller's tuning[7].

1.2 Fuzzy Logic in PID Control Systems

The most common control algorithm in the industry is the PID control, it has a simple structure, good reliability and is easy to adjust, reason why it has been widely used. In order for the PID control to enter in a complex environment of parameters adjustment, intelligent PID control arises at the historic moment.

The most common intelligent PID control methods are: fuzzy PID control, neural network PID control, genetic algorithm PID control and so on, but the

F. Castro, A. Gelbukh, and M. González (Eds.): MICAI 2013, Part II, LNAI 8266, pp. 225–232, 2013.
© Springer-Verlag Berlin Heidelberg 2013

most common is fuzzy PID control[2]. However, for the velocity control generally is used a conventional PID[1].

Fuzzy tuning of PID control is the outcome combination of the fuzzy theory, the fuzzy technology and PID control algorithm. The fuzzy tuning system of the flexible adaptable advantage with PID control structure, which are simple high control's accuracy characteristics[6].

Fuzzy Logic control (FLC) has proven effectiveness for complex non-linear and imprecisely processes, for which standard model based control techniques are impractical or impossible. Fuzzy Logic, deals with problems that have vagueness, uncertainty and use membership functions [5]. Below in Figure 1 is the structure of a fuzzy tuning of PID control model:

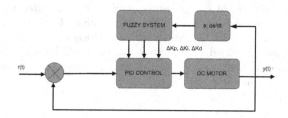

Fig. 1. Block diagram of fuzzy tuning and PID controller

The traditional PID algorithm, for a control non linear system is not easy for adjusting the control parameters and the online settings. For this type of problems, is better to use the fuzzy control theory which has a great ability and processing power. The traditional PID control, through the regulation of the control PID parameters, reaches the stability of the system, in order for the fuzzy tuning system to perform the establishment of the online parameters, setting rules in the fuzzy control chart which will connect the error derivative signal with the exchange rate of the error derivative signal and the three parameters of the PID, in the precisely moment in which the control parameters are established.

2   System Description

The fuzzy tuning of PID controller would be implemented in a Microcontroller (MCU), the challenge of the MCU is that it hosts the controller and the fuzzy system, because we are trying to make a full embedded system.

The aim is to design a fuzzy tuning of PID controller for the position of a DC motor. For this objective we follow the scheme in Figure 2: Output of Arduino is connected to the motor, the motor shaft is connected to a potentiometer for position feedback and another potentiometer would bring the desire position to the MCU.

For our purpose we are considering a simple PID controller, Figure 3, with one output gave by the Arduino Development Board we can change the output

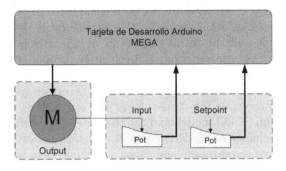

Fig. 2. Block diagram of system

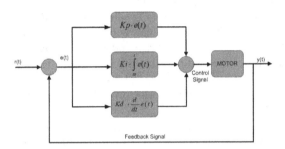

Fig. 3. Structure of a PID Controller

controller value, expecting to reach the desire value of position. The value of the output is given by three gains (Kp, Ki, Kd) and the measured values of error. The error is produced by the difference between the desire position and the actual position, but in the case of integral gain and derivative gain, the value of the error is calculated according to the request in the formula. All operations are calculated by the MCU on real time at the maximum speed of the MCU. The discrete formula of the PID, considering that the integral and derivative gain is given according to the sample period, would be:

$$u(t) = K_p e(t) + K_i T_s \sum_{i=1}^{n} e(i) + \frac{K_d}{T_s} \Delta e(t) \qquad (1)$$

where u(t) is the control signal, e(t) is the error between the reference input and the process output, T_s is the sampling period and Δ e(t) = e(t) - e(t-1). The equation 1 is used for software implementation.

The parameter of the PID controller K_p, K_i and K_d can be manipulated to provide a different response curves, it is here, when the right parameters are acquire, which are really important because we are trying to minimize the errors in the response. This errors are measured when we provide an input to the PID and wait for the stabilization.

Once the system is in steady state, we obtain the three principal qualifiers to measure the performance of the controller. The qualifiers are the errors in steady state, the overshoot and the settle time. And it is here when the intelligent systems take part of the problem, for this problem we propose the use of a fuzzy system.

The fuzzy system is in charge of minimizing the errors to the response of the PID, using a fuzzy rule set. This rule set has a structure according to the Takagi-Sugeno-Kahn (TSK) model, and the response of the defuzzifier structure would control the change of the PID controller's gains, this would be by doing some increments or decrements in the gains, searching for a better response of the system with every iteration of the fuzzy system.

The explanation of the segments in fuzzy system is listed below:

1. Fuzzifier: an input for the fuzzy system, in this case it would be the normal values (values mapped to a value between 0 and 1) of the qualifiers to the response of the PID. These values characterized the inputs in fuzzy values, which can be read in a linguistic way and classify them as follows: in very high, high, medium, low and very low. According to the value of the input, the Fuzzifier mechanism returns a membership value.
2. Knowledge base: Store IF-THEN rules provided by experts. These rules decide the behavior of the system.
3. Inference engine: collecting the membership values from the Fuzzifier and supporting with the knowledge base, this mechanism creates an output of the fuzzy system. These output is a fuzzy way.
4. Defuzzifier: the last step of the fuzzy system is the Defuzzier mechanism, the objective of this mechanism consists, in making the fuzzy output of the inference engine, understandable to mechanism that only process numeric information.

With the tools of PID Controller and the fuzzy systems, we create an intelligent system that can tune the fuzzy controller for the control's position optimum values in this DC motor and for other systems with the same characteristics. The system can be host and fully functional from a MCU with some limitations, low costs and open source development.

3   Implementation

The system proposed is a DC Motor connected to a development board Arduino MEGA through an H-bridge driver. For the signal position feedback, the shaft's transmission motor would be connected to a potentiometer, which would be the system. Also there are additional inputs, the first one consists in another potentiometer that provides a requested position (Setpoint) for the PID controller. The second input, is a selector for tuning mode, this mode begins the routine to obtain the values of gains for the PID. Once we have selected the tuning mode, the system will initiate the tuning routine, followed by a specific period of time in which the process will be concluded in order to ensure the certain optimized values of gain in the controller.

Once the system is in tuning mode, the gains of the PID controller are set to $K_p = 0.01, K_i = 0.01$ and $K_d = 0.01$. Then, the fuzzy system starts modifying them in order to obtain the optimal values, this would be through get the steady state with the actual gains, and calculate the system qualifiers that will serve like inputs for the fuzzy system. The controller has a variable sample time which is calculated in every iteration.

The TSK model is used to calculate the increments or decrements of every gain, but for this the TSK model request modify three gains, since the model is designed for only one output, we need to use three complete systems to obtain the K_p, K_i and K_d.

The fuzzy systems used in this work had three inputs, one output, and five fuzzy sets to determinate the membership function (MF), the fuzzy sets were mentioned above; Very High (VH), High (H), Medium (M), Low (L) and Very Low (VL). To allow an easy implementation, the inputs and outputs of the system were normalized between zero and one, this helps to obtain an output that can be easy escalated to wanted terms.

Next, on Table 1, a sample of the 125 rules of the knowledge base used to every gain of the PID:

Table 1. Fuzzy Rules for K_p behavior

OS	SS	ST	O
1	1	2	5
1	1	3	3
1	2	3	2
2	4	5	2
5	5	5	1

Where 1 its for Very Low (VL), 2 for Low (L), 3 for Medium (M), 4 for High (H) and 5 Very High (VH) fuzzy sets. According to the table, fuzzy rules can be read:

IF overshooting is VL, IF error in steady state is VL, IF settle time is L THEN Output it VH.
IF overshooting is VL, IF error in steady state is VL, IF settle time is M THEN Output it M.
IF overshooting is VL, IF error in steady state is L, IF settle time is M THEN Output it L.
IF overshooting is L, IF error in steady state is H, IF settle time is VH THEN Output it L.
IF overshooting is VH, IF error in steady state is VH, IF settle time is VH THEN Output it VL.

Finally, the output proposed in the defuzzifier incremented to the actual value of the gain. This will take us to find the optimal value of gain for the plant proposed.

A complete digram of the system is showed on Figure 4

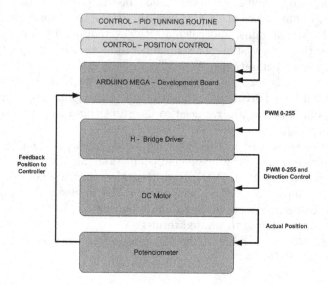

Fig. 4. Diagram of system Implemetation

Table 2. Behavior for every iteration of fuzzy tuning of PID

OS	SS	ST	Kp	Ki	Kd
-0.02	0.02	0.97	6	0.1	6
0.02	0.03	0.97	11	0.1	11
-0.02	0	0.97	16	0.1	16
-0.02	0.02	0.98	21	0.1	21
-0.02	0.01	0.98	26	0.1	26
0.38	0.39	0.98	29.14	0.1	33.85
0.38	0.39	0.98	32.27	0.1	41.75
0.47	0.47	0.98	33.65	0.1	51.16
0.47	0.47	0.98	34.99	0.1	60.53
0.2	0.21	0.98	39.17	0.1	66.28
0.2	0.21	0.98	43.29	0.1	72.04
0.21	0.22	0.98	47.33	0.1	77.95
-0.02	0.01	0.98	52.33	0.1	82.95
-0.02	0.02	0.98	57.33	0.1	87.95
-0.02	0.03	0.98	62.33	0.1	92.95

4   Experimental Results

The objective of the experiment consists in showing how a fuzzy system's implementation produces an improvement in every iteration. To show this, the system

would be tuned with an input and for every iteration, qualifier values of the system were monitored, and as a result we ensure that the fuzzy tuning of PID took the parameters to the optimal or the closest possible way. Results are showed in Table 2:

Table 2 shows how the qualifiers errors change during time, and the values of gains that were used for obtain this errors. The last values were the best values and the ones that will be used during the operation.

Finally the Figure 5 showed the response curve of the PID with the optimal values.

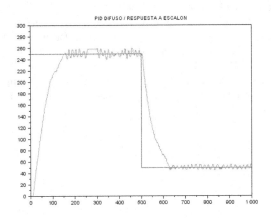

Fig. 5. Response curve to step inputs

Figure 5 is the response of DC motor for two steps, green line is position feedback and red line is the setpoint required along time, every 10 ms.

5   Conclusion

The implementation of a fuzzy tuning of PID Control is plenty justified, because of the nonlinearity response of the parameters. There is a lot of works using this type of control, but there are only a few with all control embedded in a commercial MCU with limited resources, which show a good performance in this application, even though the control of position for DC motors is a really fast process and require a faster response of the system.

This paper can be used as a base to develop future work like involving another Intelligent System for the PID tuning, or making a reduced fuzzy system that let us embedded easily these kind of systems.

References

1. Al-Mashakbeh, A.S.O.: Proportional integral and derivative control of brushless dc motor. European Journal of Scientific Research 35, 198–203 (2009)
2. Bai, R.L., Jiang, L.F., Wang, J.: The study of fuzzy self-tuning pid controller based on fpga. Chinese Journal of Scientific Instrument 8, 833–838 (2005)
3. Gu, J.J., Zhang, Y.J., Gao, D.: Application of nonlinear pid controller in main steam temperature control. In: Asia Pacific Power and Energy Engineering Conference, Wuhan, Chine, pp. 1–5 (2009)
4. Aydogdu, O., Korkmaz, M.: A simple approach to design of variable parameter nonlinear pid controller. In: International Conference on Electrical Engineering and Applications, Wuhan, China, pp. 81–85 (2011)
5. Arulmozhiyal, R., Baskaran, K.: Implementation of fuzzy pi controller for speed control of induction motor using fpga. Journal of Power Electronics 10, 65–71 (2010)
6. Zheng, Y.Y., Chen, Z.L.: Application and research of fuzzy theory. Journal of Soochow University 2, 53–57 (2011)
7. Ping, Z.W., Chao, D.Y., Zhou, Y.: Small unmanned helicopter longitudinal control pid parameter optimization based on genetic algorithm. In: ICACTE 2010, Chengdu, Chine, pp. 142–145 (2010)

A Note on Parameter Selection
for Support Vector Machines

Igor Braga, Laís Pessine do Carmo,
Caio César Benatti, and Maria Carolina Monard

Instituto de Ciências Matemáticas e de Computação
Universidade de São Paulo – São Carlos, SP – Brasil
{igorab,mcmonard}@icmc.usp.br, {lais.carmo,caiocesar}@usp.br

Abstract. Parameter selection greatly impacts the classification accuracy of Support Vector Machines (SVM). However, this step is often overlooked in experimental comparisons, for it is time consuming and requires familiarity with the inner workings of SVM. Focusing on Gaussian RBF kernels, we propose a grid-search procedure for SVM parameter selection which is economic in its running time and does not require user intervention. Based on probabilistic assumptions of standardized data, this procedure works by filtering out parameter values that are not likely to yield reasonable classification accuracy. We instantiate this procedure in the popular WEKA data mining toolbox and show its performance on real datasets.

1   Introduction

Support Vector Machines (SVM) [1] is a supervised learning method that has been used to achieve state-of-the-art classification results in many domains of application. It is usually among the methods that are experimentally evaluated when a new application or learning method is being proposed.

A crucial step when applying SVM is the selection of its parameters. In order to do it properly and efficiently, it is required an understanding of how these parameters affect SVM classification. Hence, users not familiarized with SVM tend to skip parameter selection, often resorting on default parameters of the implementations of their choice. The problem with this approach is that there are no default parameters for SVM.

There has been some effort to introduce procedures for SVM parameter selection that are both easy-to-use and principled [2,3]. However, they currently involve checking a large range of parameter candidates, which can be quite time consuming. What is more, there is an emphasis in fine-grained parameter selection, which may be overkill.

In this work we intend to make SVM parameter selection automatic and economic in its running time. In order to do that, we try to exclude parameter values that are not likely to provide good classification accuracy. After that, we try to investigate parameter candidates that are essentially different, that is, lead to different classification results. A key step to our procedure is data

F. Castro, A. Gelbukh, and M. González (Eds.): MICAI 2013, Part II, LNAI 8266, pp. 233–244, 2013.

standardization, which is a common data pre-processing task that is also useful for bringing all data features (attributes) to the same scale.

The machine learning community has much aided users by making available a wide variety of learning algorithms through open source packages. A popular environment which is widely used by machine learning experts and non-experts is the Waikato Environment for Knowledge Analysis (WEKA) [4]. It contains a wide variety of machine learning methods and also provides graphical user interfaces for easy access. Due to its popularity, we use it in this work to instantiate and illustrate the proposed SVM parameter selection procedure.

The remainder of this paper is organized as follows. In Section 2 we review SVM parameters and how they affect classification performance. In Section 3 we express caution on the use of default parameters in SVM. In Section 4 we present the proposed parameter selection procedure for SVM. In Section 5, we instantiate the proposed procedure in WEKA and conduct illustrative experiments. We conclude in Section 6.

2   Essential Parameters of SVM

This section reviews the parameters that most affect the generalization ability of Support Vector Machines[1]. It is not intended to be a tutorial on SVM classification, as good references on the subject already exist [5].

Given n training examples $(x_1, y_1), \ldots, (x_n, y_n)$, where $x \in R^d$ and $Y = \{+1, -1\}$, the optimization problem that emerges from SVM is usually written as follows

$$\max_{\alpha_1, \ldots, \alpha_n} \quad \sum_{i=1}^{n} \alpha_i - \tfrac{1}{2} \sum_{i=1}^{n} \sum_{j=1}^{n} \alpha_i \alpha_j y_i y_j \, k(x_i, x_j)$$
$$\text{subject to} \quad \sum_{i=1}^{n} \alpha_i y_i = 0,$$
$$0 \leq \alpha_i \leq C,$$

where the constant $C > 0$ and the kernel function $k(x, x')$ are parameters to be defined. After solving this problem for fixed C and k, the output variables α_i are used to derive the function $f(x)$ used to classify unseen data

$$f(x) = \text{sign} \left(\sum_{i=1}^{n} \alpha_i y_i \, k(x, x_i) + b \right), \tag{1}$$

where b is also computed from α_i.

Let us first tackle the so-called *generalization parameter* C. When a learning algorithm selects a function $f(x)$ from a set of functions $\mathcal{F}$ using training examples, it does so by means of an inductive principle. In the case of SVM, induction is performed by the Structural Risk Minimization principle [6], which controls

---

[1] Besides the parameters discussed in this section, there may be other parameters related to specific SVM solvers that do not greatly affect generalization.

two factors: 1) the number of training errors made by $f(x)$ and 2) the capacity (diversity) of the set of functions $\mathcal{F}$. In order to obtain a function $f(x)$ that delivers good classification accuracy on test examples, both factors should be small. As these factors are contradictive, a balance has to be found by controlling the parameter C.

The effect of C in SVM is clearer from its primal optimization problem, which for simplicity we show for the linear case

$$\min_{w,b,\xi_1,\dots,\xi_n} \quad \|w\|^2 + C \sum_{i=1}^{n} \xi_i$$
$$\text{subject to} \quad y_i(w \cdot x_i + b) \geq 1 - \xi_i,$$
$$\xi_i \geq 0.$$

Note that large values of C put more emphasis on the minimization of the slack variables ξ_i, which leads to correct separation of the training examples but risks overfitting. On the other hand, small values of C put more emphasis on the minimization of $\|w\|$, which leads to maximization of the margin of separation and, consequently, minimization of the capacity of the set of functions being considered [6]. This latter case, however, may lead to underfitting. Figure 1 illustrates this trade-off.

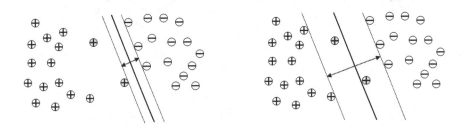

Fig. 1. Typical linear SVM scenario. The value of C used in the left is larger than the one used in the right.

We now turn our attention to the kernel function parameter $k(x, x')$, which induces the set of functions $\mathcal{F}$ from where the function $f(x)$ is picked. Two kinds of kernel functions have been extensively employed: the Gaussian RBF and the linear types. Since most domains require non-linear classification, the former is often more appropriate[2]. Another important property of the Gaussian RBF type is its universal function approximation ability [7].

In fact, Gaussian RBF kernels form a family of kernel functions parameterized by a parameter $\gamma > 0$

$$k(x, x') = \exp\left(-\gamma \|x - x'\|^2\right).$$

---

[2] An exception occurs when the number of dimensions d (features) of the training examples greatly exceeds the number of training examples n $(d \gg n)$.

This means that by choosing γ, we are effectively choosing a kernel function for SVM. The effect of choosing increasingly larger values of γ is to make the kernel an identity evaluator, that is

$$k(\boldsymbol{x}, \boldsymbol{x}') = 1, \text{ if } \boldsymbol{x} = \boldsymbol{x}',$$
$$k(\boldsymbol{x}, \boldsymbol{x}') \approx 0, \text{ if } \boldsymbol{x} \neq \boldsymbol{x}'.$$

On the other hand, choosing very small values of γ has the effect of making $k(\boldsymbol{x}, \boldsymbol{x}') \approx 1$ for any $\boldsymbol{x}$ and $\boldsymbol{x}'$. Figure 2 illustrates the effect of γ in SVM. Note how a large value of γ allows for more diversity in the set of functions implemented by SVM.

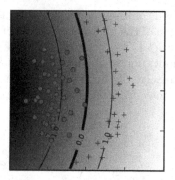 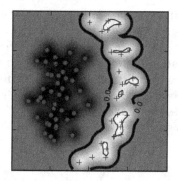

Fig. 2. SVM decision function using Gaussian RBF kernels. The value of γ used in the right is larger than the one used in the left. (Source: [3])

3   A Word of Caution about Default Parameters

The aim of machine learning algorithms is the autonomous building of models from datasets. However, learning algorithms do not necessarily provide good results without being properly tuned. In other words, besides choosing an appropriate learning algorithm for the specific learning domain, it is also necessary to set the algorithm parameters. Nevertheless, manual tuning of the algorithm parameters can frequently be very time-consuming, as well as requiring good knowledge of the learning algorithm.

As there is an increasing number of non-expert users of machine learning tools who require off-the-shelf solutions, these environments always offer default parameter values to execute the algorithms. However, while the default parameter values may be reasonably appropriate for some learning algorithms such as decision trees, in which, for example, the generalization default parameter (confidence limit[3]) is usually set to 25%, this is not the case for most learning algorithms. For example, most implementations of the standard k-NN algorithm usually take $k = 1$ as the default number of neighbors. As the learning domain

---

[3] The smaller the confidence limit, the higher the chances of pruning the tree.

is not known in advance and $k = 1$ entails less running time, this is the usual default value used in most implementations, although other values can dramatically improve the results.

This is also the case of other algorithms, such as SVM, which also strongly depends on parameter selection. It is worth noting that quite different default values are used in different implementations. For example, in WEKA and LIB-SVM[4][8,2] the default value of C is 1. In SVMlight[5] the default value is the average of $(\boldsymbol{x} \cdot \boldsymbol{x})^{-1}$, while in SVMTorch[6][9], the default value is 100. Moreover, WEKA and SVMlight use the linear kernel as default, while LIBSVM uses RBF.

In other words, default values are offered such that non-expert users can initially experiment how the software performs right out of the box. However, a typical machine learning scientist would at least try to improve the expected performance of a learning algorithm over a few parameters. In case there is a need of an optimal model, the search should be conducted over all possible parameters.

To illustrate our point, let us consider UCI's Monk-1 and Monk-2 artificial datasets [10], both from the same domain, with no missing feature values. Each dataset consists of 432 examples described by 7 features and classified as $\oplus$ or $\ominus$. Monk-1 is a balanced dataset (50% $\oplus$, 50% $\ominus$), while Monk-2 is slightly unbalanced (67% $\oplus$, 33% $\ominus$). Thus, the error of the simplest algorithm that always predicts the majority class will be 0.50 for Monk-1 and 0.33 for Monk-2. Using WEKA, we executed John C. Platt's Sequential Minimal Optimization (SMO) algorithm for training a support vector machine [11]. SMO was executed with its default parameters, which are the linear kernel and $C = 1$. We randomly select 2/3 of the corresponding dataset as a training set and 1/3 as a test set. The results are shown in Table 1, where Error is the error rate (proportion of correctly classified instances); B.Error is the balanced error (mean of the positive and negative error rates), and AUC is the area under the ROC curve [12]. Recall that AUC = 0.5 correspond to random guessing. Thus, no realistic classifier should have an AUC less than 0.5.

Table 1. Results of SVM classification using the default parameters in WEKA — linear kernel and $C = 1$

Dataset	Error	B.Error	AUC
Monk-1	0.340	0.341	0.659
Monk-2	0.340	0.500	0.500

It can be observed that the results are poor for Monk-1 and extremely poor for Monk-2. Trying to improve these results, several other values of the parameter

---

[4] A Library for Support Vector Machines
  http://www.csie.ntu.edu.tw/~cjlin/libsvm/
[5] http://svmlight.joachims.org/
[6] http://www.torch.ch/

Table 2. Results of SVM classification using the Gaussian RBF kernel and parameters $(C = 64, \gamma = 0.1)$

Dataset	Error	B.Error	AUC
Monk-1	0.088	0.087	0.913
Monk-2	0.150	0.172	0.828

C in $[10^{-6}, 10^{-5}, \ldots, 10^{6}]$ were tested, but without success. The reason is that for both datasets the relationship between class values and features is nonlinear. This situation cannot be handled by a linear kernel.

In such situations, a kernel which nonlinearly maps examples into a higher dimensional space must be used. Several nonlinear kernels have been proposed in the literature. Among them, the Gaussian RBF kernel is a reasonable choice as explained in Section 2. Table 2 shows the results of using the RBF kernel in WEKA with the assignment of parameters $C = 64$ and $\gamma = 0.1$.

Comparing the results from Table 1 and 2, the improvement obtained by using RBF with a good pair of (C, γ) values is extremely high. Observe that for Monk-1, the error went from 0.340 down to 0.088, 3.86 times lower. For Monk-2 the error went from 0.340 down to 0.150, 2.27 times lower. Moreover, for Monk-1 and Monk-2 respectively, the B.Error was 3.92 and 2.91 times lower. Furthermore, the AUC improved 38% and 67% respectively.

Considering that the RBF kernel can handle datasets having linear as well as non-linear relationship between class values and features, non-expert SVM users may be tempted to report SVM classification results using the RBF kernel with default parameter values. To illustrate the significant differences while using default and optimized SVM-RBF parameters (C, γ), we execute SMO again on datasets Monk-1 and Monk-2, and add two other real world binary datasets: Parkinson and Ionosphere [10]. The first one consists of 197 examples (25% $\oplus$, 75% $\ominus$) described by 23 features, and the second one consists of 351 examples (64% $\oplus$, 36% $\ominus$) described by 34 features. Thus, the majority error rate will be 25% for Parkinson and 36% for Ionosphere.

As before, the experiments were carried out using 2/3 of the corresponding dataset as training set and 1/3 as test set. Table 3 shows the results obtained by executing SMO using the RBF kernel with WEKA default parameters, as well as with other parameters that showed better results.

Table 3. Results of SVM classification using the Gaussian RBF kernel with the default values in WEKA $(C = 1, \gamma = 0.01)$ and with other parameter values

Dataset	Error	B.Error	AUC	Error	B.Error	AUC	(C, γ)
Monk-1	0.510	0.493	0.507	0.088	0.087	0.913	$(64, 0.1)$
Monk-2	0.340	0.500	0.500	0.150	0.172	0.828	$(64, 0.1)$
Parkinson	0.212	0.500	0.500	0.091	0.120	0.838	$(64, 10)$
Ionosphere	0.322	0.424	0.576	0.076	0.082	0.918	$(2, 1000)$

As it can be observed, the improvement obtained by SMO using RBF with other parameters (C, γ) is exceedingly good. For Monk-1 and Monk-2, using the RBF kernel with WEKA default parameters yields an accuracy that is not better than the majority error classifier. For Monk-1, the error went from 0.510 down to 0.088, 5.80 times lower, and the B.Error went from 0.493 down to 0.087, 5.67 times lower. For Monk-2 the error went from 0.340 down to 0.150, 2.27 times lower, and the B.error went from 0.500 down to 0.172, 2.91 times lower. Moreover, for Monk-1 and Monk-2 the AUC improved 80% and 67% respectively.

Also for Parkinson and Ionosphere, SMO with default parameters does not do better than the majority error classifier. However, the classification results yielded by the other parameters are very good. For Parkinson, the error and the B.Error were 2.33 and 4.24 times lower respectively, while the AUC improved 67%. For Ionosphere, the error and the B.Error were 2.66 and 4.24 times lower, while the AUC improved 59%

4   Economic Grid-Search Procedure

It was shown in the last section that using default SVM parameters may yield unsatisfactory classification accuracy. This fact is well-known within the SVM community. As a consequence, for a fixed kernel function, it is desirable to investigate the accuracy provided by SVM with respect to several parameter candidates of C. As to the kernel function, the Gaussian RBF is usually recommended, as explained in Section 2. This way, it is also desirable to investigate the accuracy provided by different candidates of the RBF parameter γ.

The most used method for selecting parameter candidates in the SVM-RBF context is the grid-search procedure with k-fold cross-validation [2,3]. Given a set $\mathcal{C} = \{C_1, C_2, \ldots, C_m\}$ of m candidates of C and a set $\Gamma = \{\gamma_1, \gamma_2, \ldots, \gamma_\ell\}$ of ℓ candidates of γ, an accuracy figure is obtained on the training data for each parameter combination $(C_i, \gamma_j) \in \mathcal{C} \times \Gamma$ through k-fold cross-validation. The pair with the highest cross-validation accuracy is then selected and an SVM classifier trained with this parameter combination is used for classifying unseen data.

Despite its popularity in the SVM community, the described procedure poses a computational problem, since $k \times m \times \ell$ calls to an SVM solver (*e.g* SMO) need to be made, with k generally equal to 10. The problem is worsened when each call to the solver is already expensive, for instance when tens of thousands of examples are available and/or data is very high-dimensional. This means that the candidate sets should be chosen very carefully as to have as few effective candidates as possible.

In what follows, we propose sets of 5 candidates each, which amounts to 25 parameter combinations. Computationally speaking, this is a much better scenario than what is usually considered. For instance, in [2] the following candidate sets are suggested for a coarse grid-search procedure: $\mathcal{C} = \{2^{-5}, 2^{-3}, \ldots, 2^{15}\}$ and $\Gamma = \{2^{-15}, 2^{-13}, \ldots, 2^3\}$, which amounts to 110 combinations.

4.1 Candidates of γ

In order to choose candidates of γ, the distribution of the values $\|x_i - x_j\|^2$ should be taken into consideration. One possible approach is to pick candidates that revolve around the *inverse* of the mean value of $\|x_i - x_j\|^2$. This way, we avoid choosing a too small or too large candidate of γ. In this work we take advantage of a data pre-processing step to approximate such mean value using a formula, thus avoiding its calculation from data.

When employing SVM classification using RBF kernels, it is very desirable to bring all features of the dataset to the same scale, since features ranging in larger intervals tend to dominate the calculation of distances in the RBF kernel. A popular procedure to tackle the scaling problem is data *standardization*: for each feature, the mean and standard deviation value is computed; then, each feature value is subtracted by the corresponding mean and divided by the corresponding standard deviation. The effect of conducting this procedure on data is that every feature will have an average value of $\hat{\mu} = 0$ and standard deviation $\hat{\sigma} = 1$. By assuming that each feature follows a Normal distribution with mean $\mu = 0$ and variance $\sigma^2 = 1$, we can come up with an approximation for the mean value of $\|x_i - x_j\|^2$.

Proposition. *Let $x = (x^1, \dots, x^d)$ and $z = (z^1, \dots, z^d)$ be two random vectors such that x^j and z^j follow a Normal distribution with mean $\mu = 0$ and variance $\sigma^2 = 1$ (standard Normal variables). Then the random variable $\|x - z\|^2$ follows a Gamma distribution with shape parameter $s = \frac{d}{2}$ and scale parameter $\theta = 4$.*

Proof. If x^j and z^j are standard normal variables, then the random variable $(x^j - z^j)$ follows a Normal distribution with mean $\mu = 0$ and variance $\sigma^2 = 2$. Thus, $\left(\frac{x^j - z^j}{\sqrt{2}}\right)$ is also a standard normal variable. By definition, the sum of the squares of d independent standard normal variables follows a Chi-squared distribution with d degrees of freedom — $\chi^2(d)$. Thus, the random variable $A = \sum_{j=1}^{d} \left(\frac{x^j - z^j}{\sqrt{2}}\right)^2$ is $\chi^2(d)$. Note that

$$\|x - z\|^2 = \sum_{j=1}^{d} \left(x^j - z^j\right)^2 = 2A.$$

The Chi-squared distribution and the Gamma distribution are related in the following way: if B is $\chi^2(\nu)$ and $c > 0$, then cB is distributed according to a Gamma distribution with shape parameter $s = \frac{\nu}{2}$ and scale parameter $\theta = 2c$. As $\|x - z\|^2 = 2A$ and A is $\chi^2(d)$, it follows that $\|x - z\|^2$ is distributed according to a Gamma distribution with $s = \frac{d}{2}$ and $\theta = 4$. $\square$

When a random variable follows a Gamma distribution, its mean value corresponds to the product $s\theta$. Under the conditions stated in the aforementioned proposition, it follows that the mean value of $\|x - z\|^2$ is $2d$. Thus, whenever we standardize the features of our dataset, we expect the average value of $\|x_i - x_j\|^2$ to be about twice the number of features in the dataset.

Considering $u = \frac{1}{2d}$, we propose as candidates of γ the values $\frac{u}{4}, \frac{u}{2}, u, 2u, 4u$. For $d \geq 4$, this range of values is enough to cover at least 90% of the distribution of $\|x_i - x_j\|^2$ when the features are standardized. This means that our parameter candidates effectively iterates over the range of most probable values of $\|x_i - x_j\|^2$.

4.2 Candidates of C

Now, let us consider the candidates of C. It can be observed from the general SVM optimization problem in Section 2 that this parameter is an upper bound on the values of the α_i variables. In Equation (1), we see that these α_i variables are used to calculate the decision function. Note that if C is too small, say 2^{-5}, the product $\alpha_i y_i\, k(x, x_i)$ will also be very small, since $0 \leq k(x, x_i) \leq 1$ when $k(x, x_i)$ is a Gaussian RBF. Under usual conditions, the sum over i will also be small, that is, far from either $+1$ or -1. Thus, the SVM solver will set b so as to classify every training example to the majority class, which results in underfitting. That way, it makes sense to remove from our candidate list small values of C.

We propose considering $C = 2^0$ as the first candidate, and the subsequent candidates $2^1, 2^2, 2^3, 2^4$. We stop at 2^4 for the following reason. If we used $C = 2^4$, then, for any x_j and x_i such that $k(x_j, x_i) = \exp(-\gamma \|x_j - x_i\|) \geq 2^{-4}$, it would be feasible to have the product $\alpha_j y_j\, k(x_j, x_i)$ close to either $+1$ or -1. Considering the probabilistic setting described previously and the proposed candidate set Γ, we would expect $k(x_j, x_i) \geq 2^{-4}$ to occur at least 90% of the time when $d \geq 4$. Thus, we would see little difference in the way the training examples are classified by taking $C = 2^5$ or a larger value.

5   Illustrative Experiments in Weka

In what follows, we instantiate our procedure for SVM parameter selection in the WEKA data mining environment[7]. Given training examples $(x_1, y_1), \ldots, (x_n, y_n)$ and test data $x_1^*, \ldots, x_m^*$, where $x \in R^d$ and $Y = \{+1, -1\}$, the two steps of the procedure are:

Data standardization. For each feature value x_i^j of the example x_i in the training set, the corresponding standardized value is computed as $\frac{x_i^j - avg(x^j)}{std(x^j)}$. For each feature value x_i^{*j} of x_i^* in the test set, the corresponding standardized value is computed as $\frac{x_i^{*j} - avg(x^j)}{std(x^j)}$. Note that the scaling factors used to standardize the test set are those of the training set.

Grid-search. Given $\mathcal{C} = \{2^0, 2^1, 2^2, 2^3, 2^4\}$ and $\Gamma = \{\frac{u}{4}, \frac{u}{2}, u, 2u, 4u\}$, where $u = \frac{1}{2d}$, a grid-search procedure with cross-validation is performed on the candidate pairs in $\mathcal{C} \times \Gamma$.

---

[7] We use version 3.6.9 of WEKA.

These two steps can be easily carried out using WEKA on a wide variety of datasets (including datasets with categorical features, which are automatically transformed into numerical ones by the SMO implementation in WEKA). After loading the training and the test set into WEKA, we choose the meta-classifier `GridSearch`. Figure 3 shows how to configure `GridSearch` to perform our parameter selection procedure for SVM. Among these settings, there is an option that enables data standardization as described previously.

Alternatively, the user may download the configuration file at

$$\text{``http://www.icmc.usp.br/~igorab/gridSearchSMO.conf''.}$$

It can be loaded using the `Open` button on the configuration window of `GridSearch`. After that, it remains to set the option `YBASE` to the value $\frac{1}{2d}$, where d is the number of features (excluding the class attribute) in his/her dataset.

Now, we illustrate our procedure for parameter selection in WEKA. For comparison, we run the same experiments using the candidate values suggested in [2] for a coarse grid-search procedure over a large range of values. The candidates

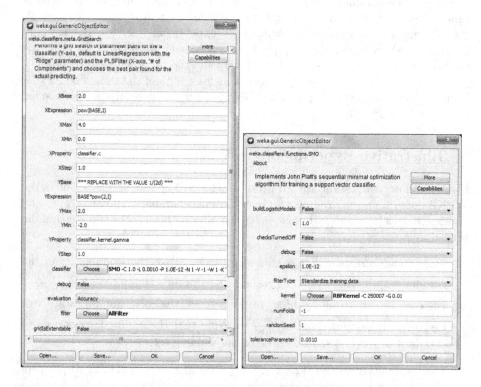

Fig. 3. Configuration options for instantiating the proposed procedure of SVM parameter selection using the `GridSearch` meta-classifier. Note that both standardization and the RBF kernel should be enabled on SMO configuration window.

Table 4. Results of SVM classification after parameter selection using the coarse grid-search suggested in [2] (110 candidate pairs) and the procedure proposed in Section 4 (25 candidate pairs)

Dataset	Coarse Grid-Search				Our Procedure			
	Error	B.Error	AUC	(C, γ)	Error	B.Error	AUC	(C, γ)
Monk-1	0.000	0.000	1.000	$(2^{15}, 2^{-03})$	0.000	0.000	1.000	$(2^4, 1.67\,\mathrm{E}^{-1})$
Monk-2	0.184	0.246	0.754	$(2^{15}, 2^{-01})$	0.150	0.172	0.828	$(2^4, 3.33\,\mathrm{E}^{-1})$
Parkinson	0.076	0.100	0.900	$(2^{15}, 2^{-03})$	0.076	0.100	0.900	$(2^4, 9.10\,\mathrm{E}^{-2})$
Ionosphere	0.067	0.071	0.929	$(2^{15}, 2^{-03})$	0.101	0.110	0.890	$(2^4, 1.47\,\mathrm{E}^{-2})$
Monk-3	0.000	0.000	1.000	$(2^{15}, 2^{-03})$	0.007	0.006	0.994	$(2^4, 8.33\,\mathrm{E}^{-2})$
Arcene	0.191	0.193	0.807	$(2^{15}, 2^{-15})$	0.191	0.189	0.811	$(2^4, 1.25\,\mathrm{E}^{-5})$
Breast-colon	0.019	0.019	0.981	$(2^{01}, 2^{-15})$	0.019	0.019	0.981	$(2^3, 1.14\,\mathrm{E}^{-5})$
Lung-uterus	0.129	0.130	0.870	$(2^{15}, 2^{-15})$	0.118	0.118	0.882	$(2^4, 1.14\,\mathrm{E}^{-5})$

are $C = \{2^{-5}, 2^{-3}, \ldots, 2^{15}\}$ and $\Gamma = \{2^{-15}, 2^{-13}, \ldots, 2^3\}$, which amounts to 110 parameter pairs. Everything else is kept intact, including data standardization.

In addition to the datasets used in Section 3, we use another four datasets, all of them with no missing attribute values: Monk-3, from the same domain as Monk-1 and Monk-2, consisting of 432 examples (47% $\oplus$,53% $\ominus$) described by 7 features; Arcene [10], consisting of 200 examples (44% $\oplus$, 56% $\ominus$) described by 10000 features; Breast-colon, consisting of 630 examples (54% $\oplus$, 46% $\ominus$), and Lung-uterus, consisting of 250 examples (50% $\oplus$, 50% $\ominus$), both described by 10937 features and fetched from the Gene Expression Machine Learning Repository (GEMLeR[8]). As before, each dataset is randomly split in a training set containing 2/3 of the examples and a test set containing 1/3 of the examples.

Note from Table 4 that in most datasets our procedure of parameter selection yields practically equal or better accuracy than the coarse grid-search procedure of [2]. Only in one dataset, Ionosphere, does our procedure perform worse. On the other hand, our procedure performs better in Monk-2. The small improvements observed in Arcene and Lung-uterus can be credited to the fine-grained nature of our parameter search.

The selected value of γ for each dataset is not so different across the two selection procedures, which shows that our strategy for selecting candidates of γ is working well. However, for Ionosphere, our strategy did not include a candidate of γ as good as the best one found by the coarse grid-search procedure. Nevertheless, when dealing with large datasets, our strategy is justified even if the results are not optimal, since a more exhaustive search may be unfeasible.

It is important to observe that in [2] it is advocated to perform a fine-grained grid-search with candidates revolving around the best parameter found by the coarse grid-search procedure. What we are effectively showing with our results is that such a coarse grid-search procedure, which is time consuming, can be avoided by previously selecting the candidates through a careful analysis of how the parameters affect SVM classification.

---

[8] http://gemler.fzv.uni-mb.si/

6   Conclusion

In this work we proposed an economic grid-search procedure for SVM parameter selection using Gaussian RBF kernels. This procedure works by first standardizing the data and then using probabilistic assumptions to select five candidates of the generalization parameter C and five candidates of the RBF parameter γ. By considering all combinations of candidates, our procedure investigates 25 candidate pairs, which is a small number compared to the number of candidate pairs usually suggested in the literature.

We instantiated our procedure in the WEKA data mining toolbox, making it very easy to be used by non-experts. Using the same environment, we conducted experiments on several datasets. The results show that our procedure for parameter selection was as effective as a traditional grid-search procedure, though using less computational resources.

As future work, we intend to investigate a smarter way of selecting parameter candidates of C. Currently, the candidates of C do not change when we consider different candidates of γ. However, we believe it is possible to select better and fewer candidates of C if this selection is done after we fix a candidate of γ.

Acknowledgments. We would like to thank the anonymous reviewers for their helpful comments. This work is supported by grant #2009/17773-7, São Paulo Research Foundation (FAPESP).

References

1. Cortes, C., Vapnik, V.: Support vector networks. Machine Learning 20(3), 273–297 (1995)
2. Hsu, C.W., Chang, C.C., Lin, C.J.: A practical guide to support vector classification. Technical report (2003),
   http://www.csie.ntu.edu.tw/~cjlin/papers/guide/guide.pdf
3. Ben-Hur, A., Weston, J.: A user's guide to support vector machines. Methods in Molecular Biology 609, 223–239 (2010)
4. Witten, I.H., Eibe, F., Hall, M.H.: Data Mining: Practical Machine Learning Tools and Techniques, 3rd edn. Morgan Kaufmann Publishers Inc. (2010)
5. Burges, C.J.C.: A tutorial on support vector machines for pattern recognition. Data Mining and Knowledge Discovery 2(2), 121–167 (1998)
6. Vapnik, V.: Statistical Learning Theory. Adaptive and Learning Systems for Signal Processing, Communications, and Control. Wiley-Interscience (1998)
7. Steinwart, I.: On the influence of the kernel on the consistency of support vector machines. Journal of Machine Learning Research 2, 67–93 (2001)
8. Chang, C.C., Lin, C.J.: LIBSVM: A library for support vector machines. ACM Transactions on Intelligent Systems and Technology
9. Collobert, R., Bengio, S.: SVMTorch: Support vector machines for large-scale regression problems. Journal of Machine Learning Research 1, 143–160 (2001)
10. Bache, K., Lichman, M.: UCI machine learning repository (2013)
11. Platt, J.C.: Fast training of support vector machines using sequential minimal optimization. MIT Press (1999)
12. Fawcett, T.: An introduction to ROC analysis. Pattern Recognition Letters 27(8), 861–874 (2006)

Reinforcement Learning Method for Portfolio Optimal Frontier Search

Jonathan Arriaga-González and Manuel Valenzuela-Rendón

Tecnológico de Monterrey, Campus Monterrey,
Av. Eugenio Garza Sada 2501 C.P. 64849 Monterrey, N.L. México
jonathan.arriaga@exatec.itesm.mx, valenzuela@itesm.mx

Abstract. In the financial field, the selection of a Portfolio of assets is a problem faced by individuals and institutions worldwide. Many portfolios at different risk aversion levels have to be considered before taking the decision to buy a specific Portfolio. Throughout this paper we present a reinforcement learning method to select risk aversion levels to populate the portfolio efficient frontier using a weighted sum approach. The proposed method selects an axis of the Pareto front and calculates the next risk aversion value to fill the biggest gap between points located in the efficient frontier. The probability of selecting an axis is updated by a reinforcement learning mechanism each time a non-dominated portfolio is found. By comparing to a strategy which selects risk aversion levels at random, we found that a quick initial efficient frontier is found faster by the proposed methodology. Real world restrictions such as portfolio value and rounded lots are considered to give a realistic approach to the problem.

Keywords: Reinforcement Learning, Efficient Frontier, Portfolio optimization.

1 Introduction

The Markowitz mean-variance model was the first approach to solve the portfolio optimization problem, it is a powerful framework for asset allocation under uncertainty [10]. This model defines the optimal portfolios as those that maximize return while minimizing risk; the solution is an efficient frontier, a smooth non-decreasing curve representing the set of Pareto-optimal non-dominated portfolios. This problem belongs to the area of Multi-objective optimization (MO), two objectives need to be optimized at the same time. Some problems arise with this model, the shape of the efficient frontier is non-linear and feasible portfolios are more dense in some regions of the pareto frontier. We propose a method to explore the efficient frontier which aims to find portfolios in all the regions, making more effort to search in the less populated zones but also to maintain a good performance in the quantity of portfolios found.

Quadratic Programming (QP) optimization has been used to solve the problem and is reported commonly as a benchmark to compare different approaches.

F. Castro, A. Gelbukh, and M. González (Eds.): MICAI 2013, Part II, LNAI 8266, pp. 245–255, 2013.
© Springer-Verlag Berlin Heidelberg 2013

QP solves this model in an efficient and optimal way if all the restrictions given are linear. When real world non-linear constraints are considered such as asset cardinality, transaction costs, minimum and maximum weights, the problem becomes more difficult and can not be solved by the QP approach. To overcome these limitations, metaheuristic search methods have been applied to the portfolio selection problem with different objectives and have proven to be successful in finding solutions. These methods are not affected by the underlying dynamics of the problem, so they can fulfill different objectives without implicit changes in its structure. An approach to solve the problem is to use the weighted sum model which transforms the multi objective problem into a single objective problem. Both QP and metaheuristic search methods can obtain the portfolio efficient frontier by solving the optimization model repeatedly with different values of the weighting parameter.

Some examples of metaheuristic search methods which have been used to solve the portfolio selection problem are genetic algorithms (GA) [1], memetic algorithms [2], simulated annealing, particle swarm optimization [6], differential evolution [12] and tabu search [4,17]. New methods have been developed to solve this problem such as the hybrid local search algorithm introduced in [11] and the Velocity Limited Particle Swarm Optimization presented in [18]. Other approaches have been reported in the literature as the Bayesian portfolio selection [8]. An overview of the use of metaheuristic optimization for the portfolio selection problem can be found in [9]. The Markowitz mean-variance model assumes a normal distribution, in [13] theoretical return distribution assumptions are compared against empirical distributions using memetic algorithms as the portfolio selection method. Different ways to measure risk are widely used such as in [16], where a memetic algorithm is used for the portfolio selection problem while considering Value at Risk (VaR) as the risk measure.

Multi-objective evolutionary algorithms have been widely reported in the literature. In [5,7], a Pareto frontier is generated using a MO evolutionary algorithm; later in [7] robustness of the portfolio is included as another objective. A review of MO evolutionary algorithms in economics and finance applications can be found in [14].

The rest of the paper is organized as follows: Section 2 describes the model for portfolio optimization. Section 3 presents the efficient frontier search method proposed in this paper. The setup used for experiments, and how the proposed approach will be compared against other methods is presented in section 4. Finally, in section 5 the results of this paper are discussed and final conclusions are presented.

2   The Portfolio Optimization Model

To solve the portfolio optimization problem by means of metaheuristic search algorithms, we first present the optimization model for the unconstrained and constrained problem.

2.1 Unconstrained Problem

The Markowitz portfolio selection model to find the Unconstrained Efficient Frontier (UEF) [10] is given by:

$$\min \sigma_P^2 \tag{1}$$

$$\max \mu_P \tag{2}$$

subject to

$$\sigma_P^2 = \sum_{i=1}^{N} \sum_{j=1}^{N} w_i w_j \sigma_{ij} \tag{3}$$

$$\mu_P = \sum_{i=1}^{N} \mu_i w_i \tag{4}$$

$$\sum_{i=1}^{N} w_i = 1 \tag{5}$$

where $w_i \in \mathbb{R}_0^+ \forall i$, μ_P is the portfolio expected return, N is the total number of assets considered, μ_i is the mean historical return of asset i, σ_{ij} is the covariance between historical returns of assets i and j, and w_i is the weight of asset i in the portfolio.

With this framework, the identification of the optimal portfolio structure can be defined as the quadratic optimization problem of finding the weights w_i that assure the least portfolio risk σ_P^2 for an expected portfolio return μ_P. This model assumes a market where assets can be traded in any fraction, without taxes or transaction costs and no short sales.

2.2 Constrained Problem

As pointed out in [4] the formulation for the Constrained Efficient Frontier (CEF) problem can formulated by the introduction of zero-one decision variables as:

$$z_i = \begin{cases} 1 \text{ if any of asset } i \text{ is held} \\ 0 \text{ otherwise} \end{cases} \tag{6}$$

where $(i = 1, \ldots, N)$. The objective and constraints are given by:

$$\min \sum_{i=1}^{N} \sum_{j=1}^{N} w_i w_j \sigma_{ij} \tag{7}$$

subject to the same constraints as for the UEF plus

$$\sum_{i=1}^{N} z_i = K \tag{8}$$

$$\varepsilon_i z_i \leq w_i \leq \delta_i z_i, \; i = 1, \dots, N \tag{9}$$

$$z_i \in \{0, 1\}, \; i = 1, \dots, N \tag{10}$$

where ε_i and δ_i are the minimum and maximum weights allowed in the portfolio for asset i.

Rounded Lots. When purchasing shares, commissions fees are usually charged per transaction and often a percentage of the total price is also considered. To reduce the average commission cost, shares are bought in groups commonly known as *lots*. A group of 100 shares is known as a *rounded lot*, an *odd lot* is a group of less than 100 shares even as small as 1 share. We introduce this restriction to the portfolio optimization problem as follows:

$$l_i = \frac{w_i A}{p_i L} \tag{11}$$

where $l_i \in \mathbb{Z}^+$, A is the portfolio value in cash with no stock holdings, L is the lot size, p_i and l_i are the price and number of equivalent rounded lots of asset i respectively. The number of shares is given by $q_i = w_i/p_i$.

Thus, we incorporate this restriction in the portfolio selection problem by re-interpreting the weights of the assets in the portfolio. In order to do so, we first calculate the quantity of integer lots that can be bought with the proportion of cash destined to asset i in the portfolio, see Eq. 11. Then the actual weight of the asset in the portfolio is determined with the following equation

$$w_i' = l_i \frac{p_i L}{A} \; . \tag{12}$$

where w_i' is the weight of asset i after being rounded down to the nearest lot. The remaining cash not invested in any asset is assumed to be risk-free. With the reinterpreted weights of the assets in the portfolio, we proceed to obtain the respective portfolio expected return μ_P and risk σ_P^2.

2.3   Efficient Frontier

With the QP equations 1–5 the efficient frontier can be found by solving repeatedly for different values of μ_P as the solution objective; this efficient frontier represents the set of Pareto-optimal portfolios. Another approach is to trace out the efficient frontier by optimizing the weighted sum of the portfolio's risk and expected return:

$$\max \left[(1 - \lambda)\mu_P - \lambda\sqrt{\sigma_P^2} \right] \tag{13}$$

where λ ($0 \leq \lambda \leq 1$) is the weighting parameter. The resulting portfolio's return and risk have an inverse non-linear relationship with this parameter, so a better selection criteria is needed.

2.4 Steepest Ascent Hill Climbing for Portfolio Selection

In [3] the performance of Steepest Ascent Hill Climbing (SAHC), in spite of its simplicity, is reported to provide good solutions while solving the portfolio selection problem. The same approach is used to optimize portfolios following the weighted sum model. To comply with the cardinality restriction of the CEF in which K assets compose the portfolio, the structure of the portfolio in the solution will be represented by K assets and K weights as in [4]. A minimum weight ε_i is set for each asset i in the solution, with the constraint $\sum_i^K \varepsilon_i < 1$. The remaining fraction of the portfolio is left for the algorithm to be optimized, so weights are normalized to $1 - \sum_i^K \varepsilon_i$. This solution structure is similar to the approaches reported in [4,17].

3 Efficient Frontier Search Methods

We propose a method to populate the efficient frontier by properly selecting λ values so that the non-dominated portfolios obtained have its parameters of risks and expected returns distributed along their respective axes. These procedures rely on the portfolio optimization algorithm, two portfolios obtained with the same λ value may not be exactly the same. They may have similar values, but result in two different points around the same Pareto coordinates, not always efficient or non-dominated. The same is true for the case of two equal portfolios obtained with different values of λ, often there is a limit in the non-dominated portfolios obtained by this parameter, the quantities in one axis can be times larger than the other and increasing or decreasing values in the weighting factor can not generate new portfolios.

3.1 The Distributed Strategy

In the Distributed Strategy (DS), the axes of Risk and Expected Return are used to generate new values of λ that generate non-dominated portfolios. This method aims to fill the biggest gaps in the axes of the Pareto frontier by looking for non-dominated portfolios in the mid-point of these gaps. The shape of the portfolio efficient frontier is known to be irregular, depending on conditions of the market and stocks involved. Some zones have more concentration of non-dominated points, while others have fewer feasible portfolios and are less populated. Exploration of the Pareto front is distributed across its axes, in a hope to cover most of the possibilities, while still giving chance to cover all the range of the λ values. The method is constantly exploring all places of the efficient frontier using random values with a low probability. This method of exploring the efficient frontier is similar to the one presented in [15], which also converts the MO problem to a single objective problem to search for points in the Pareto front. In this paper, the new weight of the model is adaptively determined by accessing newly introduced points at the current iteration and the non-dominated points so far.

Each time a new λ value needs to be selected, the following procedure is executed. First, to generate an initial set of points in the efficient frontier 10 linearly spaced values of λ are used as reference. The basis for generating the new λ value is selected from the data of the non-dominated portfolios already available. The algorithm selects among the axes of the Pareto front, the vector of λ values or a random value. If any of the axes of the Pareto front is selected, the algorithm generates the vector of values of risk or expected return from the non-dominated portfolios already available. This vector is sorted and the points that make the biggest gap are selected, the next value of λ is interpolated as the mid-point of the λ values used to find the corresponding portfolios. If the vector of λ is selected as the basis, the next value is the middle of the biggest gap after the vector is sorted. In this implementation, selecting the axes of the Pareto front as the basis have a fixed probability of 40% each, 10% for the λ vector and 10% for a random value.

3.2   Distributed Strategy with Reinforcement Learning Component

The main issues that affect the performance of the DS method are the irregular shape of the efficient frontier and the feasibility to find non-dominated portfolios in a certain region of the Pareto front. Once a region of the Pareto front has been filled with portfolios, the chances of obtaining more non-dominated portfolios in the neighborhood decrease. To overcome these problems, the Distributed Strategy with Reinforcement Learning (DRL) is proposed as a better search method that adapts to these conditions to improve the search.

This method follows the same procedure as the DS method to generate new λ values from the data of non-dominated portfolios already found. A reinforcement learning component is added to update the probabilities of selecting the different basis that guide the search for non-dominated portfolios. These probabilities never drop to zero, but are kept to a minimum value to allow the algorithm to switch to other when the dominating basis has been completely explored. The performance of each basis in finding non-dominated portfolios is the decisive factor to increase or decrease the times it is selected.

Each basis is represented by a variable which holds its points, with an initial value of 1 point each. The reinforcement mechanism only activates when a non-dominated portfolio is found. A payment of one point is given to variable representing the basis that was used to generate the last non-dominated portfolio. A discount of 5% of the points is penalized to all the variables, including the one that received the payment, this limits the points of any variable to converge to a maximum value of 19. In order to maintain learned weights, there is no penalty when the search is not successful; failed attempts are not considered. Figure 1 shows the process diagram of the DRL method.

4   Experimental Setup

In this section we report the results obtained by the aforementioned methods for different problems. To measure the performance of the DS and DRL methods,

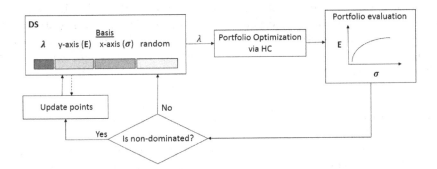

Fig. 1. Flowchart diagram of the DRL method

we compare them against other two methods, a random selection of λ values and a set of linearly spaced values through all the range of λ, known as the linspace function.

4.1 Data and Parameters

The components of three market index were considered as problems: the NAS-DAQ index (100 assets), the IPC index (28 assets) and the DAX index (30 assets). Data was obtained from the `yahoo.finance.historicaldata` datatable using the Yahoo! Query Language (YQL). Daily returns were considered, from 25-Jun-2012 to 31-Dec-2012, a lot size of $L = 100$ was set for all problems. The cardinality constraint was relaxed by taking K as the upper limit of the quantity of assets in the portfolio. In the solution structure weights for the same asset are added, the total of weights are normalized such that $\sum_i^K w_i = 1$. There are no preferences or restrictions for any of the assets, all weights in the portfolio are allowed to be $w_i \in [0,1]$. We set the maximum portfolio size to 5 assets, small portfolios are easy to manage and track its performance over time. Values for the selection of assets in the solution were the components of each index, weights for assets had a resolution of 0.01 (1%) the range 0-1. Settings for the SAHC algorithm were 10 initial random solutions. The number of iterations I of the algorithm was chosen empirically, we tested increasing values of this parameter to solve the IPC problem with the DS method until the quality of results was no longer improved, which happened at $I = 10$ iterations. The number of values that will be tested for each element of the solution was set to $V = 10$. As there are 100 possible values for the weights and 100 values for the problem with most assets, $V = 10$ means that 10% of the possible values will be tested in each element of the solution. There is a high probability that all possible values are tested for each element of the solution with similar or repeated values of λ. With these parameters we expect to obtain near-optimal portfolios for each value of λ.

Optimization of portfolios was carried out 5,000 times, with the values of λ generated by each method to explore the efficient frontier. This procedure was repeated 10 times for each problem for a more reliable analysis. The DS and DRL methods take about an hour to find the efficient frontier on a workstation with Intel Core i5-760 processor running at 2.80GHz. With respect to the number of non-dominated portfolios, we take as a benchmark the method of generating λ values with the linspace function because is a deterministic method.

4.2   Results

For the NASDAQ, the random and linspace methods obtained around 350 non-dominated portfolios at the end of the run, while an average of nearly 500 and 600 non-dominated portfolios with the DS and DRL methods respectively, see figure 2a. Weights of the DRL method switch among the vectors of risk, expected return and risk aversion to generate λ values; except for the random basis, which is increasing most of the time as can be seen in figure 2b.

The number of non-dominated portfolios found with the IPC components was 400, in this case all methods, except the DS, obtained around 410 portfolios at the end of the 5,000 optimization iterations. Initially the DS and DRL methods found more non-dominated portfolios than the random selection method, the DRL starts giving more chances to use the expected return of the non-dominated portfolios as a basis to generate new λ values. The DS began to lag around the 2,500 iterations, the DRL method reacts at this point and increases the exploration of the efficient frontier with λ values generated at a random basis more frequently. This behavior is illustrated in figures 2c and 2d.

For the DAX problem, the random and linspace methods obtained nearly the same number of non-dominated portfolios, both the DS and DRL methods got a little more portfolios. The behavior of points obtained by each basis in the DRL method is very similar to the IPC problem, see figure 2f. The reason that the frontier size obtained by the proposed methods in these two problems is nearly the same to the linspace and random approaches, is because the shape of the efficient frontier is regular in all its range.

In figure 3 is shown the portfolio efficient frontier obtained by the method of random λ values next to the one obtained by the DRL method. This serves as a comparison of the regions of the Pareto front covered by both, bigger gaps can be observed when the random approach is followed. The DRL method covers almost all the efficient frontier, except for the region with low risk and an expected return of almost 0.0025, not covered either by the other method; generating non-dominated portfolios may be unfeasible in this region.

Selecting values at random is close to a brute force approach because the resolution of points is much smaller than the linspace approach. However, the distribution of values for λ selected by these methods is flat in all its range, which leads to find efficient frontiers with similar features. By searching points in the Pareto frontier using a list of linearly spaced values, we find that most of the risk aversion values result in dominated points. Only a small range of values in the λ vector correspond to most of the portfolios found. The main reason to plot the size of the efficient frontier found by the linspace method is because it

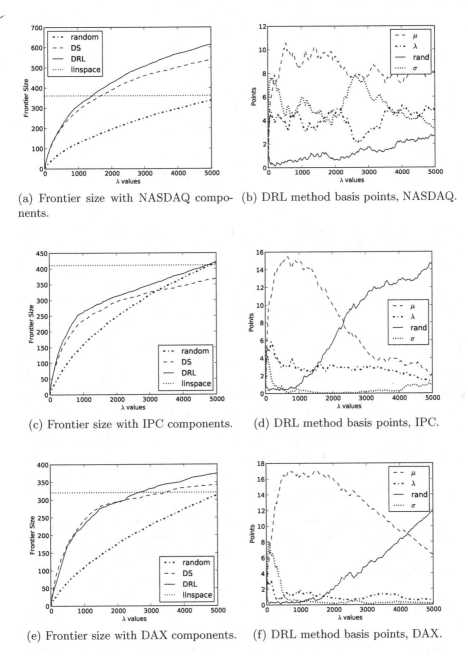

(a) Frontier size with NASDAQ components.

(b) DRL method basis points, NASDAQ.

(c) Frontier size with IPC components.

(d) DRL method basis points, IPC.

(e) Frontier size with DAX components.

(f) DRL method basis points, DAX.

Fig. 2. Figures (a), (c) and (e) show the number of non-dominated portfolios found against the number of λ values evaluated by each of the selected methods, while (b), (d) and (f) show the points of each basis in the DRL method against the number of λ values evaluated

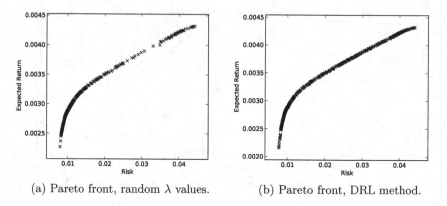

(a) Pareto front, random λ values.   (b) Pareto front, DRL method.

Fig. 3. Portfolio Efficient Frontier obtained with the components of the NASDAQ index by using random λ values (a) and the Distributed method with Reinforcement Learning (b)

depends on the order the values are selected; as it selects always the same values, the result will be very similar in every realization.

5   Conclusions

Throughout this paper we have presented the DS and DRL methods to explore the portfolio efficient frontier following a weighted sum model. The DRL approach complements the DS method with a Reinforcement Learning component, which is a big advantage when the shape of the efficient frontier is irregular and exploration in a particular zone starts to be unsuccessful. This method generates new λ values based in the characteristics of the non-dominated portfolios and adapts its search by updating the chances of selecting these features. The experimental comparison of the proposed methods against simpler approaches demonstrate its advantage at finding non-dominated portfolios.

The implementation of the DRL algorithm to cover MO problems with more than two dimensions is a tentative next step in its development. Also, testing the performance of method with other shapes of the Pareto frontier is left as a future work.

References

1. de Castro Aranha, C., Iba, H.: A tree-based ga representation for the portfolio optimization problem. In: Proceedings of the 10th Annual Conference on Genetic and Evolutionary Computation, GECCO 2008, pp. 873–880. ACM, New York (2008)
2. de Castro Aranha, C., Iba, H.: Using memetic algorithms to improve portfolio performance in static and dynamic trading scenarios. In: Proceedings of the 11th Annual Conference on Genetic and Evolutionary Computation, GECCO 2009, pp. 1427–1434. ACM, New York (2009)

3. Arriaga, J., Valenzuela-Rendón, M.: Steepest ascent hill climbing for portfolio selection. In: Di Chio, C., et al. (eds.) EvoApplications 2012. LNCS, vol. 7248, pp. 145–154. Springer, Heidelberg (2012)

4. Chang, T.J., Meade, N., Beasley, J., Sharaiha, Y.: Heuristics for cardinality constrained portfolio optimisation. Computers and Operations Research 27, 1271–1302 (2000)

5. Chiam, S., Al Mamun, A., Low, Y.: A realistic approach to evolutionary multiobjective portfolio optimization. In: IEEE Congress on Evolutionary Computation, CEC 2007, pp. 204–211 (September 2007)

6. Gao, J., Chu, Z.: An improved particle swarm optimization for the constrained portfolio selection problem. In: International Conference on Computational Intelligence and Natural Computing, CINC 2009, vol. 1, pp. 518–522 (June 2009)

7. Hassan, G., Clack, C.D.: Multiobjective robustness for portfolio optimization in volatile environments. In: Proceedings of the 10th Annual Conference on Genetic and Evolutionary Computation, GECCO 2008, pp. 1507–1514. ACM, New York (2008)

8. Lu, J., Liechty, M.: An empirical comparison between nonlinear programming optimization and simulated annealing (sa) algorithm under a higher moments bayesian portfolio selection framework. In: 2007 Winter Simulation Conference, pp. 1021–1027 (December 2007)

9. Maringer, D.: Heuristic optimization for portfolio management [application notes]. IEEE Computational Intelligence Magazine 3(4), 31–34 (2008)

10. Maringer, D.: Portfolio management with heuristic optimization. Advances in computational management science, vol. 8. Springer, Heidelberg (2005)

11. Maringer, D., Kellerer, H.: Optimization of cardinality constrained portfolios with a hybrid local search algorithm. OR Spectrum 25, 481–495 (2003), doi:10.1007/s00291-003-0139-1

12. Maringer, D., Parpas, P.: Global optimization of higher order moments in portfolio selection. Journal of Global Optimization 43, 219–230 (2009), doi:10.1007/s10898-007-9224-3

13. Maringer, D.G.: Distribution assumptions and risk constraints in portfolio optimization. Computational Management Science 2, 139–153 (2005), doi:10.1007/s10287-004-0031-8

14. Ponsich, A., Jaimes, A., Coello, C.: A survey on multiobjective evolutionary algorithms for the solution of the portfolio optimization problem and other finance and economics applications. IEEE Transactions on Evolutionary Computation 17(3), 321–344 (2013)

15. Ryu, J.H., Kim, S., Wan, H.: Pareto front approximation with adaptive weighted sum method in multiobjective simulation optimization. In: Winter Simulation Conference, WSC 2009, pp. 623–633. Winter Simulation Conference (2009)

16. Winker, P., Maringer, D.: The hidden risks of optimizing bond portfolios under var. Journal of Risk 9(4), 1–19 (2007)

17. Woodside-Oriakhi, M., Lucas, C., Beasley, J.: Heuristic algorithms for the cardinality constrained efficient frontier. European Journal of Operational Research 213(3), 538–550

18. Xu, F., Chen, W.: Stochastic portfolio selection based on velocity limited particle swarm optimization. In: The Sixth World Congress on Intelligent Control and Automation, WCICA 2006, vol. 1, pp. 3599–3603 (2006)

Weighed Aging Ensemble of Heterogenous Classifiers for Incremental Drift Classification

Michał Woźniak and Piotr Cal

Department of Systems and Computer Networks
Wroclaw University of Technology
Wyb. Wyspianskiego 27, 50-370 Wroclaw, Poland
{michal.wozniak,piotr.cal}@pwr.wroc.pl

Abstract. Nowadays simple methods of data analysis are not sufficient for efficient management of an average enterprize, since for smart decisions the knowledge hidden in data is highly required, among them methods of collective decision making called classifier ensemble are the focus of intense research. Unfortunately the great disadvantage of traditional classification methods is that they "assume" that statistical properties of the discovered concept (which model is predicted) are being unchanged. In real situation we could observe so-called concept drift, which could be caused by changes in the probabilities of classes or/and conditional probability distributions of classes. The paper presents extension of Weighted Aging Classifier Ensemble (WAE), which is able to adapt to the changes in data stream. It assumes that the classified data stream is given in a form of data chunks, and the concept drift could appear in the incoming data chunks. Instead of drift detection WAE tries to construct self-adapting classifier ensemble. Therefore on the basis of the each chunk one individual is trained and WAE checks if it could form valuable ensemble with the previously trained models. The presented extension uses the ensemble of heterogeneous classifiers, what boosts the classification accuracy, what was confirmed on the basis of the computer experiments.

Keywords: machine learning, classifier ensemble, data stream, concept drift, incremental learning, forgetting.

1 Introduction

The market-leading companies desire to exploit strength of machine learning techniques to extract hidden, valuable knowledge from the huge databases. One of the most promising directions of that research is classification task, which is widely used in computer security, medicine, finance, or trade. Designing such solutions we should take into consideration that in the modern world the most of the data arrive continuously and it causes that smart analytic tools should respect this nature and be able to interpret so-called data streams. Unfortunately most of the traditional classifiers do not take into consideration that:

F. Castro, A. Gelbukh, and M. González (Eds.): MICAI 2013, Part II, LNAI 8266, pp. 256–266, 2013.

- the statistical dependencies between the observations of a given objects and their classifications could change,
- data can come flooding in the analyzer what causes that it is impossible to label all records.

1.1 Concept Drift

This work focuses on the first problem called *concept drift* [18]. Analyzing the rapidity of concept drift, we can mainly distinguish the sudden shift and the gradual drift. Each of them can cause an accuracy deterioration as is depicted in Fig.1 for the sudden appearance of distribution change.

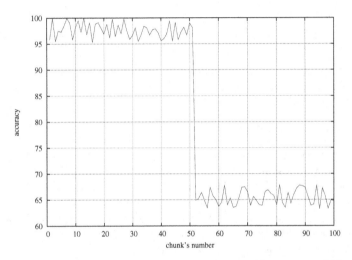

Fig. 1. Deterioration of a classification accuracy after a sudden concept drift appearance

In general, we can consider the following approaches which allow us to deal with the concept drift problem:

- Rebuilding a classification model if new data becomes available, but this solution is a quite expensive and usually impossible from a practical point of view, especially if the concept drift occurs rapidly.
- Detecting concept changes in new data and if these changes are sufficiently "significant", then rebuilding the classifier.
- Adopting an incremental learning algorithm for the classification model.

We focus on the incremental learning [11], where the model is either updated (e.g., neural networks) or needs to be partially or completely rebuilt (as CVFDT algorithm [5]). This approach assumes that the data stream is given in a form of data chunks (windows). When dealing with the sliding window the main question is how to adjust the window size. On the one hand, a shorter window allows focusing on the emerging context, though data may not be representative for a longer lasting context. On the other hand, a wider window may result in mixing the instances representing different contexts. Therefore, certain advanced algorithms adjust the window size dynamically depending on the detected state (e.g., FLORA2 [18]) or use an active learning approach to minimize the labeling cost [10]. An exemplary dependency between window size and classification accuracy is depicted in Fig.2.

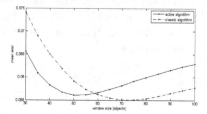 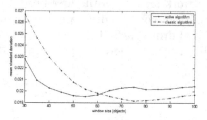

Fig. 2. Dependency between windows size, classification error and standard deviation for sliding window approach (Iris dataset) [10]

1.2 Classifier Ensemble

One of the important group of algorithms dedicated to stream classification exploits strength of ensemble systems, which work pretty well in static environments [9], because according to Wolpert's "no free lunch theorem" [19] there is not a single classifier that is suitable for all the tasks, since each of them has its own domain of competence. A strategy for generating the classifier ensemble should guarantee its diversity improvement therefore let us enumerate the main propositions how to get a desirable committee:

- The individual classifiers could be train on different datasets, because we hope that classifiers trained on different inputs would be complementary.
- The individual classifiers can use the selected features only.
- Usually it could be easy to decompose the classification problem into simpler ones solved by the individual classifier. The key problem of such approach is how to recover the whole set of possible classes.
- The last and intuitive method is to use individual classifiers trained on different models or different versions of models.

It has been shown that a collective decision can increase classification accuracy, because the knowledge that is distributed among the classifiers may be more comprehensive [15]. Usually, a diversity may refer to the classifier model, the feature set, or the instances used in training, but in a case of data stream classification diversity can also refer to the context, but the problem how the diversity of the classifier ensemble should be measured still remains. Brown et al. [3] notice that we can ensure diversity using implicitly or explicitly diversity approaches. The first group of methods includes techniques of independently generated individual classifiers, usually based on random techniques, while the second group focuses on optimization of an ensemble line-up using diversity metric. For the second case, individual classifiers are trained in a dependent manner and the aim of the optimization process is to exploit the strengths (consider a given diversity) of valuable members of the classifier pool.

Several strategies are possible for a data stream classification:

1. Dynamic combiners, where individual classifiers are trained in advance and their relevance to the current context is evaluated dynamically while processing subsequent data. The level of contribution to the final decision is directly proportional to the relevance [6]. The drawback of this approach is that all contexts must be available in advance; emergence of new unknown contexts may result in a lack of experts.
2. Updating the ensemble members, where each ensemble consists of a set of online classifiers that are updated incrementally based on the incoming data [2].
3. Dynamic changing line-up of ensemble e.g., individual classifiers are evaluated dynamically and the worst one is replaced by a new one trained on the most recent data.

Among the most popular ensemble approaches, the following are worth noting: the Streaming Ensemble Algorithm (SEA) [16] or the Accuracy Weighted Ensemble (AWE)[17]. Both algorithms keep a fixed-size set of classifiers. Incoming data are collected in data chunks, which are used to train new classifiers. All the classifiers are evaluated on the basis of their accuracy and the worst one in the committee is replaced by a new one if the latter has higher accuracy. The SEA uses a majority voting strategy, whereas the AWE uses the more advanced weighted voting strategy. A similar formula for decision making is implemented in the Dynamic Weighted Majority (DWM) algorithm [8].

In this work we propose the dynamic ensemble model called WAE (Weighted Aging Ensemble) which can modify line-up of the classifier committee on the basis of diversity measure. Additionally the decision about object's label is made according to weighted voting, where weight of a given classifier depends on its accuracy and time spending in an ensemble. The detailed description of WAE is presented in the next section. Then we present preliminary results of computer experiments which were carried out on SEA dataset and seem to confirm usefulness of proposed algorithm. The last section concludes our research.

2 Weighted Aging Ensemble Algorithm

Let's propose the idea of the WAE (*Weighted Aging Ensemble*), which was firstly presented in [20], then its modification will be presented. We assume that the classified data stream is given in a form of data chunks denotes as $\mathcal{DS}_k$, where k is the chunk index. The concept drift could appear in the incoming data chunks. We do not detect it, but we try to construct self-adapting classifier ensemble.

Therefore on the basis of the each chunk one individual is trained and we check if it could form valuable ensemble with the previously trained models. In our algorithm we propose to use the Generalized Diversity (denoted as $\mathcal{GD}$) proposed by Partridge and Krzanowski [12] to assess all possible ensembles and to choose the best one. $\mathcal{GD}$ returns the maximum values in the case of failure of one classifier is accompanied by correct classification by the other one and minimum diversity occurs when failure of one classifier is accompanied by failure of the other.

$$\mathcal{GD}(\Pi) = 1 - \frac{\sum_{i=1}^{L} \frac{i(i-1)p_i}{L(L-1)}}{\sum_{i=1}^{L} \frac{ip_i}{L}} \tag{1}$$

where L is the cardinality of the classifier pool (number of individual classifiers) and p_i stands for the probability that i randomly chosen classifiers from Π will fail on randomly chosen example.

Lets $P_a(\Psi_i)$ denotes frequency of correct classification of classifier Ψ_i and $itter(\Psi_i)$ stands for number of iterations which Ψ_i has been spent in the ensemble. We propose to establish the classifier's weight $w(\Psi_i)$ according to the following formulae

$$w(\Psi_i) = \frac{P_a(\Psi_i)}{\sqrt{itter(\Psi_i)}} \tag{2}$$

This proposition of classifier aging has its root in object weighting algorithms where an instance weight is usually inversely proportional to the time that has passed since the instance was read [7] and Accuracy Weighted Ensemble (AWE)[17], but the proposed method called Weighted Aging Ensemble (WAE) incudes two important modifications:

1. classifier weights depend on the individual classifier accuracies and time they have been spending in the ensemble,
2. individual classifier are chosen to the ensemble on the basis on the non-pairwise diversity measure.

In this work we propose to use the heterogenous ensemble instead of homogenous one, because we believe that it could boost the diversity of the classifier ensemble, what could lead to increasing the adaptation ability of the ensemble. The pseudocode of the WAE is presented in Alg. 1. The crucial element of WAE algorithm is choosing the valuable classifier ensemble (see lines 9-11). We have to emphasize that such proposition causes computation load increasing, because we have to train more than one classifier model for each chunk. Additional, choosing new ensemble is more complicated, because we have much more possible ensembles to analyze and compare the much more potential ensembles to choose as the final one. The original version of WAE algorithm [20] considers L possible ensemble, but the proposed method should evaluate $\binom{L}{k}$ ensembles, where k is the number of the possible training methods (i.e., number of classifiers trained on the basis on new data chunk).

Algorithm 1. Weighted Aging Ensemble (WAE) based on heterogenous classifiers

---

Require: input data stream,
      data chunk size,
      k classifier training procedures,
      ensemble size L

1: $i := 1$
2: $\Pi = \emptyset$
3: **repeat**
4:     collect new data chunk DS_i
5:     **for** $j := 1$ **to** k **do**
6:        $\Psi_{i,j} \leftarrow$ classifier training procedure (DS_i, j)
7:        $\Pi := \Pi \cup \{\Psi_{i,j}\}$ to the classifier ensemble Π
8:     **end for**
9:     **if** $|\Pi| > L$ **then**
10:       choose the most valuable ensemble of L classifiers using (1)
11:     **end if**
12:     $w := 0$
13:     **for** $j = 1$ **to** L **do**
14:       calculate $w(\Psi_i)$ according to (2)
15:       $w := w + w(\Psi_i)$
16:     **end for**
17:     **for** $j = 1$ **to** L **do**
18:       $w(\Psi_i) := \frac{w(\Psi_i)}{w}$
19:     **end for**
20:     $i := i + 1$
21: **until** end of the input data stream

---

3   Experimental Investigations

The aims of the experiment were to assess if the proposed method of weighting and aging individual classifiers in the ensemble is valuable proposition compared with the methods which do not include aging or weighting techniques.

3.1   Set-Up

All experiments were carried out on the SEA dataset describes in [16]. Each object belongs to the on of two classes and is described by 3 numeric attributes with value between 0 and 10, but only two of them are relevant. Object belongs to class 1 (TRUE) if $arg_1 + arg_2 < \phi$ and to class 2 (FALSE) if $arg_1 + arg_2 \geq \phi$. ϕ is a threshold between two classes, so different thresholds correspond to different concepts (models).Thus, all generated dataset is linearly separable, but we add 5% noise, which means that class label for some samples is changed, with expected value equal to 0. The number of objects, noise and the set of concepts are set by user. We simulated drift by instant random model change.

For each of the experiments we decided to form homogenous ensemble i.e., ensemble which consists of the classifier using the same model. We repeated experiments for Naïve Bayes, decision tree trained by C4.5 [14], and SVM with polynomial kernel trained by the sequential minimal optimization method (SMO) [13]. The ensemble was compared with the heterogenous ensemble contains the classifier trained on the basis of above mentioned models.

During each of the experiment we tried to evaluate dependency between data chunk sizes (which were fixed on 50, 100, 150, 200) and overall classifier quality (accuracy and standard deviation) for the following ensembles:

1. $w0a0$ - an ensemble using majority voting without aging.
2. $w1a0$ - an ensemble using weighted voting without aging, where weight assigned to a given classifier is inversely proportional to its accuracy.
3. $w1a1$ - an ensemble using weighted voting with aging, where weight assigned to a given classifier is calculated according to (2).

Method of ensemble pruning was the same for each ensembles and presented in Alg.1. All experiments were carried out in the Java environment using Weka classifiers [4].

3.2   Results

The results of experiments are presented in Fig.3-6. Fig. 3 presents overall accuracy and standard deviation for the heterogenous ensemble and how they depend on data chunk size. Fig.4-6 present the aforementioned dependency for the homogenous ensembles. Unfortunately, because of the space limit we are not able to presents all extensive results, but they are available on demand from corresponding author.

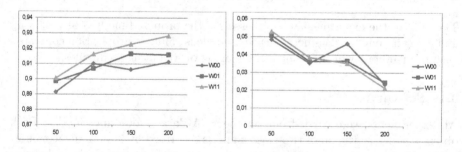

Fig. 3. Classification accuracy (left) and standard deviation (right) for the WAE using heterogenous ensemble

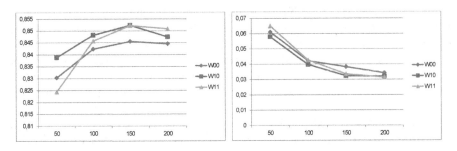

Fig. 4. Classification accuracy (left) and standard deviation (right) for the WAE using homogenous ensemble consists of C4.5 (decision tree)

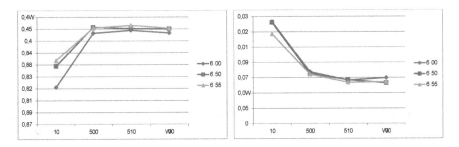

Fig. 5. Classification accuracy (left) and standard deviation (right) for the WAE using homogenous ensemble consists of SVM classifiers

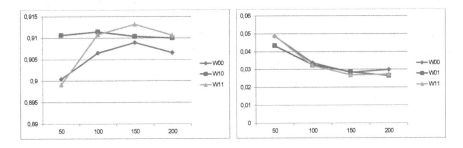

Fig. 6. Classification accuracy (left) and standard deviation (right) for the WAE using homogenous ensemble consists of Naïve Bayes classifiers

3.3   Discussion

On the basis of presented results we can formulate several observations. It does not surprise us that quality improvements for all tested method according to increasing data chunk size. The heterogenous ensemble works pretty well, and it outperforms each homogenous ensembles. Additionally, it is the most stable model (comparing to the rest of analyzed models). Usually the WAE outperformed others, but the differences are quite small and only in the case of ensemble built on the basis of Naïve Bayes classifiers the differences are statistical significant (t-test) [1] i.e., differences among different chunk sizes. The observation is useful because the bigger size of data chunk means that effort dedicated to building new models is smaller because they are being built rarely.

Another interesting observation is that the standard deviation is smaller for bigger data chunk and usually standard deviation of WAE is smallest among all tested methods. It means that the concept drift appearances have the weakest impact on the WAE accuracy.

We realize that the scope of the experiments we carried out is limited and derived remarks are limited to the tested methods and one dataset only. In this case formulating general conclusions is very risky, but the preliminary results are quite promising, therefore we would like to continue the work on WAE in the future.

4   Conclusions

The paper presented the original classifier for data stream classification tasks. Proposed WAE algorithm uses dynamic classifier ensemble i.e., its line-up is formed when new data chunk is come and the decision which classifier is chosen to the ensemble is made on the basis of General Diversity (diversity measure). The decision about object's label is made according to weighted voting where weight assigned to a given classifier depends on its accuracy (proportional) and how long the classifier participates in the ensemble (inversely proportional). The experiments conformed that proposed method can adapt to changing concept returning stable classifier. According to the obtained results we can confirm that for this model the heterogenous ensemble is the best model. But we have to notice the limitation of such approach. Such heterogenous ensemble does not allow to use more sophisticated combination method based on support functions, as aggregating. In this case only homogenous ensemble could be used, or at least ensemble of classifiers which produce the same type of support functions.

We would like to emphasize that we presented preliminary study on WAE which is a starting point for the future research. In the near future we are going to:

- carry out experiments on the wider number of datasets,
- evaluate usefulness of the other diversity measures for WAE's classifier ensemble pruning,
- assess more sophisticated combination rules based on support functions of individual classifiers.

Acknowledgment. The work was supported by the statutory funds of the Department of Systems and Computer Networks, Wroclaw University of Technology and by the Polish National Science Center under a grant N N519 650440 for the period 2011-2014.

References

1. Alpaydin, E.: Introduction to Machine Learning, 2nd edn. The MIT Press (2010)
2. Bifet, A., Holmes, G., Pfahringer, B., Read, J., Kranen, P., Kremer, H., Jansen, T., Seidl, T.: MOA: A real-time analytics open source framework. In: Gunopulos, D., Hofmann, T., Malerba, D., Vazirgiannis, M. (eds.) ECML PKDD 2011, Part III. LNCS, vol. 6913, pp. 617–620. Springer, Heidelberg (2011)
3. Brown, G., Wyatt, J.L., Harris, R., Yao, X.: Diversity creation methods: a survey and categorisation. Information Fusion 6(1), 5–20 (2005)
4. Hall, M., Frank, E., Holmes, G., Pfahringer, B., Reutemann, P., Witten, I.H.: The weka data mining software: an update. SIGKDD Explor. Newsl. 11(1), 10–18 (2009)
5. Hulten, G., Spencer, L., Domingos, P.: Mining time-changing data streams. In: Proceedings of the Seventh ACM SIGKDD International Conference on Knowledge Discovery and Data Mining, pp. 97–106 (2001)
6. Jacobs, R.A., Jordan, M.I., Nowlan, S.J., Hinton, G.E.: Adaptive mixtures of local experts. Neural Comput. 3, 79–87 (1991)
7. Klinkenberg, R., Renz, I.: Adaptive information filtering: Learning in the presence of concept drifts, pp. 33–40 (1998)
8. Kolter, J.Z., Maloof, M.A.: Dynamic weighted majority: a new ensemble method for tracking concept drift. In: Third IEEE International Conference on Data Mining, ICDM 2003, pp. 123–130 (November 2003)
9. Kuncheva, L.I.: Combining Pattern Classifiers: Methods and Algorithms. Wiley-Interscience (2004)
10. Kurlej, B., Wozniak, M.: Active learning approach to concept drift problem. Logic Journal of the IGPL 20(3), 550–559 (2012)
11. Muhlbaier, M.D., Topalis, A., Polikar, R.: Learn^{++}.nc: Combining ensemble of classifiers with dynamically weighted consult-and-vote for efficient incremental learning of new classes. IEEE Transactions on Neural Networks 20(1), 152–168 (2009)
12. Partridge, D., Krzanowski, W.: Software diversity: practical statistics for its measurement and exploitation. Information and Software Technology 39(10), 707–717 (1997)
13. Platt, J.C.: Fast training of support vector machines using sequential minimal optimization. In: Advances in Kernel Methods, pp. 185–208. MIT Press, Cambridge (1999)
14. Quinlan, J.R.: C4.5: Programs for Machine Learning. Morgan Kaufmann Series in Machine Learning. Morgan Kaufmann Publishers (1993)
15. Shipp, C.A., Kuncheva, L.: Relationships between combination methods and measures of diversity in combining classifiers. Information Fusion 3(2), 135–148 (2002)
16. Nick Street, W., Kim, Y.: A streaming ensemble algorithm (sea) for large-scale classification. In: Proceedings of the Seventh ACM SIGKDD International Conference on Knowledge Discovery and Data Mining, KDD 2001, pp. 377–382. ACM, New York (2001)
17. Wang, H., Fan, W., Yu, P.S., Han, J.: Mining concept-drifting data streams using ensemble classifiers. In: Proceedings of the Ninth ACM SIGKDD International Conference on Knowledge Discovery and Data Mining, KDD 2003, pp. 226–235. ACM, New York (2003)

18. Widmer, G., Kubat, M.: Learning in the presence of concept drift and hidden contexts. Mach. Learn. 23(1), 69–101 (1996)
19. Wolpert, D.H.: The supervised learning no-free-lunch theorems. In: Proc. 6th Online World Conference on Soft Computing in Industrial Applications, pp. 25–42 (2001)
20. Woźniak, M., Kasprzak, A., Cal, P.: Weighted aging classifier ensemble for the incremental drifted data streams. In: Larsen, H.L., Martin-Bautista, M.J., Vila, M.A., Andreasen, T., Christiansen, H. (eds.) FQAS 2013. LNCS, vol. 8132, pp. 579–588. Springer, Heidelberg (2013)

Similarity Based on Data Compression

Michal Prílepok, Jan Platos, and Vaclav Snasel

Department of Computer Science, FEECS
IT4 Innovations, Centre of Excellence
VSB-Technical University of Ostrava
17. listopadu 15, 708 33, Ostrava Poruba, Czech Republic
{michal.prilepok,jan.platos,vaclav.snasel}@vsb.cz

Abstract. Similarity detection is one of the most important areas in document processing. The applications of it starts in spam detection and goes through identification of plagiarism in the web, bachelor or master thesis and ends at identification of copied scientific papers. This paper presents an improvement of a plagiarism detection algorithm which is based on the Lampel and Ziv dictionary based compression algorithm by application of stop words removing and tests this algorithm on real dataset. Moreover, a visualization of the plagiarized documents relationship is also presented. The algorithm confirms its ability in detection of the plagiarized parts of text and also the achieved improvement when the suggested improvements are applied.

Keywords: plagiarism, compression, similarity detection, visualization.

1 Introduction

The growing number of documents, tests, books and scientific papers brings new challenges in the area of content mining, text precessing and understanding and author identification or confirmation. One of the interesting task is also a plagiarism detection. This problems is actual in many areas such as patent applications, program's source codes copying, image usage without permission, DNA processing, and many others.

This paper is focusing of the ability of the data compression to detect plagiarized texts of their parts. This task is investigated very long time but it becomes even more actual with the massive expansion of the personal computers in the world. The plagiarism may be defined using several definition but we are following this one: The plagiarism detection is the identification of highly similar sections in texts or other objects [1]. Other definitions may be fond in the literature such as this [2]. The plagiarism detection may be divided into two major areas - external and intrinsic [1]. The External plagiarism is defined as an identification of the part of the document d which exists in any of the document in the document collection D. The Intrinsic plagiarism detection is a method which detects the possibly plagiarized parts of the document just from the document itself. The second one is the more complicated.

F. Castro, A. Gelbukh, and M. González (Eds.): MICAI 2013, Part II, LNAI 8266, pp. 267–278, 2013.
© Springer-Verlag Berlin Heidelberg 2013

This paper is organized as follows. The second section contains description of the previous and related work. Section 3 describes the setup of the experiment and section 4 contains achieved results including the visualisation of the distances between similar documents. The last section contains the conclusion of the paper.

2   Current Related Work

Data compression can be used for measurement similarity of texts. There are many data compression algorithm [3] for small text file.

2.1   Similarity of the Texts

The main property in the similarity is a measurement of the distance between two texts. The ideal situation is when this distance is a metric [4]. The distance is formally defined as a function over Cartesian product over set X with non-negative real value [5] and [6]. The metric is a distance which satisfy three conditions for all $x, y, z \in X$:

1. $D(x, y) = 0$ if and only if $x \equiv y$
2. $D(x, y) = D(y, x)$
3. $D(x, y) \leq D(x, y) + D(y, z)$

The condition 1 is called identity, condition 2 is called symmetry and condition three is the triangle inequality. This definition is valid for any metric, e.g. Euclidean Distance, but the application of this principle into document or data similarity is much complicated.

The basic ideas were suggested and defined in related works by Li et al. [6], and Cilibrasi and Vitanyi [5]. They defined the so-called Normalized Information Distance (NID). The NID is based on the definition of the Kolmogorov complexity (KC). The Kolmogorov complexity $K(x)$ of the string $x = \{0, 1\}^*$ is the length of the shortest binary program with no input that outputs x [5]. The Kolmogorov complexity of the two strings may be expressed as follows: The Kolmogorov complexity of x given y is the length of the shortest binary program, for the reference universal prefix Turing machine, that on input y outputs x; it is denoted as $K(x \mid y)$ [5]. The NID is then defined as follows:

$$NID(x, y) = \frac{\max \{K(x \mid y), K(y \mid x)\}}{\min \{K(x \mid y), K(y \mid x)\}}$$

Unfortunately, the Kolmogorov complexity function is non-computable. But Li et al. and Cilibrasi reformulated this problem into a computable form using the replacement of the Kolmogorov complexity by using data compression [5,6]. The metric developed from their work is a Normalized Compression Distance.

2.2   Normalized Compression Distance

The Normalized Compression Distance (NCD) is based on Kolmogorov complexity. It makes use of standard compressors in order to approximate Kolmogorov complexity. Several papers have already used this similarity in order to compare texts of different kinds and in different ways. The NCD has been used for text retrieval [7], text clustering, plagiarism detection [8], music clustering [9,10], music style modeling [11], automatic construction of the phylogeny tree based on whole mitochondrial genomes [12], the automatic construction of language trees [13,6], and the automatic evaluation of machine translations[14].

The NCD is a mathematical way for measuring the similarity of objects. Measuring of similarity is realized by the help of compression where repeating parts are suppressed by compression. NCD may be used for comparison of different objects, such as images, music, texts or gene sequences. The NCD has several requirements to the used compressor [5]. The most important requirement is that the compressor must meets the condition $C(x) = C(xx)$ within logarithmic bounds [15] (see definition of $C(x)$ below). We may use NCD for detection of plagiarism and visual data extraction[16,5].

The resulting rate of probability distance is calculated by the following formula:

$$NCD = \frac{C(xy) - \min\left(C(x), C(y)\right)}{\max\left(C(x), C(y)\right)}$$

Where:

- $C(x)$ ist he length of compression of x.
- $C(xy)$ is the length of compression concatenation of x and y.
- $\min\{x, y\}$ is the minimum of values x and y.
- $\max\{x, y\}$ is the maximum of values x and y.

The NCD value is in the interval $0 \leq NCD(x, y) \leq 1 + \epsilon$. If $NCD(x, y) = 0$, then files x and y are equal. They have the highest difference when the result value of $NCD(x, y) = 1 + \epsilon$. The constant ϵ describes the inefficiency of the used compressor. The NCD is not a metric. It is an approximation of the NID. The computation of the NCD is very efficient because we do not need to create the output itself. We compute only the size of the output. A study of the efficient implementation of the compression algorithms may be found in [17].

2.3   Plagiarism Detection by Compression

The main idea is to use Lempel-Ziv (LZ) compression method. Principle of the method is the fact that for the same sequence of data the compression becomes more efficient. Lempel-Ziv compression method is now mostly used on data compression of various kind of data like texts, images, audio [18,19]. This compression was used to detection of plagiarized text and measurement of the similarity [20].

Creating Dictionary of Document. Creating dictionary is one of the parts of the encoding process Lempel-Ziv 78 method [21]. The dictionary is created from input text, which is splitted into separate words. If current word from the input is not in the dictionary, then this word is added. If current word is contained in dictionary, a next word from the input is added from the input to it. This will create sequence of words. If this sequence is in dictionary, the sequence is extended with the next word from input in a similar way. If the sequence is not in the dictionary, it is added to dictionary with the incrementation of the number of sequences property. The process is repeated until we reach the end of input text.

Comparison of the Documents. The comparison of the documents is the main task. One dictionary is created for each of the compared files. Then the dictionaries are compared to each other. The main property for comparison is the number of common sequences in the dictionaries. This number is represented by the parameter sc in the following formula, which is a metric of similarity two documents.

$$SM = \frac{sc}{min(c_1, c_2)}$$

- sc - count of common word sequences in both dictionaries.
- c_1, c_2 - total count of word sequences in dictionary of the first or the second document.

The SM value is in the interval $0 \leq SM \leq 1$. If $SM = 1$, then the documents are equal and they have the highest difference when the result value of $SM = 0$.

3   Experimental Setup

We used The PAN plagiarism corpus 2012 (PAN-PC-11) [22] dataset for confirmation of our algorithm. This is a corpus for the evaluation of automatic plagiarism detection algorithms. The PAN-PC-11 dataset contains 22.730 source documents based on on books from the Project Gutenberg in English (22.000), German (520) and Spanish (210) language. The plagiarized suspicious documents does not contains any real plagiarism cases. All of the annotated plagiarism cases are either artificial, i.e., generated by a computer program, or simulated, i.e., purposefully made by a human.

From this dataset we selected randomly 150 suspicious documents, 80 (53.33%) suspicious with plagiarized parts of text and 70 (46.76%) suspicious documents without plagiarized parts. Then we selected all the corresponding annotated source documents to these randomly selected suspicious documents and we added another 20% randomly selected source documents. We used 150 suspicious and 223 source documents for confirmation of our algorithm.

The comparison of the whole documents where only a small part of the document may be plagiarized is useless, because other characteristics and text of the new whole document may hide or suppress the characteristic of the plagiarized part. Therefore, we suggest to split the documents into paragraphs. We choose paragraphs, because we think that they are better than sentences. They contain more words and should be not so affected by the common words such as preposition, conjunctives, etc. The Paragraphs were separated by an empty line between them. We created a dictionary using method described in section 2.3 for each paragraph from the source document. As a results of the fragmentation of the source documents we get 108.374 paragraphs and their corresponding dictionaries. These paragraphs dictionaries serve as a reference dictionaries, against which we compare paragraph dictionaries from suspicious documents.

The set of suspicious documents was processed in a similar way. Each suspicious document was fragmented into paragraphs. The we create a corresponding dictionary using the same algorithm. Then we compared this dictionary with the dictionaries from the source documents. To improve the speed of the comparison, we choose only subset of dictionaries for comparison. The subset is chosen according the size of particular dictionary with tolerance of $\pm20\%$, e.g. when the dictionary of the suspected paragraphs contains 122 phrases, we choose all dictionaries with number of phrases between 98 and 146. This 20% tolerance significantly improve the speed of the comparison and, moreover, we believe, does not affect the overall efficiency of the algorithm. We pick up the paragraph with the highest similarity to the each paragraph of the tested paragraph.

3.1   A Modification without Stop Words

The original approach uses all words from the paragraphs from the source and suspicious documents. But we think that this is highly affected by the presence of stop words which are common to any text. Therefore, we suggest the second round of experiments which process files without these stop words. As a source of stop words we have used Full-Text stop words from MySQL[1]. The list contains 543 stop words. The algorithm defined in 2.3 is modified in a way that after the fragmentation of the text, all words from the list are removed form the paragraphs and the rest of it is then processed by the same algorithm.

4   Results

The plagiarism dataset and experiments were described in the previous section. Before we present the results achieved on the whole dataset in Table 1. In our meaning we will consider as a plagiarized document a document in which managed to find all plagiarized parts from the attached annotation XML file. Partially plagiarized document is a document in we did not detect successful all plagiarized part from annotation XML file, for example 3 from 5 parts in annotation XML file. A non plagiarized documents is a document, which did not have in the XML file annotated plagiarized part of text.

---

[1] `http://dev.mysql.com/doc/refman/5.5/en/fulltext-stopwords.html`

Table 1. Document successful rate results

	Successful rate	
	All words	Stop words
Plagiarized documents	30.67%	32.67%
Partially plagiarized documents	22.67%	20.67%
Non plagiarized documents	46.67%	46.67%

In our experiments with used all words we found 30.67% plagiarized documents, 22.67% partially plagiarized document and 46.67% non plagiarized documents. In the other approach, with removed stop word, we achieved following results. We found 32.67% plagiarized, 20.67% partially plagiarized and 46.67% non plagiarized documents.

In the case of partially plagiarized documents we could find suspicious paragraph in another document, or we found a paragraph with higher similarity as a paragraph with the same content. this cases can occurs if one of the paragraphs is shorter as the other. To illustrate this case we mention a brief example. We have two paragraphs. The first paragraph has 15 word sequences in the dictionary, the other paragraph has 13 word sequences. This paragraphs are different in 2 word sequences and have 6 same word sequences. After calculating the similarity we get value of similarity 46.15%. This similarity is higher than in the case if both paragraphs have the same number of word sequences in the dictionary. In this case, when number of word sequences is equal, we get 40% similarity. This example is depict in Table 2.

We will show the example of the algorithm on the two similar paragraphs in 4.1.

Table 2. Examples of changes in similarities

Word sequences paragraph 1 ($c1$)	15	15
Word sequences paragraph 2 ($c2$)	13	15
Equal word sequences (sc)	6	6
Similarity (SM)	46.15%	40.00%

4.1   Result Example

This first paragraph comes from one of the suspicious documents collections. Paragraph consists of two sentences.

```
Most amiable and seated he looks,
that little Johnnie he,
while foul distant behind his heels
is little Sallie she.
With flaxen curls and laughing eyes,
this complex girl we greet,
cry, "how fair is Johnnie he!
And sallie she, how sweet!"
```

The second paragraph was taken as the most similar paragraph from the source documents collection. This paragraph has the greatest similarity $SM = 0.82352$ when using all the words and similarity $SM = 0.76471$ without stop words.

```
Most amiable and fair he looks,
That little Johnnie He,
While following close behind his heels
Is little Sallie She.
With flaxen curls and laughing eyes,
This little girl we greet,
Exclaim, "How fair is Johnnie He!
And Sallie She, how sweet!"
```

The difference between exemplary paragraphs is not big. The second paragraph has changed a few words in sentences against first paragraph. Number of words in both paragraphs is the same, and, Semantically, these paragraphs can be identical.

Results of the example are summarized in the Table 3.

Table 3. Results of the example

	All words	Without stop words
Words count	42	42
Suspicious paragraph sequences ($c1$)	36	19
Source paragraph sequences ($c2$)	34	17
Common sequences(sc)	28	13
Similarity (SM)	0.82352	0.76471

As may be seen, the algorithm detect the similarity of these paragraphs very well.

4.2   Visualization of the Similarity of Documents

The previous section confirms that the method is able to detect similarity of the two paragraphs. More complicated situation appears when more than two paragraphs should be compared together. The methods may computes a similarity matrix when it compares each pair of paragraphs together, but the interpretation of such matrix is not easy task. One possibility is the usage of the clustering algorithm, but it must deals with the vectors in very high dimension. Another possibility is to reduce the the dimension or to map the paragraphs and their distance into lover dimensional space.

The second approach was heavily studied in the past, but one of the interesting approach was defined by Sammon [23]. The mapping defined in that paper is non-linear and its only feature is the Error function based on the distances between point in the original space and the point in the new space. The error function is defined as follows:

$$E = \frac{1}{\sum\limits_{i<j} D_{ij}} \sum\limits_{i<j}^{N} \frac{(D_{ij} - d_{ij})^2}{D_{ij}}$$

where the N is the number of objects, i, j are indices which go through all objects in the set, i.e. $i, j = 1 \ldots N$, D_{ij} is the distance between objects i and j in the original space and d_{ij} is the distance of the same objects in the new space. The new space usually has dimension 2 or 3.

Such mapping as was proposed by Sammon is very useful for interpretation of the results of highly dimensional data processing, because it enables its visualization with preserving the distances between objects.

To demonstrate the visualization of similarity between objects we create an artificial example. We take the four independent texts from the Canterbury Compression Corpus [24]. first two text were first and second chapter of the file *alice29.txt* - Alice's Adventures in Wonderland from Lewis Carroll. The other two was two shortened chapters from the file *plrabn12.txt* - a poem Paradise Lost by John Milton. Each file was shortened to have around 10 kB in size. The we automatically generated for version of each where we took 20, 40, 60 and 80 percent form the original text and then we added a absolutely independent text take from the original files from the dataset. The final size of the file was always size of the original text +- 20% in size. The files used as a filling were completely independant. The we make a similarity matrix for all these files, 4 original and to each 4 plagiarized files. So the final matrxi has dimension of 20×20. First, we used the algorithm described in section 2.3. Then we used also a NCD measure, which was described in section 2.2 and as a compression method we used a GZIP algorithm[2] in version 1.2.4. Because NCd is disimilarity measure and our algorithm is a similarity measure, I convert the results of our algorithm into disimilarity by subtraction the results from 1. When we take the disimilarity as a distance between objects and small numbers means higher similarity. These matrices were processed by the Sammon algorithm and the result images are depicted in Figure 1 for our algorithm and in Figure 2.

As a distance measure in the new 2-dimensional space we used standard Euclidean distance. As may be seen, four groups may be detected on each image, where they may be interpreted as a four original texts. The different position of the groups is caused by the random initialization of the initial position of the points in new space. Both pictures demonstrates the ability of the LZ Dictionary based similarity to distinguish between similar or plagiarized objects, because text with higher percentage of similarity are closer than files wit lower similarity. The pictures also demonstrates that the proposed algorithm is able to identified similarity in similar way as it is a NCD measure.

---

[2] http://www.gzip.org/

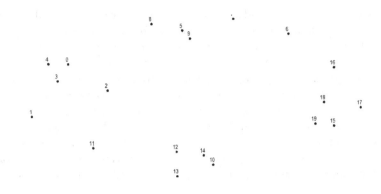

Fig. 1. Mapping of the similar text with the LZ Dictionary similarity measure

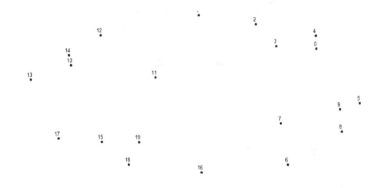

Fig. 2. Mapping of the similar text with NCD similarity measure

4.3   Results on the Dataset

To test the ability of the algorithm described in previous section on real larger dataset, we process experiments with the dataset which was described in previous section. Before we depict the results, a discussion on results similarity measure *SM* is necessary. The higher *SM* means higher similarity between paragraphs. When $SM = 0.3$ means that only 30% of the phrases in the dictionary are the same for both dictionaries. This is really small number especially when stop words were not removed from the text. Other similar words may be common words, which are not stop words but are also very frequent, e.g. verbs, adjectives etc. Paragraphs that have a value $SM \geq 0.5$ can be considered as more similar. They have most words, groups of words and sequences identical. When value of the *SM* is very close to one, the paragraphs are almost identical and it means two things. First, the paragraphs are really the same and are plagiarized. Second, paragraphs are the same but they are common features like content, preface, chapter numbering, or frequently used idioms.

On histograms (Figure 3 and Figure 4) we can see the quantity distribution of the paragraphs similarities of the document. On both histograms we can see the quantity distribution of the similarities of the same document. The first histogram (Figure 3) belongs to an algorithm, which uses all words from paragraph. The other histogram (Figure 3) belongs to an algorithm, which removes stop words from paragraph. Removing stop words caused the spreading of a large group values in the range between 0.25 and 0.45 in the first histogram to a larger interval in the second histogram. After removing stop words appeared higher number of paragraphs with a higher similarity. after removing stop words, we can better recognize plagiarized paragraphs from the original source paragraphs, because the similarity values between paragraphs have considerable differences.

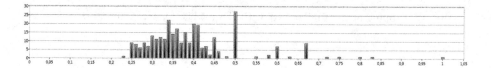

Fig. 3. Histogram of paragraph similarities with all words

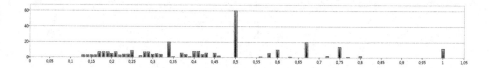

Fig. 4. Histogram of paragraph similarities without stop words

In both algorithm possibilities occurred two same problems, that have simple solutions. The first problem occurs in short sections that make up the chapter titles. These are the chapter titles such as content, preface, conclusion or numbering of chapters, for example Chapter I. In these parts of the text occurs the maximum value of similarity ($SM = 1.0$). Although the are not suspected parts of the text. This unwanted effect can be eliminated by the list of forbidden terms. This terms will not be added into the dictionary.

The second problem occurs in short paragraphs with a few simple short sentences. This paragraph types may appear in many documents although they are not plagiarized. The solution to this second problem is the appropriate text division into larger text parts.

5   Conclusion

In this paper, we applied a new similarity detection algorithm on a real dataset with additional speed improvements. We also confirms the ability to detect plagiarized parts of the documents. Moreover, a visualization of the similarity between documents was introduced. The algorithm for similarity measurement based on the Lampel Ziv compression algorithm and its dictionaries was very efficient in detection of the plagiarized parts of the documents. All plagiarized documents in a dataset were marked as plagiarized and in most cases all plagiarized parts were identified as well as their original version. Better results were achieved when a a removing of stop words was applied before the plagiarized documents were checked. This also significantly reduces the speed of the detection process and memory requirements.

Acknowledgment. This work was partially supported by the Grant Agency of the Czech Republic under grant no. P202/11/P142, and by the Grant of SGS No. SP2013/70, VŠB - Technical University of Ostrava, Czech Republic, and was supported by the European Regional Development Fund in the IT4Innovations Centre of Excellence project (CZ.1.05/1.1.00/02.0070) and by the Bio-Inspired Methods: research, development and knowledge transfer project, reg. no. CZ.1.07/ 2.3.00/20.0073 funded by Operational Programme Education for Competitiveness, co-financed by ESF and state budget of the Czech Republic.

References

1. Potthast, M., Stein, B., Eiselt, A., Barrón-cedeño, A., Rosso, P.: P.:Overview of the 1st international competition on plagiarism detection. In: SEPLN 2009 Workshop on Uncovering Plagiarism, Authorship, and Social Software Misuse (PAN 2009), pp. 1–9. CEUR-WS.org (2009)
2. Maurer, H., Kappe, F., Zaka, B.: Plagiarism - a survey
3. Platos, J., Snásel, V., El-Qawasmeh, E.: Compression of small text files. Advanced Engineering Informatics 22(3), 410–417 (2008)
4. Tversky, A.: Features of similarity. Psychological Review 84(4), 327–352 (1977)
5. Cilibrasi, R., Vitányi, P.M.B.: Clustering by compression. IEEE Transactions on Information Theory 51(4), 1523–1545 (2005)
6. Li, M., Chen, X., Li, X., Ma, B., Vitányi, P.M.B.: The similarity metric. IEEE Transactions on Information Theory 50(12), 3250–3264 (2004)
7. Granados, A.: Analysis and study on text representation to improve the accuracy of the normalized compression distance. AI Commun. 25(4), 381–384 (2012)
8. Chen, X., Francia, B., Li, M., McKinnon, B., Seker, A.: Shared information and program plagiarism detection. IEEE Transactions on Information Theory 50(7), 1545–1551 (2004)
9. Cilibrasi, R., Vitnyi, P., de Wolf, R.: Algorithmic clustering of music based on string compression. Computer Music Journal 28(4), 49–67 (2004)
10. González-Pardo, A., Granados, A., Camacho, D., De Borja Rodríguez, F.: Influence of music representation on compression-based clustering (2010)
11. Dubnov, S., Assayag, G., Lartillot, O., Bejerano, G.: Using machine-learning methods for musical style modeling. Computer 36(10), 73–80 (2003)
12. Li, M., Badger, J., Chen, X., Kwong, S., Kearney, P., Zhang, H.: An information-based sequence distance and its application to whole mitochondrial genome phylogeny. Bioinformatics 17(2), 149–154 (2001)
13. Benedetto, D., Caglioti, E., Loreto, V.: Language trees and zipping. Physical Review Letters 88(4), 487021–487024 (1996)

14. Väyrynen, J.J., Tapiovaara, T., Kettunen, K., Dobrinkat, M.: Normalized compression distance as an automatic MT evaluation metric. In: Proceedings of MT 25 Years, Cranfield, UK, November 21–22, 2009 (to appear)
15. Sculley, D., Brodley, C.: Compression and machine learning: A new perspective on feature space vectors, pp. 332–341 (2006)
16. Vitányi, P.M.B.: Universal similarity. CoRR, abs/cs/0504089 (2005)
17. Walder, J., Krátký, M., Baca, R., Platos, J., Snásel, V.: Fast decoding algorithms for variable-lengths codes. Inf. Sci. 183(1), 66–91 (2012)
18. Kirovski, D., Landau, Z.: Generalized lempel-ziv compression for audio. In: 2004 IEEE 6th Workshop on Multimedia Signal Processing, pp. 127–130 (2004)
19. Crnojevic, V., Senk, V., Trpovski, Z.: Lossy lempel-ziv algorithm for image compression. In: 6th International Conference on Telecommunications in Modern Satellite, Cable and Broadcasting Service, TELSIKS 2003, vol. 2, pp. 522–525 (2003)
20. Chudá, D., Uhlík, M.: The plagiarism detection by compression method. In: Rachev, B., Smrikarov, A. (eds.) CompSys Tech, pp. 429–434. ACM (2011)
21. Ziv, J., Lempel, A.: Compression of individual sequences via variable-rate coding. IEEE Transactions on Information Theory 24(5), 530–536 (1978)
22. Potthast, M., Stein, B., Barrón-Cedeño, A., Rosso, P.: An Evaluation Framework for Plagiarism Detection. In: Huang, C.-R., Jurafsky, D. (eds.) 23rd International Conference on Computational Linguistics (COLING 2010), pp. 997–1005. Association for Computational Linguistics, Stroudsburg (2010)
23. Sammon, J.: A nonlinear mapping for data structure analysis. IEEE Transactions on Computers C-18(5), 401–409 (1969)
24. Arnold, R., Bell, T.: A corpus for the evaluation of lossless compression algorithms, pp. 201–210

Pattern Recognition
with Spiking Neural Networks

Israel Tabarez Paz, Neil Hernández Gress, and Miguel González Mendoza

Universidad Autónoma del Estado de México
Blvd. Universitario s/n, Predio San Javier Atizapán de Zaragoza, México
itabarezp@uaemex.mx
http://www.uaem.mx/cuyuaps/vallemexico.html
Tecnológico de Monterrey, Campus Estado de México,
Carretera Lago de Guadalupe km 3.5 Col. Margarita Maza de Juarez,
Atizapán de Zaragora, México
{ngress,mgonza}@itesm.mx
http://www.itesm.edu

Abstract This manuscript is focused on some applications of method Spikeprop of Spiking Neural Networks (SNN) using an especific hardware for parallel programming in order to measure the eficience. So, we are interested on pattern recognition and clustering, that are the main problems to solve for Artificial Neural Networks (ANN). As a result, we are going to know the considerations,its limitations and advantages, that we have to take into account for applying SNN. The main advantage is that the quantity of applications can be expanded for real applications linear or non linear, with more than one attribute, and big volume of datas. In contrast, other methods spend a lot of memory to process the information, which computational complexity is propotional to the volume and quantity of attributes of datas, also is more difficult to program the algorithm for multiclass database. However, the main limitation of SNN is the convergence, that tends forward a Local minimum Value. This implies a high dependency on the configuration and proposed architecture. On the other hand, we programmed the algorithm of SNN in a GPU model NVIDIA GeForce 9400 M. In this GPU we had to reduce parallelism in order to increase quantity of layers and neurons in the same hardware in spite of contains 60000 threads, they were not enought. On the otrher hand, the divergence is reduced when the database is bigger for database multiclass.

Keywords: GPU, FPGA, Artificial Neural Networks, Spiking Neural Networks, Image Recognition, Clustering.

1 Introduction

This paper show us some applications of method Spikeprop of Spiking Neural Network (SNN). Firstly, we propose characters recognition looking upon only the five vowels, however this problem can be extended for more letters and numbers.

F. Castro, A. Gelbukh, and M. González (Eds.): MICAI 2013, Part II, LNAI 8266, pp. 270–288, 2013.
© Springer-Verlag Berlin Heidelberg 2013

The result let us to see that this metholology is very good for this applications, but also to know that there are some issues in the future. On the other hand, we apply some real database about patients in a hospital for classification according to some proposed characteristics. In this point, Olaf proposed characters recognition through its pronuntiation [4], however he says that this application is a very difficult because of encoding the datas and spent memory. The most of techniques for image recognition apply known typical techniques as contour detections, image segmentation mathematics tools. Also, traditionals Artificial Neural Networks as Perceptron and Backpropagation have beem used to pattern recognition.

There are others important methologies such as Quadratic Programming (QP) and Sequential Minimal Optimization (SMO) [15], from Support Vector Machine (SVM) [5] they both, also Izhikevich model [7] and Hodgkin – Huxley model [18], from Spiking Neural Networks (SNN) they both. First Support Vector Machine (SVM) has been used for regression, database classification or progression, but its quadratic or cubic computational complexity consumes so much of memory. On the other hand, SNN has been used for speech recognition but there are no reference about applications respect to big databases or image recognition. So, the main motivation of this work starts from knowing the applications areas of SNN in order to measure the efficiency of the method. This methodology was developed in 2003, and was called Spike Response Model (SRM) (Bohte [3], Olaf [4]). Respect to Izhikevich model [7], this is the reduced model of Hodgkin–Huxley integrated of two differential equations that explain behavior of mammal neurons.

On the other hand, parallel programming [12] consists on solving large problems by parts. However, there are several different forms of parallel computing such as bit level, instruction level, and task parallelism. This paper is focused on instruction level as in the figure 1 [10], where it is shown the principle of parallel computing. Problems of parallel programming are solved in language C for CUDA.

This paper is distributed as follows: in section 2 refers to relating works, also section 3 contains aspects related to principles of SNN and its parallelization, the architecture of the network and other considerations are included, also contains the found limitations during programming. On the other side, in section 4 treatment of image is presented. Finally, in section 5 the experiments are shown and section 6 we discuss the conclusions.

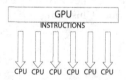

Fig. 1. Parallel programming

2   Relating Works on Spiking Neural Networks

The related works about SNN are shown in the following table 1. The most of authors are focused on the learning time to compare the speed between CPU and GPU, but nobody programmed the optimization QP.

Table 1. State of the Art

AUTHOR	DESCRIPTION OF THE PAPER	DATE
Arash [1]	Compared the speed between CPU and GPU with Izhike-vich"s model	2011
Izhikevich [8]	Designed an hybrid model of SNN for numeric methods.	2010
Bhuiyan [2]	Compared the Izhikevich and Hodgkin Huxley model applied to character recognition.	2010
Scanzio [17]	Compared the speed of processing in CUDA of algorithms feedfordward and backpropagation	2010
Xin Jin [9]	Applied a SpiNNaker chip to compare with MatLab. He evaluated the actualization of a neuron, arrangement of entry	2010
Nageswaran [11]	Presented a compilation of the Izhikevich"s models.	2009
Thomas and Luk [17] [19]	Simulated the Izhikevich"s model in a FPGA	2009
Stewart [18]	Applied Runge – Kutta"s method for Izhikevich and Bair [18] and Hodgkin Huxle"s model	2009
Prabhu [16]	Applied GPU for image recognition. He focuses on the degree of parallelism of a problem. The maximum size of image was 256 MB, and in a video memory GPU of 768 MB. As a result, author compares Dual -- Core AMD processor with a Geforce 6150 GPU, and when number of patterns increase, the CPU is linearlly slower than GPU. But when the network size increase then curve is not linear.	2008
Philipp [14]	Implemented SNN in a FPGA to simulate thousands of neurons.	2007
Pavlidis [13]	Applied evolution algorithms in SNN.	2005
Olaf [4]	Theory about SNN and codification of the entries are studies.	2004
Bohte [3]	Compared other algorithms with Spikeprop but author does not show the learning time, but presents differences between traditional ANN and SNN.	2003
Izhikevich [7]	Simulated in MatLab the Hodgkin — Huxley"s model. Also, he executes maximum 10000 neurons and 1 000 000 of sinapsys.	2003

3   Parallel Programming in SNN

The architecture of SNN consists in a set of neurons what contains delays as in the figure 2 (Olaf [4]).

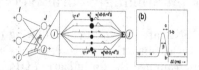

Fig. 2. Conectividad de las SNN

A neuron j, that belongs to a set Γ_j ('pre– synaptic neuron') [4], is fired when the output reaches the threshold θ after receiving a set of pulses in the time $t_i, i\epsilon\Gamma_j$. So, the dynamic of the variable $x_j(t)$ is given by the impulse response $\varepsilon(t)$ where w_{ij} are the weights from conection i to j:

$$x_j(t) = \sum_{i\epsilon\Gamma_j} w_{ij}\varepsilon(t - t_i) \tag{1}$$

The synaptic potential can be defined by the equation (2):

$$\varepsilon(t) = \frac{t}{\tau}e^{1-\frac{t}{\tau}} \tag{2}$$

The constant τ controls the width of the pulse. So, the equation (3) describes the quantity of synaptic conexions of a neuron j:

$$x_j(t) = \sum_{i\epsilon\Gamma_j}\sum_{k=1}^{m} w_{ij}^k y^k(t) \tag{3}$$

A output of a neuron is described by 4:

$$y_j^k(t) = \varepsilon(t - t_i - d_k) \tag{4}$$

Where, d_k is the delay time of a conection k fired from the pre – synaptic neuron to the rise time of the post – synaptic neuron.

Finally, equation 5 represents the output potential $u_j(t)$ for a j nauron:

$$u_j(t) = \sum_{t_j^{(f)}\epsilon F_j} \eta(t - t_j^{(f)}) + \sum_{i\epsilon\Gamma_j}\sum_{t_i^{(g)}} w_{ij}\varepsilon(t - t_i^{(g)} - d_{ij}) \tag{5}$$

Where

$$F_j = \{t^{(f)}; 1 \le f \le n\} = \{t|u_j(t) = \vartheta\} \tag{6}$$

And n is the quantity of pulses.

Parallel programming in a GPU involves to solve the problem of configuration of hardware GPU [10]. In case of SNN, is necessary to programme a kernel in three dimensions. In contrast, the simplest configuration in one or two dimensions is used in the perceptron method. In other words, all outputs of neurons per layer can be calculated at the same time because of the simple form of its activation function. However, the activation function of SNN is more complex due to exponential form, which time variable is calculated with mathematic, approximation methods, as a consecuense the outputs of neurons are not always calculated at the same time. In this case, with GPU used we got a near solution because of float presicion, but in case of SVM we need a double presicion to get the best solution.

In a GPU, parameters of the hardware architecture to be considered are threads, blocks and grids [12]. In case of SNN, each block can represent only one neuron, because of computational resources are not enough for database bigger. The main problem of SNN is to calculate the value of threshold in amplitude and time because of this implies that many values of time are needed, as well as, maybe hundreds or thousands columns per block. So, neuron is represented as a grid in tree dimensions, where each row can represent a previous neuron to be added for one output of the following neuron. This method requires good memory resources. Therefore, sometimes it is not recommended to parallel more than hardware features allow you to do.

The arrange of figure 3 represents a configuration of the GPU device in three dimensions. This is a solution for parallelizing SNN algorithm. The cube showed in this figure is only a neuron of a hidden or output layer. There are cubes as neurons are required. Each cube is divided in blocks, what depend on the length of time in the input [4]. All neurons per layer can be calculated in parallel, but a disadvantage is that this procedure requires many resources of memory. So, the time into a block depends on the length between input time and output time.

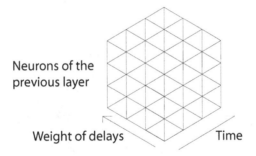

Fig. 3. Parallelization of SNN in 3D

The time is defined in the GPU as a time interval. This model card contains 255 threads por block and 235 blocks, so the total quantity of threads in the card is 60000, aproximately. Configuration of blocks in three dimension is in the equation 7:

$$threadx = \frac{SIZE}{(NN[num\_cap])(NN[num\_cap + 1])} \tag{7}$$

Where $threadx$ is the time t; $SIZE$ is threads per block; $NN[num\_cap]$ is the number of neurons in the layer where we want to get the output; $NN[num\_cap+1]$

is the number of neurons in the next layer. We can see that delays are not taking into account for parallel programming, so they are applied sequentially because of memory limitations. Also, if the time exceeds the quantity of threads per block, so we have to add more bloks, but this was encodes sequentially which affects the time processing.

On the other hand, in the figure 4 the vowals in format bmp are shown. But the image can be in other format or it can be a photo. Also, in the figure 5 the architecture of the network is shown, so the quantity of neurons in the input layer is the quantity of pixels of the image. The quantity of neurons of the hidden layer was limited to the hardware.

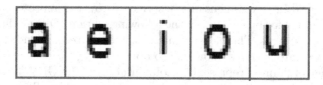

Fig. 4. Image vowals in format bmp (size 5 x 5 pixels)

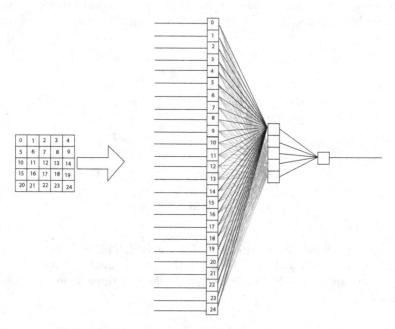

Fig. 5. Architecture of the SNN for image recognition

A big disadvantage of GPU's is the limitation of the hardware, however the parallelism can be reduced or other model of GPU could be considered.

4   Processing of the Image

There are some factors to take into account to get good results, for example the light, color of the objects, noise in the figure 6.

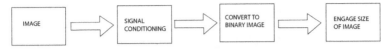

Fig. 6. Processing Image

The size of the image had to be reduced to 5 x 5 pixels because of limitations of the memory of hardware, even thought is not necesary to have so much accuracy because of image procceing. In this case, the architecture of the network depends on the size of image, so the quantity of pixels represents the quantity of the input neurons. The size of image can not be bigger because of the configuration in the blocks is according to figure 3, so the time axis needs to be large enough which consumes many threads. We used MATLAB to get the right image to be recognized. According to equation (7), it was necessary to reduce the size of image to 5 x 5 pixels, because of the quantity of neurons in the input layer must not to be more than 25 neurons.

5   Experiments

Results of character recognition is presented in this section. In the figure 7 learning stage is presented. It takes approximately two hours to achieve 4 of 5 successes and 9.937205 of quadratic medium error. It would be interesting to achieve more than five neurons in the hidden layer in order to get more efficiency and accuracy. It took aproximately two hours in the learning time. In this case, there are some peaks non desired, so the convergence depends on architecture of the GPU kernel. It would be interesting to increase the quantity of neurons in the layers in order to get better results, but the main problem are the limitations of the GPU and the difficulty to find the optimal architecture of the network and the best values of parameters.

In case of patients of a hospital for classification. We only took a sample 500 patients from 80 000 because it was no possible to take all datas because of memory limitations. This database consist of identify patients with tubeculosis which attributes refers to basical personal information of them.

The attributes are CONSECUTIVE ESTUDY CONTACT, SEX, AGE >20 (18 YES, 20 NO), EXAMINE, EXAMINE 1, EXAMINE 2, EXAMINE 3, CASE (18 YES, 20 NO). The output what we considered was QUIMIOPROFILAXIS (18 YES, 20 NO). In this application, from 500 datas we got 372 success in 21 iterations with 2.3103 73 of quadratic medium error. Time learning was 292237.156250 miliseconds. However, we can select other output attribute according to we need. Also, the name of each patient and ID of tubersculosis was omited of the traning stage because of simplify.

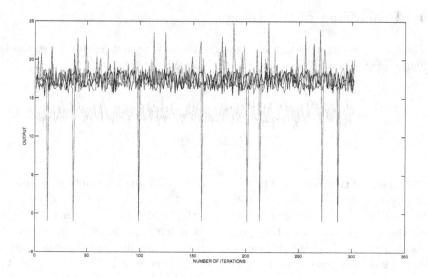

Fig. 7. Learning stage

In the figure 8, we see the convergence of the solution translated to the reduction of the quadratic medium error. However, we can see after fifth iteration
the reduction of the error is slower, so after that quantity of successes do not
increase as fast as we hope, in fact, solution tends to keep on 372 successes after
fifth iteration. This is the main disadvantage of the SNN methology.

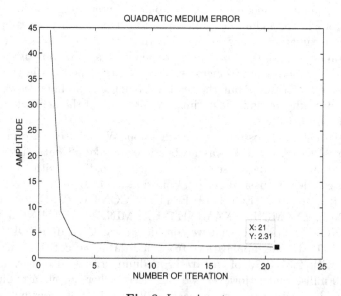

Fig. 8. Learning stage

Finally, we shows efficiency in the table 2.

Table 2. Efficiency of SNN

INPUT DATAS	SUCCESS	EFFICIENCY %
VOWELS	4	80
HOSPITAL DATAS	372	74.4

6 Conclusions

In this paper we conclude that parallelism in SNN increase speed of learning time. However, algorithm SNN has to be improved to converge forward the best solution. We propone to reduce parallelism according to architecture of the card. However, we considered that the best hardware to parallize SNN is FPGA [19], [6] to eliminate problems of copying from host to device and viceversa, what represents to increase learning time. Although, other important problem to get good results is encoding input values in the time. Results and learning time depends on encoding input values and parameters on activation function. Also, with this information is possible to know what applications are the most appropriates for SNN. As a future work, there are other technologies to use for getting good results, as SNN in a FPGA.

References

1. Ahmadi, A., Soleimani, H.: A gpu based simulation of multilayer spiking neural networks. In: 2011 19th Iranian Conference on Electrical Engineering (ICEE), pp. 1–5 (May 2011)
2. Bhuiyan, M.A., Pallipuram, V.K., Smith, M.C.: Acceleration of spiking neural networks in emerging multi-core and gpu architectures. In: 2010 IEEE International Symposium on Parallel & Distributed Processing, Workshops and Phd Forum (IPDPSW), pp. 1–8 (April 2010)
3. Bohte, S.M.: Spiking neural networks. Unpublished doctoral dissertation, Centre for Mathematics and Computer Science, Amsterdam (2003)
4. Booij, O.: Temporal pattern classification using spiking neural networks. Unpublished master's thesis, University of Amsterdam (August 2004)
5. Cortes, C., Vapnik, V.: Support-vector networks. Machine Learning 20(3), 273–297 (1995)
6. Fidjeland, A.K., Roesch, E.B., Shanahan, M.P., Luk, W.: Nemo: A platform for neural modelling of spiking neurons using gpus. In: 20th IEEE International Conference on Application-specific Systems, Architectures and Processors, ASAP 2009, pp. 137–144 (July 2009)
7. Izhikevich, E.M.: Simple model of spiking neurons. IEEE Transactions on Neural Networks 14(6), 1569–1572 (2003)
8. Izhikevich, E.M.: Hybrid spiking models. Philosophical Transactions of the Royal Society A: Mathematical, Physical and Engineering Sciences 368(1930), 5061–5070 (2010)

9. Jin, X.: Parallel Simulation of Neural Networks on Spinnaker Universal Neuromorphic Hardware. PhD thesis, University of Manchester (2010)
10. Kirk, D.B., Wen-mei, W.H.: Programming massively parallel processors: a hands-on approach. Morgan Kaufmann (2010)
11. Nageswaran, J.M., Dutt, N., Krichmar, J.L., Nicolau, A., Veidenbaum, A.V.: Efficient simulation of large-scale spiking neural networks using cuda graphics processors. Neural Networks, 791–800 (June 2009)
12. NVIDIA. NVIDIA CUDA C BEST PRACTICES GUIDE DG–05603–001v5.0, dg–05603–001v5.0 ed. (May 2012)
13. Pavlidis, N., Tasoulis, O., Plagianakos, V.P., Nikiforidis, G., Vrahatis, M.: Spiking neural network training using evolutionary algorithms. In: Proceedings of the IEEE International Joint Conference on Neural Networks, IJCNN 2005, vol. 4, pp. 2190–2194. IEEE (August 2005)
14. Philipp, S., Grübl, A., Meier, K., Schemmel, J.: Interconnecting VLSI spiking neural networks using isochronous connections. In: Sandoval, F., Prieto, A.G., Cabestany, J., Graña, M. (eds.) IWANN 2007. LNCS, vol. 4507, pp. 471–478. Springer, Heidelberg (2007)
15. Platt, J.C.: Sequiential minimal optimization: A fast algorithm for tarining support vector machines
16. Prabhu, R.D.: Somgpu: An unsupervised pattern classifier on graphical processing unit. In: IEEE Congress on Evolutionary Computation, CEC 2008 (IEEE World Congress on Computational Intelligence), pp. 1011–1018, 1–6 (June 2008)
17. Scanzio, S., Cumani, S., Gemello, R., Mana, F., Laface, P.: Parallel implementation of artificial neural network training, pp. 4902–4905
18. Stewart, R.D., Bair, W.: Spiking neural network simulation: numerical integration with the parker–sochacki method. Journal of Computational Neuroscience 27(1), 115–133 (2009)
19. Thomas, D.B., Luk, W.: Fpga accelerated simulation of biologically plausible spiking neural networks. In: 17th IEEE Symposium on Field Programmable Custom Computing Machines, FCCM 2009, pp. 45–52 (April 2009)

Subjective Evaluation of Labeling Methods for Association Rule Clustering

Renan de Padua[1], Fabiano Fernandes dos Santos[1], Merley da Silva Conrado[1],
Veronica Oliveira de Carvalho[2], and Solange Oliveira Rezende[1]

[1] Instituto de Ciências Matemáticas e de Computação,
USP - Universidade de São Paulo, São Carlos, Brazil
{padua,fabianof,merleyc,solange}@icmc.usp.br
[2] Instituto de Geociências e Ciências Exatas,
UNESP - Univ Estadual Paulista, Rio Claro, Brazil
veronica@rc.unesp.br

Abstract. Among the post-processing association rule approaches, clustering is an interesting one. When an association rule set is clustered, the user is provided with an improved presentation of the mined patters. The domain to be explored is structured aiming to join association rules with similar knowledge. To take advantage of this organization, it is essential that good labels be assigned to the groups, in order to guide the user during the association rule exploration process. Few works have explored and proposed labeling methods for this context. Moreover, these methods have not been explored through subjective evaluations in order to measure their quality; usually, only objective evaluations are used. This paper subjectively evaluates five labeling methods used on association rule clustering. The evaluation aims to find out the methods that presents the best results based on the analysis of the domain experts. The experimental results demonstrate that there is a disagreement between objective and subjective evaluations as reported in other works from literature.

1 Introduction

Association rule mining (ARM), introduced in [1], is an important task of data mining. ARM aims to "find all co-occurrence relationships, called associations, among data items" [11].

Association rules have been successfully applied for decision support (such as the cross-marketing, attached mailing applications, catalog design, add-on sales, store layout, and customer segmentation based on buying patterns) [3], for applications of telecommunications alarm diagnosis and prediction [2], for inter-disciplinary domains beyond data mining (such as indexing and similarity search of complex structured data, spatio-temporal and multimedia data mining, stream data mining, web mining, software bug mining, and page-fetch prediction) [8], and for disease prediction [17].

When generating association rules, it is necessary to deal with a huge amount of rules since the number of rules grows exponentially with the number of items in

F. Castro, A. Gelbukh, and M. González (Eds.): MICAI 2013, Part II, LNAI 8266, pp. 289–300, 2013.

the data set [9]. Many algorithms have been developed to overcome the problem of dealing with these generated rules. These algorithms follow one of these post-processing approaches: Querying (Q), Evaluation Measures (EM), Pruning (P), Summarizing (S), or Grouping (G) [5,22,14,10]. The algorithms that belong to the approaches of Q, P, and S aid the exploration process by reducing the exploration space (RES); the ones that belong to EM approach explore the process by directing the user to what is potentially interesting (DUPI); and, finally, the algorithms of G approach explore the process by structuring the domain (SD).

Grouping is a relevant approach related to SD, since it organizes the rules in groups that contain, somehow, similar knowledge. These groups improve the presentation of the mined rules, providing the user a view of the domain to be explored [18,19]. A methodology was found in the literature for post-processing association rules that utilizes the grouping approach. This methodology, called PAR-COM [5], combines clustering and objective measures to direct the user to what is potentially interesting and, consequently, reduces the association rule exploration space. Thus, the user only needs to explore a small subset of the groups that contain the potentially interesting knowledge. However, it is essential that groups be represented by labels that may provide the user a view of the subjects contained in the exploration space, helping to guide its search.

Although some methods have been proposed to label document clusters in Text Mining (TM) and Information Retrieval (IR) [13,12,16], there are few researches in the literature that deal with selecting labels for association rule clustering. Padua et al. [15] and Carvalho et al. [4] assess some labeling methods using objective evaluations. Chang et al. [7] discuss about a disagreement between objective and subjective evaluation results in a topic extraction context. The latter found that some results of objective measures are not always a good predictor of human judgments regarding the terms selected as labels for the topic extraction task. The same problem is found here since the label selection task is similar to topic extraction and association rule clustering approaches.

Considering that, we use a subjective methodology to evaluate label sets obtained by labeling methods for association rule clustering. For that, this paper presents an adapted version of the subjective evaluation methodology proposed in [7] (details in Section 3). The evaluation was applied in five labeling methods for association rule clustering in order to identify which one obtains suitable label sets according to the

The proposal of an evaluation methodology adapted from [7] is introduced and adjusted for an environment that considers clusters of association rules obtained from structured data. Specifically, the proposed evaluation methodology is based on a task named *word intrusion*. The word intrusion task, proposed in [7], consists of identifying a spurious word inserted into a set of words[1] that represent the extracted topic. The *word intrusion* task was initially proposed to evaluate whether an extracted topic has human-identifiable semantic coherence.

---

[1] In this work, a set of words represents the labels of a group.

This paper is organized as follows. The labeling methods used in this work are presented in Section 2. The subjective evaluation methodology is described in Section 3. The configuration of the experiments are introduced in Section 4 and the results are discussed in Section 5, arguing about the differences obtained between the subjective and the objective analysis. Finally, the related works are presented in Section 6 and conclusions in Section 7.

2   Labeling Methods

Although the organization of association rules through clustering provides some important clues for user, the exploration task remains a challenge since there is no explicit information about the subject of each cluster. Even in a small data set, it is not easy to define a main idea that links the association rules in each cluster. However, the cluster may be represented by a set of meaningful labels. Therefore, it is important to find a good set of labels for each cluster. In this paper, five labeling methods (LM) for association rule clustering, briefly described below, were selected and implemented to be subjectively evaluated. These labeling methods were the ones indicated by [4,6,15] as good solutions to this kind of problem (for details, please, see the references).

LM-M (*Labeling Method Medoid*) selects as labels of each cluster the items in the rule that is more similar to all the other rules in the same cluster (the cluster's medoid). The method computes the accumulated similarity of each rule considering its similarity with respect to all the other rules; then, the one with the highest value is selected. Therefore, the labels of each cluster are built by the items that appear in the cluster's medoid.

LM-T (*Labeling Method Transaction*) builds the clusters labels by selecting the items in the rule that covers the largest number of transactions. A rule covers a transaction t if all the rule items are contained in t. Therefore, this method counts the number of transactions each rule covers and selects the rule that covers the largest number of transactions. In the end, the rule items are considered as the clusters labels.

In **LM-S** (*Labeling Method Sahar* due to its reference to [19]), a simplified version of the process described in [19], the labels of each cluster are built as follows: (i) considering a set $I = \{i_1, ..., i_m\}$ containing all the distinct cluster items, a set $R = \{r_1, ..., r_n\}$ containing all the possible relationships $a \Rightarrow c$, where $a, c \in I$ – each one of these relationships represents a rule pattern; (ii) the number of rules that each pattern $r_i \in R$ covers is computed (N_c); a pattern $a \Rightarrow c$ covers a rule $A \Rightarrow C$ if $a \in A$ and $c \in C$; (iii) the pattern with the highest cover is selected; in the event of a tie all tied pattern are selected; (iv) all the selected patterns compose a set $P \subseteq R$; (v) in the end, all the distinct items in P compose the labels.

In **LM-PU** (*Labeling Method Popescul and Ungar* due to its reference to [16]), the labels of each cluster are built by the N items in the cluster that present the best tradeoff between frequency and predictiveness; formally we have: $f(i_n|C_n) * \frac{f(i_n|C_n)}{f(i_n)}$. The $f(i_n|C_n)$ measure computes the frequency f of each item

i_n in its cluster C_n. The $\frac{f(i_n|C_n)}{f(i_n)}$ measure computes the frequency f of each item i_n in its cluster C_n divided by the item frequency in all the clusters. The i_n items are all the distinct items that are present in the rules of the cluster. Each time an item i_n occurs in a rule its frequency is incremented by one. Therefore, the labels are built by the N items that are more frequent in their own cluster.

In **GLM** (*Genetic Labeling Method* [15]), the labels of each cluster are chosen by optimizing two measures, Precision and Repetition Frequency [4]. The Precision measure (P) computes the number of rules the labels cover in their own cluster and divides by the number of rules in that cluster. A rule is covered by the clusters labels if one or more items in the labels are part of the rule. The Repetition Frequency (RF) measures how different the labels are among the clusters by counting the number of items that are repeated in different cluster labels and dividing this value by the number of distinct items in all the labels. Values near 0 show that there are few repetitions among the labels while values near 1 indicate that the labels are very similar. It was considered, during the optimization process, $RF = 1.0 - RF$ so that both P and RF were maximized. GLM is a genetic algorithm approach that aims to ensure a good tradeoff between P and RF. The fitness function of an individual is defined by $Fitness(I) = (P+RF) - \left(\frac{Max(P,RF)}{Min(P,RF)} * 10^{-5}\right)$, where 10^{-5} indicates the minimal possible value the measures may get, $(P + RF)$ show how good are the measures according to the labels and $\left(\frac{Max(P,RF)}{Min(P,RF)} * 10^{-5}\right)$ the penalty proportional to the distance between P and RF. Initially, the method randomly selects the labels of each cluster among the rule items in each cluster. Thereafter, the population of labels undergoes crossover until it reaches a given number of generations.

3   Item Intrusion Task: The Subjective Evaluation Methodology

In order to subjectively evaluate the labels obtained by each labeling method described in Section 2, we implemented the *item intrusion task*, which was adapted from [7]. As proposed in [7], the users' task is to find the item, among a set of items, that is out of place or does not relate with the others, i.e., *the intruder*. The methodology works as follows:

Step A. The n best items and the m worst items in each cluster are selected according to each labeling method described in Section 2. n and m are numbers to be chosen. The n best items in each cluster represents the labels of the clusters. The m worst items, called here as intruders, are the m least items to be selected as labels and, also, the ones that appear in some of the other clusters. The last condition ensures an item will not be selected as a bad item due solely to its rarity. The process is illustrated in Figure 1. In this example, considering $n = 5$, the best ranked items, that compose the labels of the cluster k, are "Item 1", "Item 2", "Item 3", "Item 4", and "Item 5". On the other hand, considering $m = 5$, the worst ranked items that also occur in the other clusters are "Item j", "Item j-2", "Item j-4", "Item j-6", and "Item j-8". The underlined and emphasized items are considered to be present only in the current cluster. The rank is based on the criteria used on a given LM.

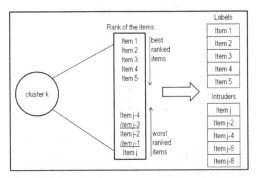

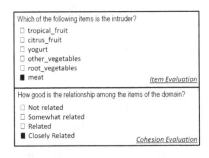

Fig. 1. The selection process of the n best items and the m worst items

Fig. 2. Illustrative example of the evaluation process

Step B. A intruder i is picked up at random from a pool built with the m items identified in [Step A].

Step C. The n items plus the intruder i are shuffled and presented to the user, as in Figure 2. In this example, the user is asked to identify the intruder, i.e., the item that should not be selected as label. It is expected that the user chooses the item i. The authors of [7] claim that when the set of labels minus the intruder i makes sense together, then the subject should easily identify the intruder.

Step D. Finally, as seen in Figure 2, the user is also asked about the cohesion of the set of labels minus the intruder i. The cohesion in this work is evaluated through four available options: "not related", "somewhat related", "related", and "closely related". The options are associated with values ranging from 1 to 4 – 1 regarding the "not related" option until 4 regarding the "closely related" option. The cohesion value may be used to determine if a labeling method is selecting the labels in a random way. When combined with the results of [Step C], the cohesion value improves the evaluation regarding the coherence of the set of labels.

It is important to mention that the methodology here presented is primarily an adaptation of the one presented in [7] for an environment that considers clusters of association rules obtained from structured data. The major difference is [Step D]. Therefore, the main contribution of this work is the subjective evaluation of labeling methods for association rule clustering. However, the presented methodology is also another contribution, since it discusses a standardized assessment process to the context of association rule clustering.

4   Experiments

Experiments were carried out to subjectively evaluate the five labeling methods applied in the context of association rule clustering (see Section 2). Thereby, this section is divided in three parts: one related to the criteria used to evaluate the obtained results, one that describes the data sets used and, finally, the one that discuss the experimental setup.

4.1   Evaluation Criteria

Based on the methodology described in Section 3, the evaluation of the results was done considering two different aspects: (i) percentage of correct answers (PCA) and (ii) cohesion (Co).

In the first aspect, the quality of the labels is measured by the rate of correct answers given by the subjects regarding the intruder selection method [Step C]. In high quality label sets the relationship of selected items presents a good summary of the cluster content. Also, the intruder item can be easily identified in the label sets with high quality. Thus, PCA metric may be expressed by $PCA = \frac{\#\ of\ correct\ answers}{\#\ of\ clusters}$. In this case, the metric checks how many times the user identifies the intruder i in each of the clusters, related to a given association rule clustering, and divides it by the total number of clusters in the clustering. A $PCA = \frac{5}{10} = 50\%$ indicates that the clustering has 10 clusters and in 5 of them the user identified, among the labels, the intruder item.

In the second aspect, the cohesion metric aims to measure how correlated the labels are without the intruder i in the subject opinion. However, in this case, a mean of the cohesions is obtained. Thus, this metric may be expressed by $Co = \frac{\sum_{i=1}^{\#\ of\ clusters} Co_i}{\#\ of\ clusters}$. In this case, the metric sums the cohesions assigned to each of the clusters by the user, related to a given association rule clustering, and divides it by the total number of clusters in the clustering. A $Co = \frac{4+3+2+4+2}{5} = 3.0$ indicates that the clustering has 5 clusters and, in average, a cohesion of 3.0.

4.2   Data Sets

Four data sets (DS) were considered to run the experiments: Adult (48842;115), Income (6876;50), Groceries (9835;169), and Sup (1716;1939). The numbers in parenthesis indicate, respectively, the number of transactions and the number of distinct items in each data set. The first three are available through the package "arules"[2]. The last one was donated by a supermarket located in São Carlos city, Brazil. All the transactions in Adult and Income contain the same number of items (named here as standardized data sets (SDS)), different from Groceries and Sup (named here as non-standardized data sets (NSDS)), whereupon each transaction contains a distinct number of items. Thus, the experiments considered different data types. The rules, in each data set, were mined using

---

[2] http://cran.r-project.org/web/packages/arules/index.html.

an *Apriori* implementation[3] with a minimum of 2 and a maximum of 5 items per rule. From the Adult set 6508 rules were extracted using a minimum support (min-sup) of 10% and a minimum confidence (min-conf) of 50%; Income 3714 rules with min-sup=17%, min-conf=50%; Groceries 2050 rules with min-sup=0.5%, min-conf=0.5%; Sup 7588 rules with min-sup=0.7%, min-conf=0.5%. The parameters were set experimentally.

4.3   Experimental Setup

Initially, in order to apply the five labeling methods described in Section 2 to perform the subjective analysis, the rule sets, related to each data set, were clustered. The clusterings were obtained using the Ward Link algorithm [21] and, as similarity measure, J-RT (see Section 6). This configuration, clustering algorithm + similarity measure, was selected because, as shown by [6], it obtains the best results when the clustering is done in the post-processing phase. Each one of the dendrograms were cut with a threshold of 0.2^4 (the value was obtained experimentally). Based on these cuts, 12 groups were obtained for the Adult data set, 5 for Income, 33 for Groceries, and 10 for Sup.

After clustering the rule sets, all the five labeling methods were applied to each clustered set. The methodology described in Section 3 was then executed in each considered configuration, i.e., labeling method + data set. In total, 20 experiments were done (20 = 5 LM × 4 DS). The values of $n = 5$ and $m = 5$ were considered to apply the subjective evaluation (see Section 3).

Once subjective evaluations are often expensive due to the large amount of data available and to the limited available time of the evaluators, a sampling of clusters was considered in each data set in all the LM. Thus, in this work, we randomly selected 20% of the clusters in each clustered rule set. Therefore, 2 groups were considered for Adult in each LM, 1 for Income, 6 for Groceries, and 2 for Sup. These selected groups, for each data set, in each LM, were the ones presented to the users as shown in Figure 2.

All the users assessed the same clusters, and also the items in the groups, in the same sequence, because as the users' interaction with the system improves, he/she may change the choices and, consequently, the results. The sequence of presentation was set randomly. However, each user evaluated only one data set of each type, i.e., one group of users evaluated the results related to Adult and Sup data sets and the other the ones related to Groceries and Income. This split was done aiming to lower the number of questions each subject should answer and to force each subject to evaluate both a standardized and a non-standardized data set.

Finally, it is important to mention that a warm-up step was considered during the experiments. In this phase, two more groups were selected to be initially presented to the users (so in Adult, for example, 4 groups were selected in the

---

[3] http://www.borgelt.net/apriori.html [Christian Borgelt's Web Page].
[4] Considering dendrograms with maximum height of 1. The root node is close or equal to 1.

total). These 2 additional groups were used as a training phase, aiming to introduce the validation process to the subjects. In this stage, the user learns how the environment works and how to interact with it. In this phase, right and wrong answers may not represent the user knowledge. These initial groups were not considered in the final results.

The Groceries and Sup data sets were evaluated by 5 users, each one having a good knowledge of the domain. The Adult and Income data sets were also evaluated by 5 users, but in this case the users did not have a good knowledge of the domain (related to customer's profile).

5   Results and Discussion

As mentioned before, to analyze the obtained results the metrics PCA and Co (Section 4) were used. The results are presented in the Tables 1 and 2 for Groceries and Sup data sets and in the Tables 3 and 4 for Adult and Income data sets. The results express the averages of PCA and Co obtained from the assessments of all the users in the analyzed clusters in each data type.

The highest values in each of the tables, regarding each one of the metrics, are marked with ▲ in each considered data set. For the Groceries data set, for example, the best value for PCA is the one related to GLM (51.43% (Table 1)); for Co also the one related to GLM (3.43 (Table 2)). It may be noted that, regarding the NSDS (Tables 1 and 2):

PCA **aspect:** according to the results obtained by [15], LM-PU is the more suitable method to be used according to objective evaluations; however, in this subjective evaluation:

- GLM is the more suitable LM to be used according to the user views;
- LM-M obtained good results;
- LM-PU and LM-S present the worst results.

Thus, there is a disagreement between the two evaluations, as noted by [7] for the topic extraction task.

Co **aspect:** following the same reasoning, it may also be observed the same disagreement regarding this other aspect:

- although GLM presents the highest value in only one data set (Groceries), in the other data set the values are more closely, indicating that GLM is also the more suitable LM to be used according to the user views considering this criterion;
- the values for Groceries have a low variation among the LM, except for GLM that presents a high value – mean of 3.26;
- the values for Sup also have a low variation among the LM, except for LM-PU that presents the worse value – mean of 3.20.

The analysis of the tables also shows interesting behaviors. In cases of high Co and low PCA values, such as in LM-S on Sup data set (3.50 x 0%), it is understandable that the method failed to distinguish the groups, i.e., the labels of the clusters were not specific enough to describe their own groups and, consequently, to distinguish each one from the others. On the other hand, in cases of low Co and high PCA values, such as in LM-PU on Sup data set (2.70 x 40%), it is understandable that the method obtained less correlated labels, but it was successful on selecting labels that best represent each group, making it easier for the subjects to find the intruder. Finally, Figure 2 shows an example of an answer given by an user regarding a group related to the Groceries data set. In this case, considering this unique group, $PCA = 1$ and $Co = 4$.

On the other hand, regarding the SDS, the users did not have a good knowledge of the domain (related to customer profile) and, therefore, the results were much worse. It may be noted that (Tables 3 and 4):

PCA **aspect:** according to the results obtained by [15], GLM is the more suitable method to be used according to objective evaluations; however, in this subjective evaluation:

  – the number of low PCA values is high, being some of them 0%. Thus, although LM-T presents the highest value in only one data set (Income), it is the only method that has an uniform behavior in both data sets. Therefore, it may be assumed that LM-T is the more suitable LM to be used according to the user's views.

  Thus, there is a disagreement between the two evaluations, as noted by [7] for the topic extraction task.

Co **aspect:** following the same reasoning, it may also be observed the same disagreement regarding this other aspect:

  – Both data sets had high Co values according to the subject's opinion, contrasting to the low PCA values.

Table 1. PCA results related to NSDS

Data set	LM-M	LM-T	LM-PU	LM-S	GLM
Groceries	46.67%	20%	11.43%	11.43%	51.43%▲
Sup	50%	50%	40%	0%	70%▲

Table 2. Co results related to NSDS

Data set	LM-M	LM-T	LM-PU	LM-S	GLM
Groceries	3.23	3.23	3.29	3.14	3.43▲
Sup	3.30	3.30	2.70	3.50▲	3.20

Table 3. *PCA* results related to SDS

Data set	LM-M	LM-T	LM-PU	LM-S	GLM
Adult	30%	40%	50%▲	30%	10%
Income	0%	40%▲	0%	0%	20%

Table 4. *Co* results related to SDS

Data set	LM-M	LM-T	LM-PU	LM-S	GLM
Adult	3.0	3.1▲	3.0	2.9	3.0
Income	3.6	3.8▲	3.6	3.4	3.8▲

6 Related Works

Since this paper aims to evaluate labeling methods for association rule cluster-ing, in this section, we briefly review some papers related to association rule clustering, mentioning their labeling methods and the methodologies used to evaluate the methods.

The aim of the clustering approach in the post-processing phase is to improve and organize the presentation of the obtained association rules. The result of this process is a structured view of domain to be explored. In [20] the authors propose a similarity measure based on transactions and apply a density clus-ter algorithm to group the association rules. They also present an evaluation in a small set of the rules to motivate the research with association rule clus-tering approach. The approach proposed in [10] explores the lexical features of the rules, rather than their statistical properties, for structuring the rule space. They explored hierarchical cluster algorithms in the evaluations using Jaccard as the similarity measure. In [10], the Jaccard value between two rules r and s, expressed by J-RI$(r,s) = \frac{|\{items\ in\ r\} \cap \{items\ in\ s\}|}{|\{items\ in\ r\} \cup \{items\ in\ s\}|}$, is calculated considering the items the rules share. The authors of [18] compare two kinds of clustering meth-ods, partitional and hierarchical, also using Jaccard as the similarity measure. However, in this case, the Jaccard value between two rules r and s is expressed by J-RT$(r,s) = \frac{|\{t\ matched\ by\ r\} \cap \{t\ matched\ by\ s\}|}{|\{t\ matched\ by\ r\} \cup \{t\ matched\ by\ s\}|}$, where t is the common transac-tions the rules match. In [10] and [18], the labels of each group are compound of the items that are presented in the rule that is more similar to all the other rules in the group (the medoid of the group). Toivonen et al. [20] do not mention how the labels are found, but provide some clues that the labels represent the most frequent and distinct items in the group.

In all the cases, the authors are mainly concerned with the domain organiza-tion and do not present a deeper evaluation of the labels. In [15], an interesting labeling method based on genetic algorithm is proposed. A comparison of label methods for association rule clustering is presented by [4]. The authors of [4] evaluate the method ideas presented in [20,10,18]. They also use an adaptation of an idea presented by [19] and the method proposed in [16] applied in the con-text of the document cluster. More detailed results may be found in [6]. Finally, to objectively evaluate labeling methods for association rule clustering, [4] propose two measures, P and RF, the ones used by [15] and, therefore, described in Section 2.

7   Conclusions

In this paper, we performed a subjective evaluation of labeling methods used for association rule clustering. The results show that the GLM method is the most suitable method to be used for NSDS according to the user's views. On the other hand, LM-T is the most suitable method to be used for SDS according to the user's views. However, in the last case, the results obtained from the evaluation suggests that it is more difficult to identify the intruder in standardized data sets. This result may be explained due to the fact that the users did not have a good knowledge of the domain (related to customer profile) but more experiments are necessary to identify the causes of this behavior.

Considering all the results, we may affirm that a good objective evaluation does not imply in a good subjective evaluation. As noted by [7] for the topic extraction task, there is, with a certain frequency, a high disagreement between the two kinds of evaluation. The results also indicate that the organization of the data set has a high impact on the quality of the results.

As future works, we intend to evaluate hybrid labeling methods that combine objective and subjective aspects.

Acknowledgements.   Grants 2009/16142-3, 2010/07879-0, 2011/19850-9, 2013/12383-0, São Paulo Research Foundation (FAPESP) and Coordenação de Aperfeiçoamento de Pessoal de Nível Superior (CAPES) (Grants DS-6345378/D, DS-8434242/M).

References

1. Agrawal, R., Imielinski, T., Swami, A.N.: Mining association rules between sets of items in large databases. In: Proceedings of the ACM SIGMOD International Conference on Management of Data, pp. 207–216 (1993)
2. Agrawal, R., Mannila, H., Srikant, R., Toivonen, H., Verkamo, A.I.: Fast discovery of association rules. In: Advances in Knowledge Discovery and Data Mining, pp. 307–328. AAAI Press (1996)
3. Agrawal, R., Srikant, R.: Fast algorithms for mining association rules. In: Proceedings of the 20th International Conference on Very Large Data Bases, pp. 487–499 (1994)
4. Carvalho, V.O., Biondi, D.S., Santos, F.F., Rezende, S.O.: Labeling methods for association rule clustering. In: Proceedings of the 14th International Conference on Enterprise Information Systems, pp. 105–111 (2012)
5. Carvalho, V.O., Santos, F.F., Rezende, S.O.: Post-processing association rules with clustering and objective measures. In: Proceedings of the 13th International Conference on Enterprise Information Systems, pp. 54–63 (2011)

6. Carvalho, V.O., Santos, F.F., Rezende, S.O.: Agrupamento de regras de associação no pré-processamento e no pós-processamento: O que vale mais a pena? Technical Report 381, Instituto de Ciências Matemáticas e de Computação - ICMC - USP (2012)
7. Chang, J., Boyd-Graber, J.L., Gerrish, S., Wang, C., Blei, D.M.: Reading tea leaves: How humans interpret topic models. In: Neural Information Processing Systems, pp. 288–296 (2009)
8. Han, J., Cheng, H., Xin, D., Yan, X.: Frequent pattern mining: Current status and future directions. Data Mining and Knowledge Discovery 15(1), 55–86 (2007)
9. Hipp, J., Mangold, C., Güntzer, U., Nakhaeizadeh, G.: Efficient rule retrieval and postponed restrict operations for association rule mining. In: Chen, M.-S., Yu, P.S., Liu, B. (eds.) PAKDD 2002. LNCS (LNAI), vol. 2336, pp. 52–65. Springer, Heidelberg (2002)
10. Jorge, A.: Hierarchical clustering for thematic browsing and summarization of large sets of association rules. In: Proceedings of the 4th SIAM International Conference on Data Mining, 10 p. (2004)
11. Liu, B.: Association rules and sequential patterns. In: Web Data Mining, pp. 17–62 (2011)
12. Manning, C.D., Raghavan, P., Schütze, H.: An Introduction to Information Retrieval. Cambridge University Press, 544 p.(2009)
13. Moura, M.F., Rezende, S.O.: A simple method for labeling hierarchical document clusters. In: Proceedings of the 10th IASTED International Conference on Artificial Intelligence and Applications, pp. 336–371 (2010)
14. Natarajan, R., Shekar, B.: Interestingness of association rules in data mining: Issues relevant to e-commerce. SĀDHANĀ – Academy Proceedings in Engineering Sciences (The Indian Academy of Sciences) 30(Parts 2&3), 291–310 (2005)
15. de Padua, R., de Carvalho, V.O., de Souza Serapião, A.B.: Labeling association rule clustering through a genetic algorithm approach. In: Catania, B., Cerquitelli, T., Chiusano, S., Guerrini, G., Kämpf, M., Kemper, A., Novikov, B., Palpanas, T., Pokorny, J., Vakali, A. (eds.) New Trends in Databases and Information Systems. AISC, vol. 241, pp. 45–52. Springer, Heidelberg (2014)
16. Popescul, A., Ungar, L.: Automatic labeling of document clusters. Unpublished manuscript (2000), http://www.cis.upenn.edu/popescul/~Publications/popescul00labeling.pdf
17. Rathinasabapathi, R., Ramesh, G.: Comparison of association rules and decision trees for disease prediction and data mining for improved cardiac care. International Journal of Computer Science and Management Research 2, 1716–1721 (2013)
18. Reynolds, A.P., Richards, G., de la Iglesia, B., Rayward-Smith, V.J.: Clustering rules: A comparison of partitioning and hierarchical clustering algorithms. Journal of Mathematical Modelling and Algorithms 5(4), 475–504 (2006)
19. Sahar, S.: Exploring interestingness through clustering: A framework. In: Proceedings of the IEEE International Conference on Data Mining, pp. 677–680 (2002)
20. Toivonen, H., Klemettinen, M., Ronkainen, P., Hätönen, K., Mannila, H.: Pruning and grouping discovered association rules. In: Workshop Notes of the ECML Workshop on Statistics, Machine Learning, and Knowledge Discovery in Databases, pp. 47–52 (1995)
21. Xu, R., Wunsch, D.: Clustering. IEEE Press Series on Computational Intelligence. Wiley (2008)
22. Zhao, Y., Zhang, C., Cao, L.: Post-mining of Association Rules: Techniques for Effective Knowledge Extraction, 372 p. Information Science Reference (2009)

An Algorithm of Classification for Nonstationary Case

Piotr Kulczycki[*], and Piotr Andrzej Kowalski[*]

Polish Academy of Sciences, Systems Research Institute
{kulczycki,pakowal}@ibspan.waw.pl

Abstract. The paper deals with the classification task, where patterns are nonstationary. The method ensures the minimum expected value of misclassifications and is independent of patterns' shapes. This procedure eliminates elements of patterns with insignificant or even negative influence on the results' accuracy. Appropriate modifications follow the classifier parameters, which increases the effectiveness of procedure adaptation for nonstationary patterns. The number of patterns is not methodologically limited in the presented concept.

Keywords: data analysis, classification, pattern nonstationarity, pattern size reduction, classifier adaptation.

1   Introduction

Classification constitutes one of the basic procedures of data analysis and exploration [Han and Kamber, 2001]. In most of the methods used today, one assumes stationarity (unchanged by time) of patterns characterizing particular classes. However, more and more often, as models have become more accurate, and investigated phenomena have become more complex [Kulczycki et al, 2007], in particular those in which new – with the most current being the most valuable – elements are continuously added to patterns, this assumption is successfully ignored.

The concept of the method for classification with nonstationary patterns proposed in this paper was conceived on the basis of the sensitivity method used in artificial neural networks. As a result of its operation, particular elements of patterns receive weights proportional to their significance for correct results. Elements of the smallest weights are eliminated. For the sake of the patterns' nonstationarity, their elements whose weights are currently small but increase successively are kept. In addition a procedure is proposed ensuring that an adaptation to changing conditions is obtained by correcting classifier parameters values. Its formula is based on the Bayes approach, providing a minimum of potential losses arising from incorrect classification. It is also possible to introduce preferences for those classes whose elements – due to potential nonsymmetrical conditioning of the task – especially should not be mistakenly assigned to others. The classifier was constructed applying the statistical kernel estimators methodology, thus freeing the above procedure from arbitrary assumptions

---

[*] Also: Cracow University of Technology, Department of Automatic Control and Information Technology .

F. Castro, A. Gelbukh, and M. González (Eds.): MICAI 2013, Part II, LNAI 8266, pp. 301–313, 2013.

regarding patterns' shapes – their identification is an integral part of the algorithm presented here.

The first sections of this paper, i.e. 2-7, briefly describe mathematical apparatus and component procedures used in the main part – Section 8 – to synthesize of the algorithm for classification with nonstationary case investigated here. The numerical verification and comparison with the similarly conditioned support vector machine concept [Krasotkina et al, 2011] is the subject of Section 9, followed by final comments and remarks.

A preliminary version of this paper was presented in part as [Kulczycki and Kowalski, 2013a].

2   Statistical Kernel Estimators

Consider the n-dimensional random variable X, with a distribution characterized by the density f. Its kernel estimator $\hat{f}: \mathbb{R}^n \rightarrow [0, \infty)$ is calculated on the basis of the random sample

$$x_1, \ x_2, \ldots, x_m \quad , \tag{1}$$

and defined – in the basic form – by the formula

$$\hat{f}(x) = \frac{1}{mh^n} \sum_{i=1}^{m} K\left(\frac{x - x_i}{h}\right) \quad , \tag{2}$$

where the positive coefficient h is known as a smoothing parameter, while the measurable function $K: \mathbb{R}^n \rightarrow [0, \infty)$ symmetrical with respect to zero, having at this point a weak global maximum and fulfilling the condition $\int_{\mathbb{R}^n} K(x) \, dx = 1$ is termed a kernel. The monographs [Kulczycki, 2005; Silverman, 1986; Wand and Jones, 1995] contain a detailed description of the above methodology.

In this paper the generalized (one-dimensional) Cauchy kernel is applied, in the multidimensional case generalized by the product kernel concept [Kulczycki, 2005 – Section 3.1.3; Wand and Jones, 1995 – Sections 2.7 and 4.5]. For calculation of the smoothing parameter, the simplified method assuming the normal distribution [Kulczycki, 2005 – Section 3.1.5; Wand and Jones, 1995 – Section 3.2.1] can be applied, thanks to the positive influence of this parameter correction procedure, presented below in Section 7. For general improvement of the kernel estimator quality the modification of the smoothing parameter [Kulczycki, 2005 – Section 3.1.6; Silverman, 1986 – Section 5.3.1] will be applied, with the intensity $c \geq 0$; as its initial standard value $c = 0.5$ can be assumed.

Details are found in the monographs [Kulczycki, 2005; Silverman, 1986; Wand and Jones, 1995].

3   Bayes Classification

Consider J sets consisting of elements of the space $\mathbb{R}^n$:

$$x_1', \; x_2', \ldots, x_{m_1}' \tag{3}$$

$$x_1'', \; x_2'', \ldots, x_{m_2}'' \tag{4}$$

$$\vdots$$

$$x_1^{'''\cdots}, \; x_2^{'''\cdots}, \ldots, x_{m_J}^{'''\cdots} \;, \tag{5}$$

representing assumed classes. The sizes m_1, $m_2, \ldots, m_J$ should be proportional to the "contribution" of particular classes in the population under investigation. Let now $\hat{f}_1$, $\hat{f}_2, \ldots, \hat{f}_J$ denote kernel estimators of a probability distribution density, calculated successively based on sets (3)-(5) treated as random samples (1) – a short description of the methodology used for their construction is contained in Section 2. In accordance with the classic Bayes approach [Duda et al, 2001], ensuring a minimum of expected value of losses, the classified element $\tilde{x} \in \mathbb{R}^n$ should then be given to the class for which the value

$$m_1\hat{f}_1(\tilde{x}), \; m_2\hat{f}_2(\tilde{x}), \ldots, m_J\hat{f}_J(\tilde{x}) \tag{6}$$

is the greatest. The above can be generalized by introducing to expressions (6) the positive coefficients z_1, $z_2, \ldots, z_J$:

$$z_1 m_1\hat{f}_1(\tilde{x}), \; z_2 m_2\hat{f}_2(\tilde{x}), \ldots, z_J m_J\hat{f}_J(\tilde{x}) \;. \tag{7}$$

Taking as standard values $z_1 = z_2 = \ldots = z_J = 1$, formula (7) brings us to (6). By appropriately increasing the value z_i, a decrease can be achieved in the probability of erroneously assigning elements of the i-th class to other wrong classes (although the danger does then exist of increasing the general number of misclassifications). Thanks to this, it is possible to favor classes which are in some way noticeable (e.g. in diagnostics, those representing faults causing large losses) or more heavily conditioned. For the classification task considered here, these are in natural way classes defined by nonstationary patterns – in the case of a significant difference in the speed of their changes, it is worth increasing coefficients relating to more varying patterns. The initial value 1.25 can be proposed for further research.

4   Discrete Derivative

The task of computing the value of the discrete derivative of the function $g : \mathbb{R} \to \mathbb{R}$ consists in calculating the quantity $g'(t)$ based on values of this function obtained for a finite number of the arguments $t_1, t_2, \ldots, t_k$. For the problem under investigation a backward derivative will be used, that is where $t = t_k$. As the task considered here does not require the differences between subsequent values $t_1, t_2, \ldots, t_k$ to be equal, it is therefore advantageous to apply interpolation methods. In the procedure worked out here, favorable results were achieved using a classic method based on Newton's interpolation polynomial. Detailed formulas are found in the survey article [Venter, 2010]. For the purposes of the procedure investigated in this paper, $k = 3$ can be taken as a standard value.

5   Sensitivity Analysis for Learning Data

When modeling multidimensional problems using artificial neural networks, particular components of an input vector most often are characterized by diverse significance of information, and in consequence influence variously the result of the data processing. In order to eliminate superfluous – from the point of view of the investigated task – input vector components, a sensitivity analysis of the network with respect to particular learning data can be performed. As a result one obtains the parameters $\overline{S}_i$ describing proportionally the influence of the particular inputs ($i = 1, 2, \ldots, m$) on the output value, and then the least significant inputs can be eliminated.

Detailed description of the above procedure is found in the publications [Engelbrecht et al, 1995; Zurada, 1992].

6   Reducing Patterns' Size

In practice, some elements of sets (3)-(5), constituting patterns of particular classes, may have insignificant or even negative – in the sense of classification correctness – influence on quality of obtained results. Their elimination should therefore imply a reduction in the number of erroneous assignments, as well as decreasing calculation time. To this aim the sensitivity method for learning data, used in artificial neural networks, briefly noted in the previous section, will be applied.

To meet the requirements of this procedure, the definition of the kernel estimator will be generalized below with the introduction of the nonnegative coefficients w_1, $w_2, \ldots, w_m$, normed so that $\sum_{i=1}^{m} w_i = m$ and mapped to particular elements of random sample (1). The basic form of kernel estimator (2) then takes the form

$$\hat{f}(x) = \frac{1}{mh^n} \sum_{i=1}^{m} w_i K\left(\frac{x - x_i}{h}\right) .$$ (8)

The coefficient w_i value may be interpreted as indicating the significance (weight) of the i-th element of the pattern to classification correctness.

The procedure for reducing patterns sets (3)-(5) consists – in its basic form – of two phases: of calculating the weight w_i, and then removing those elements of random sample (1), for which the respective weights have the lowest values. These tasks will subsequently be presented in the next two subsections.

6.1   Calculation of Weights w_i

In the method designed here, for the purpose of reduction of sets (3)-(5), separate neural networks are built for each investigated class.

The constructed network has three layers and is unidirectional, with m inputs (corresponding to particular elements of a pattern), a hidden layer whose size is equal to the integral part of the number $\sqrt{m}$, and also one output neuron. This network is submitted to a learning process using a data set comprising of the values of particular kernels for subsequent pattern elements, while the given output constitutes the value of the kernel estimator calculated for the pattern element under consideration. The network's learning is carried out using backward propagation of errors with momentum factor. On finishing this process, the thus obtained network undergoes sensitivity analysis on learning data, in accordance with the method presented in the previous section. The resulting coefficients $\overline{S}_i$ describing sensitivity, calculated in this way, constitute the fundament for calculating the preliminary values

$$\tilde{w}_i = \left(1 - \frac{\overline{S}_i}{\sum_{j=1}^{m} \overline{S}_j}\right) ,$$ (9)

after which they are normed to

$$w_i = m \frac{\tilde{w}_i}{\sum_{i=1}^{m} \tilde{w}_i} .$$ (10)

The shape of formula (9) results from the fact that the network created here is the most sensitive to atypical and redundant elements, which – taking into account the form of kernel estimator (8) – implies a necessity to map the appropriately smaller values $\tilde{w}_i$, and in consequence w_i, to them. Coefficients (10) represent – as per the idea presented while introducing the generalized form (8) – the significance of particular elements of the pattern to accuracy of the classification process.

6.2   Removal of Pattern Elements

Empirical research confirmed the natural assumption that the pattern set should be relieved of those elements for which $w_i < 1$. (Note that, thanks to normalization made by formula (10), the mean value of the coefficients w_i equals 1.)

7   Correcting the Smoothing Parameter and Modification Intensity Values

The classic universal methods of calculating the smoothing parameter value are often not proper for the classification task. This paper will propose a procedure suited to the conditioning of the investigated method of classification for nonstationary patterns, in particular those enabling successive adaptation with regard to the occurring changes.

Thus, it can be proposed to introduce $n+1$ multiplicative correcting coefficients for the values of the parameter defining the intensity of modification procedure c and smoothing parameters for particular coordinates h_1, $h_2,...,h_n$, with respect to optimal ones calculated using the integrated square error criterion. Denote them as $b_0 \geq 0$, b_1, $b_2,...,b_n > 0$, respectively. It is worth noticing that $b_0 = b_1 = ... = b_n = 1$ means in practice no correction. Next through a comprehensive search using a grid with a relatively large discretization value, one finds the most advantageous points regarding minimal incorrect classification sense. The final phase is a static optimization procedure in the $(n+1)$-dimensional space, where the initial conditions are the points chosen above, while the performance index is given as the number of misclassifications. This is an integer – to find the minimum a modified Hook-Jeeves algorithm [Kelley, 1999] was applied.

Following experimental research it was assumed that the grid used for primary searches has intersections at the points 0.25, $0.5,...,1.75$ for every coordinate. For such intersections the value of the performance index is calculated, after which the obtained results are sorted, and the 5 best become subsequent initial conditions for the Hook-Jeeves method, where the value of the initial step is taken as 0.2. After finishing every one of the above 5 "runs" of this method, the performance index value for the end point is calculated, and finally among them the one with the smallest value is shown.

Apart from the first step, the above procedure can be used in the simplified version, to successively specify current values for the correcting coefficients b_0, $b_1,...,b_n$ as part of adaptation to changes in nonstationary conditions. To this end the Hook-Jeeves algorithm is used only once, taking the coefficients' previous values as initial conditions.

Finally it is worth noting that the correction of classification parameters is not necessary in this procedure. It does, however, increases classification accuracy and furthermore enables the use of a simplified method for calculation of smoothing parameters values, proposed in Section 2.

8   Classification Method for Nonstationary Patterns

This section, the most essential in this publication, presents the classification method for the nonstationary case, that is when all or some patterns of classes undergo significant – considering the investigated task – changes. Here, material presented in Sections 2-7 will be used. A block diagram of the calculation procedure is shown in Fig. 1. Blocks symbolizing operations performed on all elements of patterns (3)-(5) jointly are drawn with a continuous line, while a dashed line denotes operations on particular classes, and a dotted line – separate operations for each element of those patterns.

First one should fix the reference sizes of patterns (3)-(5), hereinafter denoted by m_1^*, $m_2^*,...,m_J^*$. The patterns of these sizes will be the subject of a basic reduction procedure, described in Section 6. The sizes of patterns available at the beginning of the algorithm must not be smaller than the above referential values. These values can however be modified during the procedure's operation, with the natural condition that their potential growth does not increase the number of elements newly provided for the patterns. For preliminary research, $m_1^* = m_2^* =...= m_J^* = 25 \cdot 2^n$ can be proposed. Lowering these values may worsen the classification quality, whereas an increase results in an excessive calculation time.

The elements of initial patterns (3)-(5) are provided as introductory data. Based on these – according to the procedures mentioned in Section 2 – the value of the parameter h is calculated (for the parameter c it is initially assumed to be equal 0.5). Figure 1 shows this action in block A. Next corrections in the parameters h and c values are made by taking the coefficients b_0, $b_1,...,b_n$, as described in Section 7 (block B in Fig. 1).

The next procedure, shown by block C, is the calculation of the parameters w_i values mapped to particular patterns' elements, separately for each class, as in Section 6.1. Following this, within each class, the values of the parameter w_i are sorted (block D), and then – in block E – the appropriate m_1^*, $m_2^*,...,m_J^*$ elements of the largest values w_i are designated to the classification phase itself. The remaining ones undergo further treatment, denoted in block U, which will be presented later, after Bayes classification has been dealt with.

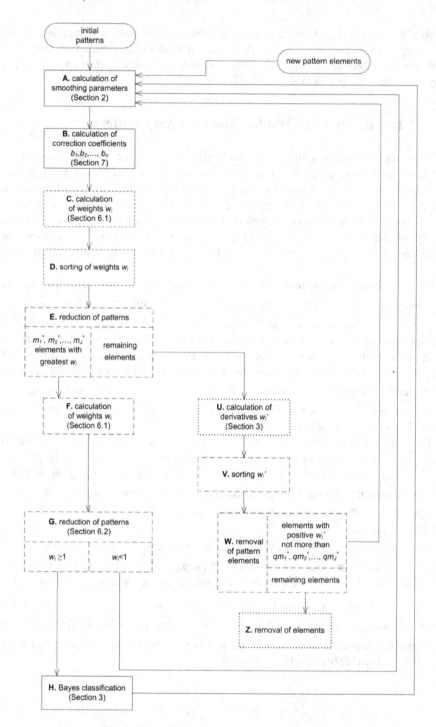

Fig. 1. Block diagram for classification algorithm

The reduced patterns separately go through a procedure newly calculating the values of parameters w_i, presented in Section 6.1 and depicted in block F. According to Section 6.2, as block G in Fig. 1 denotes, these patterns' elements for which $w_i \geq 1$ are submitted to further stages of the classification procedure, while those with $w_i < 1$ are sent to block A for further processing in the next steps of the algorithm, after adding new elements of patterns. The final, and also the principal part of the procedure worked out here is Bayes classification, presented in Section 3 and marked by block H. Obviously many tested elements $\tilde{x}$ can be subjected to classification separately. After the procedure has been finished, elements of patterns which have undergone classification are sent to the beginning of the algorithm to block A, to further avail of the next steps, following the addition of new elements of patterns.

Now – in reference to the end of the paragraph before the last – it remains to consider these patterns' elements, whose values w_i were not counted among the m_1^*, $m_2^*, \ldots, m_J^*$ largest for particular patterns. Thus, within block U, for each of them the derivative w_i' is calculated. If the element is "too new" and does not possess the $k - 1$ previous values w_i, then the gaps are filled with zeros (because the values w_i generally oscillate around unity, such behavior significantly increases the derivative value, and in consequence ensures against premature elimination of this element). Next for each separate class, the elements w_i' are sorted (block V). As marked in block W, the respective

$$q m_1^*, \quad q m_2^*, \ldots, q m_J^* \tag{11}$$

elements of each pattern with the largest derivative values, on the additional requirement that the value is positive, go back to block A for further calculations carried out after the addition of new elements. If the number of elements with positive derivative is less than $q m_1^*, \quad q m_2^*, \ldots, q m_J^*$, then the number of elements going back may be smaller (including even zero). The remaining elements are permanently eliminated from the procedure, as shown in block Z. In the above notation q is a positive constant influencing the proportion of patterns' elements with little, but successively increasing meaning. The standard value of the parameter q can be proposed to be close to $k/2$, where k denotes the order of a discrete derivative, multiplied by the number of new elements added to the algorithm divided by the reference values, such however that $q \geq 0.05$; an increase in the parameter q value allows more effective conforming to pattern changes, although this potentially increases the calculation time, while lowering it may significantly worsen adaptation. In the general case this parameter can be different for particular patterns – then formula (11) takes the form

$$q_1 m_1^*, \quad q_2 m_2^*, \ldots, q_J m_J^*, \tag{12}$$

where $q_1, q_2, \ldots, q_J$ are positive.

The above procedure is repeated following the addition of new elements (block A in Fig. 1). Besides these elements – as has been mentioned earlier – for particular patterns respectively m_1^*, $m_2^*, ..., m_J^*$ elements of the greatest values w_i are taken, as well as up to qm_1^*, $qm_2^*, ..., qm_J^*$ (or in the generalized case $q_1m_1^*$, $q_2m_2^*, ..., q_Jm_J^*$) elements of the greatest derivative w_i', so successively increasing its significance, most often due to the nonstationarity of patterns.

9   Empirical Verification and Comparison

The correct functioning and properties of the concept under investigation have been comprehensively verified numerically, and also compared with results obtained using a related procedure based on a support vector machine (SVM) method. Research was carried out for data sets in various configurations and with different properties, particularly with nonseparated classes, complex patterns, multimodal and consisting in detached subsets located alternately. Nonstationarity increased successively either in steps or periodically. The standard values of the parameters previously proposed in this paper were obtained through research carried out for verification purposes.

The following are the results obtained for a simple but representative case, enabling a telling illustration and interpretation of the procedure summaries in Section 8. For visual purposes the two dimensional space ($n = 2$) and the two classes ($J = 2$) will be used. For both classes, the patterns begin with 100 elements ($m_1 = m_2 = 100$), obtained using a generator with normal distribution with the unique variance. The expected value of the first – stationary – class is located permanently in the origin of the space $\mathbb{R}^2$, while for the second – nonstationary – following an initial period of no movement, encircles it with the radius 3, adding 10 new elements every 10 degrees before coming to a stop in its original location. According to the suggestions formulated earlier, it was also assumed $m_1^* = m_2^* = 100$ and $q = 0.2$.

Figure 2 illustrates the number of misclassifications in a typical course of a procedure created in this paper. From the beginning, up to step 18, the second class is invariable. First a slight increase in the number of erroneous classifications occurs – in every step around 10% new elements of patterns are added, which worsens the working conditions for the neural network. Finally, however, once the patterns are stabilized, the number of misclassifications settles at the level 0.08. In step 18 the aforementioned orbital movement of the second class begins. First the number of erroneous classifications rises to around 0.12, and then – after the kernels, which were not previously removed due solely to a positive derivative w_i', have received the appropriate meaning – the number of misclassifications drops and levels off at 0.105. In step 54, where the second class stops, occurrences similar to the above take place, when the number of classification errors returns to its initial level of 0.08.

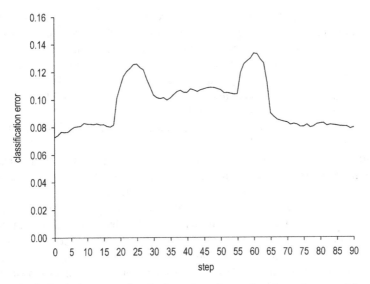

Fig. 2. Typical course using the investigated procedure ($z_1 = 1$, $z_2 = 1$)

Thanks to the generalization of formula (6) to (7), the classification quality can increase by mapping to the classes with nonstationary patterns greater values of the coefficients z_i . Figure 3 shows the results obtained with $z_1 = 1$ and $z_2 = 1.25$. It is worth noting that the total number of misclassifications lowered with respect to that obtained for the basic case in Fig. 2. This especially concerns local maximums existing after the second class starts and stops moving (steps 18 and 54).

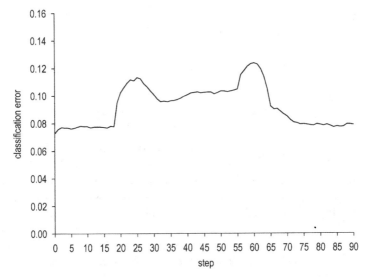

Fig. 3. Course with differing values of the coefficients z_i : $z_1 = 1$, $z_2 = 1.25$

The procedure worked out and described here was compared with a method based on the support vector machine (SVM) concept, presented in the publication [Krasotkina et al, 2011], taken as the closest regarding the conditioning considered in this paper research task. The obtained results are shown in Fig. 4 – they were achieved in conditions identical to Fig. 3, with which they will be compared. Although in conditions of stationarity of the second pattern (steps before 18 and after 54) the number of misclassifications leveled off at 0.08, in the case using the SVM, however, starts at 0.10, instead of 0.07 as in the procedure investigated here (compare Fig. 3 and 4). When the second pattern changes (steps 18-54) the amount of errors generated by the SVM settles at the level 0.12, or even slightly higher than that of local maximums appearing in the method presented in this paper after steps 18 and 54 (compare again Fig. 3 and 4). It should be underlined, though, that when the second class is moving, the number of misclassifications does not fall to the level $0.1-0.105$ (Fig. 4), as is the case with the procedure worked out here (Fig. 3). Thus one can see that the concept method in this paper has an advantage over the SVM procedure, especially in conditions of gradual change. Taking into account the fact that its idea is based on derivatives of a predictive nature, this observation is completely understandable.

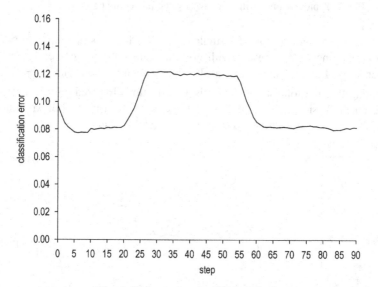

Fig. 4. Course using the SVM method

To summarize: numerical testing wholly confirmed the positive features of the method worked out. In particular, the results show that the classifying algorithm can be used successfully for inseparable classes of complex multimodal patterns as well as for those consisting of incoherent subsets at alternate locations. The examined nonstationarity increased successively, and was periodical as well as occurring in steps. For the former type, the procedure presented in this paper proved to be particularly advantageous and useful.

10   Final Comments and Remarks

This paper presented a classification procedure which allows for nonstationarity of patterns and successive supply of new elements to them. Neither the number of classes itself, nor the number of nonstationary ones are methodologically limited. The concept is based on the Bayes approach, which allows for the minimization of expected loss value arising from erroneous classifications, as well as actively influencing the proportion of probabilities of classification errors between particular classes. The use of kernel estimators frees the algorithm from patterns' shapes. The procedure operation is based on the sensitivity method used with artificial neural networks. It enables the removal of those elements of patterns, which are of insignificant or even negative influence on accuracy of results. However, it retains for further calculation some of these elements which due to nonstationarity successively increase their positive impact. Appropriate adaptation is also performed on classifier parameters.

A broad description of the presented method – in particular the full set of formulas – is contained in the paper [Kulczycki and Kowalski, 2013b] which will appear soon.

References

1. Duda, R.O., Hart, P.E., Storck, D.G.: Pattern Classification. Wiley, New York (2001)
2. Engelbrecht, A.P., Cloete, I., Zurada, J.: Determining the Significance of Input Parameters Using Sensitivity Analysis. In: Sandoval, F., Mira, J. (eds.) IWANN 1995. LNCS, vol. 930, pp. 382–388. Springer, Heidelberg (1995)
3. Han, J., Kamber, M.: Data Mining: Concepts and Techniques. Wiley, New York (2001)
4. Kelley, C.T.: Iterative Methods for Optimization. SIAM, Philadelphia (1999)
5. Krasotkina, O.V., Mottl, V.V., Turkov, P.A.: Bayesian Approach to the Pattern Recognition Problem in Nonstationary Environment. In: Kuznetsov, S.O., Mandal, D.P., Kundu, M.K., Pal, S.K. (eds.) PReMI 2011. LNCS, vol. 6744, pp. 24–29. Springer, Heidelberg (2011)
6. Kulczycki, P.: Estymatory jadrowe w analizie systemowej. WNT, Warsaw (2005)
7. Kulczycki, P., Hryniewicz, O., Kacprzyk, J. (eds.): Techniki informacyjne w badaniach systemowych. WNT, Warsaw (2007)
8. Kulczycki, P., Kowalski, P.A.: Bayes classification of imprecise information of interval type. Control and Cybernetics 40, 101–123 (2011)
9. Kulczycki, P., Kowalski, P.A.: Klasyfikacja Bayesowska przy Niestacjonarnych Wzorcach. In: Proceedings of the 11th International Conference on Diagnostics of Processes and Systems, Lagow Lubuski, Poland, September 8-11, paper_4 (2013a)
10. Kulczycki, P., Kowalski, P.A.: Bayes Classification for Non-Stationary Patterns (in press, 2013b)
11. Silverman, B.W.: Density Estimation for Statistics and Data Analysis. Chapman and Hall, London (1986)
12. Venter, G.: Review of Optimization Techniques. In: Encyclopedia of Aerospace Engineering, pp. 5229–5238. Wiley, New York (2010)
13. Wand, M.P., Jones, M.C.: Kernel Smoothing. Chapman and Hall, London (1995)
14. Zurada, J.: Introduction to Artificial Neural Neural Systems. West Publishing, St. Paul (1992)

Using NIAR *k*-d Trees to Improve the Case-Based Reasoning Retrieval Step

Fernando Orduña Cabrera[1] and Miquel Sànchez-Marrè[2]

[1] ITESCA Instituto Tecnológico Superior de Cajeme
[2] KEMLG Group, Universitat Politècnica de Catalunya-BarcelonaTech.
Barcelona, Catalonia
forduna@itesca.edu.mx, miquel@lsi.upc.edu

Abstract. Case retrieval is one important step in the case-based reasoning cycle. Up to now, several algorithms have been proposed for the indexing of cases, since the original indexing approach of *k*-d trees came up in literature. Main approaches propose the use a precomputed binary search tree to get an average logarithmic time effort in searching. The proposal presented in this paper consists of an indexing algorithm based on the principle of binary search trees for efficient case retrieval according to a given similarity measure called *sim*. The proposed NIAR *k*-d tree algorithm embodies two main steps based on the computation of the average value of the corresponding attribute among the subtree cases, and selecting for that attribute, the value of the Nearest Instance/case to the Average as the Root (partition value). Experimental results with some databases have shown that the retrieval step in NIAR *k*-d tree is faster than the standard *k*-d tree approach. The time efficiency, the depth and breadth in both trees are analyzed. The results obtained depict a significant difference of levels in the trees. The presented approach is implemented within a current research work on introspective reasoning framework for case-based reasoning in continuous domains.

Keywords: Retrieval, Indexing, Binary Search Trees; *k*-d Trees.

1 Introduction

The retrieving of similar cases is one of the key steps in the case-based reasoning (CBR) paradigm [Kolodner *et. al*, 1985]. The case base must be analyzed to detect a set of potentially useful cases for adaptation purposes. Commonly, there is a distinction between *surface* and *structural similarity* [Holyoak & Koh, 1986]. Structural similarity computation is normally quite expensive, because all available knowledge of the domain must be taken into account. On the contrary, the retrieval step should manage the similarity computation of all cases in the case base as fast as possible. Therfore, this task can only rely on the comparison of syntactical features, i.e., surface similarity [Gentner & Forbus, 1991]. In addition, in the CBR literature there can be distinguished two different approaches about similarity assessment [Althoff & Wess, 1992]: the *representational approach* [Kolodner, 1980] and the *computational*

F. Castro, A. Gelbukh, and M. González (Eds.): MICAI 2013, Part II, LNAI 8266, pp. 314–325, 2013.
© Springer-Verlag Berlin Heidelberg 2013

approach [Aha, 1991]. The former is based on using a structured memory of cases, and the later is based on the computation of an explicit similarity measure called *sim*. The work presented in this paper is based on the computational approach.

In a relatively small case base scenario, the similarity computation of all cases can performed through a sequential process by comparing each case, in the case base, against the current problem. This strategy is reasonable given that its computational time effort is linear ($O(n)$, being *n* the number of cases), but it is not feasible for larger case bases. Several strategies have been proposed to improve the retrieval step for large case bases. Some approaches use massively parallel computer hardware to speed up the similarity assessment process. Others are based in the pre-computation of efficient indexation schemes, which improve the efficiency of the retrieval step. In this sense, a new strategy following these later approaches will be explained in this contribution.

Additionally, some indexation schemes were designed in order to find the *m* most similar cases (*m* nearest neighbours, or *m*-NN) such as in [Friedmann et al. 1977, Wess et al. 1993], while others focused on the one most similar case (nearest neighbor or 1-NN) [Bentley 1975, Arya et al. 1993]. In our work, we have taken the second option (the similarity). The most similar case is the aim of the retrieval process. However, having in mind that the value *m* normally is low, in these case the most similar cases are needed, and depending on the minimum number of cases in the leaves of the indexing tree (*bucket size*), the 1-NN indexing strategies can also provide the *m*-NN without exploring other subspaces of the indexing tree.

In CBR applications, sometimes the cases can be represented in a structured way by a set of independent features. Similarly, other applications require more sophisticated case representations when attribute dependent cases exists; and normally they also cover a subspace rather than a point in the problem-solution space. The former are named as *point cases*, and the later as *generalized cases*. Most of the indexing approaches in the CBR literature have dealt with point cases [Bentley, 1975, Friedman et al., 1977, Wess et al., 1993, Arya et al., 1993], but also some compute scientists have focused their contributions on the attribute dependent generalized cases [Bergmann & Tartakovski, 2009]. In this paper, the point case representation will be addressed.

Cases can be considered as points within a multidimensional search space, where each attribute is one dimension that can be explored with an associative search. The idea of our approach is to structure the search space according to the observed statistical distribution of the values of the attributes, and using this computation in advance to improve the case retrieval process according to a given similarity measure *sim* [Stottler et al., 1989]. Our approach is based on the earlier concept of a multidimensional (*k* dimensions) binary search tree, i.e. a *k*-d tree [Bentley 1975, Friedman et al. 1977, Broder 1990]. The rationale behind is to try to get the subtrees of each internal node as much balanced as possible, in order to reduce the number of tree levels, and consequently, increase the retrieval speed. A *k*-d tree is similar to a discrimination tree/network [Kolodner 1993, Charniak and McDermott 1985]. Major differences rely on how to decide which attribute must be the discriminator one at each internal node of the tree. In discrimination trees, there are some heuristic approaches to derive which are the most discriminant attributes. For instance, an expert-based discrimination list or some other automatic procedures such as using unsupervised feature- weighting techniques [Núñez and Sànchez-Marrè 2004].

This contribution is organized as follows, in the Section 2 the fundamentals of k-d trees will be explained. In Section 3 the NIAR k-d tree approach will be detailed. The experimental work done to evaluate the proposal and the results will be discussed in Section 4. Finally, the conclusions and future research work will be outlined in Section 5.

2 k-d Trees

One of the most solicited indexing methods for a case base was based on the database query approach applying a k-d tree proposed by [Bentley 1975] and [Friedman et al. 1977].

The fundamental idea behind a standard k-d tree is to partition a k-dimensional attribute space into some simpler subspaces and to search for the nearest neighbors in the corresponding subspaces. These subspaces are k-dimensional cubes having faces parallel to the coordinate planes. A k-d tree is a binary search tree very similar to a decision tree. The internal nodes are labeled with *attribute names* and the edges with *partition values*. The leave nodes are labeled with a disjoint subset of the cases (*bucket of cases*). Every node of a k-d tree represents a subset of the case base. The root node represents the whole case base. Each internal node partitions the represented set of cases into two disjoint subsets. The left subtree contains the subset of cases with a value for the *discriminator attribute* of the node less or equal than the *partition value*. The right subtree contains the subset of cases with a value for the *discriminator attribute* of the node greater than the *partition value*.

The construction of the k-d tree is recursive. Beginning with a root node, the represented set of cases is partitioned according to a chosen *discriminator attribute* and a chosen *partition value*. This recursive procedure ends when a certain *termination criterion* is fulfilled, such as the number of cases in a subset is less or equal than the *bucket size*.

The retrieval task in a k-d tree is a recursive traversal search of the tree, starting from the root node and following the corresponding subtree until a leaf is reached. At each internal node, it descends the tree following the branch whose constraint on the discriminator attribute of the node ($\leq$ or $>$) is matched by the attribute value in the query case. When a leaf is reached, the similarity measure *sim* between the query case and the cases in the bucket is computed.

The average computational time for retrieving the most similar case is $O(\log_2 n)$ (being n the number of cases) if the tree is optimally organized, such as in discrimination trees. For the worst case, the retrieval cost is $O(n)$. Thus, on average, it really improves the case retrieval of a sequential linear procedure for computing the similarity value for each one of the cases in the case base.

The different approaches based on the use of k-d trees differ in how the *discriminator* attribute is determined, and how the *partition value* is selected at each internal node of the tree. The original k-d tree formulation [Bentley, 1975] proposed to choose the discriminator attribute *cycling over the list of the attributes*, and selecting the partition value at *random*. The standard *k*-d tree approach [Friedman et al. 1977] suggests to select the attribute with the *highest spread* (range) in values, and the *median* of the attribute value distribution.

The application of *k*-d trees for similarity-based retrieval in CBR was first proposed by [Wess et al. 1993]. They explored four approaches for selecting the attributes: the Category-utility of CobWeb [Fisher 1987], Entropy measuring proposed by [Quinlan 1983], selecting the attribute maximizing the dispersion (interquantile distance) with respect to the similarity measure *sim*, and selecting the attribute which maximizes the average similarity within partitions and buckets. This later strategy was the best according to the experimentation undertaken by authors.

In addition, in the work by [Bergmann and Tartakovski, 2009] which addresses the generalized cases retrieval, it is proposed to select the discriminator attribute as the one maximizing the dispersion of projections of cases, as well as to take into account the length and intersection of projected case intervals.

All contributions previously cited above and others such as [M. Hapala, 2011] and [A. Franco-Arcega, 2012] have shown that the standard *k*-d tree approach is feasible to be improved, and until now, standard *k*-d tree approach was improved in different ways as described in literature mentioned above. In our contribution, a new proposal to improve the standard *k*-d tree approach has been formulated. The results obtained have shown that the NIAR *k*-d tree is an efficient case retrieval method. The proposed indexing technique is a fast indexing strategy and the generated trees are well balanced according to the results obtained.

3   The NIAR *k*-d Tree Approach

As explained in the previous sections, the different approaches based on the standard *k*-d tree approach as an associative retrieval procedure differ both in the selection criteria for the discriminating attributes and in the selection of the partition value. All proposed strategies try to improve the retrieval time for query cases through the generation of well-balanced binary trees. A balanced tree is a very compact tree where the number of cases represented by each subtree is nearly the same than in the other subtree. This guarantees a stable retrieval time independently of the distribution of the query cases.

Our proposal performs quite similar to the standard *k*-d tree, by selecting the discrimination attributes cycling major through he list of attributes, but differs of standard *k*-d tree approach in the technique of selecting the split value for each attribute at the internal nodes. The proposed partition value is the attribute value more similar to the average value of the attribute values from the instances in the corresponding node. The technique proposed is explained below.

The name *NIAR* means that the attribute value of the Nearest Instance to the Average will be the Root node partition value. To find this split value, the process proposed is as follows:

1. Compute the average value Att_l^i of the corresponding attribute i among the instances in the current node l.

Let be $\{X_j\}_{j=1,n}$ the case base composed of n cases. Each case X_j could be described with the set of k attributes: $X_j = (X_j^1, X_j^2, ..., X_j^k)$.
Let be I_l the set of instances represented by the Node(l):

$$I_l = \{X_j | X_j \in Node(l)\} \quad l = 1, ... \tag{1}$$

The computation of the average value of attribute i among the instances at node l, Att_l^i is defined by the following equation:

$$Att_l^i = \frac{1}{\#I_l}\left(\sum_{j=1}^{\#I_l} X_j^i\right) \tag{2}$$

2. Find the Nearest Instance attribute value to the Average value ($X_{NIARoot}^i$) of the attribute values from the instances (I_l) in the corresponding node l, which will be the Root partition value.

Once computed the mean of the corresponding attribute, the next step is to find the nearest instance to the mean value obtained. The average value computed probably does not really exist in the list of instances given that it is not a true split value. This average value can't be taken as the final split value because is a virtual value so far and thus, the partition value would be virtual and would increase the number of levels of the tree. To reduce the number of levels in the tree, the Nearest Instance to the average value of the attribute must be located within all the instances (I_l) of the corresponding node l:

$$NIARoot = Arg\ Max_{j=1,\#I_l}sim^i\left(Att_l^i, X_j^i\right) \tag{3}$$

where sim^i is the similarity measure on the dimension of the attribute i. Then, finally the partition value is $X_{NIARoot}^i$

3. Once the partition value is found, all the node l instances with lower or equal values than the partition value will be the instances of the left subtree, constituting the new node ($2*l$), and, all the node l instances with higher values than the partition value will be the instances of the right subtree, constituting the new node ($2*l+1$).

4. Recursively, continue generating the tree for the left *son* node, and for the right son node, until the number of instances of a node is lower or equal than the bucket size (m cases)

The procedure for generating the NIAR k-d tree is detailed in the following algorithm:

```
Input: case base CB, discriminator attribute i, total num-
ber of attributes k, bucket size m. Output: NIAR k-d tree
root node.
procedure GenNIARtree (CB, i, k, m)
```

```
var
n, sum, ni, atti, NIARoot, partitionValue, lowerPart, upperPart
begin
  n := count(CB); {number of cases of CB}
  if n > m then {cases do not fit in one bucket}
    sum := 0;
    for j:= 1 to n do
      sum := sum + consult(CB,j,i) {value i of case j}
    end;
    atti:= sum / n; {Average value of attribute i}
    maxsim := - infinity; {is the minimum possible value of simi function i.e., 0}
    for j:= 1 to n do
      if simi(Atti, consult(CB,j,i)) > maxsim then
        maxsim := simi(Atti, consult(CB,j,i));
        NIARoot := j;
      end {if}
    end {for}
    partitionValue := consult(CB,NIARoot,i);
    lowerSon := Ø; upperSon := Ø;
for j:= 1 to n do
 if consult(CB,j,i) <= partitionValue then
    lowerPart := lowerPart + case(CB,j)else
    upperPart := upperPart + case(CB,j)end {if}
end {for}
    ni = i mod k + 1; {next indexing attribute}
return (make-
node(i,partitionValue,GenNIARtree(lowerPart,ni,k,m),
  GenNIARtree(upperPart,ni,k,m))) else
    return (makeLeaf(CB,n.m)){make a bucket of n cases}
  end {if} end {GenNIARtree}
```

The procedure count(CB) computes the number of cases in CB. The procedure consult(CB,j,i) provides the value of the attribute i in the case j of the CB. The procedure simi(Atti, consult(CB,j,i)) computes the similarity measure between *Atti* (the average of the attribute i) and the value of the attribute i in the case j. The procedure case(CB,j) returns the case j of CB. The procedure makeNode(i,partitionValue,lowerSon,upperSon)) returns an internal node including the discrimination attribute i, the splitting value parti-tionValue, and two pointers to the nodes of the subtrees lowerSon and upper-Son. The procedure makeLeaf(CB,n.m) returns a leaf node with a bucket filled with the cases in CB.

The average computational time for generating a NIAR k-d tree is $O(n*\log_2 n)$, being n the number of cases, and $O(n^2)$ for the worst case, improving the effort for generating the k-d tree of some of the standard k-d trees, as its cost does not depend on the number of attributes k.

4   Experimental Evaluation and Results

All k-d trees can only cope with numerical or categorical ordered attributes, where an order relation exists. This means that the splitting process, separating two sets according to the order relation of all cases/instances is possible. K-d trees are not initially suitable for unordered categorical attributes.

Experiments on eight databases from UCI Machine Learning repository [Frank and Asuncion 2010] were conducted. The databases selected were *Abalone, Car, Ecoli, Glass, Ionosphere, Pima, Letter and Waveform*. All the databases have numerical attributes or categorical ordered attributes, which can be transformed to a numerical ordered attribute. In *Abalone* database, one unordered categorical was transformed into a numerical one to test some future research work on this specific usage in the NIAR k-d trees. In table 1 there is the description of all databases used in the experimental evaluation.

Table 1. Description of databases used in the experimentation

Database	Short Name	#Inst	#Cont	#CatOrd	#CatNOrd	#Classes
Abalone	AB	4177	7	0	1	29
Car Eval.	CA	1728	0	6	0	4
Ecoli	EC	336	7	0	0	8
Glass	GL	214	9	0	0	7
Ionosphere	IO	351	34	0	0	2
Pima	PI	768	8	0	0	2
Letter Rec.	LE	20000	16	0	0	26
Waveform	WA	5000	21	0	0	3

It was aimed in this experimental setting, to assess both the retrieval CPU time effort, the depth of the generated trees, and the distribution of cases at the tree levels. We compared the standard k-d tree approach using the median value as the partition value at each internal node against the NIAR k-d tree approach. Authors wanted to compare also their approach with the best experimental approach proposed by [Weiss et al 1993] based on selecting the attribute which maximizes the average similarity within partitions and buckets. This later strategy was the best one according to the experimentation undertaken by them. Unfortunately, authors were not able to get the necessary algorithmic details from the original source to reproduce it.

Each experimental test retrieved the same cases in both trees, and computed the retrieval time in both approaches. The experimental validation was done by taking random samples from the *test set* with a number of cases equal to the 15% of data in each database.

Each experimental validation was conducted in the following way:

- The cases to be retrieved are randomly selected from the database.
- Case retrieval for each query test case was executed for both tree approaches and the retrieval time was computed.

- The mean time of all query cases retrieval in *test set* was computed for each *k*-d tree approach.
- Searching for accurate results, a multiple validation process was performed. Each experiment was repeated twelve times in both trees. Once computed the 12 runs for each database with both approaches, the maximal and minimal time consumed were excluded to get more stable results. Thus, finally only 10 runs were considered.
- With the ten time mean values obtained before, a final time average over all runs was calculated and this value was the best estimation of a general case retrieval time consumed by the CPU.

The whole experiment cycle was repeated for each database. A Phenom II and Quad Core processor computer workstation with 8 GB of RAM was used to conduct the complete experiment.

The table 2 depicts the average CPU processing time for a case retrieval using the two approaches, and for all the databases tested. The time computed is expressed in *nanoseconds*. The time reduction percentage is between the two methods is presented for comparative purposes.

Table 2. Average CPU Time (in ns) for case retrieval

Database	*k*-d Tree	NIAR *k*-d Tree	Time Reduction (%)
Glass	1745	1558	10,72
Ecoli	1794	1428	20,4
Ionosphere	1909	1740	8,9
Pima	1935	1584	18,13
Car	2808	1997	28,88
Abalone	2596	1714	33,98
Waveform	2577	1926	25,26
Letter	3942	2764	29,88
Mean	*2413.25*	*1838.875*	*22*

The results shown in table 2 and figure 1 shows a difference in time consuming when a search is implemented. It seems that the proposed NIAR *k*-d tree strategy is more efficient in retrieving information. The comparison between NIAR *k*-d tree algorithm and standard k-d tree approach is that NIAR-Tree is on average 22% faster retrieving information than the standard approach according to the experimental results obtained.

The second dimension used to assess the performance of the NIAR *k*-d tree proposal was the evaluation of the *tree depth* and the distribution of nodes at the different levels of the tree. The table 3 shows significant differences in the number of tree levels in both trees, for all the databases. It is seen that the NIAR *k*-d tree approach builds trees with a significant reduction of levels, and the standard *k*-d tree builds trees with more levels that cause a more expensive time in the retrieval.

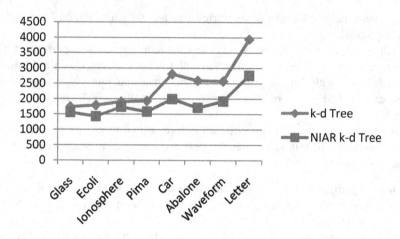

Fig. 1. Comparison of retrieval time in both approaches

Table 3. Depth of trees generated using both approaches

Data Base	*k*-d Tree Depth	NIAR *k*-d Tree Depth
Waveform	26	13
Glass	14	11
Pima	21	11
Ecoli	26	13
Ionosphere	16	13
Abalone	46	14
Car	37	16
Letter	62	41

Abalone, Letter and Car databases are the databases show a higher reduction in the depth of the tree (32, 21 ad 21 levels reduction) despite that they are the largest databases (4177, 20000 and 1728 respectively). The other large database is Waveform with a reduction of 13 levels. Not surprisingly, these four databases are the ones were the time retrieval reduction was higher. This fact means that the reduction in time retrieval is directly correlated with the decrease in the number of levels in the trees.

Thus, it is very interesting to try to find out to which factor is due the reduction of levels. A reasonable answer is that the trees would be more balanced, i.e. the number of nodes in the tree will be more uniformly distributed along the different levels of the tree. In order to check this hypothesis a third dimension was analized: the expanded nodes at each level. This means that the tree should be expanded uniformly in breadth not to generate extra levels in the tree increasing the depth of the tree.

To illustrate this fact in table 4 is detailed for the database Abalone, the number of nodes expanded at each level for both approaches in comparison with the complete (maximum) number of nodes that will generate the most compact possible tree. The results show why the NIAR k-d tree has a better performance than the standard k-d tree.

Table 4. Distribution of expanded nodes by level in both approaches and compared with the most compact possible binary tree, for the Abalone database

Level	Most compact tree	*k*-d tree	NIAR *k*-d tree
0	**1**	1	**1**
1	**2**	2	**2**
2	**4**	4	**4**
3	**8**	8	**8**
4	**16**	15	**16**
5	**32**	22	**32**
6	**64**	38	**64**
7	**128**	53	**128**
8	**256**	71	**256**
9	512	92	502
10	1024	124	940
11	2048	149	1271
12	4096	163	829
13	8192	197	122
14	16384	216	2

In the first eight levels, the NIAR *k*-d tree has expanded the maximum nodes, as would do the most compact tree. On the contrary, the *k*-d tree has a different situation: starting at level 4 and going on, it has not expanded all the nodes that would be desirable. For example, at level 4, only 1 node has been missed, but at level 8, 185 nodes have not been expanded. In the 14th level of NIAR *k*-d tree, which is the last level for this approach, the last 2 nodes have been expanded while in the *k*-d tree 216 nodes have been expanded. This table outlines the fact that the NIAR *k*-d tree provides a more structured and breadth-balanced tree than a standard *k*-d tree.

The Wilcoxon Signed-Range Test [Wilcoxon 1945] was used to determinate differences in the time retrieval from the two approaches (data from table 2). The Wilcoxon signed-rank test is a non-parametric statistical hypothesis test used when comparing two related samples, matched samples, to assess whether their population mean ranks differ (i.e. it is a paired difference test). It can be used as an alternative to the paired Student's t-test when the population cannot be assumed to be normally distributed. We used it, in order not to assume any restrictive hypothesis on the sample like normality.

The *p* value reported by the this statistical test was 0.0078, which is less than the critical value tabulated for a sample of 8 individuals (4 at 95%, 2 at 98%). Thus, at a 95% of confidence or even at a 98% of confidence, the difference between the paired samples is significant. This means that the NIAR *k*-d tree approach provides faster case retrieval time than the standard *k*-d approach.

5   Conclusions and Future Work

NIAR k-d tree algorithm was tested in 8 different databases from the UCI repository. Several dimensions have been evaluated: retrieval time, depth of the generated trees, and breadth-distribution of the nodes of the trees. Experimental results showed a re-duction in the retrieval time, which was confirmed as statistically significant using the Wilcoxon Signed-Range Test at 98% level of confidence. It was shown that the tree structure obtained by NIAR k-d tree proposal reduces the number of levels of the indexing tree, with a consequently time reduction. This reduction of levels is related to a better distribution of the nodes of the tree. The NIAR k-d tree proposal expands more nodes per level than the standard k-d approach. This fact generates a reduction in the number of levels in the tree. It is conjectured that the motivation, which makes the reduction in the number of levels in the tree, is the use of the actual average value of the discriminator attribute among the cases in each node. This partition value is an actual value of the distribution of values within the cases, and cause that the partition are almost equally sized, which causes a more compact and balanced tree, reducing the depth of the indexation tree.

This method proposed is part of a set of policies and strategies which are being de-veloped and implemented in an introspective reasoning framework for CBR in conti-nuous domains [Orduña and Sànchez-Marrè, 2009].

A future research work on unordered categorical attributes and its usage in the NIAR k-d trees will be undertaken.

Another interesting line of research is to afford the incremental problem in the building of k-d trees, especially when facing continuous domains, where a lot of new cases are generated and must be stored incrementally in the case base. The indexing strategies should be analyzed and modified to show reasonable time in the updating of the case base indexation.

Acknowledgments. The authors wish to thank to Felix F. Gonzalez N., for his sup-port in reviewing the document and his punctual comments.

References

1. Aha, D.W.: Case-Based Learning Algorithms. In: Bareiss, R. (ed.) Proceedings: Case-Based Reasoning Workshop. Morgan Kaufman Publishers (1991)
2. Althoff, K.-D., Weß, S.: Case-Based Reasoning and Expert System Development. In: Schmalhofer, F., Strube, G., Wetter, T. (eds.) GI-Fachtagung 1991. LNCS, vol. 622, pp. 146–158. Springer, Heidelberg (1992)
3. Sunil, A., Mount, D.M.: Algorithms for Fast Vector Quantization. In: Proc. of DCC 1993: Data Compression Conference, pp. 381–390. IEEE Press (1993)
4. Bentley, J.L.: Multidimensional binary search trees used for associative searching. Com-munications of the ACM 18(9), 509–517 (1975)
5. Bergmann, R., Tartakovski, A.: Improving KD-Tree Based Retrieval for Attribute Depen-dent Generalized Cases. In: Proceedings of the Twenty-Second International FLAIRS Conference, pp. 319–324. Association for the Advancement of Artificial Intelligence (2009)
6. Broder, A.J.: Strategies for Efficient incremental Nearest Neighbor Search. Pattern Recog-nition 23, 171–178 (1990)
7. Charniak, E., McDermott, D.: Introduction to Artificial Intelligence. Addision-Wesley (1985)

8. Fisher, D.: Cobweb: Knowledge Acquisition via Conceptual Clustering. Machine Learning 2, 139–172 (1987)
9. Frank, A., Asuncion, A.: UCI Machine Learning Repository. University of California, School of Information and Computer Science, Irvine, CA (2010), http://archive.ics.uci.edu/ml
10. Friedman, J.H., Bentley, J.L., Finkel, R.A.: An Algorithm for Finding Best Matches in Logarithmic Expected Time. ACM Trans. Math. Software 3, 209–226 (1977)
11. Gentner, D., Forbus, K.D.: MAC/FAC: a Model of Similarity-Based Retrieval. In: Proceedings of the 13th Annual Conference of the Cognitive Science Society, pp. 504–509 (1991)
12. Holyoak, K.J., Koh, K.: Analogical Problem Solving: Effects of Surface and Structural Similarity in Analogical Transfer. In: Midwestern Psychological Association (ed.) Proceedings of the Conference of the Midwestern Psychological Association (1986)
13. Kolodner, J.L.: Retrieval and Organizational Strategies in Conceptual Memory. Ph.D. Thesis, Yale University (1980)
14. Kolodner, J.L., Simnpson, R.L., Sycara, K.: AProcess Model of Case-Based Reasoning in Problem Solving. In: IJCAI (ed.) Proc. of IJCAI 1985, pp. 284–290. Morgan Kaufmann Publishers, Los Angeles (1985)
15. Kolodner, J.L.: Case-Based Reasoning. Morgan Kaufmann (1993)
16. Núñez, H., Sànchez-Marrè, M.: Instance-based Learning Techniques of Unsupervised Feature Weighting do not perform so badly! In: Proceedings of 16th European Conference on Artificial Intelligence (ECAI 2004), pp. 102–106. IOS Press, València (2004)
17. Orduña Cabrera, F., Sànchez-Marrè, M.: Dynamic Adaptive Case Library for Continuous Domains. In: Sandri, S., Sànchez-Marrè, M., Cortés, U. (eds.) Proc. of 12th International Conference of the Catalan Association of Artificial Intelligence (CCIA 2009), Cardona, Barcelona, Catalonia. Frontiers in Artificial Intelligence and Applications Series, vol. 202, pp. 157–166 (2009)
18. Quinlan, J.R.: Learning efficient Classification procedures and Their Application to Chess Endgames. In: Michalski, R., Carbonell, J., Mitchell, T. (eds.) Machine Learning. Tioga Press (1983)
19. Stottler, R.H., Henke, A.L., King, J.A.: Rapid retrieval Algorithms for Case-Based Reasoning. In: Proceedings of the 11th International Conference on Artificial Intelligence, IJCAI 1989, Detroit, Michigan, USA, pp. 233–237 (1989)
20. Wess, S., Althoff, K.-D., Derwand, G.: Using k-d Trees to Improve the Retrieval Step in Case-Based Reasoning. In: Wess, S., Althoff, K.-D., Richter, M.M. (eds.) EWCBR 1993. LNCS, vol. 837, pp. 167–181. Springer, Heidelberg (1994)
21. Wilcoxon, F.: Individual comparisons by ranking methods. Biometrics Bulletin 1(6), 80–83 (1945)
22. Hapala, M., Havran, V.: Review: Kd-tree Traversal Algorithms for Ray Tracing. Computer Graphics Forum 30(1), 199–213 (2011)
23. Franco-Arcega, A., Carrasco-Ochoa, J., Sanchez-Diaz, G., Martinez-Trinidad, J.: Building fast decision trees from large training sets. Intelligent Data Analysis 16, 649–664 (2012)

Weighting Query Terms towards Multi-faceted Information Fusion of Market Data

Rajendra Prasath[1], Philip O'Reilly[1], and Aidan Duane[2]

[1]University College Cork, Cork, Ireland
[2]Waterford Institute of Technology, Waterford, Ireland
{R.Prasath,Philip.OReilly}@ucc.ie, aduane@wit.ie

Abstract. This paper presents a framework that uses information fusion to capture similar contexts, and then apply these to learn similar instances from a knowledge base in an unsupervised way. These experiments are part of an initiative to build an intelligent business information system with capabilities for multi-faceted repeatable data analysis and decision making. The proposed framework consists of three components: *Query Understanding*, *Information Fusion* and *Reasoning & Learning*. As part of the proposed framework, we present a new approach to performing the weighting of query terms which is aimed at improving our understanding of a user's query intent. The proposed query terms weighting method captures the key contexts of the user's query intent using evidence from corpus statistics. By way of example, the datasets used in our experiments consist of the information retrieved from different sources pertaining to Mobile Payments, a rapidly evolving sector of the Financial Services industry. We illustrate the performance of the proposed information retrieval system using the new query terms weighting approach on three different datasets. Our experiments illustrate that the proposed query terms weighting approach significantly improves the retrieval of texts with a greater variety of contextual information.

1 Introduction

Users identify their information needs in the form of specific query keywords. Users consider these keywords to be an expression of their exact information needs at that given moment. A query can be expressed in a number of different ways, using different views of the same information, yet ultimately it seeks the same result. In the Financial Services sector, a number of organizations have expressed an interest in analyzing the positives and negatives of applying different business models to new products/services prior to their development and launch. The commercial importance for businesses in devising and adopting the most profitable, cost effective, and appropriate product/service business model is critical for organizational performance and success. To adopt and implement an appropriate product/service business model, it is necessary for organizations to have an in-depth knowledge of the existing marketplace and commercial environment, and to learn from their own previous successful launches of products/ services [8]. To the best of our knowledge, and the knowledge of our Financial Services industry research partners, there is no

F. Castro, A. Gelbukh, and M. González (Eds.): MICAI 2013, Part II, LNAI 8266, pp. 326–337, 2013.
© Springer-Verlag Berlin Heidelberg 2013

commercially available Decision Support Application (DSA) that enables these organizations to research the specifics of the marketplace in which they operate in order to develop, test, and validate appropriate business models for proposed new products/services. However, given the multi-faceted nature of data, developing, testing, and validating an appropriate business model for a new product/service is a complicated process. It is extremely time-consuming for business executives engaged in critical decision making to process and analyze each and every piece of information pertaining to their decision making task. To simplify this task, it is essential to develop an "Intelligent" system that learns the contextual meaning of the data using a wide variety of textual data, and then applies this learning to similar instances that arise, thus, providing the business executive with more vital observations and trends pertaining to their decision making task. With this in mind, our proposed framework will enable decision makers to enter a specific set of keywords related to their decision making task; perform information fusion to capture similar contexts by retrieving and fusing multi-faceted information pertaining to their task; before outputting the results in a structured format. Thus, this paper specifically focuses on how to achieve a better understanding of the users exact query intent by weighting their query terms.

2 Motivation

The volume of information available on the World Wide Web is growing exponentially. Research [6] has illustrated that ninety percent of the information in the world today has been created in the last two years alone. Indeed, with this explosion in online information, McKinsey estimates that by 2018, U.S. businesses will need 1.5 million new data managers and analysts to manage and process this data [4]. Thus, the volume of online information has become an issue for many organizations, as trying to mine this web-based information and stay abreast of developments, has become a very time consuming and difficult process. With significant levels of valuable information typically hidden in this textual content, the inability to review such content is highly disadvantageous to many organizations as they are unable to use it to support complex business decision making. Therefore, a significant opportunity exists to develop a method for mining contextual data from free text content.

In the computer science literature, Chang *et* al. [2] proposed an interactive reasoner called *PEQULIAR* that applies progressive query language and interactive reasoning (cum learning) for information fusion support. However, this research is limited in that the reasoner is guided by humans to elaborate the query by means of some rule and then a query processor uses this to produce a more informative answer. Therefore, this work is motivated by an organizations needs to learn from previous cases and experiences, especially in relation to designing and commercializing new products and services. By fusing an organizations internal knowledge with that from external sources, organizations would have a greater insight on the market and would be in a position to learn and apply similar contexts to solve similar problems which they currently face. In order to assist organizations with this dilemma, we have derived a framework that uses information fusion to capture similar contexts and then applies these to learn similar instances from a knowledge base in an unsupervised way, similar to a Pseudo-Relevance Feedback (PRF) approach.

3   Information Fusion Based Text Retrieval

Reasoning about data with varying dynamics is vital for many applications where the basic data sources come from different types and the generated data is heterogeneous. Data obtained from such sources is often ambiguous and associated with certain levels of uncertainty. To derive acceptable results from the analysis of such data, information fusion is used. In this experiment, we use information from a wide variety of web sources to resolve ambiguity and to provide market and organizational knowledge to the user, enabling better decision making. The derived reasoner is capable of choosing distinct aspects of the query from the external data and the query processor executes on these aspects to form an expanded query that retrieves a set of more informative answers to the specific users decision making task. We plan to capture the aspects of the query using the Clustering-by-Directions (CBD) [3] approach but in a unsupervised way. Using these aspects of the query, probable relevant information is retrieved. The Reasoner then accepts this information fused from multiple sources and identifies similar text/cases that may potentially represent similar contexts. The Learner is then applied to these text segments to perform context sensitive assessments, updating both the learning experience and the knowledge base.

3.1   The System Design

The proposed framework, as shown in Figure. 1, consists of three major components: *Query Understanding*, *Information Fusion* and *Reasoning and Learning*.

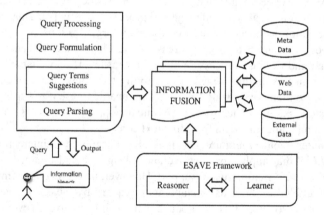

Fig. 1. The Proposed Framework

Query Understanding: User query terms are processed to get associated aspects (each aspect is assumed to represent a "facet") and then the query term weighting is applied to identify their individual weights depending on the corpus statistics. The query term weighting technique used in this paper, puts more weight on the query terms relating to entities / services rather than other associated terms. For example, consider the query: *countries adopting mobile payments*. In this query "countries" is the main focus and it might represent the number of countries adopting mobile payments, or name of the countries adopting mobile payments or type of payment services in countries adopting mobile payments. We obtain the weight for each of these query terms [its weight, in brackets] as follows: payments [2.0595], adopting [4.2886], countries[6.3057], mobile [1.0530]. In this paper, we considered the effects of the proposed query weighting technique in the retrieval of textual descriptions.

Algorithm 1. Retrieving Potential Textual Descriptions

Require: A Search Interface that obtains the user query and performs the retrieval of textual descriptions
Input: Query Q having a sequence of keywords: $q_1, q_2, \cdots, q_n$
Description:

1: **Input:** Enter the user query into the system
2: **Query Terms Weighting:** Extract the query terms and use corpus statistics to determine their individual weights as follows:

$$score(q_i) = averageTF(q_i) * IDF(q_i), \forall i \in [1, n]$$

where $averageTF(q_i)$ is computed as the ratio between the total number of occurrences of the given query term across the textual descriptions in the collection and the total number of textual descriptions (in terms, the total number of textual descriptions in which the term occurs) and $IDF(q_i) = \log(\frac{N}{df(q_i)})$ where N = total number of textual descriptions and $df(q_i)$ = frequency of textual descriptions given the query term q_i.
3: **Text Retrieval:** Compute $cosine(Q, T)$ using cosine similarity and retrieve all textual descriptions
4: **Re-Rank:** Sort texts in the decreasing order of their similarity scores and choose top k textual descriptions
5: **return** top k textual descriptions ($k \leq n$)
Output: The ranked list of top $k \leq n$ textual descriptions as potential informative pertaining to the user query

---

Information Fusion: This component uses the expanded query to retrieve information from multiple sources and applies fusion to rank them in the order of their contextual similarity. This produces a set of top ranked pieces of information pertaining to the user query. In this work, we have evaluated the retrieval effectiveness of the given queries on different datasets. This component is yet to mature to infuse information extracted from different sources to get single combined results.

Reasoning and Learning: This component is yet to mature for reporting. However the idea behind the Reasoner is that the top ranked list of text segments are processed to identify similar patterns. These patterns are then sent to the Learner with the actual user information need. The Learner is supposed to perform context sensitive assessments between the patterns and the actual information needs. The knowledge gained through learning will be reused to solve similar such scenarios as guided by Case Based Reasoning (CBR) [1,5].

The pseudo code of the proposed approach is illustrated in Algorithm. 1. The proposed system works as follows: A user enters their information needs in the form of a query. The system receives this query and applies the proposed query terms weighting approach using corpus statistics to understand the level of importance of these query terms in order to identify the precise intended context of the user's query. Using the weight computed for each query term, the system reformulates the given query into the weighted query. This weighted query is used to retrieve documents from the search system. By default, we use standard cosine similarity as the scoring function. Results are retrieved from multiple sources, evaluated, and then fused to get a combined list of the most relevant textual descriptions pertaining to the context of the given query. In this specific study, the tasks of retrieval and evaluation have been performed. This research is evolving towards the goal of developing a more sophisticated fusion approach that combines the results obtained from multiple sources.

4   Experimental Results

4.1   Datasets

We have prepared three different types of market data from the web resources.

META Dataset: This collection consists of the structured data, manually crafted from the profiles of several Financial Services companies in the form of attribute-value pairs. We specifically focused on ten Financial Services companies involved in Mobile Payments, viz., *Octopus*, *Square Up*, *Visa*, *iZettle*, *Paypal*, *ISIS*, *Groupon*, *Mastercard*, *Oyster* and *American Express*. We manually extracted the key elements of various factors associated with the business models of each of these services.

Table 1. Statistics of the Datasets

Dataset	Coverage	Types of Data
META	60 Documents with 14 topics	Company Profiles, Annual Reports and Business News
WEB	671 Documents	Web Documents from Financial Services
WIKI	867 English Wiki Pages	Wikipedia Articles [from enwiki dumps]

WEB Dataset: We collected seed URLs of Web documents/reports associated with Financial Services companies specifically involved in Mobile Payments, using popular search engines like Google, Bing and Yahoo!. We used seven different types of user queries related to Mobile Payments to crawl 671 web documents from various Financial Services associated sources.

WIKI Dataset - External Knowledge Data: We used Wikipedia - the largest open source multilingual repository to extract useful information associated with various Mobile Payment services. Using the May 2013 snapshot of the English Wikimedia dump[1], we extracted data associated with the various activities of the selected ten

---

[1] Downloaded from http://dumps.wikimedia.org

Financial Services companies listed above. The WIKI documents extracted need to be parsed at a more granular level of information, for example, extracting the elements of the *infobox* has to be improved. The statistics of all these tiny datasets are given in Table. 1

The queries used in the experiment specifically relate to an analysis of Mobile Payments for the Financial Services sector, and are listed in Table. 2

Table 2. List of Queries

QID	Queries
Q1	What percentage of consumers adopt mobile payments?
Q2	In which countries are mobile payments adopted?
Q3	In which countries are mobile payments available?
Q4	What mobile payment models exist?
Q5	Who are the main mobile payment providers?
Q6	Who are the main mobile payment operators?
Q7	Are consumers willing to pay for mobile payments?

Even though, the above listed queries represent questions and look like they are seeking answers, as in Q&A systems, the primary focus is on retrieving textual descriptions, where the context matches the actual context of the given query. By matching the "context" of the query, we mean different aspects pertaining to the focused information need of the given query. For example, consider query - Q4 (Table. 2) which searches for Mobile Payment models. The retrieved textual descriptions contain details associated with Mobile Payment models currently used in the market, but can also contain services/business models considered relevant to the context of the query.

Evaluation Methodology. We used the following steps for the subjective evaluation to test the quality of the content retrieved:

- The focus is on evaluating the quality or goodness of the document content in terms of the coverage of informative subtopics pertaining to the query.
- We used three evaluators to judge the quality of the content in the top twenty results retrieved from two systems: the baseline system with the *vector space model* (VSM) [7] and the system with the proposed query terms weighting approach.
- The evaluator reviewed one query at a time and from top twenty ranked documents.
- Each evaluator picked up the top twenty ranked textual descriptions retrieved for a specific query and evaluated the results by analyzing the context of the textual descriptions. The number of facets covered by each document pertaining to the query is identified. Then, depending on the variety of facets and their importance pertaining to the query, the quality of the content is scored using the three point scale as outlined in Table. 3.
- Final scores are used to compute $p@d$ [precision at top d documents] for both lists.

While evaluating the pieces of information retrieved by the base line and the proposed systems, the evaluators are instructed to focus on the relevance of the textual descriptions retrieved with respect to the query context. We do not apply deep natural language parsing on the textual content (except sentence level parsing with '.' as the sentence marker). In this work, we try to get probable text fragments that could represent the intended context of the users information needs(especially queries relating to Mobile Payments for the Financial Services sector).

The following scale is applied during the evaluation:

Table 3. Guidelines for the subjective evaluation

Score	Description
1.0	Many aspects of the query context
0.5	Partial information of the query context
0	Noisy / irrelevant information

We applied the following evaluation measure: $p@d$ to evaluate the ranked list of top d (= 5, 10, 20) results retrieved for each query. We used three different tiny datasets for this experiment with the same set of queries listed in Table. 2. The top 5, 10 and 20 results were manually evaluated and the observations relating to the retrieved textual descriptions are discussed in the subsequent section.

5   Discussion

In this section, we present our key observations on the nature of the textual descriptions retrieved for the specific information needs expressed using the Mobile Payment queries. Figures. 2, 4 and 6 show the performance of textual descriptions retrieval using the vector space model based approach with META, WIKI and WEB datasets respectively.

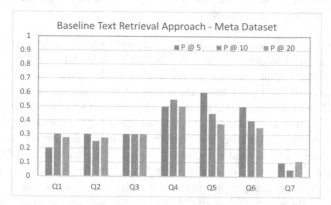

Fig. 2. Baseline system with *META* dataset

With the META dataset, the baseline approach performed well for two queries: Q4 and Q5 in which the textual descriptions retrieved have partial query contexts for the top

5 results. It performed poorly for queries related to consumer focused factors, especially with queries: Q1 and Q7. Using the META dataset, the proposed system identified several key pieces of information pertaining to the methods of Mobile Payments offered by influential Financial Services companies in this area, and also revealed that PayPal and iZettle provide mobile payment services that customers are actually willing to pay for. Table. 4 provides an analysis of the retrieval efficiency of the proposed approach based on an evaluation of the META dataset results.

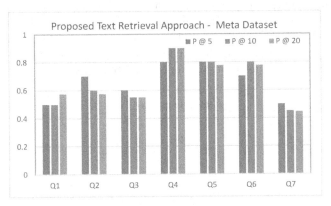

Fig. 3. The Proposed System with *META* dataset

Table 4. Retrieval efficiency of the proposed approach with META dataset

QID	Abstract of the text retrieved with META Dataset
Q2	One additional record was returned which provided much greater insight.
Q3	All records were relevant: with 128 million active accounts in 193 markets and 25 currencies around the world, PayPal enables global commerce, processing more than 7.6 million payments daily.
Q4	More precise records retrieved and a greater number of highly relevant content: Isis is a joint venture between AT&T, T-Mobile and Verizon Wireless in the mobile payment space
Q5	Retrieved texts have much greater precision: O2 in the UK; ISIS, Square cash and PayPal offer Mobile payment services
Q7	PayPal & iZettle offer mobile payment services that customers are willing to pay

With the WIKI dataset (4), the base line approach performed better for two queries: Q4 and Q5, retrieving specific information which appeared in the the top 10 results. Using the WIKI dataset in Query 2, the proposed system performed well in retrieving a greater depth of information pertaining to companies involved in Mobile Payments. For other queries using the WIKI dataset, the proposed system performed moderately. However, there is a huge fall in precision for Query Q4 which seeks information on different Mobile Payment models. To summarize, for customer related queries, the proposed system performed much better than the baseline system.

With the WEB dataset (6), the base line system performed well for product oriented user queries. However, the performance of the system is poor with strategy oriented queries (i.e., queries - Q1 and Q6). However, the standard approach performed consistently well in capturing different models of the Mobile Payment services. Figure. 5 and 7 show the performance of textual descriptions retrieval using the proposed query terms weighting approach. For Query Q3, most of the records retrieved were relevant. Some of the results revealed specific analytical data that incorporated statistics on the number of payments made on a daily basis using mobile phones. For Query Q4, the proposed system captured partner information related to joint ventures in the Mobile Payment sector. Similar observations were noted for Q5 and Q6. For customer oriented queries, using the META dataset, the proposed system captured information on users' willingness to pay for Mobile Payments.

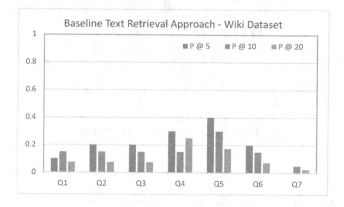

Fig. 4. Baseline system with *WIKI* dataset

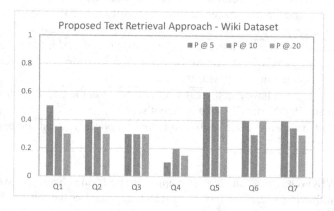

Fig. 5. The Proposed System with *WIKI* dataset

With the WEB dataset, the proposed system performed exceptionally well, and captured textual descriptions incorporating company oriented information. A snapshot of the retrieved information using the proposed approach with the WEB dataset is illustrated in Table 6. The following paragraph reveals, on a query by query basis,

Table 5. Retrieval efficiency of the proposed approach with WIKI dataset

QID	Abstract of the text retrieved with WIKI Dataset
Q2	O2 and Barclays offer Mobile payments in the UK
Q3	Some minor additional information on payment method and providers
Q4	Zoompass is a mobile payment service allowing users to send, request and receive money via their mobile phones.
Q5	O2 in the UK provide mobile payments
Q6	Some minor additional information: O2 in the UK provide mobile payments
Q7	Retrieved some minor additional information on payment method and providers

the performance of the system in terms of the quality of information retrieved. For query Q1, the proposed system retrieved a greater depth of information with more insights on Mobile Payments. It also revealed valuable insights, such as, 53 percent of mobile service provider's predict that retail payments drive consumers to adopt Mobile Payments, and that only 12 percent of mobile phone users have made Mobile Payments in the past twelve months. For query Q2, the proposed system revealed a few

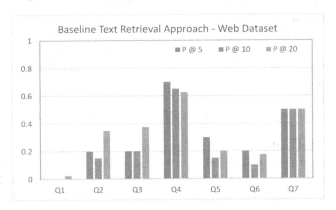

Fig. 6. Baseline system with *WEB* dataset

countries have already adopted Mobile Payments, while also identifying countries such as Kenya and South Africa where such Mobile Payment services are currently being incorporated. The precision of information retrieved for Query Q2 is consistent across the Top 100 results. A similar scenario was observed for Query Q3. For Query Q4, the system performed a perfect retrieval of textual descriptions, in much higher numbers, and with greater relevance to the query context. For Query Q5, the proposed system retrieved the names of the companies involved in providing Mobile Payment services.

For the query Q6, we have noticed query drift at the top order of the retrieved textual descriptions. This is due to the fact that the system was unable to disambiguate the operators involved in the Mobile Payments sector. Finally, for the customer oriented Query Q7, the proposed system revealed specific information, such as, 6% of customers

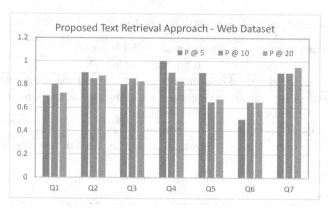

Fig. 7. The Proposed System with *WEB* dataset

Table 6. Retrieval efficiency of the proposed approach with WEB dataset

QID	Abstract of the text retrieved with WEB Dataset
Q1	53 percent of mobile industry leaders predict that retail payments will be the thing that drives consumers to adopt mobile payments. Only 12 percent of mobile phone users reporting that they made a mobile payment in the past 12 months.
Q2	Mobile payments are already the norm in other countries such as Japan, Canada, Europe, and Kenya; Kenya and South Africa are among the countries where mobile payments are drawing previously unbanked people into the modern banking system.
Q3	Mobile payments are available in 74 Countries; iZettle mobile payments are now available in 7 E.U. countries; RFID has been used in Japan and South Korea.
Q4	PayPal, ClickandBuy are mobile payment models; In Europe, NFC mobile payment business models have yet to materialize; Two different types of payment models exist for mobile environments: carrier centric models and payment service provider (PSP) centric models.
Q5	Square, Intuit GoPayment, VeriFone Sail, and PayAnywhere are some of the main mobile payment providers; MasterCard centered on mobile payments across the globe.
Q6	Square, Intuit GoPayment, VeriFone Sail, and PayAnywhere are some of the main mobile payment providers
Q7	The percentage of customers willing to pay for Mobile Payments; 6% of respondents in a recent survey reported that it is easier to pay with other methods.

consider Mobile Payment services as the easiest method to make their payments, and that there is a growing number of customers willing to make Mobile Payments.

To summarize, our analysis reveals that using the proposed approach, the observed quality and relevance of the retrieved texts was much better than the baseline results.

Specifically, the evaluators stated that the information retrieved was very useful in providing insights on Mobile Payment revenue models and providers. Indeed, they noted that if such an approach was incorporated into a commercially available software offering, they would be interested in utilizing they system on an ongoing basis.

6 Conclusion

In this paper, we propose a framework that uses information fusion to capture similar contexts and deep insights from textual data. These experiments are part of our efforts to design an intelligent business information system with multi-faceted repeatable data analysis and decision making capabilities. The proposed framework consists of three components: *Query Understanding, Information Fusion* and *Reasoning & Learning*. We present a new method to perform query term weighting using corpus statistics to capture contextual factors, which is aimed at improving our understanding of a user's query intent. The effects of the proposed query term weighting method are illustrated using three different tiny datasets, consisting of information retrieved from different sources pertaining to Mobile Payments, a rapidly evolving sector of the Financial Services industry. We demonstrate, using a number of queries pertaining to Mobile Payments, that the proposed query term weighting method proficiently captures the key context of each query, using data arising from multiple sources. We also show that the textual descriptions retrieved using the proposed method significantly improves the retrieval of texts, contain a greater variety and quality of relevant contextual information, than the base line results. To support our findings, we present the querywise performance of the base line and the proposed system.

Acknowledgments. A part of this work is supported by B-MIDEA project.

References

1. Aamodt, A., Plaza, E.: Case-based reasoning: Foundational issues, methodological variations, and system approaches. AI Commun. 7(1), 39–59 (1994)
2. Chang, S.K., Jungert, E., Li, X.: A progressive query language and interactive reasoner for information fusion support. Inf. Fusion 8(1), 70–83 (2007)
3. Kaczmarek, A.: Interactive query expansion with the use of clustering-by-directions algorithm. IEEE Transactions on Industrial Electronics 58(8), 3168–3173 (2011)
4. Manyika, J., Chui, M., Brown, B., Bughin, J., Dobbs, R., Roxburgh, C., Byers, A.H.: Big data: The next frontier for innovation, competition, and productivity (May 2011), http://www.mckinsey.com/insights/business_technology/ big_data_the_next_frontier_for_innovation
5. Öztürk, P., Aamodt, A.: A context model for knowledge-intensive case-based reasoning. Int. J. Hum.-Comput. Stud. 48(3), 331–355 (1998)
6. Rasmusse, M.B., Madsbjerg, C.: Big data gets the algorithms right but the people wrong (July 2013), http://www.businessweek.com/articles/2013-07-16/ big-data-gets-the-algorithms-right-but-the-people-wrong
7. Salton, G., Wong, A., Yang, A.C.S.: A vector space model for automatic indexing. Communications of the ACM 18, 229–237 (1975)
8. Teece, D.J.: Business models, business strategy and innovation. Long Range Planning 43(2-3), 172–194 (2010)

An Agents and Artifacts Approach
to Distributed Data Mining

Xavier Limón[1], Alejandro Guerra-Hernández[1], Nicandro Cruz-Ramírez[1],
and Francisco Grimaldo[2]

[1] Universidad Veracruzana, Departamento de Inteligencia Artificial, Sebastián
Camacho No 5, Xalapa, Ver., México 91000
xavier120@hotmail.com, {aguerra,ncruz}@uv.mx
[2] Universitat de València, Departament d'Informàtica, Avigunda de la Universitat,
s/n, Burjassot-València, España 46100
francisco.grimaldo@uv.es

Abstract. This paper proposes a novel Distributed Data Mining (DDM)
approach based on the Agents and Artifacts paradigm, as implemented
in CArtAgO [9], where artifacts encapsulate data mining tools, inherited from Weka, that agents can use while engaged in collaborative, distributed learning processes. Target hypothesis are currently constrained
to decision trees built with J48, but the approach is flexible enough to
allow different kinds of learning models. The twofold contribution of this
work includes: i) JaCA-DDM: an extensible tool implemented in the
agent oriented programming language Jason [2] and CArtAgO [10,9] to
experiment DDM agent-based approaches on different, well known training sets. And ii) A collaborative protocol where an agent builds an initial
decision tree, and then enhances this initial hypothesis using instances
from other agents that are not covered yet (counter examples); reducing in this way the number of instances communicated, while preserving
accuracy when compared to full centralized approaches.

Keywords: Multi-Agent System, Distributed Data Mining, CArtAgO,
Jason, Collaborative Learning.

1   Introduction

As the amount of data produced by the everyday systems grows and distribute,
the problems faced by Data Mining also grows. Being this the case, Data Mining as a research field needs to keep the pace. Distributed Data Mining (DDM)
addresses the problem of mining huge amounts of distributed, even geographically, data. From the point of view of software engineering, DDM systems need to
exhibit various desirable characteristics, such as scalability, configuration flexibility and reusability [7]. Multi-Agent Systems (MAS) are inherently decentralized
and also distributed systems, being a good option to implement DDM systems
that cope with the requirements. Nowadays, agent-based DDM is growing in
popularity [14].

F. Castro, A. Gelbukh, and M. González (Eds.): MICAI 2013, Part II, LNAI 8266, pp. 338–349, 2013.

In this work we present JaCA-DDM, a novel approach to DDM based on the Agents and Artifacts paradigm, as implemented in CArtAgO [9]. Agents in the system are implemented in the well known agent oriented programming language Jason [2]. CArtAgO artifacts play a big role in our approach, for obtaining a modular, scalable, distributed Java based architecture, easy to design, implement and maintain. We also present a distributed learning strategy that borrows ideas from collaborative concept learning in MAS [3]. This strategy is an incremental collaborative protocol that tries to enhance a model created with few instances, by means of contradictory instances provided by the agents on the system. In this way, it is possible to reduce the number of instances communicated, while at the same time maintaining the accuracy of a centralized approach.

This paper presents a work in progress aimed to develop an agents & artifacts competitive approach for DDM. To this end, JaCA-DDM is used to create an experimental setting aimed to test the differences in accuracy and number of training examples used between our strategy and a traditional centralized strategy. Being this comparison our main concern, we put aside many efficiency aspects for the moment, but the main strategy and system architecture are open enough to allow further efficiency enhancements.

This paper is organized as follows. Section 2 introduces the background for this paper, this includes: DDM, agent based DDM, and CArtAgO environments. Section 3 introduces JaCA-DDM and describes the generalities of our leaning strategy. In section 4 the experimental setting and results obtained are addressed. Finally, section 5 closes with a conclusion and future work.

2   Background

Data mining is a discipline that merges a wide variety of techniques intended for the exploration and analysis of huge amounts of data, with the goal of finding patterns and rules somewhat hidden in it [13]. Since data mining is about data, it is important to know the origin and distribution of this data in order to exploit it efficiently. A traditional way of doing data mining is using a centralized schema. In this way, all the data and learned models are on the same site. With the ubiquitous presence of computational networks, it is common to find data belonging to the same system spreaded in various sites, even in sites that are geographically far away from each other. From the data mining point of view, some questions may arise in these distributed scenarios: Which is the best strategy for constructing learning models that take into account the data from all the sites?, What is the best way to face heterogeneous databases?, How can the communication of the data and the data mining process be optimized?, How can the privacy of the data be preserved?, Is there some efficient way to treat cases where the data changes and grows constantly?

A lot of systems devoted to DDM have been created. According to the strategy that they implement, those systems can be classified into two major categories [7]: centralized learning strategies, and meta-learning strategies. In the centralized strategies, all the data is moved to a central site, and when all data is merged together, data mining algorithms are applied sequentially to produce a single learning model. In general, the centralized strategy is inapplicable because of the cost of data transmission. Meta-Learning refers to a general strategy that seeks to learn how to combine a number of separate learning processes in an intelligent way [4]. The idea behind Meta-Learning is to collect locally generated classification models and from there generate or simulate a single learning model. To accomplish this, it is necessary to collect the prediction of the local classification models on a validation data set, and then create a meta-level training data set from the predictions of the locally generated classification models. To generate the final meta-level classification model from the meta-level training data set, voting, arbitrating and combining techniques can be used [6]. Meta-learning is an efficient and scalable way to do DDM since the data transmitted is limited and the process is parallel, with a good load balance. Nevertheless, it is not as efficient as its centralized counterpart when a new instance needs to be classified. This is because the classification process is not direct, the classification query has to traverse a decision process that maybe has various classification models involved. Centralized learning is also simpler, to setup a meta-learning system can be more difficult. Another disadvantage of distributed meta-learning is that, because classifiers are not built globally on data, the model's performance may suffer as a result of incomplete information [11].

We propose an alternative learning strategy borrowed from SMILE [3], a setting for collaborative concept learning in MAS, designed for maintaining the consistency of the learned hypothesis when facing new evidence. A concept has to be consistent with respect to a set of examples that can be received from the environment or from other agents. The hypothesis is kept consistent through a series of incremental revisions. In this way, the hypothesis is incrementally enhanced through a process that involves the use of counter examples (examples not covered by the current hypothesis). We took this idea and translate it to DDM terms.

Data mining is applied to a variety of domains that have their own particularities, making it difficult to come with a general way of treating all scenarios. MAS are a straight and flexible way to implement DDM systems since they are already decentralized distributed systems. Each agent can do various tasks concurrently and it can be seen as an independent process. The location of the agents is in some degree irrelevant and transparent. The communication between agents is done in a high abstract level, that makes it easy to implement sophisticated protocols and behaviors. Some agent-based DDM systems [14] had been done in the past with successful results, e.g., JAM [12], a Meta-learning agent based DDM system, is one of the most influential. Our approach is closer to centralized distributed DDM systems. The challenges of agent based DDM are discussed in detail in [8].

A fundamental part of a MAS is the environment where it is deployed. It is important to adequately model the environment such that the agents can be able to perceive it, modify it, and exploit it. CArtAgO is an infrastructure and architecture based on artifacts used for modeling computational environments in multi-agent systems. With CArtAgO the concept of environment is simplified, the environment is a set or artifacts.

An artifact is a first order abstraction used for modeling computational environments in MAS. Each artifact represents an entity of the environment, offering services and data structures to the agents in order for them to improve their activities, especially the social ones. Artifacts are also of great value in the design and reutilization of multi-agent systems since their structure is modular, based on object-oriented concepts. Artifacts are conceived as function-oriented computational devices, functionality that the agents may exploit in order to fulfill their individual and social activities. The vision proposed by CArtAgO impacts directly in the agent theories about interaction and activity. Under this vision a MAS is conceived as a set of agents that develop their activities in three distinct ways: computing, interacting with other agents and using shared artifacts that compose the computational environment.

Artifacts can be the objective of the agent activity as well as the tool the agents use to fulfill their activities, reducing the complexity of their tasks. Since the environment is composed by artifacts, the state of each artifact can be perceived by the interested agents. The infrastructure of CArtAgO was designed having in mind distributed environments. It is possible to define work-spaces to determine the context where an artifact exists and can be perceived and used. The distributed environment is transparent for the agent, the later is one of the most valuable characteristics of CArtAgO. In this work, CArtAgO plays an important role, and is one of the base technologies used to support JaCA-DDM.

3 JaCA-DDM: A Jason Multi-Agent System for DDM

JaCA-DDM (Jason & CArtAgO for DDM) is a Multi-Agent System implemented in Jason and situated in a CArtAgO environment. JaCA-DDM is used to create and run distributed learning experiments that are based on the collaborative learning strategy explained later. Currently it supports J48 decision trees, but it can easily be extended to support other classification learning approaches. The artifacts provided by this environment encapsulate data mining tools as implemented by WEKA[5]. In what follows, the artifacts, agents, and the workflow are described in detail.

The MAS is composed by a coordinator agent and n workers. There are three main types of artifacts used by the agents: Oracle, InstancesBase and ClassifierJ48. The coordinator uses the Oracle to extract information about the learning set and split it among the workers and itself. Each agent stores its training examples in an InstancesBase artifact. Instances distribution is shown in figure 2 (page 344). The coordinator induces an initial model with its instances using ClassifierJ48. Then it asks for contradictory instances as shown in figure 3 (page 345). The interactions amongst the artifacts are shown in figure 1. In what follows, a more detailed account for each artifact is presented.

Since the main goal of JaCA-DDM is to experiment distributed learning scenarios, we are interested in partitioning existing training data sets in a controlled way to enable comparisons with centralized scenarios. The single `Oracle` artifact creates random stratified data partitions and distributes them among the agents. An agent can use the `Oracle` artifact to: obtain the attributes information, as described in the ARFF file; restart the artifact for a new running of the system; recreate the artifact to run a new round in the cross-validation process; get the number of instances stored in the artifact; and reinitialize the artifact with a new training set. The `port1` is used to get other artifacts linked with this one. Usually `InstancesBase` artifacts are linked via this port to get set of instances.

`ClassifierJ48` is a single artifact in charge managing and creating the learning model. An agent can execute a set of operations (∘) on an instance of this artifact to: add a new training instance to the artifact; build a J48 classifier with the instances stored in the artifact; print the tree representation of the computed classifier; classify an instance; and restart the artifact for running a new experiment. An agent can also link other artifacts to this one, so that the linked artifacts can execute linked operations (⋄) on the `Classifier48` for: getting the J48 classifier; and classifying an instance. Observe that the artifact is used to classify instances in two ways: i) An agent executes `classifyInstance` over a string representing the instance to be classified, obtaining an integer representing the instance class as defined in WEKA; ii) Another artifact executes `classifyInstance` to classify an instance stored in that artifact. The `port1` is used to link other artifacts linked to this one. Usually `InstancesBase` artifacts are linked via this port to classify instances.

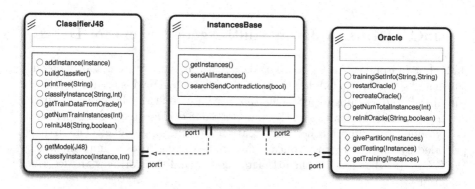

Fig. 1. The main artifacts used in JaCA-DDM

`InstancesBase` is an artifact class implementing local repositories of instances for the agents, so each agent has control of a InstancesBase artifact. Such an artifact can be linked with an `Oracle` artifact, via `port2`, in order to execute the linked operation `givePartition` to obtain a set of instances. It can be also linked to a `ClassifierJ48`, via `port1`, in order to search for a contradiction in the local repository and add it to the `ClassifierJ48`. A contradiction is an instance wrongly classified by the current model.

Other artifact related to the experimental setting provided by JaCA-DDM include: the GUI artifact is a front end for launching experiments and setting the different parameters for the experiment; the Evaluator artifact performs statistical operations with the results gathered, this operations include standard deviation, medias and paired T-test.

The collaborative learning strategy proposed has the following characteristics: there exists a central site, in this site the data is controlled by a special agent known as the coordinator. In this central site a base model is induced using the instances of the site, this base model serves as the first model that presumably needs enhancement since it maybe was induced with few instances. The base model can be shared between the different sites. The coordinator agent also is in charge of the experiment control, initialization of artifacts, control of the learning process, and managing the results. In each of the other sites, a worker agent resides, this agent manages the data of its corresponding site and runs a process with the purpose of finding contradictions between the base model and the instances of the site. A contradiction exists when the model does not predict the instance class correctly. The contradictory instances are sent to the central site enhancing the base model in a posterior induction. The process repeats itself until no contradictions are found.

To run the experiments we used a single computer to simulate different distributed scenarios consisting of various sites, the number of sites is configurable. Despite using a single computer for the experiments, the system architecture is flexible, it can also be applied in a true distributed environment without any major change.

Before an experiment begins, the parameters for the experiment are set through the GUI, those parameters include: database path, number of worker agents (in this manner simulating various sites) and type of model evaluation (hold-out or cross validation with its respective parameters). An experiment has the following general workflow: first, the coordinator determines which agents are going to participate in the experiment (currently all the agents participate). Then the coordinator creates the artifacts needed passing the relevant parameters. From there, each agent sends a request to Oracle, asking for its data partition. The coordinator sends all its examples to ClassifierJ48 in order to create the base model. Next, the coordinator begins the social process, asking to each worker, one by one, if it has contradictory examples. If a worker finds a contradiction, the contradictory example is sent to ClassifierJ48. When a worker finishes sending all the contradictions, the coordinator may issue an induction request to ClassifierJ48, the frequency of this induction request can be tuned in order to increase efficiency. This process continues until no more contradictions are found.

The interaction diagrams in figures 2 (data distribution) and 3 (learning process) summarizes the workflow described earlier. These figures omit the InstancesBase artifacts for the sake of readability. Remembering that each agent has an InstancesBase associated for the storage and administration of its instances.

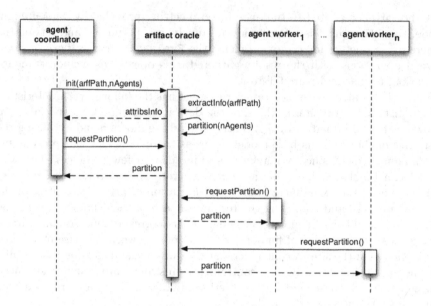

Fig. 2. Data distribution

Our current learning strategy is linear in the sense that only one worker agent at a time searches and sends contradictions. We are not exploiting yet the concurrent and parallel facilities that the architecture of JaCa-DDM provides.

4 Experiments and Results

JaCa-DDM was used to create a series of experiments to compare our collaborative learning strategy and a traditional centralized strategy. This comparison takes into account the number of examples used for training, classification accuracy and time. Since we ran the experiments in a single multi-core computer and not in a distributed system, the time results may not be fair because the cost of communication is not present, nevertheless, for the sake of completeness, we also show time results. A set of ten databases of the UCI repository [1] was used, giving consistent results. Table 1 lists the five most representative databases that are reported in the present.

A randomized stratified policy was used to distribute the data among the agents. Stratification ensures that each data partition conserves the ratio of class distribution. Stratified cross validation with 10 folds and 10 repetitions was applied. For each database, experiments were done with 1, 10, 30, 50 and 100 worker agents. For comparison, the same data partitions were used for both strategies. Two tailed paired T test with 0.05 degrees of significance are used to verify if there are significant differences between both strategies. The results are presented confronting the collaborative model against the centralized one (CollvsCen column in table 3) and the collaborative model against the base

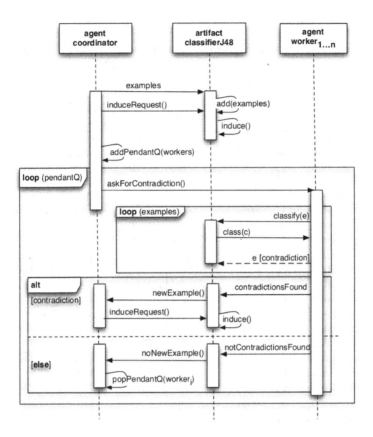

Fig. 3. Learning process

Table 1. Data Sets

Data Set	Instances	Attributes	Classes
adult	48842	15	2
german	1000	21	2
letter	20000	17	26
poker	829201	11	10
waveform	5000	41	3

model (CollvsBas column in the same table). 0 means there is not significant difference; 1 means that the first strategy paired won; and -1 means that the first strategy lost. J48 was used with pruning and the rest of the WEKA options set to default.

Table 2 shows the number of examples used to learn. For the collaborative model (Collab), the standard deviation is also shown, because of the variations in each experiment (100 runs). This table shows that our strategy definitely reduces the number of training examples used to induce the model. This can be seen for example in the results for the adult database (except for 1 worker agent) where

Table 2. Number of instances used to learn

Data Set	Wks	Total	Centralized	Base	Collab
adult	1	48842	43957	21978	27468.85 ± 107.53
adult	10	48842	43957	3996	16121.10 ± 147.73
adult	30	48842	43957	1417	15162.07 ± 142.62
adult	50	48842	43957	861	15403.52 ± 163.40
adult	100	48842	43957	435	16063.00 ± 221.61
german	1	1000	900	450	698.20 ± 15.68
german	10	1000	900	81	613.64 ± 13.94
german	30	1000	900	29	614.03 ± 16.20
german	50	1000	900	17	618.74 ± 15.94
german	100	1000	900	8	629.59 ± 16.10
letter	1	20000	18000	9000	11803.68 ± 164.30
letter	10	20000	18000	1636	8349.14 ± 217.90
letter	30	20000	18000	580	8259.17 ± 238.86
letter	50	20000	18000	352	8389.38 ± 227.43
letter	100	20000	18000	178	8628.10 ± 284.24
poker	1	829201	746280	373140	374100.00 ± 14.24
poker	10	829201	746280	67843	71419.50 ± 150.61
poker	30	829201	746280	24073	38988.50 ± 1750.09
poker	50	829201	746280	14632	48773.50 ± 994.89
poker	100	829201	746280	7388	81041.50 ± 1141.97
waveform	1	5000	4500	2250	3836.38 ± 33.40
waveform	10	5000	4500	409	3534.60 ± 34.54
waveform	30	5000	4500	145	3523.18 ± 34.12
waveform	50	5000	4500	88	3543.13 ± 34.50
waveform	100	5000	4500	44	3561.68 ± 37.20

only about 35% of the instances where used for training in our strategy. The standard deviation results show that our strategy is stable enough. Base reports the number of examples used to construct the initial model. Total reports the number of available examples.

Table 3 reports the accuracy of the obtained models. This table also shows, as mentioned, the results for paired T-test. Standard deviation is due to data random distribution for each experiment. Our approach (Collab) maintains a similar accuracy when compared with the centralized strategy. Even in the cases where our approach loses, the difference is very small, e.g., the poker database. There are significant differences in those cases because the standard deviation of the centralized strategy is small.

Finally, table 4 shows the mean time (ms) for inducing a model. From this results it is obvious that our strategy has its process overhead, this is more noticeable in small databases like german. Nevertheless, as the database grows, the advantages of our strategy begin to show up. This is specially true for the poker database, where the time efficiency actually improves. This boost in the time efficiency occurs because as the data grows it is more efficient to do multiple inductions with a small amount of data, rather than doing a single induction with

Table 3. Accuracy results

Data Set	Wks	Centralized	Base	Collab	CollvsCen	CollvsBas
adult	1	86.00 ± 0.44	85.78 ± 0.48	86.32 ± 0.45	1	1
adult	10	85.97 ± 0.44	84.75 ± 0.57	86.22 ± 0.56	1	1
adult	30	85.99 ± 0.43	83.84 ± 0.73	86.25 ± 0.57	1	1
adult	50	86.02 ± 0.44	83.54 ± 0.89	86.28 ± 0.51	1	1
adult	100	85.98 ± 0.43	82.20 ± 1.58	86.30 ± 0.52	1	1
german	1	72.05 ± 3.73	71.33 ± 4.05	71.82 ± 4.02	0	0
german	10	71.57 ± 3.74	68.38 ± 3.81	71.73 ± 3.78	0	1
german	30	71.83 ± 4.11	68.14 ± 3.89	71.18 ± 4.00	0	1
german	50	71.75 ± 4.0	66.56 ± 5.56	71.51 ± 3.96	0	1
german	100	72.50 ± 3.73	65.36 ± 7.94	71.79 ± 4.09	-1	1
letter	1	87.98 ± 0.76	83.74 ± 0.87	88.18 ± 0.74	1	1
letter	10	88.07 ± 0.70	69.28 ± 1.35	88.26 ± 0.70	1	1
letter	30	87.96 ± 0.80	57.86 ± 1.69	88.23 ± 0.84	1	1
letter	50	88.09 ± 0.73	51.26 ± 2.23	88.26 ± 0.80	1	1
letter	100	88.02 ± 0.67	40.35 ± 3.11	88.26 ± 0.76	1	1
poker	1	99.78 ± 0.01	99.76 ± 0.010	99.79 ± 0.01	0	0
poker	10	99.78 ± 0.01	99.06 ± 0.11	99.74 ± 0.01	-1	0
poker	30	99.79 ± 0.01	96.47 ± 0.25	99.76 ± 0.01	-1	0
poker	50	99.79 ± 0.01	92.22 ± 1.36	99.33 ± 0.02	-1	0
poker	100	99.79 ± 0.01	87.99 ± 0.40	98.99 ± 0.79	-1	1
waveform	1	75.35 ± 1.87	74.77 ± 2.03	75.24 ± 1.75	0	1
waveform	10	75.36 ± 1.99	70.89 ± 2.22	75.08 ± 1.88	0	1
waveform	30	75.35 ± 1.90	67.52 ± 3.03	74.69 ± 2.09	-1	1
waveform	50	75.05 ± 1.74	65.44 ± 3.26	74.85 ± 1.94	0	1
waveform	100	75.21 ± 1.99	62.76 ± 4.54	74.99 ± 2.04	0	1

a big amount of data. Since our strategy pretends to be applied in scenarios where the amount of data is really big, this result is very promising.

As we continue to develop our approach, a more in depth analysis about the results and consequences of our collaborative learning strategy will be done. For the present paper, we limited our analysis to the most noticeable facts as an evidence of the plausibility of the approach.

5 Conclusions and Future Work

In this paper we presented JaCa-DDM, an extensible tool that we proposed to run a series of experiments of DDM. The principles entailed by JaCa-DDM make it easy to extend and improve it. This is due to the modular nature of the system and the fact that agents and artifacts raise the level of abstraction, so we can think naturally in terms of shared services, communication and workflow.

As the results in the previous section show, our learning strategy is promissory. Our initial expectation of reducing the number of training instances used to train the model while conserving the accuracy of a traditional centralized strategy was fulfilled. Now we have the challenge to improve the learning strategy to

Table 4. Processing time in milliseconds

Data Set	Wks	Centralized	Collab	Data Set	Wks	Centralized	Collab
adult	1	1393.97	5913.78	letter	1	795.76	5435.10
adult	10	1419.80	14191.26	letter	10	816.49	17850.55
adult	30	1435.85	15167.84	letter	30	813.13	18120.53
adult	50	1441.34	12626.48	letter	50	826.68	14723.98
adult	100	1465.65	9720.67	letter	100	848.36	11643.36
german	1	10.14	68.16	poker	1	143236.00	180256.00
german	10	7.70	264.52	poker	10	147610.00	120582.00
german	30	6.70	385.76	poker	30	145595.00	53229.00
german	50	6.73	402.97	poker	50	148476.00	54364.50
german	100	6.89	546.88	poker	100	147646.00	54837.00
waveform	1	372.84	3330.27				
waveform	10	370.02	9056.13				
waveform	30	377.05	9371.32				
waveform	50	390.79	6669.84				
waveform	100	399.83	6933.90				

enhance efficiency as well as to do a more in depth analysis of the benefits and consequences of this approach. This analysis has to take into account more databases with a wide range of characteristics as well as more classification techniques, and not only J48. As it was mentioned earlier, we ran the experiments in a single computer, simulating various distributed sites. In the future, we hope to do experiments in a true distributed setting. In this way, we can have a better account of time results that will help us to move forward in the efficiency enhancements that we want to implement.

Acknowledgements. First author was supported by the Conacyt scholarship 320544. Second author was supported by the Conacyt project 78910.

References

1. Bache, K., Lichman, M.: UCI machine learning repository (2013)
2. Bordini, R.H., Hübner, J.F., Wooldridge, M.: Programming multi-agent systems in Agent Speak using Jason, vol. 8. Wiley-Interscience (2007)
3. Bourgne, G., El Fallah Segrouchni, A., Soldano, H.: SMILE: Sound multi-agent incremental learning. In: Proceedings of the 6th International Joint Conference on Autonomous Agents and Multiagent Systems, p. 38. ACM (2007)
4. Chan, P.K., Stolfo, S.J.: On the accuracy of meta-learning for scalable data mining. Journal of Intelligent Information Systems 8(1), 5–28 (1997)
5. Hall, M., Frank, E., Holmes, G., Pfahringer, B., Reutemann, P., Witten, I.H.: The weka data mining software: an update. ACM SIGKDD Explorations Newsletter 11(1), 10–18 (2009)
6. Prodromidis, A., Chan, P., Stolfo, S.: Meta-learning in distributed data mining systems: Issues and approaches. Advances in Distributed and Parallel Knowledge Discovery 3 (2000)

7. Rao, V.S.: Multi agent-based distributed data mining: An overview. International Journal of Reviews in Computing 3, 83–92 (2009)
8. Rao, V.S., Vidyavathi, S., Ramaswamy, G.: Distributed data mining and agent mining interaction and integration: A novel approach (2010)
9. Ricci, A., Piunti, M., Viroli, M.: Environment programming in multi-agent systems: an artifact-based perspective. Autonomous Agents and Multi-Agent Systems 23(2), 158–192 (2011)
10. Ricci, A., Viroli, M., Omicini, A.: Construenda est CArtAgO: Toward an infrastructure for artifacts in MAS. Cybernetics and Systems 2, 569–574 (2006)
11. Secretan, J.: An Architecture for High-Performance Privacy-Preserving and Distributed Data Mining. PhD thesis, University of Central Florida, Orlando, Florida (2009)
12. Stolfo, S., Prodromidis, A.L., Tselepis, S., Lee, W., Fan, D.W., Chan, P.K.: Jam: Java agents for meta-learning over distributed databases. In: Proceedings of the 3rd International Conference on Knowledge Discovery and Data Mining, pp. 74–81 (1997)
13. Witten, I.H., Frank, E.: Data Mining: Practical machine learning tools and techniques. Morgan Kaufmann (2005)
14. Zeng, L., Li, L., Duan, L., Lu, K., Shi, Z., Wang, M., Wu, W., Luo, P.: Distributed data mining: a survey. Information Technology and Management 13(4), 403–409 (2012)

Evaluating Business Intelligence Gathering Techniques for Horizon Scanning Applications

Marco A. Palomino[1], Tim Taylor[1], and Richard Owen[2]

[1] European Centre for Environment and Human Health
University of Exeter Medical School
Truro, TR1 3HD, United Kingdom
[2] University of Exeter Business School
Exeter, EX4 4PU, United Kingdom
{m.palomino,timothy.j.taylor,r.j.owen}@exeter.ac.uk

Abstract. Business intelligence systems exploit futures and foresight techniques to assist decision makers in complex and rapidly changing environments. Such systems combine elements of text and data mining, forecasting and optimisation. We are particularly interested in the development of horizon scanning applications, which involve the systematic search for incipient trends, opportunities, challenges and constraints that might affect the probability of achieving management goals. In this paper, we compare and contrast a couple of case studies that we have carried out in collaboration with Lloyd's of London and RAL Space to evaluate the use of various information retrieval techniques to optimise the collection of Web-based information. Also, we discuss the implementation of potential improvements to our previous work which aim to develop a semi-automated horizon scanning system.

1 Introduction

Fundamental developments in data mining, classification, clustering and trend analysis have been gaining increasing attention for futures research over the past few years [1, 2]. The use of the World Wide Web for the extraction of information, and its eventual use in futures research, has been increasing too [3–5]. Regrettably, organisations keep making mistakes and realising later on, in hindsight, that they neglected important information [6]. According to a survey conducted by the *Fuld-Gilad-Herring Academy of Competitive Intelligence*, two-thirds of 140 corporate strategists admitted that their organisations have been surprised by as many as three high-impact events in the past five years. Moreover, the vast majority of them—to be precise, 97%—stated that their organisations have no early warning system in place [7]. Unsurprisingly, organisations continue to be blindsided, despite the abundance of business intelligence methods to detect *warning signals* [8].

Warning signals frequently appear in the form of disconnected data that at first resemble background noise, but which can then be recognised as part of a

F. Castro, A. Gelbukh, and M. González (Eds.): MICAI 2013, Part II, LNAI 8266, pp. 350–361, 2013.

larger pattern when viewed through a different frame or by connecting it with other pieces of information [9]. Recognising them involves knowing where to look for clues, how to interpret weak signals and when to discard or act on faint and ambiguous stirrings. *Horizon scanning*, which is the focus of this paper, has proved to improve an organisation's resilience against high-impact events that are not necessarily in the immediate environment.

Horizon scanning has been defined as *"the systematic search for incipient trends, opportunities, challenges and constraints (henceforth 'issues') that might affect the probability of achieving management goals and objectives* [10]. *Objectives of horizon scanning are to anticipate issues, accumulate reliable data and knowledge about them, and thus inform policy making and implementation"* [11].

At present, horizon scanning is used by some governments across the world [12]. The interest in horizon scanning stems from the rapid pace at which change is occurring, and the difficulties governments face in anticipating it and keeping their policies and strategies current [13]. Performance among organisations, from corporations to hospitals, has improved with horizon scanning, particularly when it is performed continuously [14]. In the UK, the importance of horizon scanning has been highlighted by a series of perceived failures in science and policy—for instance, the UK Government was insufficiently prepared and reacted poorly to the outbreak of the foot/hoof and mouth disease in 2001.

Horizon scanners—dedicated analysts responsible for scanning the horizon— make frequent use of search engines to retrieve information [15]. Indeed, search engine results play a significant part in the elaboration of the reports that horizon scanners communicate to decision makers. Thus, we propose the development of a semi-automated horizon scanning system that employs search engines' APIs. By leveraging the existing infrastructure of proven search engines, our system aims to automate the human-intensive process of detecting and summarising emerging trends. We realise that the results yielded by the most popular search engines are often inconsistent, obsolete and redundant [16]; yet, we compare and contrast API data with other sources of information, rather than simply aggregating and displaying their results as in the case of a meta search engine.

The remainder of this paper is organised as follows: Section 2 reviews related work. Section 3 details the implementation of a horizon scanning prototype system that we have used as a testbed for our research. Section 4 reports on the evaluation derived from our case studies, and, finally, Section 5 states our conclusions and highlights opportunities for future work.

2   Related Work

Traditional monitoring processes in organisations are largely arbitrary, depending on what concerned individuals are reading, thinking about, and sharing informally with each other. But this is insufficient: no foresight function can operate without a disciplined process [17].

SRI International—subsequently *SRI Consulting Business Intelligence* (SRIC-BI)—set the foundations for present-day horizon scanning by providing foresight capabilities for longer than 25 years—starting in 1979—to gauge changes in the commercial, technical, and cultural environments on a monthly basis. James B. Smith originally brought the scanning process to SRI International with the assistance of the futurist consulting group *Weiner, Edrich, Brown, Inc.*, which directed the first industry-wide futures research program, known as the *Trend Analysis Program of the American Council of Life Insurance*. The *SRIC-BI's Scan* program has evolved since then as a group process that relies heavily on human expertise to identify early signals of change, discontinuities, inflection points, and disruptive forces in the business environment [17].

Literature referring to the application of horizon scanning and the results of specific scans keeps growing [10, 11, 18–23], but only a few academic papers describe the methodology to carry out an automated scan [15, 24–26].

Shaping Tomorrow [27] and *Recorded Future* [28] are two private firms using Web-based scanning tools. Shaping Tomorrow uses a variety of manual, semi-manual and automated scanning processes to track and share information from around the world. It is supported by a virtual network of volunteer and client researchers who investigate items of specific interest to them. Recorded Future is established on the premise that the information available on the Web is useful to support forecasting methods, financial or otherwise. By applying *temporal analytics*—i.e., by associating timed entities with event instances to track trends, historical developments and information written about the future—Recorded Future expects to draw conclusions and gain insight [29].

As opposed to Shaping Tomorrow and Recorded Future, we are not interested in providing consumer and general scouting to particular clients. Our research is undertaken with a purely academic interest, our software is based on open source technology, and we rely on free access to search engines' APIs. Additionally, we do not intend to predict the future, but rather to improve the resilience of organisations and their capability to react to new risks and opportunities.

3 System Implementation

Until machines can read, process, integrate, and analyse the breadth of topics and treatments in a typical online document, we will need to depend on humans for scanning, particularly in the case of intelligence gathering systems [17]. Such systems need to be able to identify new patterns as well as track existing ones that evolve over time. Realistically, what we expect to deliver at this stage is a system that utilises data from the past to shed light on the future and makes the scanners work more efficient. We have developed a system that builds upon the suggestions documented by Nie *et al.* to collect information that is relevant to the issues of concern within an organisation [30]. Although Nie *et al.*'s approach is limited to electronic journals, we follow their recommendations to use the entire Web as an information source, and we describe this process of information retrieval, analysis and communication as *Web-based horizon scanning* [15].

Web-based horizon scanning comprises several components, as described by Palomino *et al.* [15]: emerging information which is relevant to an organisation is retrieved manually or otherwise from a variety of Web-based sources—for instance, online scientific, peer-reviewed literature, news and other websites, and online databases. Key parts of the retrieved information may be extracted and later on categorised in some way—in its simplest form grouped within a specific topic area. Afterwards, the information is often archived in a database. Periodically, outputs are presented to decision makers or more generally through one or more communication mechanisms—typically a report or newsletter. Figure 1 shows a generalised approach to Web-based horizon scanning for strategic decision support. It emphasises the iterative nature of horizon scanning, noting that the processes of information retrieval and information extraction and archival are repeated continuously.

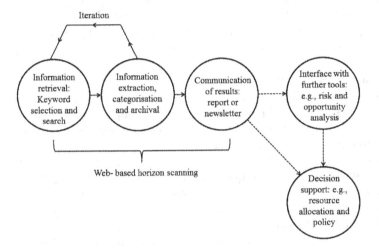

Fig. 1. A generalised approach to Web-based horizon scanning for decision support—Adapted from Palomino, *et al* [15]

At the moment, we refer to the implementation of our horizon scanning system as a *prototype*, in the sense that it is an early sample built as a proof-of-concept demonstration to test our ideas. The first component of our system is related to the selection of keywords.

3.1   Keywords

To bootstrap the search for emerging information on the Web, a suitable set of *keywords* has to be selected. Keywords are descriptive words or phrases that are mentioned consistently in relation to the issues of concern which will lead the search for emerging information and may help to better characterise them.

Our selection of keywords is supported by keyword extraction software, and requires the additional choice of a reputable source, which may be a keynote, a journal paper or a website from which the keywords will be extracted. We refer to this source as the *seed*, since it provides the starting point for the whole scanning process. We have implemented our own keyword extraction software and it is based on *TextRank* [31], derived from Google's *PageRank* [32], which determines the importance of a word by the number of words with which it co-occurs, and the relative importance of those co-occurring words.

Once keywords have been selected, the next step in our search for emerging information consists of using keyword combinations to produce queries that are automatically submitted to commercial, Web search engines.

3.2   Search Engine APIs

To automate our search for relevant information on the Web, we programmatically release queries containing combinations of keywords via *Google's Custom Search API* [33]. The inner workings of Google's APIs, as well as most of the technology and algorithms that support the operation of Google's search engine, are considered proprietary and they are not publicly available for scrutiny [34].

After experimenting with different APIs for horizon scanning purposes, we have realised that the data that they provide tend to differ from what it is reported by the traditional *Web user interfaces* of the corresponding search engines, also known as *WUIs*[1]. Consider, for example, a query including the keywords eHealth and breakthrough separated by a semicolon, to indicate that we wish to retrieve documents containing both keywords anywhere in their text. Submitting the query to *Bing's WUI* [35] on 25 July 2012 yielded 14,300 results; whereas submitting the same query, on the same date and approximately the same time, to *Bing's API* [36] yielded, exclusively, 255 results.

Table 1 shows the difference between the number of results reported by Bing's WUI and API for 26 different queries, requesting specifically that the results should be documents written in English language and published in the United Kingdom—this is achieved in the WUI by specifying results only English and only from United Kingdom; and in the API by setting the market parameter to English - United Kingdom or en-GB [36]. Table 1 also shows the total number of results reported by Bing's WUI and API on 25 July 2012 and on average over two weeks, starting on 20 July 2012 and releasing the queries once a day. We could not collect statistics for longer than two weeks, because Bing's Search API 2.0 was decommissioned in early August 2012. The latest and currently available version of Bing's API does not provide the total number of results for each query. Note that the queries that we used were meant to discover new issues in *eHealth* and *telemedicine*, and make use of a series of keywords originally identified by the UK *Defence Science and Technology Laboratory* (Dstl) as descriptors of new developments—e.g., revolutionary, paves the way, etcetera.

Bing is not the only search engine whose result counts for its WUI and API are so dissimilar. Google also appears to overestimate the result counts displayed by its WUI when compared with its own API. The extent of these differences

---

[1] For the vast majority of users, Web browsers are the primary mode of interaction with a search engine. The user interface that allows a person to interact with a search engine via a Web browser is called a Web user interface, or simply WUI.

Table 1. Differences reported by Bing's WUI and API for 26 queries that required results in **English language** published in the **United Kingdom**, exclusively, on 25 July 2012 and on average over 2 weeks

Query	Bing's WUI 25/07/2012 10:55	Bing's API 25/07/2012 10:52:58	Bing's WUI average (2 weeks)	Bing's API average (2 weeks)
ehealth; breakthrough	14,300	255	14,516	253
telemed; breakthrough	148	8	147	8
ehealth; "closer to reality"	124	2	137	2
telemed; "closer to reality"	5	0	6	0
ehealth; "first time"	25,100	29,900	25,859	25,911
telemed; "first time"	315	184	317	175
ehealth; groundbreaking	15,200	89	14,654	88
telemed; groundbreaking	95	1	94	1
ehealth; "new development"	13,300	119	12,455	123
telemed; "new development"	11	4	11	4
ehealth; "new threat"	59	0	47	0
telemed; "new threat"	2	1	2	1
ehealth; novel	37,800	24,200	38,954	29,538
telemed; novel	14,000	273	10,519	273
ehealth; "paves the way"	243	6	256	5
telemed; "paves the way"	3	1	3	1
ehealth; "previously impossible"	18	3	17	3
telemed; "previously impossible"	2	0	2	0
ehealth; "previously unknown"	184	5	198	4
telemed; "previously unknown"	1	1	1	1
ehealth; revolutionary	15,800	255	15,995	249
telemed; revolutionary	226	71	232	70
ehealth; unprecedented	12,100	339	12,186	331
telemed; unprecedented	136	89	133	88
ehealth; "world's first"	18,600	142	15,396	142
telemed; "world's first"	119	4	122	4

and, more generally, the instability of Google's search engine results for 100 days, starting on 3 August 2012, has been reported at the *10th International Workshop on Text-based Information Retrieval*—see Palomino *et al* [16]. The queries were released at approximately the same time of the day for the entire length of the experiment—between 9:00 GMT and 10:00 GMT.

On the basis of our research, result counts provided by WUIs seem to be overestimated due to their use for marketing purposes [16, 34]: search engines are economically motivated tools, and the higher the number of results they report, the larger the market they may approach. We consider the use of APIs to be a better choice than the use of WUIs, though the amount of results and information that we can derive from the APIs is smaller; yet, such results and information are more recent than those produced by the WUIs—this conclusion seems valid for Google and Bing.

4   Case Studies

In collaboration with *Lloyd's of London*, one of the global leaders in the insurance market, we carried out a study to use our horizon scanning prototype for framing decision making on novel risks—specifically risks associated with *space weather* and how these might affect terrestrial and near-Earth insurable assets. As part of this study, we benchmarked our prototype against current information retrieval practice within Lloyd's. The results highlighted the potential of Web-based horizon scanning, but also the challenges of undertaking it effectively [24].

After working with Lloyd's of London, we worked with *RAL Space*—a world-class space research centre based at the *Rutherford Appleton Laboratory* (RAL)

[37]—to undertake a review for the European Union Framework Programme 7 (FP7) project *Q Detect: Developing Quarantine Pest Detection Methods for use by National Plant Protection Organisations (NPPO) and Inspection Services* [38]. The review looked into current and future aerial platform technologies and instrumentation options for detecting and monitoring diseases in vegetation and the mapping of pests. Since decision making on the uptake and use of emerging technology for disease monitoring has to be supported by timely and high quality information, RAL Space used horizon scanning to produce the review.

Table 2 displays a summary of the case studies described above in terms of the subject, context, dates and the method that we employed to rank and select the results. Each programmatic release of queries in the Lloyd's study resulted in 9,000 to 10,000 documents being retrieved. To reduce the list of documents to a manageable size for the evaluation of Lloyd's analysts, we sorted and filtered the documents by means of a *measure of importance*. Our hypothesis, which we subsequently tested, was that the documents of most importance—i.e., those of greatest relevance—were the ones that consistently appear at the top of Google's search results. We thus presented a ranked list of documents once per iteration to Lloyd's analysts, with the ranking being based on the number of times that the document was retrieved by Google over the course of consecutive days—i.e., *cumulative retrieval occurrences* from daily programmatic releases of queries. The same approach was used in the RAL Space study, except that the length of the experiment was shorter and hence the number of programmatic releases of queries per iteration was smaller. Additionally, in the RAL Space study we employed *relevance feedback* [39].

Table 2. Case studies

	Lloyd's Study	RAL Space's Study
Subject	Space weather	Remote monitoring of plants
Context	Risk analysis in the insurance industry	Collection of reliable data and knowledge
Time	September 14th - October 12th 2010	12 - 19 October 2012
Method	Cumulative retrieval occurrences from daily programmatic releases of queries	Cumulative retrieval occurrences from programmatic releases of queries aided by relevance feedback

As part of the Lloyd's study, we identified several documents that *Lloyd's Emerging Risks Group* considered very relevant to assess insurance exposure. Nevertheless, the number of very relevant documents retrieved per week decreased as the experiment progressed, while the number of non-relevant documents increased over the same period [24].

Table 3 exhibits—in its first half—the number of very relevant, relevant and non-relevant documents retrieved per iteration in our study with Lloyd's. The second half of Table 3 shows the corresponding numbers for our study with RAL Space. Table 3 shows that the number of very relevant documents decreased by one in the second iteration with RAL Space, but then remained constant, which is an improvement over the results of the Lloyd's study, where the number of very relevant documents decreased by 10 after the first set of results and kept decreasing afterwards.

Table 3. Lloyd's evaluation results

	Lloyd's				RAL Space		
	Iteration 1	Iteration 2	Iteration 3	Iteration 4	Iteration 1	Iteration 2	Iteration 3
Very relevant	29	19	11	5	16	15	15
Relevant	66	64	74	74	15	23	24
Non-relevant	5	17	15	21	19	12	11

To further evaluate the performance of our prototype, we used *precision*, one of the most common measures for evaluating information retrieval systems [40]. Precision is defined as the fraction of retrieved documents that are relevant to the search. We computed precision by considering all the documents evaluated by the analyst as being relevant or very relevant to be at least relevant, and compared these to the total number of documents presented in each iteration— i.e., 100 in the case of Lloyd's and 50 in the case of RAL Space.

Table 4 displays the precision of our prototype per iteration in both case studies. The final column shows the overall precision value for both studies. The precision of the prototype did increase per iteration when we worked with RAL Space. Also note that the *fall-out ratio*—i.e., the number of non-relevant documents—decreased over the length of the study with RAL Space—as indicated in Table 3.

Table 4. Precision per iteration

	Iteration 1	Iteration 2	Iteration 3	Iteration 4	Overall
Lloyd's	95%	83%	85%	79%	85.5%
RAL Space	62%	76%	78%	–	72%

A possible explanation as to why the number of relevant documents decreased as the Lloyd's study progressed is related to the timescale of the evolution of space weather documents on the Web. A period of four weeks might be insufficient to capture a significant number of additional newly published documents after our first search—i.e., after the first release of queries has been made.

Even though there were reasons to justify why most of the very relevant documents retrieved in the Lloyd's study were discovered in the first iteration, one of the major goals behind our work with RAL Space was to improve the performance of our prototype to make sure that the retrieval of relevant documents remained constant over the whole length of the experiment[2].

---

[2] In the case of the two studies discussed in this paper, analysts working for Lloyd's and RAL Space followed a very specific criteria to judge the relevance of the documents— and this criteria can be consulted in [24]. Nevertheless, it is worth stating that a number of factors may affect the extent to which an analyst rates a document as "relevant" or "very relevant", including individual experience and personality.

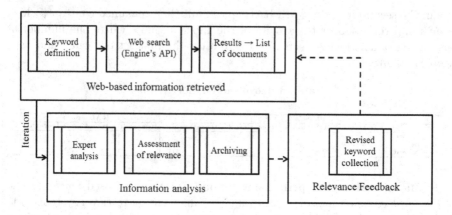

Fig. 2. A generalised Web-based horizon scanning approach using relevance feedback

During the Lloyd's study we did not modify the queries that we released daily. However, when working with RAL Space, we did want to modify these queries with every iteration, based on the feedback received from RAL Space's analysts. At the end of each iteration, we collected feedback from RAL Space's analysts by asking them to indicate, for each document in our list of results, whether it was relevant, very relevant or non-relevant. The documents that were marked as very relevant were used to extract, automatically, new keywords that were not considered in the initial queries. Similarly, documents that were considered non-relevant were used to remove from our list of keywords those that served to retrieve them. The diagram displayed in Figure 2 depicts the Web-based horizon scanning process with an added component to employ relevance feedback.

5   Conclusions

The Web offers huge potential as a global, dynamic information source for the discovery of emerging risks and opportunities, especially for the identification of novel issues that lie outside traditional search domains. However, the potential of the Web must be reconciled with critical challenges in terms of the ability to retrieve documents of high relevance and credibility.

We have presented in this paper a prototype system that illustrates the implementation of a semi-automated, Web-based horizon scanning system. This prototype has been tested in a risk analysis application for the insurance industry, and the results of this test suggested the utilisation of relevance feedback to improve its performance.

Relevance feedback provides a method for reformulating queries based on previously retrieved relevant and non-relevant documents. In view of its simplicity, we recommend that it should be incorporated into operational text retrieval for horizon scanning systems.

5.1 Future Work

The extraction of keywords from newly retrieved documents that have been considered relevant may eventually increase the number of keywords and, consequently, the number of queries, which would in turn increase the documents collected, without guaranteeing that we are actually gathering more useful information. Devising a way to adequately assign weights to keywords so that subsequent queries give higher importance to keywords with greater weights is a feature that we expect to implement in the near future.

A possible alternative to approach the association between keywords and weights might be based on the use of different locations for keywords within documents. According to Page *et al* [41], titles are more descriptive of the contents of a document than the rest of the text. Page *et al* have also stated that the text contained in the hyperlinks that point to a document, also known as the *anchor text*, *link text*, or *link title*, is greatly descriptive of the contents of the document referred to [41]. Hence, we may use the most important keywords— i.e., those extracted from documents that have been considered very relevant—to search for documents that contain them in the title, or that are referred to by anchor text containing them.

Acknowledgments. The European Centre for Environment and Human Health—part of the University of Exeter Medical School—is part financed by the European Regional Development Fund Programme 2007 to 2013 and European Social Fund Convergence Programme for Cornwall and the Isles of Scilly.

References

1. Chan, S.W.K., Franklin, J.: A text-based decision support system for financial sequence prediction. Decision Support Systems, 189–198 (2011)
2. Michalewicz, Z., Schmidt, M., Michalewicz, M.: Adaptive Business Intelligence. Springer, Heidelberg (2006)
3. Linstone, H.A., Turoff, M.: Delphi: A brief look backward and forward. Technological Forecasting and Social Change 78, 1712–1719 (2011)
4. Gheorghiu, R., Curaj, A., Paunica, M., Holeab, C.: Web 2.0 and the emergence of future oriented communities. Economic Computation & Economic Cybernetics Studies & Research 43, 1 (2009)
5. Gnatzy, T., Warth, J., von der Gracht, H., Darkow, I.L.: Validating an innovative real-time delphi approach - a methodological comparison between real-time and conventional delphi studies. Technological Forecasting and Social Change 78, 1681–1694 (2011)
6. Wissema, H.: Driving through red lights: How warning signals are missed or ignored. Long Range Planning 35, 521–539 (2002)
7. Fuld, L.: Be prepared. Harvard Business Review, 1–2 (2003)
8. Schoemaker, P.J., Day, G.S., Snyder, S.A.: Integrating organizational networks, weak signals, strategic radars and scenario planning. Technological Forecasting and Social Change 80, 815–824 (2013)

9. Ansoff, I.H.: Managing strategic surprise by response to weak signals. California Management Review 18, 21–33 (1975)

10. Sutherland, W.J., Woodroof, H.J.: The need for environmental horizon scanning. Trends in Ecology & Evolution 24, 523–527 (2009)

11. Sutherland, W.J., Aveling, R., Bennun, L., Chapman, E., Clout, M., Côté, I.M., Depledge, M.H., Dicks, L.V., Dobson, A.P., Fellman, L., Fleishman, E., Gibbons, D.W., Keim, B., Lickorish, F., Lindenmayer, D.B., Monk, K.A., Norris, K., Peck, L.S., Prior, S.V., Scharlemann, J.P., Spalding, M., Watkinson, A.R.: A horizon scan of global conservation issues for 2012. Trends in Ecology & Evolution 27, 12–18 (2012)

12. Roberts, G., Stonebridge, C.: Building policy research capacity. Technical report, The Conference Board of Canada, Canada (2007)

13. Stonebridge, C.: Horizon scanning: Gathering research evidence to inform decision making. Technical report, The Conference Board of Canada, Canada (2008)

14. Choo, C.W.: Environmental scanning as information seeking and organizational learning. Information Research 7 (2001)

15. Palomino, M., Bardsley, S., Bown, K., De Lurio, J., Ellwood, P., Holland-Smith, D., Huggins, B., Vincenti, A., Woodroof, H., Owen, R.: Web-based horizon scanning: concepts and practice. Foresight 14, 355–373 (2012)

16. Palomino, M.A., Taylor, T., McBride, G., Owen, R.: Instability in search engine results: Lessons learnt in the context of horizon scanning applications. In: 10th International Workshop on Text-based Information Retrieval, Prague, Czech Republic (in Press, 2013)

17. Patton, K.M.: The role of scanning in open intelligence systems. Technological Forecasting and Social Change 72, 1082–1093 (2005)

18. Sutherland, W.J., Clout, M., Côté, I.M., Daszak, P., Depledge, M.H., Fellman, L., Fleishman, E., Garthwaite, R., Gibbons, D.W., Lurio, J.D., Impey, A.J., Lickorish, F., Lindenmayer, D., Madgwick, J., Margerison, C., Maynard, T., Peck, L.S., Pretty, J., Prior, S., Redford, K.H., Scharlemann, J.P., Spalding, M., Watkinson, A.R.: A horizon scan of global conservation issues for 2010. Trends in Ecology & Evolution 25, 1–7 (2010)

19. Sutherland, W.J., Bardsley, S., Bennun, L., Clout, M., Côté, I.M., Depledge, M.H., Dicks, L.V., Dobson, A.P., Fellman, L., Fleishman, E., Gibbons, D.W., Impey, A.J., Lawton, J.H., Lickorish, F., Lindenmayer, D.B., Lovejoy, T.E., Nally, R.M., Madgwick, J., Peck, L.S., Pretty, J., Prior, S.V., Redford, K.H., Scharlemann, J.P., Spalding, M., Watkinson, A.R.: Horizon scan of global conservation issues for 2011. Trends in Ecology & Evolution 26, 10–16 (2011)

20. Sutherland, W.J., Bardsley, S., Clout, M., Depledge, M.H., Dicks, L.V., Fellman, L., Fleishman, E., Gibbons, D.W., Keim, B., Lickorish, F., Margerison, C., Monk, K.A., Norris, K., Peck, L.S., Prior, S.V., Scharlemann, J.P., Spalding, M.D., Watkinson, A.R.: A horizon scan of global conservation issues for 2013. Trends in Ecology & Evolution 28, 16–22 (2013)

21. Carlsson, P., Jorgensen, T.: Scanning the horizon for emerging health technologies: Conclusions from a European workshop. International Journal of Technology Assessment in Health Care 14, 695–704 (1998)

22. Douw, K., Vondeling, H., Oortwijn, W.: Priority setting for horizon scanning of new health technologies in Denmark: Views of health care stakeholders and health economists. Health Policy 76, 334–345 (2006)

23. O'Malley, S.P., Jordan, E.: Horizon scanning of new and emerging medical technology in Australia: Its relevance to medical services advisory committee health

technology assessments and public funding. International Journal of Technology Assessment in Health Care 25, 374–382 (2009)

24. Palomino, M., Vincenti, A., Owen, R.: Optimising web-based information retrieval methods for horizon scanning. Foresight 15, 159–176 (2013)

25. Palomino, M., Taylor, T., Owen, R.: Towards the development of an automated, web-based, horizon scanning system. In: Ganzha, M., Maciaszek, L.A., Paprzycki, M. (eds.) FedCSIS, pp. 1009–1016 (2012)

26. Palomino, M.A., Taylor, T., McBride, G., Owen, R.: Web-based horizon scanning: Recent development with application to health technology assessment. Business Informatics 3, 139–159 (2012)

27. Shaping Tomorrow: Shaping Tomorrow: Make better decisions today (2013), http://www.shapingtomorrow.com/

28. Recorded Future: Recorded Future: Web Intelligence for Business Decisions (2013), https://www.recordedfuture.com/

29. Truvé, S.: Big data for the future - unlocking the predictive power of the web. Technical report, Recorded Future, Cambridge, MA (2011)

30. Nie, K., Ma, T., Nakamori, Y.: An approach to aid understanding emerging research fields of the case of knowledge management. Systems Research and Behavioral Science 26, 629–643 (2009)

31. Palomino, M.A., Wuytack, T.: Unsupervised extraction of keywords from news archives. In: Vetulani, Z. (ed.) LTC 2009. LNCS, vol. 6562, pp. 544–555. Springer, Heidelberg (2011)

32. Brin, S., Page, L.: The anatomy of a large-scale hypertextual web search engine. Comput. Netw. ISDN Syst. 30, 107–117 (1998)

33. Google: Custom Search (2013), https://developers.google.com/custom-search/

34. Rayson, P., Charles, O., Auty, I.: Can google count? Estimating search engine result consistency. In: Proceedings of the 7th Web as Corpus Workshop (WAC-7), Lyon, France (2012)

35. Microsoft: Bing (2013), http://www.bing.com/

36. Microsoft: Bing API, Version 2 (2013), http://msdn.microsoft.com/en-us/library/dd251056.aspx

37. RAL Space: STFC RAL Space (2013), http://www.stfc.ac.uk/ralspace/default.aspx

38. Q-DETECT: Q-DETECT: Developing tools for on-site phytosanitary inspection (2013), http://www.qdetect.org/0_home/index.php

39. Salton, G., Buckley, C.: Improving retrieval performance by relevance feedback. Journal of the American Society for Information Science 41, 288–297 (1990)

40. Manning, C.D., Raghavan, P., Schütze, H.: Introduction to Information Retrieval. Cambridge University Press, New York (2008)

41. Page, L., Brin, S., Motwani, R., Winograd, T.: The pagerank citation ranking: Bringing order to the web. Technical report, Stanford Digital Library Technologies Project (1998)

Identification of Relations in Region Connection Calculus: 9-Intersection Reduced to 3⁺-Intersection Predicates*

Chaman L. Sabharwal and Jennifer L. Leopold

Computer Science Department, Missouri University of S&T,
Rolla, MO – 65409, USA
{chaman,leopoldj}@mst.edu

Abstract . The intersection between objects relates to a class of problems where either precise intersection is required or imprecise intersection is acceptable. The calculation of intersection between two 2D/3D objects is a computation-intensive process. For qualitative spatio-temporal reasoning, it is sufficient to know the existence of intersection instead of the precise intersection. In order to identify RCC8 relations, the 9-Intersection model considers the pairwise intersection of interiors, boundaries, and exteriors of objects. It was determined that the 9-Intersection is sufficient for identifying spatial relations. Later, it was shown that a 4-Intersection model is sufficient to achieve the same results making the definition (and implementation) of the RCC8 relations worth studying in greater detail. Herein we prove that the 9-Intersection model can be further reduced to almost three intersection predicates, producing a 3⁺-Intersection model. This results in improved algorithmic and computational efficiency as a consequence of fewer predicates and faster intersection operations.

Keywords: Spatial Reasoning, Qualitative Reasoning, Region Connection Calculus, Spatial Object Intersection.

1   Introduction

Imprecision and uncertainty are widespread in the physical world [1]. A ubiquitous task in QSR is the intersection between objects [2, 3, 4, 5]. Typically, the intersection between objects refers to a class of problems where either precise intersection is required [4] or imprecise intersection is acceptable [2, 3]. The computational complexity varies depending on the quality of intersection. The precise calculation of intersection between two 2D/3D objects is a computation-intensive process. For the qualitative spatial reasoning (QSR) domain, it is sufficient to know the existence of intersection instead of the quantity of intersection (i.e. precisely where the intersection occurs and what the intersection is). In particular, the calculation of the intersection predicate IntInt(A, B), intersection between the interiors objects A and B, is more complex than other types of intersections [6]. In this paper, we prove that

---

* The rights of this work are transferred to the extent transferable according to title 17 U.S.C. 105.

F. Castro, A. Gelbukh, and M. González (Eds.): MICAI 2013, Part II, LNAI 8266, pp. 362–375, 2013.
© Springer-Verlag Berlin Heidelberg 2013

9-Intersection model can be further reduced to almost three intersection predicates, 3^+-Intersection framework. This reduces the computation time considerably while retaining the same accuracy as the 9-Intersection model. Specifically, it not only reduces the number of intersections, it also replaces the slow intersection algorithm with a faster odd parity test to accomplish the same intersection detection task.

There is a wide class of applications for intersection detection in areas such as geometric modeling [4], virtual reality [7], and Geographical Information Systems for qualitative spatial reasoning (QSR) [2]. The determination of intersection between concave objects is much more complex than that of convex objects. Also the intersections between concave objects do not form closed algebra, as intersection between two concave objects may not result in a concave object, but rather a collection of disjoint objects violating the closedness property. Concave objects can be segmented into convex objects; this renders the task to working with convex objects only. So the finite intersection algebra is closed for convex objects. A bounded region, which is non-empty connected set, partitions the space into three parts: interior, boundary and exterior, see Fig. 1.

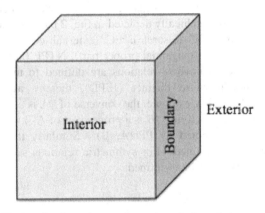

Fig. 1. The interior, boundary, and exterior of a bounded convex region

Perhaps the most well known formal model for qualitative spatial representation and reasoning is RCC8, which distinguishes spatial relations by employing first order logic [5] or a 9-Intersection model [2] that compares the intersections of one region's interior, boundary, and exterior with those of another region. In order to identify RCC8 relations, the 9-Intersection model uses nine intersection predicates, see Table 1, where shaded entries correspond to the 4-Intersection model [3]. The RCC8 distinct topological relations corresponding to the 9-Intersection model are displayed in Fig. 2. RCC8 forms a jointly exhaustive and pairwise distinct (JEPD) set of relations and a composition table provides a basis for qualitative spatial reasoning [2]. Originally the 9-Intersection model was designed independently of the logical foundations. First order logic is useful for knowledge acquisition and deriving inferences, whereas 9-Intersection is useful for knowledge representation and implementation. RCC8 may be considered as the spatial counterpart of Allen's thirteen interval relations among intervals of time [8].

Table 1. 9-Intersection 3x3 matrix and Reduced 4-Intersection 2x2 Matrix (Shaded) for Calculating RCC8 Relations

	Interior	Boundary	Exterior
Interior	Int(A)∩Int(B)	Int(A)∩Bnd(B)	Int(A)∩Ext(B)
Boundary	Bnd(A)∩Int(B)	Bnd)∩Bnd(B)	Bnd(A)∩Ext(B)
Exterior	Ext(A)∩Int(B)	Ext(A)∩Bnd(B)	Ext(A)∩Ext(B)

The paper is organized as follows: Section 2 gives a very terse description of the related work, the reader may refer to the referenced papers for details; Section 3 describes the innovation, related mathematical foundations and efficiency considerations of the authors' work, Section 4 is devoted to optimizing an application, Section 5 draws conclusions, followed by references in Section 6.

2   Background

For any two regions A and B in 2D/3D space, the spatial relation between A and B is denoted by R(A, B). As hierarchically depicted in Fig. 2 based on connectivity, there are eight RCC8 relations: DC (discrete), EC (external connection), PO (partial overlap), EQ (identical), TPP (tangential proper part), NTPP (non-tangential proper part), TPPc, and NTPPc. Converse relations are defined to make these relations jointly exhaustive and pairwise distinct (JEPD), thereby avoiding ambiguous interpretations of the data. For example, the converse of "A is a proper part of B" is "A contains B"; instead of specifying "B is a proper part of A" as PP(B, A), in RCC8 this converse relation is denoted by PPc(A, B). Similarly the TPPc(A, B) and NTPPc(A, B) relations are defined. For symmetric relations such as DC, EC, PO, EQ, no (distinct) converse relation is defined.

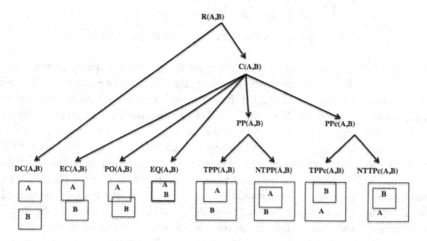

Fig. 2. Hierarchy of the RCC8 JEPD relations

Each of the RCC8 relations can be described uniquely by using a 9-Intersection matrix between two regions A and B, where symbol Int represents the region's interior, Bnd denotes the boundary, and Ext represents the exterior, see Fig. 3. For example, the predicate IntInt(A, B) is a binary relation that represents the truth value of intersection, Int(A)∩Int(B), between the interiors of region A and region B; the truth value of this function is either true (for non-empty intersection) or false (for empty intersection) for that intersection. Similarly, there are other predicates for the intersection of A's interior, boundary, or exterior with those of B.

It was established that the 9-Intersection model presents a sufficient set of intersection predicates for identifying RCC8 spatial relations [2, 5]. In qualitative spatial reasoning in 3D [6], it was observed that one of the intersection predicates does not contribute any knowledge in distinguishing the relations. This predicate was discarded from the algorithm implementation without sacrificing the accuracy in results. The implementation extensively used the remaining eight intersections, thus the name 8-Intersection. For a mathematical proof, see Theorem 1 in Section 3. Later it was observed from Table 2 and Fig. 3 and analytically proved that a 4-Intersection version yields the same results as the 9-Intersection model [3]. In Table 2, the shaded entries are sufficient to distinguish RCC8 relations. In the 8-Intersection model, there are 64 entries, whereas in the 4-Intersection model there are 32 entries; however only 26 entries (shaded) actually are used to classify all the eight relations.

Table 2. The 8-Intersection and 4-Intersection Vectors. Only the Shaded Entries are used to distinguish RCC8 Relations.

	IntInt	BndBnd	IntBnd	BndInt	IntExt	BndExt	ExtInt	ExtBnd
DC	F	F	F	F	T	T	T	T
EC	F	T	F	F	T	T	T	T
EQ	T	T	F	F	F	F	F	F
PO	T	T	T	T	T	T	T	T
TPP	T	T	F	T	F	F	T	T
NTPP	T	F	F	T	F	F	T	T
TPPc	T	T	T	F	T	T	F	F
NTPPc	T	F	T	F	T	T	F	F

In Fig. 3, this table is translated into a decision tree for visual understanding of the 4-Intersection model. In Section 3, we lay the ground work to improve the efficiency of the intersection predicates in Table 2 and Fig. 3, so as to make the most expensive Interior-Interior intersection predicate the least used, and yet achieve the same results.

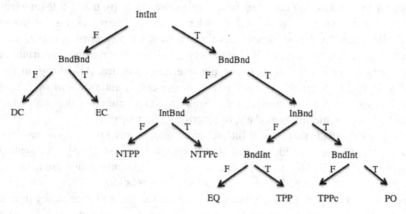

Fig. 3. Decision tree using 4-Intersection model. Each relation is determined with at most 4 predicates

3   Mathematical Analysis

3.1   Mathematical Foundations

Herein we present mathematical analysis to support the reduction in the number of required intersection predicates in RCC8 and VRCC-3D+, a region connection calculus for the 3D objects [9]. There is no need to check the predicate ExtExt(A, B), the exterior-exterior intersection predicate, to determine any relation [6]; for bounded regions, the intersection between the exteriors of two regions is always trivially non-empty and thus the intersection predicate ExtExt(A, B) contributes no knowledge in distinguishing the relations. We provide mathematical proof of this observation in Theorem 1. Note that we use the following notation in the proofs: A^i stands for the interior of set A; A^b represents the boundary of set A; A^e corresponds to the exterior of set A; A^c denotes the complement of set A, and $\bar{A}$ connotes the closure of set A.

Theorem 1. Let there be two bounded sets A and B, it is shown that $A^e \cap B^e \neq \varnothing$, (i.e., intersection predicate ExtExt(A, B) is always true).

Proof.   Since A and B are bounded, their exteriors A^e and B^e are unbounded.
The closure, $\bar{B}$, of B is bounded.
Suppose $A^e \cap B^e = \varnothing$.   Then $A^e \subseteq (B^e)^c = \bar{B}$.
This is a contradiction because A^e, which is unbounded, is a subset of $\bar{B}$ which is bounded.
Therefore the supposition is false.
Hence the theorem holds good.

This proves that the original 9-Intersection predicates can be replaced with eight intersection predicates, thus the name 8-Intersection. The next theorem shows that the predicate IntInt(A, B) is not independent of predicate IntBnd(A, B); in fact, IntBnd(A, B) implies IntInt(A, B). Similarly BndInt(A, B) implies IntInt(A, B). Thus if the value of IntBnd(A, B) or BndInt(A, B) is true, it ensures that we do not need to compute the value of predicate IntInt(A, B), it is true by *de facto*. In Table 3, the five relations entries (PO, TPP, TPPc, NTPP, NTPPc) have IntBnd(A, B) or BndInt(A, B) value true, thus IntInt(A, B) is true without computation. In the entries for relations, DC, EC, EQ, both IntBnd and BndInt are false. However BndBnd is false for DC and true for EC, and EQ. Thus BndBnd resolves identification of DC without considering IntInt. For the intersection predicate entries for two relations EQ and EC, both BndBnd and IntInt(A, B) are false. They can be simplified and made more efficient as shown in Theorem 4.

Theorem 2. For any two regions A and B, if the predicate IntBnd(A, B) is true, then the predicate IntInt(A, B) is true. That is, if $A^i \cap B^b \neq \varnothing$, then it is shown that $A^i \cap B^i \neq \varnothing$.

Proof. Let IntBnd(A, B) be true. Then $A^i \cap B^b \neq \varnothing$.

Let $x \in A^i \cap B^b$. Then $x \in A^i$ and $x \in B^b$.

Since $x \in A^i$ and A^i is an open set, there a neighborhood $N_r(x) \subset A^i$ for some positive real r, r>0.

Since $x \in B^b$ and B^b is the boundary set, then every neighborhood $N_y(x)$ of x intersects both the interior and exterior of B. That is $N_y(x) \cap B^i \neq \varnothing$ and $N_y(x) \cap B^e \neq \varnothing$. In particular, $N_r(x) \cap B^i \neq \varnothing$. Now we have $N_r(x) \subset A^i$ and $N_r(x) \cap B^i \neq \varnothing$. Therefore $N_r(x)$ has points common to A^i and B^i .

Hence $A^i \cap B^i \neq \varnothing$ and the predicate IntInt(A, B) is true

Similarly if $A^b \cap B^i \neq \varnothing$, then $A^i \cap B^i \neq \varnothing$.

Note that the converse of Theorem 2 is not true. We may have IntInt true without IntBnd(A, B) or BndInt(A, B) or both true. For example, in the case of equal objects or externally connected objects, IntInt(A, B) is true despite the fact that both IntBnd(A, B) and BndInt(A, B) can be false. Theorems 3 and 4 prove that IntInt(A, B) need not be directly calculated. So IntInt(A, B) can be replaced with a much simpler point-in-object odd-parity rule. Briefly, when IntBnd(A, B) and BndInt(A, B) are false, and BndBnd(A, B) is true, if a semi-infinite ray from the centroid C of one object, A, intersects the boundary of the other object, B, an odd number of times, then C is inside B, hence IntInt(A, B) is true. Note that the converse may not be true. Thus it simplifies the decision tree and IntInt(A, B) computation, where EC(A, B) and EQ(A, B) are special siblings, see Fig. 4(b). Those relations can be distinguished with a much simpler test than IntInt(A, B). For representing this intersection we denote it by ROI meaning "Ray-Object Intersection-ray through the interior point of one object with the boundary of the other object".

Theorem 3. If the predicate BndBnd(A, B) is true, and BndInt(A, B) and IntBnd(A, B) are false, then the predicate EQ(A, B) is true if and only if there is a point common to the interior of A and the interior of B.

Proof. Let the predicate BndBnd(A, B) be true, BndInt(A, B) and IntBnd (A, B) be false.

Therefore $A^b \cap B^b \neq \emptyset$, $A^b \cap B^i = \emptyset$ and $A^i \cap B^b = \emptyset$.

The proof is presented in two parts, using necessary and sufficient conditions.

Necessary: If $A=B$, then $A^i=B^i$. It follows that every point of A^i is in B^i, thus A^i and B^i share at least one point,

Sufficient: Let A^i and B^i have a point in common. That means $A^i \cap B^i \neq \emptyset$. We show that $A=B$.

Since $A^b \cap B^i = \emptyset$, then $B^i \subseteq (A^b)^c$. This means $B^i \subseteq A^i \cup A^e$ where $A^i \cap A^e = \emptyset$, by definition.

Since $B^i \cap A^i \neq \emptyset$ and $B^i \subseteq A^i \cup A^e$ with B^i connected and $A^i \cap A^e = \emptyset$,

we have $B^i \subseteq A^i$. Similarly we can derive that $A^i \subseteq B^i$.

Therefore $B^i = A^i$, or $A^i = B^i$. Since $A^b \cap B^i = \emptyset$ and $A^i \cap B^b = \emptyset$, $A^b = B^b$.

Now $\bar{A} = \bar{B}$. Hence we have proved that $A = B$.

Theorem 4. If predicate BndBnd(A, B) is true, and BndInt(A, B) and IntBnd (A, B) are false, then the predicate EQ(A, B) is true if and only if the predicate EC(A, B) is false.

Proof. Let predicate BndBnd(A, B) be true, BndInt(A, B) and IntBnd (A, B) be false.

That is, $A^b \cap B^b \neq \emptyset$, $A^b \cap B^i = \emptyset$ and $A^i \cap B^b = \emptyset$.

Under these conditions, using necessary and sufficient conditions we have,

(a) Necessary: Let EQ(A, B) be true. Then $A \subseteq B$ and $B \subseteq A$.

Then $A \subseteq B$ implies $A^i \subseteq B$. Since A^i is open and B^i is the largest open set contained in B, then $A^i \subseteq B^i$. Similarly $B^i \subseteq A^i$. Thus $A^i = B^i$ implying $A^i \cap B^i \neq \emptyset$, hence EC($A$, B) is false.

(b) Sufficient: Let EC(A, B) be false,

Then by definition, one of the following is true: $A^i \cap B^i \neq \emptyset$, $A^i \cap B^b \neq \emptyset$, $A^b \cap B^i \neq \emptyset$, $A^b \cap B^b = \emptyset$.

Since it is given that $A^i \cap B^b = \emptyset$, $A^b \cap B^i = \emptyset$, $A^b \cap B^b \neq \emptyset$,

the only possibility is $A^i \cap B^i \neq \emptyset$.

We have seen in Theorem 3 that if $A^i \cap B^i \neq \emptyset$, then $A=B$.

Hence the predicate EC(A, B) is false implies that predicate EQ(A, B) is true.

This completes the proof.

Note that it is also true that "EQ(A,B) is false if and only EC(A,B) true".

3.2   Efficiency Considerations

In the 4-Intersection model, four of the RCC8 relations can be identified with four intersection predicates, two of the relations can be identified with three intersection predicates, and the remaining two relations can be identified with two intersection predicates. In Table 2, it is clear from looking at the IntInt and BndBnd columns that those are the most useful predicates in the sense that they are sufficient to partition the RCC8 relations into three classes: {DC, EC}, {NTTP, NTTPc}, and {PO, EQ, TPP, TPPc}. That heuristic is the basis for the conceptual decision tree shown in Fig. 3. It was proved mathematically that all other intersections do hold good *de facto* [3].

The average number of predicate computations to determine an RCC8 relation using the 4-Intersection model is 3.25; see Table 3. Yet there is inherent inefficiency even in the 4-Intersection model. IntInt is computed and used first for the identification of every relation, and it is the most computation-intensive of all the predicates.

Theoretically the intersection predicates can be executed in any order. If we rearrange predicate computations in accordance with the result presented in Section 3.1, it improves the efficiency. Additionally, the ray-object intersection (ROI) based on the odd-parity rule can be seamlessly integrated in place of the IntInt predicate, thereby providing more efficiency. The computational cost of implementing ROI is less than half of the computation in implementing IntInt.

Table 3. Shaded Vectors Used For 4-Intersection Model, Average Computation is 3.25 Predicates Per Relation

RCC8	IntInt	BndBnd	IntBnd	BndInt
DC	F	F	F	F
EC	F	T	F	F
PO	T	T	T	T
EQ	T	T	F	F
TPP	T	T	F	T
NTPP	T	F	F	T
TPPc	T	T	T	F
NTPPc	T	F	T	F

Herein we show that the efficiency can be further enhanced in the following ways: (1) six of the RCC8 relations can be identified with at most 3-Intersection predicates (see Table 4, Fig. 4(a)) because the IntInt predicate is not necessary to determine those relations; (2) for the remaining two RCC8 relations which need to be resolved with predicate IntInt (Fig. 4(b)), we use an odd-parity rule to speed up the computation of IntInt; and (3) the average number of predicate computations for determination of an arbitrary RCC8 relation can be reduced to less than 3 (see Table 4), which results in a saving of at least 12% in computation time, see Table 5.

In Table 4, the last column is denoted by Hint in the header, hybrid intersection representing IntInt or ROI; the value of IntInt is T/F as usual, the value of ray-object intersection, ROI, is O/E for odd even parity.

In terms of tree terminology, in this case, the average distance from the root is smaller if the root predicate is "farther away" from the IntInt predicate. This is a considerable improvement in implementation performance when a test is executed thousands of times. Our observation and intuition comes from the fact, that if IntBnd is true, then IntInt is true by *de facto*.

Table 4. Shaded Vectors used for 3⁺-Intersection Model Average Computation is less than 3 Predicates Per Relation

RCC8	BndBnd	BndInt	IntBnd	Hint
DC	F	F	F	F
EC	T	F	F	E
PO	T	T	T	T
EQ	T	F	F	O
TPP	T	T	F	T
NTPP	F	T	F	T
TPPc	T	F	T	T
NTPPc	F	F	T	T

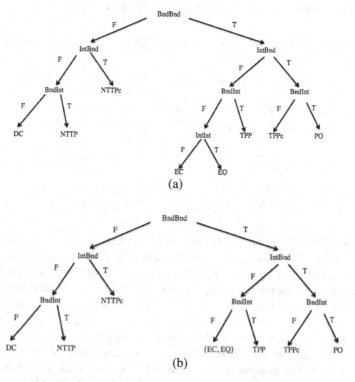

(a)

(b)

Fig. 4. (a) Modified version of 4-Intersection model with IntInt as the last test. (b) Since IntInt is the last predicate, it can be implemented with a simpler, less rigorous test.

The average number of predicate tests for a relation has been reduced to less than 3. This amounts to saving at least 12% in computation time, see Table 5.

Table 5. Percent Speedup Gain By 3^+-Intersection Model over other Models

Model	Number Of Predicates	Average Required Predicates	Percent Relative Gain
9-Intersection	9	9	210
8-Intersection	8	8	176
4-Intersection	4	3.25	12
3^+-Intersection	3^+	2.9	

3.3   Example Ray-Object Intersection, Point-in-Object Odd Parity Rule

In general, the odd parity rule to test a point inside an object is standard. However, the test for predicate IntInt(A,B) is not that trivial. Even parity may lead to IntInt(A,B) being true (Fig. 5(a,b)) or false (Fig. 5(c)), whereas odd parity also could result in IntInt(A,B) being true (Fig. 6(a,b,c)). For IntInt(A,B) we note that: (1) this parity test is inconclusive, (2) even parity is not the opposite of odd parity, and (3) there is no clear cut way to determine the test point C in A to establish the truth of IntInt(A,B). Here we describe the hurdles in the computation of the IntInt(A,B) predicate and how to circumvent them.

Example 1. *Consider the case depicted in Fig. 5: (a) the object B is inside A; (b) B overlaps A, (c) B is outside object A.* Let C be an arbitrary point in A. The semi-infinite ray CP does not intersect B in each case. The ray CQ intersects tangentially at a point (counted as double point) on B in each case. The ray CR cross intersects B at two points in each case. In each case ray-object intersection parity is even. But this does not tell anything about IntInt(A,B), which is true in Fig. 5(a,b) and false in Fig. 5(c).   In Fig. 5(a,b), if C were selected to be inside B then there is odd parity. So the problem becomes one of selecting the test point as well. This will be revisited when we analyze Example 3 and Fig 7.

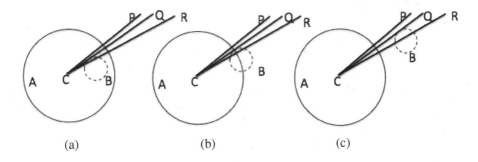

(a)   (b)   (c)

Fig. 5. Object B is inside, overlaps, and is outside of object A, in (a), (b), and (c) respectively. The ray CP does not intersect B, CQ tangentially intersects B, and CR cross intersects B at two points. In (a) and (b) IntInt(A,B) is true, whereas in (c) IntInt(A,B) is false.   Thus even parity is inconclusive.

Example 2. *Consider the case depicted in Fig. 6: (a) the object B is inside A; (b) B equals A, (c) B is contains object A.* Let C be an arbitrary point in A. In each case, the semi-infinite ray CP intersects B, ray-object intersection parity is odd and IntInt(A,B) is true. One would be tempted to think the odd parity rule works all the time. However it depends on how you select the test point C. In Fig. 5(a) and Fig. 6(a), B is inside A, the ray CP intersects B, parity is not odd (even) in Fig. 5(a), but parity is odd in Fig. 6(a). In both the cases IntInt(A,B) is true. Thus it is inconclusive to apply the parity rule unless one has selected the test point, C, appropriately.

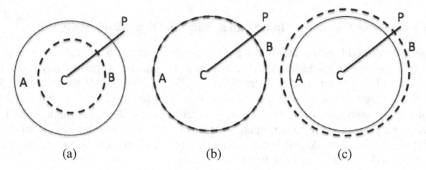

(a)   (b)   (c)

Fig. 6. Object B is inside, identical, outside of object A. The ray CP intersects all of them in one point. Odd intersection parity and IntInt(A,B) is true.

Example 3. *Consider the case depicted in Fig. 7: (a) the object B is equals A; (b) B is touches object A.* Referring back to the decision tree construction shown in Fig. 4(a, b), suppose that predicate BndBnd(A,B) is true, and IntBnd(A,B) and BndInt(A,B) are false. There are only two such configurations, examples of which are depicted in Fig. 7(a,b). The test point C can be located at any position in A. In the case Fig. 7(a) the ray-object intersection parity is odd and IntInt(A,B) is true. In Fig. 7(b) the ray-object intersection parity is even and IntInt(A,B) is false. So we arrive at the conclusion, that under these conditions, we can unambiguously apply the odd parity rule to test IntInt(A,B).

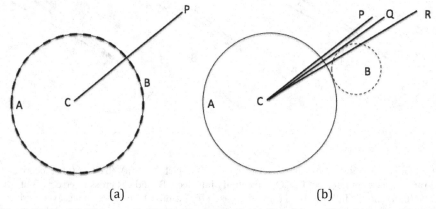

(a)   (b)

Fig. 7. BndBnd(A,B) is true, IntBnd(A,B), and BndInt(A,B) is false. The odd parity rule holds in (a) and IntInt(A,B) is true, whereas in (b) odd parity does not hold and IntInt(A,B) is false.

4   Optimizing an Application

In general, the qualitative spatial reasoning problem concerns determining the spatial relations among pairs of objects (or regions) in a given collection. Qualitative reasoning is utilized in many applications and requires computation over data sets of hundreds of thousands of 2D/3D points. Consequently, many attempts have been made to speed up the determination of RCC8 relations. VRCC-3D+, a region connection calculus for 3D objects, utilizes three of the 9-Intersection predicates (specifically, IntInt, IntBnd, and BndInt) to detect occlusion in 2D. Yet it also qualifies the connectivity between objects using the RCC8 relations, albeit considered using 3D rather than the more traditional 2D data. Here we briefly describe the historical approaches used to reduce computation time and explain how our approach extends the previous approaches to optimize algorithmic and computation time

Again the primary question is if we are presented with two spatial objects, how do we find the RCC8 relation between them? Without additional information, it is equally likely to be any one the eight JEPD RCC8 relations. Let us first enumerate some of the strategies employed in the algorithms for relation identification:

(a)   The brute force and worst case approach is to compute each of the nine intersection predicates and test each of the eight RCC8 relations to determine which one is the actual relation between the two objects (or regions) of interest.

(b)   To avoid testing all the eight relations, a composition table [2] is used to consider what is known about the spatial relations between other pairs of objects in the scene, and eliminate the impossible relations between the pair of objects of interest This reduces the number of possible relations to test. However, for each possible relation, 9-Intersection predicates still are computed.

(c)   To improve the computation time of the algorithm, Quinlan's ID3 algorithm is used to order the 9-Intersection predicates based on which predicate will provide the most information about the RCC8 relations that could hold for the pair of objects of interest (again, using knowledge of what is already known about the spatial relations between other objects in the scene) [10].   The algorithm orders the predicates, but does not necessarily reduce the number of intersection predicates that must be computed.

(d)   To reduce the computational overhead of the 9-Intersection predicates, it was determined that all the nine predicates are not necessary to distinguish the RCC8 relations [6]. The 9-Intersection predicates were replaced with 8-Intersection, then subsequently 4-Intersection predicates were determined to be sufficient for identifying any RCC8 relation [3].

Prior to and independent of steps (b)-(d), an attempt was made to sort the predicates based on complexity [11]. It was determined that such a calculation would depend on hardware implementation of the predicates (e.g., availability of

GPUs). No conclusive decision could be made as to which predicate is faster to implement and apply.

This made the problem more interesting from an algorithmic point of view and the subject of further exploration. The number of predicates used to classify a relation is of paramount importance. Even a slight speed up can make an enormous difference in the usability of an application. Each operation requires significant computation "under the hood", so our goal is to avoid it as much as possible. As shown in Section 3, we have reduced the computation of predicates without sacrificing the accuracy. One predicate IntInt was justifiably removed from the 4-Intersection decision tree, see Fig. 4(b). There are two RCC8 relations that require the IntInt predicate. But functionality of that predicate can be supported with the more efficient ray-object intersection. While there is a little conceptual difference, there is significant mathematical and computational difference.

5   Conclusion

For qualitative spatial reasoning, a major task is to compute the intersections between regions. This paper provides a shorter and more efficient path to determine RCC8 relations. Specifically we have seen that 9-Intersection was reduced to 8-Intersection, which was further reduced to 4-Intersection models in the past. In this paper we have moved a step further to reduce predicate computations to almost three intersections, 3^+-Intersection. In this way, six of the RCC8 relations are identified with at most 3-Intersections. The remaining two RCC8 relations are resolved with a 4th intersection which replaces the complex IntInt predicate with a simple point-in-object test using an odd-parity rule. The average number of predicate tests for a relation has been reduced to less than 3. This amounts to saving at least 12% in computation time, see Table 5. This is considerably more efficient than the previously used intersection frameworks, particularly when there are tens of thousands of regions to be analyzed in a dataset, and hundreds of thousands of data points. We intend to use this improved characterization in our future work in spatial reasoning, and hope others will find it useful as well.

References

[1] Dutt, S.: Approximate Spatial Reasoning Integrating qualitative and quantitative constraints. International Journal of Approximate Reasoning 5, 307–331 (1991)
[2] Egenhofer, M.J.: Deriving the Composition of Binary Topological Relations. Journal of Visual Languages and Computing 5(2), 133–149 (1991)
[3] Sabharwal, C., Leopold, J.: Reducing 9-Intersection to 4-Intersection for Identifying Relations in Region Connection Calculus. In: Proceedings of the 24th International Conference on Computer Applications in Industry and Engineering (CAINE 2011), Honolulu, Hawaii, November 16-18, pp. 118–123 (2011)
[4] Sabharwal, C.L., Factor, J.D.: Cross Intersection Between Any Two C^0 Parametric Surfaces. In: Proceedings of the International Australian Computer Graphics Conference, Ausgraph 1988, Melbourne, Australia, pp. 37–42 (1988)

[5] Randell, D.A., Cui, Z., Cohn, A.: A Spatial Logic Based on Regions and Connection. In: Proceedings of the Third International Conference on Principles of Knowledge Representation and Reasoning, pp. 165–176 (1992)

[6] Albath, J., Leopold, J., Sabharwal, C.: Visualization of Spatio-Temporal Reasoning Over 3D Images. In: Proceedings of the 2010 International Workshop on Visual Languages and Computing (in Conjunction with the 16th International Conference on Distributed Multimedia Systems), Oak Brook, IL, October 14-16, pp. 277–282 (2010)

[7] Held, M., Klosowski, J.T., Mitchell, J.S.B.: Evaluation of Collision Detection Methods for Virtual Reality Fly-Throughs. In: Gold, C., Robert, J.M. (eds.) Proc. 7th Canad. Conf. Computat. Geometry, Québec City, Québec, Canada, August 10-13, pp. 205–210 (1995)

[8] Allen, J.F.: Maintaining knowledge about temporal intervals. Communications of the ACM 26, 832–843 (1983)

[9] Sabharwal, C.L., Leopold, J.L.: Evolution of Region Connection Calculus to VRCC-3D+. In: Wang, P.P. (ed.) New Mathematics and Natural Computation (World Scientific) Cognition, Intelligence & Language. World Scientific Publishing Co. Pte. Ltd. (to appear)

[10] Eloe, N., Leopold, J., Sabharwal, C., McGeehan, D.: Efficient Determination of Spatial Relations Using Composition Tables And Decision Trees. In: IEEE Symposium on Computational Intelligence for Multimedia, Signal and Vision Processing (CIMSIVP), Singapore, pp. 1–7 (2013)

[11] Albath, J., Leopold, J., Sabharwal, C., Perry, K.: Efficient 3D Qualitative Spatial Reasoning with RCC-3D. In: Proceedings of KSEM 2010, pp. 470–481 (2010)

Fast and Robust Object Recognition Based on Reduced Shock-Graphs and Pruned-SIFT

Rafael Orozco-Lopez and Andres Mendez-Vazquez

Computer Sciences
Cinvestav Guadalajara
Jalisco, Mexico
{orozco,amendez}@gdl.cinvestav.mx

Abstract. Fast algorithms for image recogition have become a priority when the number of images to be analyzed can be counted in the number of millions. Therefore, the need for fast algorithms for image recognition. This paper describes an algorithm capable of recognize an object in an image by the fusing information from a reduced version of the Shock-Graph algorithm and the Scale Invariant Feature Transform (SIFT) points. The proposed algorithm uses the reduced Shock-Graph to obtain a skeleton of an object in order to minimize the number of SIFT points to reduce the computational complexity of object image comparison. The proposed algorithm is capable of recognizing objects in a fast way under rotation, deformation and scaling. Using a collection of shapes, we demonstrate the performance of our implementation using a combination of the reduced Shock-Graph and SIFT points.

1 Introduction

In recent years, the desire of having computers systems with object recognition abilities has been growing [1]. Mostly, because of the large amounts of images stored in the World Wide Web. Therefore, the need of new and faster algorithms for image recognition. Furthermore, this is why the field of image recognition over large data sets is being widely researched, and a lot of different methods have been proposed to solve the many problems imposed by the size of the data sets [2–16].

For example, Timothee et al. [8] have proposed an algorithm that works with the shape of a pre-segmented image. They obtain image elements called mega pixels from the object. Then, with a large data base of different poses of that object, they can associate each mega pixels (simulating a puzzle) to reconstruct the object and then recognize it. This presents a problem, if you do not have a large data base of the object in all possibly poses, this method hardly will recognize the object in question.

On the other hand, Huttenlocher et al. [7] proposed a fast way to compare objects by using the Hausdorff distance. This distance measures the scope of each point of a model set that is near to a point in an image set. This distance is used to get the degree of resemblance between two objects that will be superimposed

F. Castro, A. Gelbukh, and M. González (Eds.): MICAI 2013, Part II, LNAI 8266, pp. 376–387, 2013.

one over the other. This method can find how an image is likely similar to another, but it has the drawback that the recognition of a single object is more difficult because the comparison is done over the entire image where object is.

Still using the idea of having large database, Christopher M. Cyr and Benjamin B. Kimia [15, 16] presented a 3D recognizer that uses a large database with objects in all possibles angles. The method obtains the histograms of the elements in the database. By making a comparison between these different objects, they were able to say if objects looked similar to a target object. This is a fast, but not so accurate method, but it is still good enough when dealing with large databases of objects. Ali et al. [13] presented a different solution using saliency maps. With this approach they created a graphical representation that was compared with elements in a object database. This method presented a highly invariance to translation, rotation, scaling and occlusion of an object. Still the complexity of the algorithm makes it infeasible for large databases.

K. Siddiqi et al. [5, 6] proposed the use of Shock-Graphs for image recognition. The algorithm uses a series of complex rules and metrics for the creation and the comparison of graphs based on images. The Shock-Graphs are robust against deformation in the images. Nevertheless, it is known that this algorithm has a NP-Complete time complexity [17]. On the other hand, D. G. Lowe et al. [2] presents an algorithm based in SIFT descriptors (Scale-Invariant Feature Transform), which are invariant to translation, rotation and scaling. However, they are not robust against deformations in the images.

Each algorithm by itself has the ability to recognize an object individually, but as we have pointed out, they are slow (Shock-Graphs) or unreliable when images are deformed (SIFT descriptors). These are the reasons why in this paper, we describe the use and an implementation of the Reduced rule version of Shock-Trees and Pruned-SIFT descriptors for faster image recognition through information fusion. First, we use a reduced Shock-Trees to obtain an initial skeleton for the target object. Second, using that skeleton, SIFT descriptors are pruned to obtain the precise descriptors associated to the target object. After all this, a similarity function is applied to obtain comparative measures between different objects. Thus, the proposed algorithm has some the goodnesses of both algorithms and few of their weaknesses. This is of great importance when we look for fast and accurate algorithms for image recognition. In addition, this hierarchical process [18] resemblances the one that the human brain uses in order to recognize objects, as Siddiqi et al. mention in [6]. For example, a human being first notice the presence of an object, such as a square, before she/he realizes that it is a picture of Picasso.

The rest of this paper is structured in the following way. Section 2 describes the basic algorithms that are used in the proposed algorithm. In section 3, we describe the proposed algorithm. This section describes the way Shock-Graph and SIFT were used in the proposed algorithm. In section 4, a series of case studies are used for testing the proposed algorithm. These experiments show the benefits in speed and accuracy of object detection when fusing information coming from the reduced Shock-Graph and SIFT descriptors Finally, in the conclusion, we look at future work using the proposed algorithm.

2 Image Recognition: Shock-Graphs and SIFT Descriptors

When looking at the state of the art in computer vision [18], the task of image recognition can be decomposed as follows: First, the general shape of an object is recognized, for example a square; then, in the identification phase, the shape is identified as a paint, a glass, a book, etc. Treves et al. [18] proposed that these are the steps that the human brain uses to recognize an object, and actually these are the steps that Shock-Graph and SIFT descriptors methods follow in order to identify objects.

The Shock-Graph is a generic 2-D representation of an image [5] used to recognize an object through a special representation of the object shape. This representation is robust to deformation, scaling and occlusion. The Shock-Graph is a derivation of the concept of an skeleton of a shape, the medial axis curve. This specific curve is the set of all points within a closed Jordan curve such that a circle with center at one of these set points is contained within the curve and touches two fronts.

The Shock-Graph algorithm uses a coloring mapping method to recognize each segment to be part of the Shock-Graph [5]. There are 4 types of Shock elements, and they follow the following rules, all of which are based on a radius function from the skeleton to the perimeter of the shape (Fig. 1):

1. The 1-shock, when the radius function presents no changes, it is known as a protrusion.
2. The 2-shock, when the radius function get a strict local minimum such that if the medial axis would be disconnected the skeleton will be separated in two parts.
3. The 3-shock, when the radius function is equal along an interval.
4. The 4-shock, when the radius function gets a strict local maximum.

Once, the whole skeleton has been identified in the examined shape, the algorithm follows a series of rules to obtain the Shock-Graph of the analyzed shape. These rules can be seen in (Fig. 2).

After all these steps have been completed, images can be compared by the use of a recursive algorithm distance defined in [6]. Other examples of methods to measure similarity are: The distance among their nodes [5], the eigenvalue distance defined by Matrix representation of the graph [6] or it is even possible to combine these methods together for data fusion.

On the other hand, the SIFT descriptors describe salient points in the images, which are unique between them, when looking at a specific image. In addition, they are robust to scaling, rotation and translation. These properties make them valuables in the following way: Once the human brain recognizes an object shape,

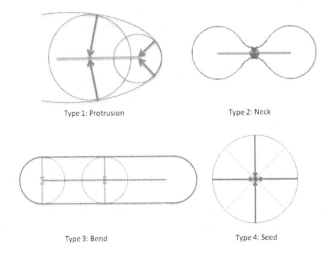

Fig. 1. Types of Shocks

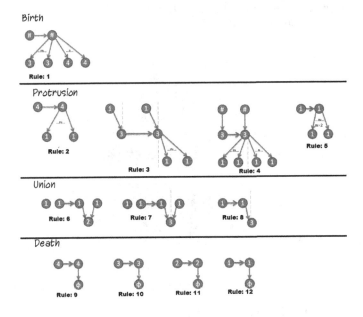

Fig. 2. The Shock Rules

it tries to identify it by using the texture of the object. Clearly, the SIFT descriptors can be used for this task.

To obtain the SIFT descriptors, it is necessary to follow the next steps: First, it is necessary to identify key locations through the use of maximum o minimum Gaussian difference [2]. Then, each point is used to generate a characteristic

vector that describes the region of the local sampled image relative to its scale
space of the frame. The result is a characteristic vector called SIFT Key[2]. These
vectors have four characteristics:

1. Position in X, position in Y, A_{ij}.
2. Gradient,

$$M_{ij} = \sqrt{(A_{ij} - A_{i+1,j})^2 + (A_{ij} - A_{i,j+1})^2}. \tag{1}$$

3. Orientation,

$$R_{ij} = a \tan 2(A_{ij} - A_{i+1,j}, A_{i,j+1} - A_{ij}) \tag{2}$$

The power of SIFT descriptors lay down in the fact that when at least three
SIFT Key are in agreement with respect to a specific object, David G. Lowe et
al.[2], there exists a strong evidence that the object is the sought one. This is
similar the triangulation process where only three satellites are needed for GPS
localization,

The SIFT approach has the main advantage of being robust to occlusion,
translation, scaling, rotation and partially to changes of illumination. This is
because the SIFT descriptors obtain salient properties directly from the image.
These are properties that are unique to an object (Fig. 3), and are found when
a high variance appears in the pixels associated to it.

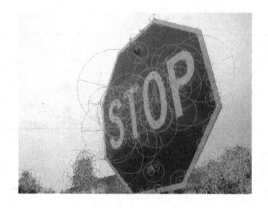

Fig. 3. Example of SIFT descriptors

3   The Proposed Algorithm

Our aim is to use a form of data fusion [19], using a proposed Reduced Shock-
Tree and Pruned-SIFT descriptors, to do image recognition. This method is
possible thanks to our approach to data fusion with the Shock-Graphs and SIFT
descriptors.

3.1   Reduced Shock-Graphs

Our approach tries to avoid the computational complexity of the shock-graph rules by reducing them only to protrusions, joints and end-points. Protrusion nodes are the edges of any skeleton, except for the first and last pixels on them. Those first and last pixels are the joint nodes or the end-point nodes. All this nodes are discovered by using the following reduced subset of rules (Fig.5).

This reduces the robustness of the Shock-Graphs because the lack of the distinctive nodes for protrusions, bend and neck. However, the proposed algorithm has a complexity of $O(n)$ and does not have the recursive loop that in some cases end in an NP complexity as in the traditional Shock-Graph algorithm. Nevertheless, the proposed algorithm does not have the same robustness as the traditional one, but this is levered by combining the reduced Shock-Graph with the SIFT descriptors in a way that will be explained in the next subsection. An example of this approach is in (Fig.4)

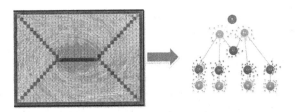

Fig. 4. Interpretation of Reduced Shock-Graphs with Pruned Sifts

After the skeleton is obtained from the pre-segmented object, the proposed algorithm will be used to compare similarities with other skeletons in a specific data set by using a Hausdorff distance [7]:

$$H(A, B) = max(h(A, B), h(B, A))   \tag{3}$$

where

$$h(A, B) = \max_{a \in A} \min_{b \in B} \|a - b\| \tag{4}$$

and $\|.\|$ is an underlying norm on the points of A and B. Using this distance allow for a fast matching among the skeleton in our data set.

The purpose of the reduced Shock-Graph is to maintain some of the robustness properties against deformation, while reducing the complexity of the original skeleton edge discovery [5]. To further reduce computational complexity, the proposed algorithm prunes the number of SIFT descriptors to the ones near to the Shock-Graph.

An example of reduced Shock-Graph is shown in (Fig. 5, and it is possible to see the structure of the Shock-Graph. There, green pixel segments are associated to green nodes representing the end points. The red pixel segments are associated to red nodes representing protrusion nodes. Finally, the blue pixel segments are associated to blues nodes representing joint nodes.

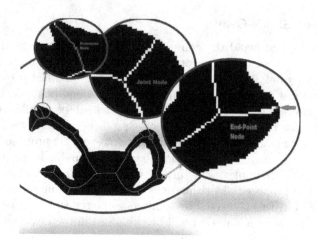

Fig. 5. Protrusion, Joint and End-Point Nodes

3.2 Pruned-SIFT Descriptors

The pruning of SIFT descriptor is based on the idea that there are no SIFT descriptor, belonging to an object, far away from the skeleton of the object. This idea takes in account that sometimes SIFT descriptors belong to other objects or are just background information,and they will not add extra information for the recognition of the object in question. This pruning is done using a arbitrary distance, "limit distance" (LD) represented by the next equation:

$$LD = MaxDistance/3, \tag{5}$$

where $Maxdistance$ is the Maximum Value among all the "distances" between all the skeleton pixels and the pixels from the shape of the object. In (Fig. 7) we can see the Pruned Sift(Center of the image) compared with the Sift Descriptors (Left of the image) in the same image. The use of LD equation was entirely proposed under our criteria, this equation shows better results without so many SIFT descriptors out of the object's body.

The entire process can be seen in (Fig. 6). In (Fig. 6 A), the original image, and in (Fig. 6 B), the segmented one. Next, the skeleton is obtained (Fig. 6 C). In the image (Fig. 6 D), it is possible to see the SIFT descriptors from the original image, and the distance of the pixels from the segmented image perimeter and the pixels from the skeleton (Fig.6 E and F). After that, the SIFT descriptors are eliminated by the defined metric the Limit Distance's Equation and we get the previously mentioned (Fig.7) SIFT descriptors. In the final step, the SIFT descriptors generated on the image will be associated with the nodes in the Reduced Shock-Graph (protrusions, joints and end-points nodes) that are near to them. An example can be seen in (Fig. 7). Once the Pruned SIFT descriptors associated with the three different nodes of the reduced Shock-Graph are identified, it is possible to save all this information, reduced Shock-Graph

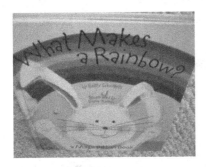

A: Original Image

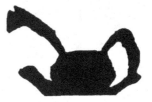

B: Segmented Image

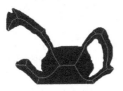

C: Image's Skeleton

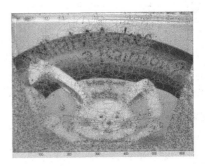

D: Image's SIFT

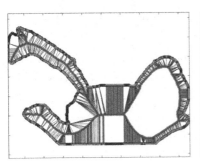

E: Representation of distance
between the skeleton
and the perimeter of the object

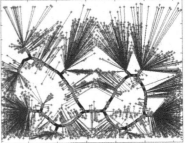

F: Representation of distance
between the skeleton
and the SIFTs

Fig. 6. Steps for pruning SIFTS

and pruned SIFT descriptors, for each image for a posterior identification using the previously defined distance.

There are two Phases for recognition of an object: The first one uses the Hausdorff distance between skeletons, thus the nearest one will be chosen as a match. Although, this first phase does not provide with a robust match between

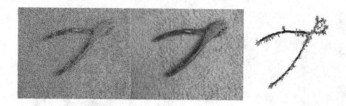

Fig. 7. SIFT associated with the Reduced Shock-Graph

	0	16.9706	255.8202	216.2082	118.532	93.3809	180	213.2836	149.8332	149.8332	144.0625	124.7878	204.7486	178.6309
	17	0	245.5219	208.8923	103.512	87.6641	167.5858	204.9415	92.1141	103.3683	128.0039	126.1428	198.6983	177.9017
	255.8202	245.5219	0	129.6534	159.325	236.7805	115.8361	193.1321	201.9431	189.0026	165.9518	212.4924	194.1649	225.1777
	207.8114	203.5903	129.6534	0	189.759	193.4994	122.6744	123.8467	122.6744	122.6744	144.0035	122.6744	142.1302	143
	118.5327	103.8123	159.9281	189.7894	0	112.8051	97.2677	132.0984	97.2677	101.0445	77.0779	98.6154	214.0841	153.5252
	93.3809	87.6641	236.7805	193.4994	112.80	0	166.0753	216.7879	166	183.3712	132.0606	155.6535	208.9593	218.2292
	180	167.5858	161.7931	180.9420	180.34	169	0	101.2423	118	106.1179	80.5047	145	127.3499	178
	215.6757	207.3379	228.9738	151.1589	297.82	237.4889	106.1179	0	125.7179	120.8305	235.7192	244.1311	171.5721	171.2921
	92.5419	92.1141	201.9431	135.2479	173.0809	152.4270	118	126.1467	0	60.8112	115.1173	123.6932	115.7670	127.2517
	106.0189	103.3683	189.0026	138.6795	180.0250	183.3712	106.1179	118.5116	60.8112	0	116.3787	135.7940	104.7855	113.8859
	144.0625	128.0039	165.9518	144.0035	105.5462	132.0606	129.1898	144.0035	74.2428	107.0561	0	122	151	154.3924
	124.7878	126.1428	212.4924	151.3209	147.9595	164.4780	145	142.6359	54.0370	98.7168	122	0	215.1279	129.0039
	180.9530	175.3283	210.6395	162.6100	214.0841	204	202.8522	127.4755	93.4773	90.5539	151	215.1279	0	160.7762
	174.4162	160.4649	225.1777	143	153.5252	216	178	132.5028	111.9464	81.6884	154.3924	113.6354	160.7762	0

Fig. 8. Table of Results from Hausdorff distance

objects, it helps to create a set of candidate images for posterior evaluation. In the second phase, the pruned SIFT descriptors associated to their respective nodes are used in order to find at least three matches between the SIFT descriptors between the image and the candidates. If a match of three SIFTs is found, there is a strong evidence that the input object and one or more objects in the data set are similar. Because of the computational complexity of the two phase process, finding similar objects is quite easy. This is shown in the following section.

4   Experiments

In (table 8), a series of comprehensive experiments with a series of objects is shown. This table was created by using the first phase of the proposed method, and each cell shows the resulting distance between different objects. It can be observed that each match of the same image with itself has a zero distance. It was found that the distance between some objects sometimes does not match perfectly as show in (table 8).

It is more, some skeletons presents more similarity to other objects than the real ones, but is enough to pick candidates among all represented objects for the next phase. There, using the pruned SIFT descriptors, it is possible to obtain a better matching. In the second study case, the two phase process for image similarity was used with following figure (Fig. 9) as input. It can be seen that except for the bird (Fig. 9G), which could only be matched by two Pruned Sifts, the rest of the objects in example where identified. For example, the couple(Fig. 9J), the sign (Fig. 9F) and the worm (Fig. 9I) match perfectly. For the other objects like clouds (Fig. 9D,Fig. 9E) and trees (Fig. 9A,Fig. 9B,Fig. 9C) and the sun (Fig. 9H) the matching was sufficiently good to identify them. Now, it is possible to see that thanks to the pruning made in the SIFTS, the mismatches are reduced from the original approach of [2]. Thus, it can be concluded that the SIFTS with the pruning are more reliable when combined with the Reduced Shock-Graphs.

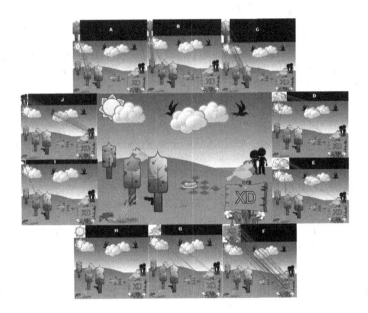

Fig. 9. Case of Study - Matching various objects in single a image

4.1   Conclusions

Although, the initial experiments gave us good results, it is necessary to add some more robustness in the reduced Shock-graph/pruned SIFT descriptor method to facilitate an initial pre-recognition. In addition, it is necessary to improve the metric for the comparison of the Shock/SIFT graphs. For this, we are looking at the use of eigenvalue based metrics or locality sensitive hashing [13]. At the same time, it is necessary to avoid increasing the computational complexity of the proposed algorithm. Finally, it is necessary to combine the proposed method with a database to do a more extensive series of experiments.

Acknowledges. We appreciate the financial support given by CONACYT. and our dear friend Daniel Madrigal and my brother Miguel Angel Orozco for making us some images for these cases of study.

References

1. Dean, T., Ruzon, M., Segal, M., Shlens, J., Vijayanarasimhan, S., Yagnik, J.: Fast, accurate detection of 100,000 object classes on a single machine. In: Proceedings of IEEE Conference on Computer Vision and Pattern Recognition, Washington, DC, USA (2013)
2. Lowe, D.G.: Distinctive image features from scale-invariant keypoints. Int. J. Comput. Vision 60, 91–110 (2004)
3. Leonardis, A., Bischof, H.: Robust recognition using eigenimages. Comput. Vis. Image Underst. 78, 99–118 (2000)
4. Murase, H., Nayar, S.: Illumination planning for object recognition using parametric eigenspaces. IEEE Transactions on Pattern Analysis and Machine Intelligence 16, 1219–1227 (1994)
5. Siddiqi, K., Shokoufandeh, A., Dickenson, S., Zucker, S.: Shock graphs and shape matching. In: Sixth International Conference on Computer Vision, pp. 222–229 (1998)
6. Siddiqi, K., Shokoufandeh, A., Dickenson, S., Zucker, S.: Shock graphs and shape matching. In: Sixth International Conference on Computer Vision, pp. 222–229 (1998)
7. Huttenlocher, D.P., Klanderman, G.A., Kl, G.A., Rucklidge, W.J.: Comparing images using the hausdorff distance. IEEE Transactions on Pattern Analysis and Machine Intelligence 15, 850–863 (1993)
8. Cour, T., Shi, J.: Recognizing objects by piecing together the segmentation puzzle. In: IEEE Conference on Computer Vision and Pattern Recognition, CVPR 2007, pp. 1–8 (2007)
9. Macrini, D., Dickinson, S., Shokoufandeh, A., Siddiqi, K., Zucker, S., Trokhimtchouk, M., Phillips, C., Dimitrov, P.: View-based 3-d object recognition using shock graphs. In: Proceedings of the Internal Conference on Pattern Recognition, pp. 24–28 (2002)
10. Boykov, Y., Kolmogorov, V.: An experimental comparison of min-cut/max-flow algorithms for energy minimization in vision. IEEE Transactions on Pattern Analysis and Machine Intelligence 26, 1124–1137 (2004)
11. Blum, H.: A Transformation for Extracting New Descriptors of Shape. Models for the Perception of Speech and Visual Form, 362–380 (1967)
12. Liu, L., Chambers, E., Letscher, D., Ju, T.: Extended Grassfire Transform on Medial Axes of 2D Shapes, Washington, WA, USA (2011)

13. Shokoufandeh, A., Dickinson, S.: Graph-theoretical methods in computer vision. In: Khosrovshahi, G.B., Shokoufandeh, A., Shokrollahi, M.A. (eds.) Theoretical Aspects of Computer Science. LNCS, vol. 2292, pp. 148–174. Springer, Heidelberg (2002)

14. Achanta, R., Estrada, F., Wils, P., Süsstrunk, S.: Salient region detection and segmentation. In: Gasteratos, A., Vincze, M., Tsotsos, J.K. (eds.) ICVS 2008. LNCS, vol. 5008, pp. 66–75. Springer, Heidelberg (2008)

15. Cyr, C., Kimia, B.: 3d object recognition using shape similiarity-based aspect graph. In: Proceedings of the Eighth IEEE International Conference on Computer Vision, ICCV 2001, vol. 1, pp. 254–261 (2001)

16. Cyr, C.M., Kimia, B.B.: A similarity-based aspect-graph approach to 3d object recognition. International Journal of Computer Vision 57, 5–22 (2004)

17. Garey, M.R., Johnson, D.S.: Computers and Intractability: A Guide to the Theory of NP-Completeness. W. H. Freeman & Co., New York (1979)

18. Treves, R., Rolls, E.T.: Computational analysis of the role of the hippocampus in memory. Hippocampus 4, 374–391 (1994)

19. Carvalho, H., Heinzelman, W., Murphy, A., Coelho, C.: A general data fusion architecture. Proceedings of the Sixth International Conference of Information Fusion 2, 1465–1472 (2003)

Matching Qualitative Spatial Scene Descriptions á la Tabu

Malumbo Chipofya*, Angela Schwering, and Talakisew Binor

Institute for Geoinformatics,
University of Münster, Germany
{mchipofya,schwering,talak}@uni-muenster.de

Abstract. Matching spatial scene descriptions requires appropriate representations and algorithms based on the application at hand. This work outlines a simple model for matching qualitatively described spatial scenes extracted from sketch maps. Standard qualitative constraint networks are combined to provide a suitable qualitative representation for a sketched spatial scene. Two scenes are then matched using an implementation of the Tabu search metaheuristic, employing standard and specialised data structures. We give a detailed description of the representation and algorithm, and examine the performance of the model using an example dataset.

Keywords: Spatial Scene Matching, Qualitative Constraint Network, Tabu Search.

1 Introduction

Matching qualitative descriptions of a pair of spatial scenes is a task that involves finding correspondences between the spatial entities in the first scene and those in the second that, in a sense, respect the spatial relations within the scenes being matched. This type of spatial scene matching has been applied in different forms in areas such as object and scene recognition in computer vision [1] and spatial information retrieval [2, 3]. The goal of the matching is to determine the similarity of the compared scenes or to determine whether one contains a copy of the other. In most cases one considers a set of spatial aspects of interest, which may include, among others, topology, directions, relative orientations, orderings, adjacencies, and distances (or proximities). As such the precise information on each of these dimensions must be abstracted into some form qualitative measure. The intuitive meaning of qualitative in this case is that no more than a finite number of distinctions can be made between the spatial relationship enjoyed by a pair of entities and the spatial relationship of any other pair of entities.

The foregoing discussion is indicative of two requirements of a solution to the matching problem. First, the input must be suitably described. This means in particular that the data used for matching must expose the most essential

---

* Corresponding author.

F. Castro, A. Gelbukh, and M. González (Eds.): MICAI 2013, Part II, LNAI 8266, pp. 388–402, 2013.

features for the task at hand. The second requirement is the design of an algorithm that performs that matching task itself. The first requirement demands a representation component and the second demands an operational component.

We consider the representation component for the task of matching sketch maps in section 3. In section 4 we present a matching algorithm that uses the tabu search metaheuristic and examine its performance on an example dataset, while proposing solutions to problems encountered during our tests. To kick-start the discussion we briefly outline some related works in section 2 which follows immediately.

2   Related Work

Although the idea of qualitative spatial information matching for information retrieval has been considered for more than a decade now [2], most work on it focused on data modeling [2, 4–6] and on finding appropriate measures of similarity [3]. The challenge to solving the problem however remained in the search domain. To that end several works have been published that attempt to solve the problem either directly or indirectly.

The work in [7] evaluated an implementation of the famous Bron-Kerbosch max-clique algorithm applied to qualitative constraint network (QCN) matching. In that implementation much effort was spent in clique enumeration since all maximal cliques had to be discovered before termination. [8] presented an algorithm for QCN matching based on the interpretation tree model matching paradigm. Search is performed by an A* algorithm using the same heuristic as that used in our work. One of the biggest drawbacks for the algorithm in [8] is the ever growing search frontier. Our algorithm overcomes this drawback by applying local search while constraining the size of the neighborhoods to explore using what we refer to as extension sets.

3   Qualitative Representation of Spatial Scenes

As noted above, qualitative representation of spatial information involves representing only the relevant distinctions in a spatial configuration. For example, orientations with a predominantly northerly heading can all be regarded as belonging to the qualitative orientation North. Qualitative representations together with logical and algebraic mechanisms for performing some useful computations on them form what are known as qualitative spatial calculi and their study as Qualitative Spatial Reasoning (QSR) [9]. A qualitative calculus formalizes the semantics of the considered distinctions by considering them as relations over the set of spatial entities for which the distinctions are considered. The spatial entities form the domain of the calculus and are usually of the same primitive type (i.e. points, line segments, lines, regions, etc.) To describe a spatial scene using a qualitative calculus, one associates with each pair of entities, a relation from the calculus. The resulting structure is what is called a Qualitative Constraint Network (QCN) [10]. Matching qualitative spatial scene descriptions can therefore be considered as the task of matching qualitative constraint networks.

3.1 Qualitative Spatial Calculi and Qualitative Constraint Networks

A qualitative calculus can be seen as a pair of algebraic structures together with a map between them. In this view, propagated by Ligozat [11, 12], a qualitative calculus is "constructed" from a partition scheme defined on the domain of interest (e.g. the set of oriented line segments in $\mathbb{R}^2$) usually called the universe of the calculus. A partition scheme is a pair $\mathfrak{C} = (U, (r_i)_{i \in I})$, where U is a non-empty *universe*, I is a finite set and $(r_i)_{i \in I}$ is a partition of $U \times U = U^2$ satisfying

1. There is an identity element $r_0 \in (r_i)_{i \in I}$ given by $r_0 = \{(u, v) \in U^2 \mid u = v\}$ denoted $1'_{\mathfrak{C}}$
2. $(\forall i \in I)\, (\exists j \in I)$ such that $r_i^{\smile} = r_j$ where $r_i^{\smile} = \{(u, v) \in U^2 \mid (v, u) \in r_i\}$

In this case the classes $(r_i)_{i \in I}$ are atomic binary relations, called the base relations of the calculus, because they form a so called jointly exhaustive pairwise disjoint (JEPD) set. For any calculus $\mathfrak{C}$ we will denote by $\mathcal{B}_{\mathfrak{C}}$ the set of base relations of $\mathfrak{C}$ and by $U_{\mathfrak{C}}$ its universe or domain. The full calculus generated by $\mathcal{B}_{\mathfrak{C}}$ is given by the set $2^{\mathcal{B}_{\mathfrak{C}}}$ which forms a boolean Algebra and to which all operations are extended in a set theoretic way. These are the general relations of the calculus. The relation $\cup_{i \in I} r_i$ is the top element and is as usual denoted $1_{\mathfrak{C}}$. The bottom element is $0_{\mathfrak{C}} = \emptyset$. A relation R is said to be a *refinement* of another relation R' if $R \subseteq R'$. Given two base relations r_i and r_j their composition is given by:

$$r_i \circ_{\mathfrak{C}} r_j = \{(x, y) \in U_{\mathfrak{C}}^2 \mid \exists z \in U_{\mathfrak{C}}\ (x, z) \in r_i,\ (z, y) \in r_j\}$$

For the sake of readability, whenever $\mathfrak{C}$ is clear from the context we will leave out the subscript. The definitions above are given in [11] where a detailed discussion on the algebraic aspects can be found.

Definition 1 (Qualitative Constraint Network). *Given a calculus $\mathfrak{C}$ and a set N of variables, a QCN over $\mathfrak{C}$ is a pair (N, C) where $C : N^2 \to 2^{\mathcal{B}}$. A QCN is called atomic if $C(\bar{a}) \in \mathcal{B}$, for every pair $\bar{a} \in N^2$.*

A QCN is a complete graph where the nodes are variables and the edges are labeled by general relations from a qualitative calculus. For this reason the variables are called nodes and pairs of nodes are called arcs or edges.

A QCN $\mathcal{N} = (N, C)$ over $\mathfrak{C}$ is said to be consistent with respect to $\mathfrak{C}$ if there is an assignment $\varphi : N \to U$ of variables to elements of the domain such that for each $i, j \in N$ and any $R \in \mathcal{B}$, $(\varphi(i), \varphi(j)) \in R$ implies $R \in C(i, j)$. Determining consistency of a network is usually hard so approximations are often used [13, 14]. One such approximation is the closure of a network. A network is said to be closed or path-consistent if every restriction of the network to three nodes is consistent. Equivalently, the network $\mathcal{N}$ is closed if for all $i, j, k \in N$

1. $C(i,i) \in \mathbf{1}'$
2. $C(i,k) \cap \big(C(i,j) \circ C(j,k) \big) \neq \emptyset$

A refinement $\mathcal{N}$ is a network $\mathcal{N}' = (N, C')$ such that $C'(i,j) \subseteq C(i,j) \; \forall i,j \in N$. We write $\mathcal{N}' \leq \mathcal{N}$ if $\mathcal{N}'$ is a refinement of $\mathcal{N}$. The closure of $\mathcal{N}$, written $cl(\mathcal{N})$ is the largest refinement of $\mathcal{N}$. $cl(\mathcal{N})$ has the same solutions as $\mathcal{N}$ [13, 14]. Notice that $\mathcal{M}$ is closed if and only if $\mathcal{M} = cl(\mathcal{M})$. There are many algorithms for computing the closure of a network, a popular one of which is Peter Van Beek's PATH-CONSISTENCY algorithm [15]. Having set the ground we will now outline some concrete qualitative calculi applied to sketch map representation.

3.2   Representation of Sketch Maps by QCNs

The main motivation for considering qualitative approaches to represent the spatial "content" of sketch maps is that sketch maps are often, if not always, distorted, schematized, and simplified [16, 17]. However, there is a certain level of generality or abstraction at which the deviation of the spatial information content of a sketch map from that of a corresponding cartographic map almost disappears [16]. This is true for example when considering coarse topological relations in RCC5 or RCC8 [18]. As such qualitative representations enable us to partially overcome the aforementioned problems. In addition, there are only a limited number of values to deal with so that computations are more transparent.

We assume that a sketch map depicts the spatial configuration of a number of geographic features. Each feature, which we call a (sketch) object is represented, geometrically, by a set of geometric primitives. As such, objects of some features types can be decomposed into primitive components. Three classes of features are considered, namely, streets, city blocks, and landmarks. Streets are lineal features. Each street consists of one or more street segments which are maximally connected components of a street that are not internally intersected by any other street segment. Street segments act as links between places of interest. A place of interest may be a landmark, an intersection of streets segments, or the interior of a city block. City blocks are regions bounded entirely by street segments and a landmark is any feature that is neither a street segments nor a city block. City blocks and landmarks are approximated by polygons while street segments are approximated by line segments.

Given the characterization above, a qualitative representation of a sketch map is a set of QCNs each specifying the spatial relations among the sketched objects for a particular aspect of space. Based on suggestions in previous works [6] our representations consist of four QCNs each: i) a QCN over RCC8 of topological relations within the combined set of landmarks and city blocks, ii) a QCN over $\mathcal{DRA}_7$ of connectivity relations between street segments, and two QCNs over a simple algebra, described below, which is used to connect iii) landmarks to street segments by capturing their proximity relations, and iv) street segments to city blocks by fixing for each street segment its left and right adjacent city block. The QCNs i and ii for the example map of Figure 1 (a) are shown in Figure 1 (c) and (b) respectively.

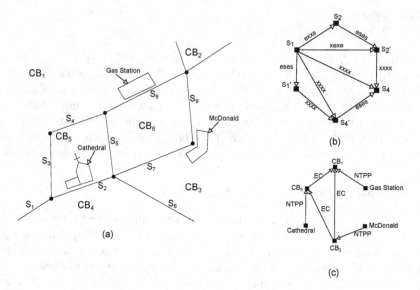

Fig. 1. An example sketch map (a) and constraint networks for topological relations involving landmarks and city blocks (b) and connectivity relations for street segments. Not all nodes and arcs are shown in the QCNs. Street segments are oriented and both orientations are indicated as in s_1 and s_1' together with their reverse segments.

For the landmark to street proximity and city block to street adjacency we build an algebra of relations as follows. Let A, B be sets and let $\{R_0, R_1\}$ be a partition of $A \times B$. Then $iR_0 = \check{R}_0$ and $iR_1 = \check{R}_1$ partition $B \times A$. We then have a partition scheme on $A \cup B$ with base relations $R_0, R_1, iR_0, iR_1, I_A \cup I_B$, and $D_A \cup D_B$, where I_A and D_A are, respectively, the diagonal and diversity relations on A, and I_B and D_B are defined similarly for B. Thus if a suitable interpretation into a class of spatial entities can be obtained we have a qualitative spatial calculus. In order to maintain a clear distinction between elements of the sets A and B the relations $I_A \cup I_B$ and $D_A \cup D_B$ must be refined into relations I_A, I_B, D_A and D_B.

We use the generic scheme above to make weak connections between landmarks and street segments on one hand, and between street segments and city blocks on the other. A landmark l is proximal to street segment s if s is in the boundary of the city block containing l and it is the nearest street segment to l. Setting A above to the set of landmarks and B to the set of street segments we let $(l, s) \in R_0$ if l is proximal to s. For a street segment s and a city block c, we similarly let $(s, c) \in R_0$ if s is a boundary segment of c. We call these two interpretations of R_0 the proximity relation and the boundary relation, respectively. Figure 2 shows example QCNs for proximity and boundary relations. This concludes the discussion on qualitative representation of sketch maps. Next we show how to match two qualitative representations by matching their corresponding QCNs.

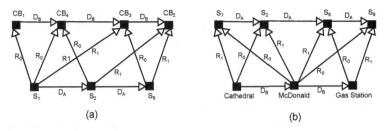

(a)   (b)

Fig. 2. Constraint networks for proximity and boundary relations for objects in the example sketch map of Figure 1. Not all nodes and arcs are shown.

4   Matching

4.1   QCN Matching

A QCN matching problem is a special case of a graph matching problem [19] where the input graphs are complete and edge labeled. A partial solution to a QCN matching problem is called a *match*. We make this precise in the following definitions.

Definition 2 (Disjoint Union of QCNs). *Let* $\mathcal{N} = (N, C)$ *and* $\mathcal{N}' = (N', C')$ *be QCNs with* $N \cap N' = \emptyset$. *The disjoint union of* $\mathcal{N}$ *and* $\mathcal{N}'$ *is the QCN* $\mathcal{N} \uplus \mathcal{N}' = (N \cup N', C'')$ *where*

$$
C''(i,j) = \begin{cases} C(i,j) & \text{if } i,j \in N \\ C'(i,j) & \text{if } i,j \in N' \\ 1 & \text{otherwise} \end{cases}
$$

The set of arcs connecting nodes from N to N' are called the joining arcs. A QCN matching problem is the problem of finding refinements of the joining arcs that maximize the number of those arcs labeled with relations under $\mathbf{1}'$, the identity relation. Formally, let $\mathbf{Id}_{\mathcal{N}} = \{(i,j) \in \mathcal{N} \mid C(i,j) \leq \mathbf{1}'\}$ denote the arcs of QCN $\mathcal{N}$ labeled with relations under $\mathbf{1}'$. The QCN matching problem is stated as follows.

Definition 3 (QCN Matching Problem). $P(\mathcal{N}, \mathcal{N}')$: *find* $\mathcal{M} \leq \mathcal{N} \uplus \mathcal{N}'$ *such that*

1. $\mathcal{M}$ *is closed,*
2. $C_{\mathcal{M}}(i,j) = C_{\mathcal{N}}(i,j)$ *whenever* $i,j \in N$,
3. $C_{\mathcal{M}}(i,j) = C_{\mathcal{N}'}(i,j)$ *whenever* $i,j \in N'$, *and*
4. *for any* $\mathcal{M}' \leq \mathcal{N} \uplus \mathcal{N}'$ *satifying 1. to 3. above,* $|\mathbf{Id}_{\mathcal{M}'}| \leq |\mathbf{Id}_{\mathcal{M}}|$.

A match is a set $m = (N \times N') \cap \mathbf{Id}_{\mathcal{M}}$ for any closed $\mathcal{M} \leq \mathcal{N} \uplus \mathcal{N}'$. Thus a solution to the QCN matching problem is a refinement of the disjoint union of the input QCNs that maximizes the possible size of a match. This characterization is based in part on [3, 8]. Now, having established that QCN matching is an optimization problem, we must proceed to establish methods for discovering the optimal solutions. As the title of this paper suggests, our method of choice is based on the so called Tabu search metaheuristic.

4.2   Tabu Search

Tabu search is a metaheuristc search scheme designed to solve typical optimization problems. Tabu search is built on two main principles, namely, local search and prohibition. As a local search algorithm, each iteration of Tabu involves searching for good solutions within the *neighborhood* of a current solution. To escape local optima and avoid cycling over small regions of the solution space, Tabu enlists the help of prohibition lists - the taboo lists (see [20–23] for an overview). The following presents a tabu based algorithm for the QCN matching problem together with detailed discussions on some of its aspects.

The Solution Space for QCN Matching. Given an instance $P(\mathcal{N},\mathcal{N}')$ of the QCN matching problem, the solution space for P is the set

$$sol(P) = \{(\mathcal{M}, m) \mid \mathcal{M} = cl(\mathcal{M}) \leq \mathcal{N} \uplus \mathcal{N}', \; m = (N \times N') \cap \mathbf{Id}_{\mathcal{M}}\}$$

Any two solutions $(\mathcal{M}, m)$ and $(\mathcal{M}', m)$ can only differ in labels on arcs in $(N \times N')\backslash m$. So we may quotient $sol(P)$ by the equivalence relation $\{(p, p\prime) \mid p = (\mathcal{M}, m), p\prime = (\mathcal{M}', m') \; : \; m = m'\}$ to get a more simplified description. It also allows us to freely refer to solutions as tuples of arcs given by the m's. So we'll write $m \in sol(P)$ for $(\mathcal{M}, m) \in sol(P)$ whenever it is convenient to do so, ensuring that we match superscripts and subscripts wherever applicable.

Neighborhoods of Solutions. For any solution m of $P(\mathcal{N},\mathcal{N}')$, the constructive and destructive neighborhoods of m are, respectively,

$$cNbh(m) = \{m' \in sol(P) \mid \exists (i, j) \in N \times N' \; : \; m' = m \cup \{(i, j)\}\}$$

$$dNbh(m) = \{m' \in sol(P) \mid \exists (i, j) \in N \times N' \; : \; m' = m\backslash\{(i, j)\}\}$$

The neighborhood of m is the set

$$nbh(m) = cNbh(m) \cup dNbh(m)$$

Moves, Move Evaluation, and Auxiliary Objectives. In local search, an algorithm progresses by iteratively making a *move* that generates a new (preferably better) solution from the current one. This is repeated for until the optimum is found or a fixed number of iterations have been executed as illustrated by the tabu search scheme that we employ (see Algorithm 1).

For the neighborhood defined above, an elementary move sets the current solution to one of its neighbors. In general, a move is a sequence of solutions $m_0 m_1 \cdots m_{k-1}$, for some $k > 1$, such that $m_i \in nbh(m_{i-1})$ for each $i < k$. A

Algorithm 1. Tabu Search for QCN Matching

---

    input : QCNs $\mathcal{N} = (N, C), \mathcal{N}' = (N', C')$, and the maximum number of
                iterations maxIter
    output: A match $(\mathcal{M}, \mathsf{m})$

    // initilization
1 iter $\longleftarrow$ 0;
2 $\mathsf{m} \longleftarrow \emptyset$;
3 extensionSet $\longleftarrow N \times N'$;
4 $(\mathcal{M}', \mathsf{m}') \longleftarrow (\emptyset, \emptyset)$;
5 $(\mathcal{M}, \mathsf{m}) \longleftarrow (\mathcal{N} \uplus \mathcal{N}', \mathsf{m})$;

    // iteration
6 **while** $|\mathsf{m}| < |N|$ *and* iter $<$ maxIter **do**
7      $(\mathcal{M}, \mathsf{m}) \longleftarrow$ bestMove$(\mathcal{M}, \mathsf{m})$;
8   **if** $|\mathsf{m}'| < |\mathsf{m}|$ **then**
9         $\lfloor$ $(\mathcal{M}', \mathsf{m}') \longleftarrow (\mathcal{M}, \mathsf{m})$;
10   updateSearchState();

---

move is called *elementary* whenever $k = 2$. In the following we are concerned only with elementary moves. The choice of the next move in each iteration is made based on the values of the following functions. Let

$$f(m_0 m_1) = |\{(i, j) \in N \times N' \mid \mathbf{1}' \cap C_{\mathcal{M}}(i, j) \neq \mathbf{0}\}| \ .$$

Then f approximates the best possible size of a match reachable from m_1. The evaluation of move $m_0 m_1$ is given by

$$e(m_0 m_1) = |m_1| \ ,$$

and the heuristic estimate on it is thus

$$h = f - e \ .$$

The approach in [8] uses the functions e and h to drive a A* search over a standard interpretation tree [1]. By contrast, the algorithm presented here (Algorithm 2) chooses the best *admissible* match in the much broader neighborhood of the current solution and moves to it. The set $cxtensionSet(m)$ contains pairs $(i, j) \in (N \times N')\backslash m$ for which $\mathbf{1}' \cap C_{\mathcal{M}}(i, j) \neq \emptyset$. First the constructive moves from m into $cNbh(m)$ are computed from $extensionSet(m)$ by removing from it all *tabu* moves. Then an estimate of the possible extension of each solution in $cNbh(m)$ is computed by the procedure $simpleForwardCheck$. The computed values are used to impose an order on $cNbh(m)$, implemented as a priority queue, by which the solutions are subsequently processed. Once the queue is filled, solutions are polled from it in order (those with highest extension first). When a solution is polled, the procedure $forwardCheck$ from [8] enforces closure on the underlying QCN and computes $h(m)$. Solutions are polled from the queue until either the queue is empty or the estimated extension of the current polled solution falls below the best value of h obtained so far. If two solutions have the same values of h and e then break ties randomly. The value of $h(m)$ is stored in $m \cdot score$.

Tabu Status and Aspiration Criteria. Since the existence of tabu moves can cause the search stall when there are no more admissible moves or indeed they may cause cycling, an aspiration criterion is introduced (lines 21 - 31). Here $cNbh(m)$ is reconstructed to include only the tabu moves that are also in $extensionSet(m)$. All moves are evaluated using $forwardCheck$. The best aspiring move is the one that has the highest value of $h(m)$, is estimated to be along the path towards a solution that is at least as good as the current best solution, and its associated pair has witnessed the least number of drop moves since the start of execution. However in order to apply aspiration only moves with an $h(m)$ value less than the length of the sequence of constructive moves executed after the last destructive.

The intuition of this choice is the following: If a move is currently tabu then it was last executed no more than $tabuTenure$ iterations ago. Since drop moves don't become tabu, the currently selected move must have been added to and dropped from the solution within this time. If the move is allowed, then we may have fallen into a cycle because possibly the same conditions hold that were true when it was last added. Since moves are always chosen to improve the value of h, setting the acceptance threshold to less than $iter - (lastDropTime + 1)$ ensures that no short cycles occur. Once a drop move is executed it will be followed by a series of drop moves until a non-tabu add move is encountered, which diversifies the search. Moreover, the converse is also true: this strategy encourages a rapid ascent into local maxima.

Finally, if aspiration failed to produce a constructive move, destructive moves are evaluated in a fashion similar to the aspiration moves. Ties are broken by giving preference to moves that correspond to deleting arcs that have been in the solution the longest.

Updating Tabus and other Data Structures. As its name suggests, the procedure $updateSearchState$ updates the sets $extensionSet(m)$ and $tabuSet$, the global variables $iter$ and $lastDropTime$, and the move specific variables $move.dropsWitnessed$ and $move.tabuTime$. The set $extensionSet(m)$ refers to the current solution and is reconstructed each iteration from what we call consistent sets. For each arc $e \in (N \times N')$,

$$consistentSet(e) = \{e' \mid \exists \mathcal{M} \leq \mathcal{N} \uplus \mathcal{N}' : e \in \mathbf{Id}_{\mathcal{M}}, C_{\mathcal{M}}(e') \cdot \mathbf{1}' \neq \emptyset\}$$

. Then $extensionSet(m)$ is defined as follows

$$extensionSet(m) = \bigcap_{e \in m} consistentSet(e) .$$

Consistent sets are updated during the execution of $forwardCheck$. All the (two) forward check procedures execute the following scheme

Algorithm 2. bestMove

---

input : Current match $(\mathcal{M}, m)$
output: The new match $(\mathcal{M}', m')$ to move to

1 $(\mathcal{M}', m') \longleftarrow (\emptyset, \emptyset)$;
2 $(\mathcal{M}', m').score \longleftarrow -1$;
3 extensibility $\longleftarrow \infty$;
4 Q $\longleftarrow \emptyset$;
5 cNbh $\longleftarrow$ extensionSet \ tabuSet;
6 **foreach** $(\mathcal{M}'', m'')$ *in* cNbh **do**   // constructive neighborhood
7 $\quad$ $(\mathcal{M}'', m'') \longleftarrow$ simpleForwardCheck$(\mathcal{M}'', m'')$;
8 $\quad$ **if** $(\mathcal{M}'', m'').score > -1$ **then** Q.offer$(\mathcal{M}'', m'')$;

9 **repeat**   // try non-tabu moves first
10 $\quad$ $(\mathcal{M}'', m'') \longleftarrow$ Q.poll();
11 $\quad$ **if** $(\mathcal{M}'', m'') == (\emptyset, \emptyset)$ **then**
12 $\quad\quad$ break;
13 $\quad$ $(\mathcal{M}'', m'') \longleftarrow$ forwardCheck$(\mathcal{M}'', m'')$;
14 $\quad$ **if** $(\mathcal{M}'', m'').score > (\mathcal{M}', m').score$ **then**
15 $\quad\quad$ $(\mathcal{M}', m') \longleftarrow (\mathcal{M}'', m'')$;
16 $\quad$ **else if** $(\mathcal{M}'', m'').score == (\mathcal{M}', m').score$ **then**
17 $\quad\quad$ **if** $\Delta(\mathcal{M}'', m'').score < \Delta(\mathcal{M}', m').score$ **then**
18 $\quad\quad\quad$ $(\mathcal{M}', m') \longleftarrow (\mathcal{M}'', m'')$;
19 $\quad\quad$ **else if** $\Delta(\mathcal{M}'', m'').score == \Delta(\mathcal{M}', m').score$ **then**
20 $\quad\quad\quad$ randomly replace $(\mathcal{M}', m')$ with $\mathcal{M}'', m''$;

21 **until** $(\mathcal{M}'', m'').score < (\mathcal{M}', m').score$;
22 **if** $(\mathcal{M}', m').score < 0$ **then**   // try tabu moves with aspiration
23 $\quad$ cNbh $\longleftarrow$ extensionSet $\cap$ tabuSet;
24 $\quad$ **foreach** $(\mathcal{M}'', m'')$ *in* cNbh **do**
25 $\quad\quad$ $(\mathcal{M}'', m'') \longleftarrow$ forwardCheck$(\mathcal{M}'', m'')$;
26 $\quad\quad$ **if** $(\mathcal{M}'', m'').score + |m''| \geqslant$ bestSoFar *and*
27 $\quad\quad$ $(\mathcal{M}'', m'').score <$ iter $-$ (lastDropTime $+1$) **then**
28 $\quad\quad\quad$ **if** $(\mathcal{M}'', m'').score > (\mathcal{M}', m').score$ **then**
29 $\quad\quad\quad\quad$ $(\mathcal{M}', m') \longleftarrow (\mathcal{M}'', m'')$;
30 $\quad\quad\quad$ **else if** $(\mathcal{M}'', m'').score == (\mathcal{M}', m').score$ **then**
31 $\quad\quad\quad\quad$ **if** $(\mathcal{M}'', m'').dropsWitnessed < (\mathcal{M}', m').dropsWitnessed$ **then**
32 $\quad\quad\quad\quad\quad$ $(\mathcal{M}', m') \longleftarrow (\mathcal{M}'', m'')$;

33 **if** $(\mathcal{M}', m').score < 0$ **then**   // try drop moves, they are never tabu
34 $\quad$ dNbh $\longleftarrow$ all matches reached by dropping a pair from $(\mathcal{M}, m)$;
35 $\quad$ **foreach** $(\mathcal{M}'', m'')$ *in* dNbh **do**
36 $\quad\quad$ $(\mathcal{M}'', m'') \longleftarrow$ simpleForwardCheck$(\mathcal{M}'', m'')$;
37 $\quad\quad$ **if** $(\mathcal{M}'', m'').score > (\mathcal{M}', m').score$ **then**
38 $\quad\quad\quad$ $(\mathcal{M}', m') \longleftarrow (\mathcal{M}'', m'')$;
39 $\quad\quad$ **else if** $(\mathcal{M}'', m'').score == (\mathcal{M}', m').score$ **then**
40 $\quad\quad\quad$ **if** $(\mathcal{M}'', m'').tabuTime < (\mathcal{M}', m').tabuTime$ **then**
41 $\quad\quad\quad\quad$ $(\mathcal{M}', m') \longleftarrow (\mathcal{M}'', m'')$;

1. set all arcs in m to $\mathbf{1}'$
2. propagate constraints
3. count arcs in $(N \times N')\backslash m$ that intersect $\mathbf{1}'$

$forwardCheck$ updates consistent sets during the counts in step 3 above. This approach to updating means that the algorithm can start with a set of empty consistent sets. Each consistent set is the populated as more knowledge is discovered during the search. Since at the start all arcs are evaluated and those with the highest estimated extension pushed through the $forwardCheck$ procedure, most of the good arcs will have their consistent set updated during the first iteration. The difference between $forwardCheck$ and $simpleForwardCheck$ is that $forwardCheck$ performs a full constraint propagation yielding a closed QCN upon exit while $simpleForwardCheck$ only runs a partial propagation that simply ensures that non-atomic arcs are consistent with the atomic arcs with which they share nodes. Consequently $forwardCheck$ is worst case $\mathcal{O}((N+N')^3)$ while $simpleForwardCheck$ requires a worst case $\mathcal{O}(N \cdot N')$ steps to termination.

5   Evaluation and Discussion

We ran the matching algorithm on six sample sketch maps, matching each sketch map to itself. The algorithm was run 10 times for each aspect and the results were tabulated as shown in table 1, which is a sample from our six tables for successful completions. The corresponding sketch map is shown in figure 3. The results are illustrative at best and by no means represent an accurate picture of the algorithmic performance. However they indicate certain aspects to be considered for an integrated solution.

Table 1. Summary of successful executions of the QCN matching algorithm for QCNs derived from an example sketch map. The optimal value is indicated in the second column

Calculus	Optimal	# Success	Iterations to Success			
			Min	Mean	St. dv.	Max
RCC8	13	7	16	254	242.45	810
$\mathcal{DRA}_7$	10	10	10	10	0	10
Proximity relation	17	5	17	258.8	261.14	764
Boundary relation	16	10	16	16	0	16

First notice that $\mathcal{DRA}_7$ and $Boundary$ always succeed and within a number of iteration equal to the size of the optimal solution. These data are appropriately constrained. Every street segment bounds only one or two city blocks. On the other hand, Proximity and RCC8 were unable to find their optima several times (table 2) and if they did they often took long (table 1).

We made the following observations on the data. The data has There are some combinations of pairs (components of a match) that are strongly coupled, with

Table 2. Summary of executions, with the best suboptimal solutions overall, of the QCN matching algorithm for QCNs derived from an example sketch map

Calculus	Best Suboptimal	# Subopt.	Iterations to best suboptimal			
			Min	Mean	St. dv.	Max
RCC8	12	2	266	332	66	398
$\mathcal{DRA}_7$	0	0	0	0	0	0
Proximity relation	14	3	116	301.33	140.2	455
Boundary relation	0	0	0	0	0	0

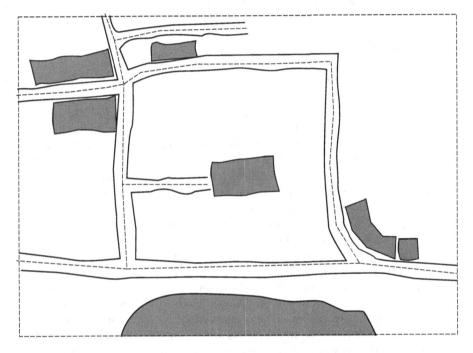

Fig. 3. One of the sketch maps used in the evaluation of the matching algorithm. Shaded regions correspond to landmarks, the inner dotted lines are streets, and the polygons formed by streets and the dotted border are the city blocks.

respect to the input data, in the sense that breaking them apart leads to a drastic drop in the heuristic estimate h. Since this is the main driver of the algorithm, it means that once a solution containing any of these strongly coupled components has been entered, it will be hard leave its neighborhood entirely. Also bad pairs may reinforce each other, in such a way that search moves from one bad solution to the next without ever touching good regions. This can lead to a phenomenon that has been described in [22] using the notion of so called *chaotic attractors*. The number of choices available for the next move are many. However only a few of them can be continued. But every drop move only drops one of the good pairs.

To solve this problem one may introduce dynamic components that may include filters to detect such events and reaction mechanisms to be triggered when such an event is detected. Three obvious events for our problem are the *hard bound*, the *wide basin*, and the *cycle* events. For a fixed given number of iterations, a hard bound is one which has not been breached during that number of iterations. This may indicate that we stumbled into a bad region. A wide basin indicates that no overall improving trend has been observed over that number of iterations and can be detected using a simple filter such as the moving average of solution sizes. Finally, a cycle event says the search is going in circles by observing the number and intervals of repeated solutions. If any of these has been encountered then diversification steps can be taken.

6   Conclusion

We have presented a model of qualitative representation and a Tabu search based algorithm for the QCN matching problem. The use of extension sets to determine the neighborhood of a given solution allows the algorithm to reduce the number of potential candidate solutions to be evaluated. However, the reduction only occurs after the first iteration. Therefore, the initial iteration takes a lot of effort to complete but the iterations after that will evaluate less points. This means that a different strategy is required to cut down the number of iterations executed at the beginning. Through the tests reported above we have learned that tabu tenure and aspiration criteria need to be adjusted dynamically as the search progresses. We have proposed event-reaction mechanisms for doing so and suggested possible implementation methods.

The matching algorithm outlined in section 4.2 above assumes only one pair input QCNs is given at a time. However, the strength our model of spatial scenes lies in part in the connections between the different aspects of space represented in the model. The extension to several QCNs is made as follows. Instead of a pair of QCNs the input becomes an array of pairs of QCNs each with an associated calculus. The match is shared by all QCNs and whenever a new pair is added to the match, all QCNs in which the pair participates are updated during *bestMove*. The choice of the best move must take into account the influence of the size of each QCN and the calculi being used, among other factors.

The grounding of the QCN matching problem in a proper mathematical framework is also essential for uncovering the underlying structure of the problem. This is can be done in the traditional way by studying the Category of QCNs. Already we may note that as in the category **Set** of sets and functions, the disjoint union defined in this paper corresponds to a coproduct of objects in the Category of QCNs. Are there constructions that characterize the chaotic attractors mentioned in section 5 above? What are they? What are their universal properties? These are part of on going work.

Metaheuristic search methods, while guaranteed to perform worse whenever efficient algorithms exist for a problem, may be surprisingly simple in form and fast and flexible in performance. Our tabu search based implementation for the

QCN matching has shown promising results albeit on a very limited sample set. For an implementation that covers a wider problem space we will require the enhancements outlined above and more. However, we believe we are making strides in the right direction.

Acknowledgments. This work is funded by the German Research Foundation (DFG) through the International Research Training Group (IRTG) on Semantic Integration of Geospatial Information (GRK 1498) and the SketchMapia project (Grant SCHW 1372/7-1).

References

1. Grimson, W.E.L.: Object Recognition by Computer – The Role of Geometric Constraints. MIT Press, Cambridge (1990)
2. Egenhofer, M.: Spatial-query-by-sketch. In: Burnett, M., Citrin, W. (eds.) IEEE Symposium on Visual Languages, Boulder, CO, pp. 60–67 (1996)
3. Nedas, K., Egenhofer, M.: Spatial-scene similarity queries. Transactions in GIS 12(6), 661–681 (2008)
4. Blaser, A.: Geo-spatial sketches. Technical report, University of Maine, Department of Spatial Information Science and Engineering and National Center for Geographic Information and Analysis, Boardman Hall 321, Orono, Maine 04469, USA (1998)
5. Kopczynski, M., Sester, M.: Representation of sketch data for localisation in large data sets. In: XXth Congress of the International Society for Photogrammetry and Remote Sensing (ISPRS), Istanbul, Turkey (2004)
6. Chipofya, M., Wang, J., Schwering, A.: Towards cognitively plausible spatial representations for sketch map alignment. In: Egenhofer, M., Giudice, N., Moratz, R., Worboys, M. (eds.) COSIT 2011. LNCS, vol. 6899, pp. 20–39. Springer, Heidelberg (2011)
7. Chipofya, M.: A qualitative reasoning approach for improving query results for sketch-based queries by topological analysis of spatial aggregation. Master's thesis, Universitat Jaume I, Universität Münster, Universidad Nova de Lisboa (2010)
8. Wallgrün, J.O., Wolter, D., Richter, K.F.: Qualitative matching of spatial information. In: Proceedings of the 18th SIGSPATIAL International Conference on Advances in Geographic Information Systems, GIS 2010, pp. 300–309. ACM, New York (2010)
9. Cohn, A.G., Renz, J.: Qualitative spatial representation and reasoning. In: van Hermelen, F., Lifschitz, V., Porter, B. (eds.) Handbook of Knowledge Representation, vol. 46, pp. 551–596. Elsevier (2008)
10. Renz, J., Schmid, F.: Customizing qualitative spatial and temporal calculi. In: Orgun, M.A., Thornton, J. (eds.) AI 2007. LNCS (LNAI), vol. 4830, pp. 293–304. Springer, Heidelberg (2007)
11. Ligozat, G., Renz, J.: What is a qualitative calculus? A general framework. In: Zhang, C., Guesgen, H.W., Yeap, W.-K. (eds.) PRICAI 2004. LNCS (LNAI), vol. 3157, pp. 53–64. Springer, Heidelberg (2004)
12. Ligozat, G.: Categorical methods in qualitative reasoning: The case for weak representations. In: Cohn, A.G., Mark, D.M. (eds.) COSIT 2005. LNCS, vol. 3693, pp. 265–282. Springer, Heidelberg (2005)

13. Montanari, U.: Networks of constraints: Fundamental properties and applications to picture processing. Information Sciences 7, 95–132 (1974)

14. Ladkin, P.B., Maddux, R.D.: On binary constraint problems. J. ACM 41(3), 435–469 (1994)

15. van Beek, P.: Reasoning about qualitative temporal information. Artificial Intelligence 58(1-3), 297–326 (1992)

16. Wang, J., Schwering, A.: The accuracy of sketched spatial relations: How cognitive errors influence sketch representation. In: Presenting Spatial Information: Granularity, Relevance, and Integration. Workshop at COSIT 2009, Aber Wrac'h, France (2009)

17. Schwering, A., Wang, J.: Sketching as interface for vgi systems. In: Geoinformatik, Kiel, Germany (2010)

18. Cohn, A.G., Bennett, B., Gooday, J., Gotts, N.M.: Qualitative spatial representation and reasoning with the region connection calculus. Geoinformatica 1, 275–316 (1997)

19. Riesen, K., Jiang, X., Bunke, H.: Exact and inexact graph matching: Methodology and applications. In: Aggarwal, C.C., Wang, H. (eds.) Managing and Mining Graph Data. Advances in Database Systems, vol. 40, pp. 217–247. Springer, US (2010)

20. Glover, F.: Tabu search – part 1. ORSA Journal on Computing 1(3), 190–206 (1989)

21. Glover, F.: Tabu search – part 2. ORSA Journal on Computing 2(1), 4–32 (1990)

22. Battiti, R., Tecchiolli, G.: The reactive tabu search. ORSA Journal on Computing 6(2), 126–140 (1994)

23. Gendreau, M., Potvin, J.Y.: Tabu search. In: Burke, E., Kendall, G. (eds.) Search Methodologies, pp. 165–186. Springer, US (2005)

Classification of Mexican Paper Currency Denomination by Extracting Their Discriminative Colors

Farid García-Lamont[1], Jair Cervantes[1], Asdrúbal López[2], and Lisbeth Rodríguez[1]

[1] Universidad Autónoma del Estado de México, Av. Jardín Zumpango s/n, Fraccionamiento El Tejocote, CP 56259, Texcoco-Estado de México, México
[2] Universidad Autónoma del Estado de México, Camino viejo a Jilotzingo Continuación Calle Rayón, CP 55600, Zumpango-Estado de México, México
{fgarcial,alchau}@uaemex.mx, {chazarra17,lisbethr08}@gmail.com

Abstract. In this paper we describe a machine vision approach to recognize the denomination classes of the Mexican paper currency by extracting their color features. A banknote's color is characterized by summing all the color vectors of the image's pixels to obtain a resultant vector, the banknote's denomination is classified by knowing the orientation of the resulting vector within the RGB space. In order to obtain a more precise characterization of paper currency, the less discriminative colors of each denomination are eliminated from the images; the color selection is applied in the RGB and HSV spaces, separately. Experimental results with the current Mexican banknotes are presented.

Keywords: Banknotes recognition, color classification, image processing.

1 Introduction

Nowadays, more and more money transactions are performed using automated machines; for example, payment of services, parking, bank operations, among others. Currently in Mexico, many money transaction processes are still in the transition to be automated, but several others have not been automated.

Automated money transactions in Mexico are necessary not only to give comfort to people, but also to speed up and increase the number of transactions, since a huge amount of monetary transactions are performed with Mexican Pesos [1]. The current technology employed is bought to foreign companies, but this technology is expensive and the recognition algorithms are not revealed due to patent rights [2], [3].

Related works on paper currency recognition have focused on the classification of Euros [4], [5] and US Dollars [6], [7]. Other related works address the recognition of the paper currency of specific countries [8]-[12], in these papers the banknotes of each country are modeled by extracting their very particular features; so, the recognition methods are customized depending on the nationality of the paper currency.

The most employed banknotes' features for recognition in related works are the texture [6], [9], [10] or both texture and size [4], [5], [11]. The disadvantages with these features are, in one hand, the banknotes with different denominations may have

F. Castro, A. Gelbukh, and M. González (Eds.): MICAI 2013, Part II, LNAI 8266, pp. 103–112, 2013.

the same size; on the other hand, usually the banknotes are mistreated because they may have hand written notes or they may be worn and torn due to daily use, so, the texture pattern of mistreated banknotes is altered, leading to inaccurate recognition [11]. Hence, it must be selected a feature to characterize the denomination of the paper currency without being affected by the size or the mistreat level of the banknotes.

Like in many other countries, in Mexico there are used different colors to distinguish the denomination classes of the banknotes easily. The advantages of using the color features are: 1) the chromaticity of the colors does not change before mistreated banknotes; 2) the colors of the banknotes are not affected by the banknotes' size.

Hence, in this paper we extract the color features, under the RGB space, of the Mexican paper currency to classify their denominations classes. In order to obtain accurate models, there are selected the discriminative colors by applying a color selection approach, separately, in two different color spaces. The banknotes' images are acquired by scanning the banknotes under the same illumination conditions.

The rest of the article is organized as follows: Section 2 presents how the color features of the banknotes are extracted. Section 3 shows the color selection approaches; Section 4 describes the tests and experimental results. Discussion in Section 5 and the paper ends with conclusions in Section 6.

2   Color Extraction

Currently the Mexican paper currency has six denomination classes: 20, 50, 100, 200, 500 and 1000 Pesos. We focus on the recognition of the first five denomination classes because they are employed for common daily transactions, see Table 1.

The banknotes have different colors distributed throughout their surfaces; the color with more occurrences is defined as the "dominant" color, which is the main feature to recognize the denomination. The dominant colors of the 20, 50, 100, 200 and 500 denominations are blue, pink, yellow, green and brown, respectively.

But the dominant color may not be the only one that characterizes the banknote's denomination, because there may be two or more colors with a similar number of occurrences that contribute with significant data about the banknote. For instance, the dominant color of the 100 Pesos banknote is yellow; however, the color of a considerable amount of the banknote's area is red. Therefore, red is also a significant color feature of this denomination that must be included for the banknote's characterization.

To model colors we use the RGB space, which is accepted by most of the image processing community to represent colors [13], it is based in a Cartesian coordinate system where colors are points defined by vectors that extend from the origin [14], where black is located in the origin and white in the opposite corner to the origin, see Fig. 1. The color vector of a pixel p is a linear combination of the basis vectors red, green and blue, written as:

$$\phi_p = r_p \hat{\imath} + g_p \hat{\jmath} + b_p \hat{k} \tag{1}$$

Where the scalars r, g and b are the red, green and blue, respectively, components of the color vector.

Table 1. Images of the Mexican banknotes denominations used for common daily transactions

Denomination	Front face	Back face
20		
50		
100 (old)		
100 (new)		
200 (old)		
200 (new)		
500 (old)		
500 (new)		

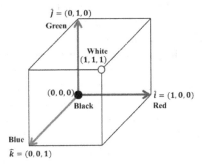

Fig. 1. RGB color space

The orientation and magnitude of a color vector defines the chromaticity and the intensity of the color, respectively [14]. If we sum two color vectors with the same orientation, then, the result is a vector with the same orientation of the two previous and its magnitude will be larger than the previous ones, that is, the resulting color has the same chromaticity but brighter. On the other hand, if two color vectors with different chromaticity are sum the resultant will have different orientation, and also larger; that is, the resulting chromaticity is a combination of the chromaticity of the previous vectors.

The addition of the color vectors of all the pixels of the image gives the resultant vector R, whose orientation may be similar to the color vector's orientation of the dominant color, where R contains data of all the color features of the banknote. Thus, a banknote can be characterized by computing R as follows.

Let $\{\phi_1, ..., \phi_N\} \subset \mathbb{R}^3$ the set of the pixels' color vectors of a given image, where N is the number of pixels of the image; the resultant vector R is computed with:

$$R = \sum_{p=1}^{N} \phi_p \tag{2}$$

Due to what it is relevant is the orientation of the vector, not its magnitude, the resultant vector is normalized:

$$u_R = \frac{R}{\|R\|} = r_u \hat{\imath} + g_u \hat{\jmath} + b_u \hat{k} \tag{3}$$

The vector u_R characterizes the color feature; later this vector is fed to a classifier for banknote recognition. Observe that the direction cosines of u_R are $\cos \alpha_R = r_u / \|u_R\|$, $\cos \beta_R = g_u / \|u_R\|$ and $\cos \theta_R = b_u / \|u_R\|$. Moreover $\|u_R\| = 1$, therefore, the components of the vector u_R are the cosines of the angles between the vector and the basis vectors. So, the orientation of R is implicit in u_R.

3   Selection of Discriminative Colors

The resulting vector includes colors that may not provide relevant data of the banknote that may alter the accuracy of the characterization; hence, there are eliminated these colors of the paper currency's image. Thus, the colors with high variance are eliminated because they are considered as not important data.

Despite we assume the illumination conditions do not vary during the image acquisition, the colors printed on the paper currency may lose their intensities because the banknotes may be worn-out or they may have dirt. Due to the RGB space is sensible to color intensity, several color preprocessing applications are performed in the Hue, Saturation and Value (HSV) color space [13], [15] because the Value component, also known as intensity, is decoupled from the chromaticity of the color. So, we apply, separately, the color selection in the RGB space and in the HSV space. This lets us compare which space is convenient to perform the color selection.

3.1   Preliminaries

Computing the mean and variance of vectors involves the following mathematical operations. Let $\{\phi_1, \dots, \phi_m\} \subset \mathbb{R}^n$ a set of vectors, the mean of the vectors is computed with:

$$\mu_\phi = \frac{1}{m} \sum_{p=1}^{m} \phi_p \tag{4}$$

The covariance matrix Ω is built:

$$\Omega = \frac{1}{m} \Phi \Phi^T \tag{5}$$

Where $\Phi = [\phi_1 - \mu_\phi, \dots, \phi_m - \mu_\phi]$; the variance value is obtained by computing the norm of the covariance matrix, that is $\sigma_\phi^2 = \|\Omega\|$. The norm of the matrix is computed with [16]:

$$\|\Omega\| = \sqrt{\lambda(\Omega^T \Omega)} \tag{6}$$

Where λ is the largest eigenvalue of the matrix obtained with $\Omega^T \Omega$.

3.2   Color Selection in the RGB Space

Before the vectors R and u_R are computed, the image is preprocessed by setting to zero the color vectors with high variance. Due to the colors in this space depend on their intensities, the color vectors are normalized and then the color vector selection is performed. Let $\{\phi_1, \dots, \phi_N\} \subset \mathbb{R}^3$ the set of the color vectors of an image, by normalizing the color vectors with $\tilde{\phi}_p = \phi_p / \|\phi_p\|$ we obtain the set $\{\tilde{\phi}_1, \dots, \tilde{\phi}_N\} \subset \mathbb{R}^3$. The color vectors with high variance are set to zero; that is:

$$\tilde{\phi}_p = \begin{cases} \tilde{\phi}_p, & \|\tilde{\phi}_p - \mu_{\tilde{\phi}}\|^2 < \sigma_{\tilde{\phi}}^2 \\ 0, & \text{otherwise} \end{cases} \tag{7}$$

Where $0 = [0,0,0]$, the mean $\mu_{\tilde{\phi}}$ and the variance $\sigma_{\tilde{\phi}}^2$ are computed as mentioned in Section 3.1. After the color selection, the vectors are processed with equations (2) and (3).

3.3   Color Selection in the HSV Space

The HSV space is cone shaped, see Fig. 2, where the hue or chromaticity is in the range $[0, 2\pi] \subset \mathbb{R}$; the saturation is the distance to the glow axis of black-white, the value is the height in the white-black axis. Both saturation and value are in the interval $[0,1] \subset \mathbb{R}$. Computing the mean and variance of the hue as a scalar value cannot be precise, because the hue data near 0 are different from the hue data near 2π, but the chromaticity in both cases is very similar. So, the hue of a pixel is represented as a two-element unit vector whose orientation is the pixel's hue data.

Let $\{\phi_1, \dots, \phi_N\} \subset \mathbb{R}^3$ the set of color vectors of an image in the RGB space, these vectors are mapped to the HSV space to form the set $\{\varphi_1, \dots, \varphi_N\} \subset \mathbb{R}^3$. Each vector φ_p has the elements hue (h), saturation (s) and value (v); i.e., $\varphi_p = [h_p, s_p, v_p]$.

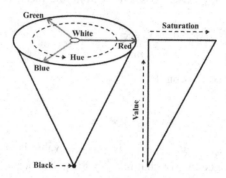

Fig. 2. HSV color space

We obtain the set $\{\psi_1, \dots, \psi_N\} \subset \mathbb{R}^2$, where $\psi_p = [\cos h_p, \sin h_p]$. Therefore, a pixel's color vector is set to zero if the hue component of its corresponding vector φ has high variance. That is:

$$\phi_p = \begin{cases} \phi_p, & \|\psi_p - \mu_\psi\|^2 < \sigma_\psi^2 \\ 0, & \text{otherwise} \end{cases} \tag{8}$$

Where the mean μ_ψ and the variance σ_ψ^2 are computed as mentioned in Section 3.1. Once the color vector selection is finished, the selected vectors are normalized and processed with equations (2) and (3). Fig. 3 (a) and (b) show the images obtained after preprocessing in the RGB and HSV spaces, respectively, of the same 20 Pesos banknote. The black pixels are the ones whose color vectors have high variance.

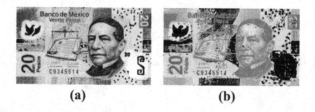

(a)   **(b)**

Fig. 3. Images (a) and (b) obtained after preprocessing in the RGB and HSV spaces, respectively, of the same 20 Pesos banknote

4 Experiments and Results

The experimental stage consists on classifying a set of 1600 banknotes, 320 banknotes per denomination class. In this set 400 images are acquired from severely mistreat banknotes and/or with handwritten notes, 80 images per denomination class; the rest of the images are obtained from banknotes with the usual mistreat level. The training set contains 16 images, for each denomination class there are employed one image of the front face and one image of the back face of the banknote. The training set is slightly imbalanced because there are two kinds of banknotes for the 100, 200 and 500 Pesos denominations; therefore, for these denominations there are employed 4 training images per class while for the 20 and 50 Pesos denominations there are employed 2 training images per class.

For classification, the Learning Vector Quantization (LVQ) networks are suitable for this purpose. A LVQ network is a supervised version of vector quantization, similar to self-organizing maps; usually, it is applied for pattern recognition or multi-class classification [17]. The employed LVQ networks have 32 neurons, the learning rate value is 0.01; the networks are trained with the Kohonen rule [17].

Note that the banknotes are characterized with three different feature vectors: u_W is obtained without image preprocessing; u_{RGB} and u_{HSV} are obtained by applying the image preprocessing in the RGB and HSV spaces, respectively. Moreover, it is possible to build "new" characterizations of the banknotes by combining, concatenating, these feature vectors.

Table 2 shows the results obtained by modeling the banknotes' colors with the feature vectors and their combinations. The rows "W", "RGB" and "HSV" show the results using the feature vectors u_W, u_{RGB} and u_{HSV}, respectively. The rows "W-RGB", "W-HSV" and "RGB-HSV" shows the results by combining the vectors u_W and u_{RGB}, u_W and u_{HSV}, u_{RGB} and u_{HSV}, respectively. Finally, the row "W-RGB-HSV" shows the results by combining the three feature vectors.

Table 2. Recognition rates (%) obtained by combining the feature vectors

Feature vector	Denomination class					Average rate
	20	50	100	200	500	
W	100	87.50	96.67	100	82.50	93.34
RGB	100	97.50	100	86.16	86.25	93.98
HSV	100	95	100	97.44	92.50	96.98
W-RGB	100	97.50	100	98.07	83.75	95.86
W-HSV	100	97.50	100	98.07	93.12	97.73
RGB-HSV	100	97.50	100	97.87	93.12	97.70
W-RGB-HSV	100	97.50	100	97.43	90	96.98

Regardless the feature vector combinations, the 20 Pesos denomination is the best classified. The recognition rate of the 100 Pesos denomination remains at 100% when at least a color selection approach is applied.

With the feature vector u_W all the 200 Pesos banknotes are successfully classified and 96.67% of the 100 Pesos banknotes are correctly identified. While the recognition rates for the 50 and 500 Pesos denominations are low, 87.50% and 82.50%, respectively. Using the feature vector u_{RGB} the recognition rates of the 50, 100 and 500 Pesos denominations are improved up to 97.50%, 100% and 86.25%, respectively. The recognition rate of the 200 Pesos denomination falls at 86.16%.

Moreover, with the feature vector u_{HSV} all the 100 Pesos banknotes are properly identified. The recognition rates of the 200 and 500 Pesos banknotes are higher than the obtained using the feature vector u_{RGB}, but the recognition rate of the 200 Pesos denomination is lower than using the feature vector u_W. Although the recognition rate of the 50 Pesos denomination is higher with respect the obtained using u_W, it is lower that the obtained using u_{RGB}.

With the combination W-RGB the recognition rates remain almost the same using the feature vector u_{RGB}; except for the 200 and 500 Pesos banknotes where the recognition rates are higher and slightly lower, respectively.

The recognition rates obtained with the combination W-HSV are slightly higher than employing the feature vector u_{HSV}; from 95% to 97.44% and 92.50% to 97.50%, 98.07 and 93.12% for the 50, 200 and 500 Pesos denominations, respectively.

The combination RGB-HSV gives almost the same recognition rates to the obtained with the combination W-HSV; except for the 200 Pesos denomination, where its recognition rate falls from 98.07% to 97.87%.

With the combination of the three feature vectors, the recognition rates are very similar to the obtained with the combination RGB-HSV, where the recognition rate of the 500 Pesos denomination is notably lower, reaching 90%.

5   Discussion

Without using color selection, most of the 50 Pesos banknotes misclassifications are recognized as 500 Pesos and viceversa. This happens because both denominations have colors in common, although such colors may not be characteristic of these denominations, therefore the feature vectors of these denominations become similar.

With the image preprocessing in the RGB space the recognition of the 50 Pesos banknotes is improved, because the non-discriminative colors of this denomination are eliminated. However, for the 500 Pesos denomination the discriminative colors cannot be selected such that to avoid being misclassified as 50 Pesos. The recognition of the 200 Pesos denomination becomes less precise because several green tonalities are eliminated; in consequence, the yellow tonalities predominate. Thus, several 200 Pesos banknotes are misclassified as 100 Pesos.

The color selection in the HSV space improved the recognition rates. The most notable result is the recognition of the 500 Pesos denomination; the colors of the 500 Pesos denomination in common with the 50 Pesos denomination are eliminated in the image preprocessing, due to these colors are not characteristic of this denomination. But the recognition rate of the 50 Pesos denomination is lower than the obtained with the RGB color selection, because the feature vector's orientation is similar to the brown hue; therefore, the 50 Pesos banknotes are misclassified as 500 Pesos.

In general, the recognition rates using any combination of feature vectors are higher than employing the feature vectors separately. The combination of the feature vectors lets to build a feature vector containing the attributes of the feature vectors that give shape. The highest rates are obtained with the combinations where the color selection is performed in the HSV space. The color selection is more precise in the HSV space because the chromatic hue is an attribute that describes a pure color; while the colors in the RGB space is represented on the spectral components of the basis colors. Besides, despite the color vectors are normalized in the color selection in the RGB space, the influence of the intensity is not totally eliminated.

In order to improve the recognition rate, it may be useful to employ other banknote's feature; for instance, the texture feature, although this feature has the drawbacks mentioned before. Another possibility is to use a fuzzy logic-based classifier, due to the fuzzy nature of the color chromaticity.

The average recognition rate of Mexican paper currency reported in [18] is 96%, using only color features, without color selection and by processing only images of banknotes with the usual mistreat level; while we obtain 97.73% without discarding any image from the image database, which contains images of severely damaged banknotes.

Though none of the reviewed papers mention their processing times, it is useful to know that because we can decide on which kind of applications the proposed approach is adequate to be employed. The processing time depends not only on the kind of mathematical operations, but also the resolution of the images and the hardware used. In this paper, the average resolution of the images of the 20, 500, 100, 200 and 500 Pesos denominations are 524×951, 522×1002, 518×1140, 518×1665 and 523×1201 pixels, respectively; the microprocessor employed is a Core i5-3310 at 2.90GHz and 4GB RAM, the algorithms are implemented in Matlab R2009a. Table 3 shows the average processing time of one image of any of the five denomination classes; from the image preprocessing up to the classification.

Table 3. Average processing time, in seconds units

Feature vector	Processing time
W	0.0656
RGB	1.6012
HSV	0.7485

It takes longer to classify a banknote when its image is preprocessed in the RGB space than on the HSV space, because the dimensions of the vectors in the RGB and HSV spaces are 3 and 2, respectively. Without color selection the processing is fast because there are performed essentially arithmetic sums. The processing time of the combinations can be computed by adding the processing times of the feature vectors that model the combinations. Given the processing times and recognition rates, this approach can be used in applications that do not require a very fast recognition; for instance, automatic vending machines. The processing time can be reduced by using either a more powerful processor or images at lower resolution.

In many other countries, as in Mexico, there are employed different colors to identify their paper currency's denominations; for instance, Euros and Pound Sterling. Our approach can also be used to classify the paper currency of countries that use colors to recognize their paper currency's denominations. Note that our proposal does not recognize counterfeits; it is beyond the scope of this paper due to counterfeit detection is country-dependable [19].

6   Conclusions

We have proposed a computer vision approach for the recognition on Mexican paper currency. The denomination classes are recognized by extracting and selecting discriminative color features of the paper currency. The banknote's color is modeled by summing all the color vectors of the image's pixels, and it is classified by knowing the location of the resulting vector within the RGB space. The recognition becomes more accurate by using the combination W-HSV; although the combination of the feature vectors RGB-HSV gives almost the same recognition rate, the processing time is larger. Severely damaged banknotes, which are difficult to find in real life, can be accurately classified.

Acknowledgments. This work was sponsored by Secretaría de Educación Pública: convenio PROMEP/103.5/13/6535.

References

1. Bank for International Settlements: Monetary and Economic Department, "Triennial central bank survey for foreign exchange and derivatives market activity in December 2010: Preliminary global results" (2010)
2. Tecnocont, http://www.tecnocont.es
3. Galantz, http://www.galantz.com.ar
4. Jae-Kang, L., Il-Hwan, L.: New recognition algorithm for various kinds of Euro banknotes. In: Conf. of the IEEE Industrial Electronics Society (IECON), pp. 2266–2270 (2003)
5. Lee, J.K., Jeon, S.G., Kim, I.H.: Distinctive Point Extraction and Recognition Algorithm for Various Kinds of Euro Banknotes. Int. J. Control Autom. Syst. 2(2), 201–206 (2004)
6. Hasanuzzaman, F., Yang, X., Tian, Y.: Robust and effective component-based banknote recognition for the blind. IEEE Trans. Syst. Man Cybern. Part C: Appl. Rev. 42(6), 1021–1030 (2012)
7. Kagehiro, T., Nagayoshi, H., Sako, H.: A Hierarchical Classification Method for US Bank Notes. Trans. Inf. Syst. E89D(7), 2061–2067 (2006)
8. Sajal, R., Kamruzzaman, M., Jewel, F.: A machine vision based automatic system for real time recognition and sorting of Bangladesh bank notes. In: Int. Conf. Computer and Information Technology (ICCIT), pp. 560–567 (2008)
9. Poorrahangaryan, F., Mohammadpour, T., Kianisarkaleh, A.: A Persian banknote recognition using wavelet and neural network. In: Int. Conf. Computer Science and Electronics Engineering (ICCSEE), vol. 3, pp. 679–684 (2012)
10. Guo, J., Zhao, Y., Cai, A.: A reliable method for paper currency recognition based on LBP. In: IEEE Int. Conf. Network Infrastructure and Digital Content, pp. 359–363 (2010)
11. Hassanpour, H., Farahabadi, P.M.: Using Hidden Markov Models for Paper Currency Recognition. Expert Syst. Appl. 36(6), 10105–10111 (2009)
12. Takeda, F., Sakoobunthu, L., Satou, H.: Thai banknote recognition using neural network and continues learning by DSP unit. In: Palade, V., Howlett, R.J., Jain, L. (eds.) KES 2003. LNCS (LNAI), vol. 2773, pp. 1169–1177. Springer, Heidelberg (2003)
13. Paschos, G.: Perceptually Uniform Color Spaces for Color Texture Analysis: An Empirical Evaluation. IEEE Trans. Image Process 10(6), 932–937 (2001)
14. Gonzalez, R.C., Woods, R.E.: Digital Image Processing, 2nd edn. Prentice Hall (2002)
15. Wang, F., Man, L., Wang, B., Xiao, Y., Pan, W., Lu, X.: Fuzzy-based Algorithm for Color Recognition of License Plates. Pattern Recognit. Lett. 29(7), 1007–1020 (2008)
16. Bronshtein, I., Semendyayev, K., Musiol, G., Muehlig, H.: Handbook of Mathematics. Springer, Heidelberg (2007)
17. Hagan, H.: Neural Network Design. PWS Publishing Company (1996)
18. García-Lamont, F., Cervantes, J., López, A.: Recognition of Mexican banknotes via their color and texture features. Expert Syst. Appl. 39(10), 9651–9660 (2012)
19. Lee, K.H., Park, T.H.: Image segmentation of UV for automatic paper-money inspection. In: Int. Conf. Control, Automation, Robotics and Vision, pp. 1175–1180 (2010)

Towards Reduced EEG Based Brain-Computer Interfacing for Mobile Robot Navigation

Mufti Mahmud[1,2,3,*] and Amir Hussain[3]

[1] Theoretical Neurobiology & Neuroengineering Lab, Department of Biomedical Sciences, University of Antwerp, 2610−Wilrijk, Belgium
http://www.tnb.ua.ac.be/
[2] Institute of Information Technology, Jahangirnagar University, Savar, 1342−Dhaka, Bangladesh
http://www.juniv.edu/iit/index.php
[3] Cognitive Signal Image and Control Processing Research (COSIPRA) Laboratory, School of Natural Sciences, University of Stirling, Stirling FK9 4LA, UK
http://cosipra.cs.stir.ac.uk/
mufti@tnb.ua.ac.be, ahu@cs.stir.ac.uk

Abstract. Rapid development in highly parallel neurophysiological recording techniques along with sophisticated signal processing tools allow direct communication with neuronal processes at different levels. One important level from the point of view of Rehabilitation Engineering & Assistive Technology is to use the Electroencephalogram (EEG) signals to interface with assistive devices. This type of brain-computer interface (BCI) aims to reestablish the broken loop of the persons with motor dysfunction(s). However, with the growing availability of of instruments and processes for implementation, the BCI is also getting more complex. In this work, the authors present a model for reduced complexity BCI based on EEG signals through a few simple processes for automated navigation and control of robotic device. It is demonstrated that not only with few number of electrodes, but also using simple features like evoked responses caused by Saccadic eye movement can be used in building robust BCI for rehabilitation which may revolutionize the development of assitive devices for the disabled.

Keywords: Brain-computer interface, Electroencephalogram, mobile robot, robot navigation, neuronal signal analysis.

1 Introduction

Increasing growth in the microtechnology has provided scientists with tools to interface with the neural process at multiple levels. Also, the availability of various efficient computational resources and improving knowledge about brain functionality and dysfunctions have allowed development of novel therapeutic and replacement strategies [1] [2]. Disorders such as Amyotrophic Lateral Sclerosis

---

* Corresponding author.

(ALS) or spinal cord injury cause communication disruption between the brain and the body resulting in loss of voluntary muscle control in patients. These patients have reduced quality of life, and are dependent on caretakers thus escalating social costs [3]. The existing assistive technology devices are either dependent on motor activities from specific body parts or use complex systems which sometimes are difficult to be used by the patients. Therefore, alternative strategies are required to better suit the needs of such patients [4].

The previous works in development of Brain-Computer Interface (BCI) show that the signal acquisition and processing are getting complicated with the growing availability of more sophisticated recording devices [5] [7] [6]. Bi et al. [8] did a review on the existing technologies to control robotic devices using EEG. Avoiding the various complexities, rather simple method may be employed in coupling neuronal signals to robotic devices as described in related previous works [9] [10] [11]. The goal of this paper is to highlight the fact that it is very much possible to create a simple BCI system using EEG signals recorded through conventional EEG acquisition devices and use these signals to command and control a robotic device's navigation. The figure 1a shows the schematic and figure 1b shows the communication cartoon of the such a reduced complexity BCI. The model was validated using EEG signals caused by eye movements to control the navigation of an educational robot, ePuck (http://www.e-puck.org/).

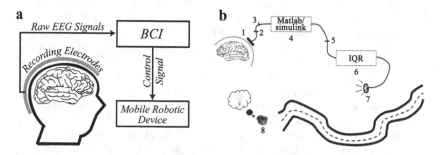

Fig. 1. (a) The schematic of the Brain-Computer interface system. The raw EEG signals are transformed into control signals which control the robotic device. (b) The communication cartoon of the BCI model. The numbers 1 to 10, each denotes an interface during the communication process. Each recording electrode (1) records signals, sends them to the multiplexer (2), where all the channels combined together are fed to the preamplifier (3) for amplification and sent to the computer (4) for analysis. The analyzed signals are sent to the UDP port (5) and then to the robot controlling computer (6), from where these received control signals are sent through Bluetooth (7) to the robot (8).

2   Methods

2.1   BCI Model Design

A two-layered approach was adhered in designing the BCI model:

– The upper layer (also first layer) contained the signal acquisition process and generated the control signals from the acquired raw EEG signals.
– The lower layer (also second layer) contained the scheme of commanding and controlling of the robotic device. This layer received the binary control signals (BCS) from the upper layer and they were sent to the robotic device to be controlled.

The two-layered approach in this case was very important as it separated two main operational paradigms of the system, namely, the signal acquisition and processing paradigm, and the robotic device commanding and controlling paradigm. This decoupling facilitated independent treatment of the two operations, one without affecting the other. The low cohesion among the two paradigms also allowed us in programming sophisticated signal processing and analysis algorithms to calculate the BCS without influencing the robot commanding process. Thus, we could keep the robotic device interfacing paradigm simplified just to respond to the BCS to command and control the robotic device which enhanced the reusability of the methods. The figure 2 shows the flowchart outlining the major steps of the BCI method. The top two boxes belong to the upper layer and the bottom two belong to the lower layer.

The EEG signal acquisition was performed using a Matlab Simulink framework (http://www.mathworks.com) and the signal processing was performed using Matlab scripting. The interfacing with the robotic device was done using an open-source program called 'IQR' [13] [14] capable of mimicking neuronal network behavior based on the BCS.

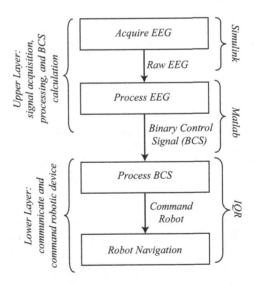

Fig. 2. Flowchart showing the major steps of the system, their input and outputs. It also indicates the two layers (left side curly braces), and the software tools used in implementing the individual steps (right side curly braces).

2.2   Electroencephalogram (EEG) Signal Acquisition

The Electroencephalogram signals are generated due to firing of neuronal populations in the brain which propagates along the cortex. By placing silver-silver chloride (Ag-AgCl) electrodes on various specific locations of the scalp, these propagated signals can be recorded. Therefore, electrodes located at a specific part of the scalp provide necessary information related to that corresponding part of the brain. For example, the visual cortex is located at the caudal portion of the brain (occipital lobe) and if one would like to get information on visual stimuli, the electrodes must be placed at the occipital region of the brain.

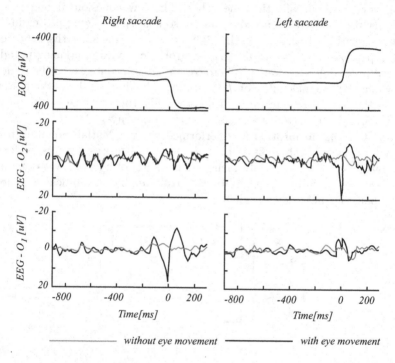

Fig. 3. EEG signals recorded by EOG and 'O$_1$', 'O$_2$' electrodes of the EEG from one subject while performing the saccadic movement during an experiment

The EEG signal were recorded using a four channel commercial EEG recording device, g$^®$.MOBIlab, manufactured by the g.tec medical engineering GmbH, Austria (http://www.gtec.at/). We used the 10-20 international system of electrode mapping [11] for placing the electrodes. Two electrodes were used in recording simultaneous signals from 'O$_1$' and 'O$_2$' and a third electrode was used as a reference, placed at 'F' or 'F$_P$' position. The model was successfully tested with the EEG signals recorded using these two electrodes. These recorded signals were event related evoked response during saccadic eye movements [12]. Traces of representative EEG signals recorded by the 'O$_1$' and 'O$_2$' electrodes are shown in figure 3 (middle and bottom panel). The top panel of the figure 3 shows recordings of Electrooculography (EOG, a method used for measuring eye movement), and demonstrates that the saccadic eye movement can be detected from the electrodes with a reasonable effort of signal processing.

2.3   Processing of EEG Signals

Preprocessing. Before extracting signal events (events caused by saccadic eye movements) from the recorded signals, artifact removal was performed on-the-fly to remove artifacts caused by eye blink, cardiac rhythms, and body movements (details on the methods applied can be found in [15] [16]). The power line noise (50-60 Hz components) was removed using stop-band filter of 50 and 60 Hz. Also, there can be other packages used for preprocessing the EEG signals [17] [18] [19].

Detection of Saccadic Events. It is vital to extract the events from the clean EEG signals. At first, signals from both channels were filtered using a band-pass filter (cut-off frequencies: 15 Hz and 100 Hz) to remove the alpha wave generated by the occipital region of the brain. Then the signals were scanned for the occurrence of the sharp change in their amplitude based on a dynamic threshold which was calculated using the standard deviation of the EEG signals with a 100 ms window. The system was trained for about 2 minutes before the start of the actual experiment to be able to adapt with the signal variability. This threshold got renewed every 100 ms by calculating the ratio between the usual electrical activity and the existing threshold.

BCS Generation. In the EEG if an event was detected, a high BCS signal (i.e., 1) was generated otherwise it remained at low (i.e., 0). These processed individual channels were then multiplexed and sent to another computer running on Linux through an User Datagram Protocol (UDP) port using a crossover ethernet cable for interfacing with the robot to control it.

2.4   Interfacing with the Robotic Device

The interfacing with the robotic device was performed at the lower layer of the BCI flow (see figure 2). To process the BCS and to command the robotic device an open source software named 'IQR' [13] [14] was used. The IQR is a flexible platform for large scale neural simulation and robust application development to interface with robotic devices. This software allows design of large scale neuronal populations, and connect them with either excitatory or inhibitory connections.

To achieve our goal of controlling the navigation of the robotic device through steering its wheels using the BCS, three modules were developed (figure 4). Two main processes were designed to receive the BCS coming from the UDP port ('simulink IN' process) and sending a command to the mobile robot ('Robot' process) (figure 4 (a)). These individual processes (figure 4 (b) and (c)) were carefully designed, each with a number of neuronal populations to perform the desired task . The 'Simulink IN' process received the inputs from each EEG channel in the upper layer (indicated by the 'M' and an inward arrow to the square boxes in figure 4 (c)); on the other hand, the 'Robot' process was designed to control the movement of the robot's wheels (the communication with the mobile robotic device is indicated by the outward arrow and 'M' at the bottom square box of figure 4 (b)). As the nature of the BCS were binary, they were used to act as synapse, either excitatory or inhibitory, to make a population of neurons active or inactive.

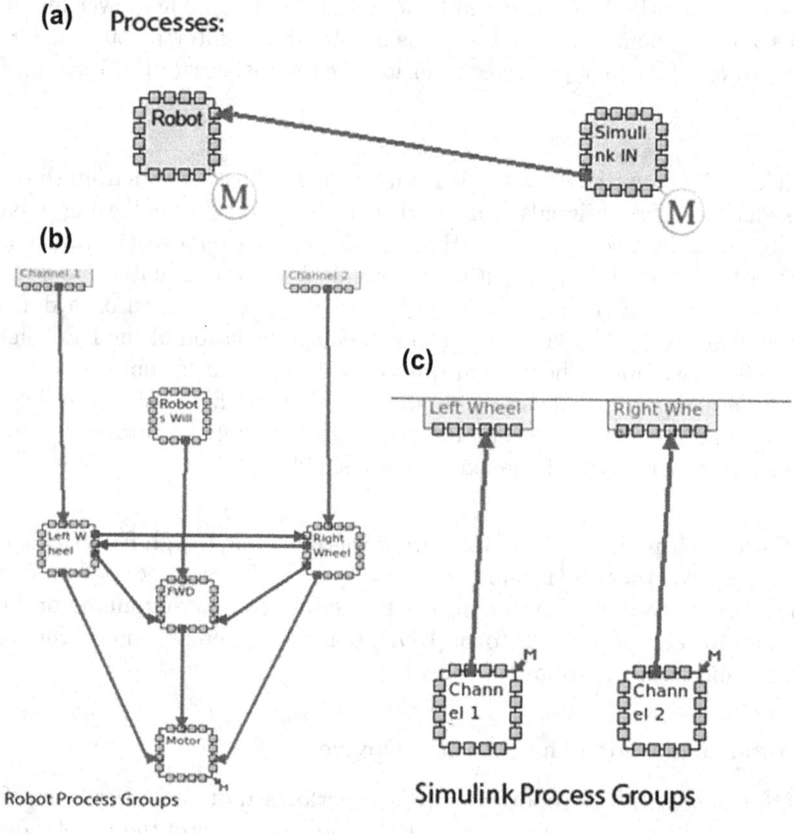

Fig. 4. IQR modules for generating and commanding the robotic device. The square boxes represent neuronal populations and the lines represent connectivity between two populations. The excitatory and inhibitory connections are shown using red and blue color lines, respectively.

The 'Simulink IN' process contained two neuronal populations: 'Channel 1' and 'Channel 2'. Each channel received input from one EEG electrode. The main purpose of this process was to continuously scan the BCS and send the relevant synaptic signal (high for 1 and low for 0) to the 'Robot' process to communicate with the mobile robotic device.

The 'Robot' process was designed to communicate and command the robotic device. This was done by five neuronal populations (as seen in figure 4 (b)). The five populations were to perform predefined tasks based on the input they received from the 'Simulink IN' process. The name and purpose of the neuronal populations are:

- **Motor:** This neuronal population represented and communicated with the motor of the robotic device. The robotic device was mainly commanded using this neuronal population.
- **Left Wheel:** This neuronal population received input from the 'Channel 1' and was connected to three other populations. It was mainly responsible to make the left wheel to move forward.
- **Right Wheel:** This neuronal population received input from the 'Channel 2' and was mainly responsible for the right wheel's forward movement.
- **Robot's Will:** This neuronal population represented the robot's will to move forward, thus, always provided high synapses to the population it was connected to (i.e., 'FWD').
- **FWD:** This neuronal population represented the combined movement of the left and the right wheels. When a synapse was made to the 'motor' neuronal population, both the wheels would move forward.

When there was no input: the Robot's will neuronal population constantly generated excitatory synapse to the Motor through the FWD neuronal population that kept the robotic device moving forward. Each time a neuronal population corresponding to a wheel fired: an excitatory synapse was sent to the Motor, an inhibitory synapse to the other wheel inactivating that wheel's activity, and another inhibitory synapse to the FWD neuronal population making the Motor to stop working for the previous command and to get ready to process the new command.

When a neuronal population corresponding to a wheel received a synaptic input, based on the channel from where it was generated the corresponding wheel's forward driving motor was activated and the other wheel was stopped. This operation caused the robot to take a turn (right or left) based on the received control signal. Once the control signal was low (i.e., 0), the stopped wheel was restarted thus continuing the forward movement.

For instance, let us assume that the Left wheel neuronal population received a synaptic input. This inactivated the 'Right wheel' and the 'FWD' neuronal populations through inhibitory synapses, and activated the 'Motor' neuronal population by an excitatory synapse; as a result, the right wheel was stopped, but the left wheel kept on rotating allowing the robotic device to turn right. Therefore, a synapse from a wheel was required to stop the other wheel to steer the robotic device to follow a predefined course by taking a left and a right turn.

3 Discussion

Though it started as a game at its beginning, gradual refinement to the signal processing algorithms and new neuronal population modeling using IQR, we demonstrated that it is not necessary to have many electrodes to interface and control robotic devices. It can very well be done using only three electrodes.

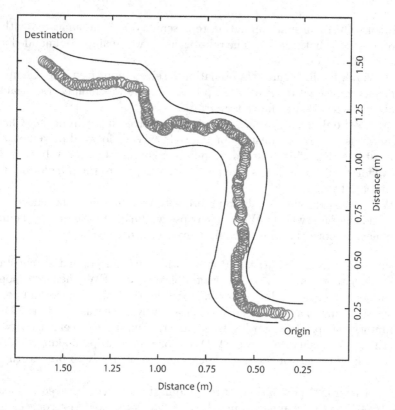

Fig. 5. Navigation result of the robotic device during an experiment to follow a pre-defined path

Healthy volunteers were plugged in with the necessary equipments of EEG signal detection. The recorded and artifact removed EEG signals related to the saccadic eye movement is shown in figure 3. The saccadic movement direction of the subject was clearly reflected through sharp changes of amplitude in recorded signals from the contralateral electrodes. The dynamic threshold detected this sharp change and generated the binary control signals which in turn triggered the activation of a particular neuronal population in the IQR modules by providing an excitatory synapse for taking a turn. The excitatory synapse from the forward movement neuronal population kept the robot moving forward; to turn the robotic device left, the left wheel was stopped through an inhibitory synapse generated by the right wheel neuronal population, and the vice-versa for a right turn. A combination of these saccadic movements can guide the robot to follow a predefined course, as seen in the figure 5.

4   Conclusion

This Brain-computer interface based on the EEG demonstrated in this paper was a proof-of-principle of reduced complexity BCI. By applying this technique it is possible to provide mobility to the people with motor dysfunction. The system was tested thoroughly using events caused by the saccadic eye movements and is to demonstrate the model's workability. It is very much possible to adapt and extend the BCI model to use any other type of signal (voluntary or involuntary) through proper signal processing techniques capable of transforming the input signal to a binary decision signal. It would be very useful to see the this model implemented to control assistive robotic devices (e.g., robotic wheelchair) for the disabled.

References

1. Mason, S., Birch, G.: A general framework for brain-computer interface design. IEEE Trans. Neural Syst. Rehabil. Eng. 11(1), 70–85 (2003)
2. Millán, J., Renkens, F., Mouriño, J., Gerstner, W.: Non-invasive brain-actuated control of a mobile robot. In: Proceedings of the 18th International Joint Conference on Artificial Intelligence, Acapulco, Mexico, pp. 1121–1126 (2003)
3. Vaughan, T.M., Heetderks, W.J., Trejo, L.J., Rymer, W.Z., Weinrich, M., Moore, M.M., Kübler, A., Dobkin, B.H., Birbaumer, N., Donchin, E., Wolpaw, E.W., Wolpaw, J.R.: Rain-computer interface technology: a review of the second international meeting. IEEE Trans. Neural Syst. Rehabil. Eng. 2(11), 94–109 (2003)
4. Fatourechi, M.: Design of a self-paced brain computer interface system using features extracted from three neurological phenomena. Ph.D. Dissertation, The University of British Colombia, Canada (2008)
5. Ferreira, A., Celeste, W., Cheein, F., Bastos-Filho, T., Sarcinelli-Filho, M., Carelli, R.: Human-machine interfaces based on EMG and EEG applied to robotic systems. Journal of NeuroEngineering and Rehabilitation 5(1), 10 (2008)
6. Moon, I., Lee, M., Chu, J.: Wearable emg-based hci for electric-powered wheelchair users with motor disabilities. In: Proceedings of 2005 IEEE International Conference on Robotics and Automation (ICRA 2005), Barcelona, Spain, pp. 2649–2654 (2005)
7. Mourino, J.: EEG-based analysis for the design of adaptive brain interfaces, Ph.D. Dissertation, Universitat Politecnica de Catalunya, Barcelona, Spain (2003)
8. Bi, L., Fan, X.A., Liu, Y.: EEG-based brain-controlled mobile robots: a survey. IEEE Trans. Human-Machine Systems 43(2), 161–176 (2013)
9. Mahmud, M., Hawellek, D., Valjamae, A.: A brain-machine interface based on EEG: extracted alpha waved applied to mobile robot. In: Proceedings of the 2009 ECSIS Symposium on Advanced Technologies for Enhanced Quality of Life (ATEQUAL 2009), Iasi, Romania, pp. 28–31 (2009)

10. Mahmud, M., Hawellek, D., Bertoldo, A.: EEG based brain-machine interface for navigation of robotic device. In: Proceedings of the 3rd IEEE/RAS-EMBS International Conference on Biomedical Robotics and Biomechatronics (BioRob 2010), Tokyo, Japan, pp. 168–172 (2010)

11. Mahmud, M., Bertoldo, A., Vassanelli, S.: EEG Based Brain Machine Interfacing: Navigation of Mobile Robotic Device. In: Bedkwoski, J. (ed.) Mobile Robots - Control Architectures, Bio-interfacing, Navigation, Multi Robot Motion Planning and Operator Training, pp. 129–144. Intech, Rijeka (2011) ISBN: 978-953-307-842-7

12. Ohno, K., Funase, A., Cichocki, A., Takumi, I.: Analysis of eeg signals in memory guided saccade tasks. In: IFMBE Proceedings of World Congress on Medical Physics and Biomedical Engineering, COEX Seoul, Korea, pp. 2664–2667 (2006)

13. Bernardet, U., Blanchard, M., Verschure, P.: IQR: a distributed system for real-time real-world neuronal simulation. Neurocomputing 44(46), 1043–1048 (2002)

14. Bernardet, U., Verschure, P.: IQR: A tool for the construction of multi-level simulations of brain and behaviour. Neurocomputing 8(2), 113–134 (2010)

15. Haas, S., Frei, M., Osorio, I., Pasik-Duncan, B., Radel, J.: EEG ocular artifact removal through armax model system identification using extended least squares. Communications in Information and Systems 3, 19–40 (2003)

16. Rohalova, M., Sykacek, P., Koska, M., Dorffner, G.: Detection of the eeg artifacts by the means of the (extended) kalman filter. Measurement Science Review 1, 59–62 (2001)

17. Mahmud, M., Bertoldo, A., Girardi, S., Maschietto, M., Vassanelli, S.: SigMate: a Matlab–based neuronal signal processing tool. In: 32nd Intl. Conf. of IEEE EMBS, pp. 1352–1355. IEEE Press, New York (2010)

18. Mahmud, M., et al.: SigMate: A Comprehensive Software Package for Extracellular Neuronal Signal Processing and Analysis. In: 5th Intl. Conf. on Neural Eng., pp. 88–91. IEEE Press, New York (2011)

19. Mahmud, M., Bertoldo, A., Girardi, S., Maschietto, M., Vassanelli, S.: SigMate: A MATLAB–based automated tool for extracellular neuronal signal processing and analysis. J. Nerusci. Meth. 207, 97–112 (2012)

Practical Speech Recognition
for Contextualized Service Robots

Ivan Vladimir Meza Ruiz*, Caleb Rascón, and Luis A. Pineda Cortes

Instituto de Investigaciones en Matemáticas Aplicdas y en Sistemas (IIMAS)
Universidad Nacional Autónoma de México (UNAM)
Ciudad Universitaria, D.F., México
ivanvladimir@turing.iimas.unam.com, caleb.rascon@iimas.unam.com,
lpineda@unam.com
http://www.iimas.unam.mx

Abstract. In this work, we present the speech recognition module of a service robot that performs various tasks, such as being a host party, receiving multiple commands or giving a tour guide. These tasks take place in diverse acoustic environments, e.g., a home or a supermarket, in which speech is one of the main modalities of interaction. Our approach relies on three strategies: 1) making the recognizer aware of the task context, 2) providing prompting strategies to guide the recognition, and 3) calibrating the audio setting specific to the environment. We provide an evaluation with recordings from real interactions with a service robot in different environments.

Keywords: speech recognition, service robots, language models.

1 Introduction

Service robots have the goal to help humans on a wide range of day-to-day activities, such as cleaning and organizing the home, shopping in a supermarket or hosting a restaurant. A natural way to interact with service robots during the realization of a task is using speech in order to indicate the room to clean, the products to shop or the order to bring. On one hand, task-based speech recognition is not as complex as open domain applications such as web search, because the language to be used is more constrained. On the other hand, the setting for a service robot imposes great challenges, since the recognition is carry out in noisy environments, in which the performance of speech recognition is affected

* We thank Lisset Salinas, Gibran Fuentes, Arturo Rodriguez, Esther Venegas, Varinia Estrada, Iván Sánchez, Mario Peña, Carlos Gershenson, Mauricio Reyes, Hernando Ortega and Joel Duran for creating the infrastructure which made possible the recollection of the Golem-II+ Log corpus. We also thank the early suggestions from Lucian Galescu for the development of our speech recognition system. Finally, we thank the support of CONACYT through the project 81965, and PAPIIT-UNAM with the project IN115710-3.

F. Castro, A. Gelbukh, and M. González (Eds.): MICAI 2013, Part II, LNAI 8266, pp. 423–434, 2013.
© Springer-Verlag Berlin Heidelberg 2013

[1]. Additionally, in order to have an autonomous robot is preferable that the microphone system is located on-board. This makes it difficult to guarantee a clean speech signal since the user cannot be expected to be close to the microphone.

In the present approach we take advantage of the structure of the task. For instance, if a robot acts as a host party there could be a part in which the guests introduce themselves, and another stage in which the robot takes an order from them. Our intuition is that the Automatic Speech Recognition (ASR) module can benefit from the task structure since the language used during a task will change dynamically. In the case of service robot the context is defined by the progress of the robot in the task, which is commonly referred as the state of the task. In particular, we propose to tie this state to a particular language model: if the robot asks *would you like to continue*, the speech recognizer module would load a language model specific for the *yes* and *no* answers. Other examples of possible language models are common names, objects, locations, etc. We call this strategy *contextualized speech recognition*.

However, there are cases in which the complexity of the environment or the task make the speech recognition fails. For these we propose complement speech recognition with *prompting strategies*: first, the robot asks the user to repeat or paraphrase what he/she has said; second, we identify whether the user speaks too low or high to be intelligible by the robot; and third, the robot provides audio feedback when the recognizer has started and stopped listening. The goal of the prompting strategies is to contextualize the user about *what*, *how* and *when* the robot is expecting an interaction.

In addition to the previous strategies, we also use a calibration procedure that is based on the signal to noise radio (SNR). It aims to identify the best setting for the microphones in order to catch an appropriate speech signal. The calibration is performed *in situ*.

In summary, the three strategies aim to take advantage of contextual aspects of the task. First, guide ASR with the changes of language during the task; second, contextualize the user with what the robot is expecting; and finally, to take into account the acoustic context. These three strategies and their evaluation are outlined as follows. In Section 2, we present an overview of previous work in robust speech recognition for service robots. In Section 3, we introduce the cognitive architecture and dialogue models that underlie the development of our system. In Section 4, we explain the contextualized speech recognition. In Section 5, we introduce the prompting strategies. In Section 6, we review our software and hardware setting. In Section 7, we present an evaluation of the proposed strategies. Finally, in Section 8, we present the conclusions of this work.

2   Previous Work

The use of speech as a mean of communication for a service robot is a current topic of research. For instance, in the RoboCup@Home competition most of the teams use a speech recognition system [2]. The main challenge is to maintain a robust performance in noisy environments using on-board microphones. The reduction on speech performance can be so significant that some developments provide alternative modalities of interaction [3].

Doostdar et. al. [4] propose parallel decoding approach, called dual in their work. They focus on the decoding techniques for the language model. In their case, they use a finite state grammar (FSG) and a trigram model in parallel; FSGs have a high accuracy but are too constrained for natural language expressions, while the trigram models are more flexible. *Heinrich and Wermter* ([5]) extend this idea by using a multipass decoder which uses also a combination of a FSGs and a trigram model. In their work, they also present a comparison between headset, ceiling and on-board microphones.

Ishi et. al. [6] present a rich speech module setting in their robot. Their system uses an array of twelve omnidirectional microphones arranged in a T-shape, to track the audio signal in front the robot. The signal is cleaned by using feature-space single-channel noise suppression. The clean signal is passed on a voice activity detection phase and reach the speech recognizer when required. This work also presents the use of parallel decoding for adults and children speech. However, this setting faced difficulties in a field trial at a train station [7].

Our work differs from previous research in two ways: 1) we trigger different decoders for different context of the task, instead of using parallel decoding 2) we do not pre-process the speech signal to track it or clean it. We rely in a calibration done *in situ* to reach a good quality of speech from a user in front of the robot. Additionally, we explore the use of prompting strategies, which help to reach a satisfactory interaction. All this while keeping the number of microphones involved in speech recognition on board at a minimum (1 microphone).

3 Cognitive Architecture and Dialogue Models

The behavior of our robot, Golem-II+, is regulated by the Interaction-Oriented Cognitive Architecture (IOCA, [8]). IOCA coordinates the different skill-modules of the robot in order to perform a task. IOCA relies on a reactive and an interpretation cycle (see Figure 1). In the reactive cycle, the recognition and the rendering modules interact together to produce a specific reaction to an input. For instance, obstacle avoidance can be implemented in this fashion. In this case, the obstacle recognition module detects obstacles in certain positions and interacts directly with the navigation module to avoid them.

For the interpretation cycle, IOCA proposes three stages: *recognition - interpretation, dialogue management* and *specification - rendering*. In the stage of recognition - interpretation, the external stimulus is interpreted in the context of the task. For instance, if the user asks the robot *go and clean the kitchen* such speech is interpreted as *clean(kitchen)*. The dialogue management stage relates such interpretation with the corresponding actions. For our example, the dialogue management stage might choose to execute the actions *navigate(Place)* and *clean(Place)*. Finally, the specification-rendering stage will perform such actions.

Dialogue models are used by the dialogue management stage to control the flow of the interaction. A dialogue model represents the structure of task and

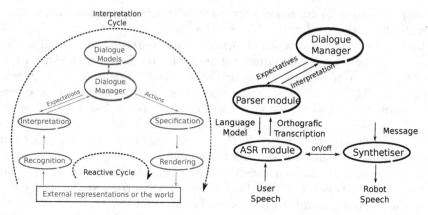

Fig. 1. Interaction Oriented Cognitive Architecture and Speech module (ASR module)

is composed by situations, expectations and actions. Situations abstract over stages on the realization of a task in which the robot has a set of expectations codified in advance in the dialogue model.

In particular, the speech recognition module takes part in both the reactive and interpretation cycles. In the former cycle, it interacts with the synthesizer to prevent voice synthesis when the speech module is on, or vice versa. As a part of the interpretation cycle, the speech recognition module is in charge of producing an orthographic transcription which is further parsed and interpreted. Figure 1 illustrates the speech recognition module in the context of the IOCA architecture.

4   Contextualized Speech Recognition

A common strategy to boost speech recognition performance in service robots is to handcraft the language models specific to the task rather than using general purpose speech recognition [12,9]. Indeed, from previous experience in the field of dialogue systems, we know that contextualized language models improve the performance of such systems [10,11].

In the present framework, we constrain the model of the expected phrases depending on the context. The context is defined by the state of the task. In the IOCA architecture, this strategy is straightforward to implement. The expectations, which are tied to situations, are passed top-down to the parser module to trigger a specific language model to be used in the speech recognizer (ASR) as illustrated in Figure 1. Table 1 illustrates some examples of the expectations and their associate language models. In case there is more than one expectation for a situation (e.g., a *yes/no* answer) a combination of two or more language models is triggered.

Table 1. Language models for specific expectations

Expectations	Utterance examples
yes	*yes,okay,all right, . . .*
no	*no,don't, do not, . . .*
navigate(X)	*go to the kitchen, go to the living room, go to the bedroom, . . .*

5   Prompting and Recovery Strategies

The success of contextualized recognition and interpretation relies on identifying the correct language models for the different contexts. In order to guide the user about what the robots expects, we incorporate prompting strategies in the definition of dialogue models. So far, we have analyzed three prompting cases:

1. Beep sounds to signal when the recognizer is listening.
2. A module which monitors the volume of the user speech.
3. Asking the user what to repeat or paraphrase when the speech recognition fails.

In the first case, the speech recognizer module provides feedback through two different beep sounds. The first indicates when to start speaking; the robot is programmed to wait up to two seconds for a user utterance, otherwise the robot claims it did not listen anything. The second beep indicates the user when the speech recognizer is switched off paying attention (other robots follow a similar strategy [13].)

For the second case, we implement a module which we named *LoudSystem*. This module monitors the sound and provides an assessment of the speech loudness. This assessment is used by the dialogue model to provide feedback if the user is speaking too loud or too soft. This module assumes that the magnitude of the energy of the background noise is -58 dB (because of the calibration of the volume settings as described in section 6). Under this assumption, a real-time estimation of the signal to noise ratio (SNR) is computed using the energy values obtained while the user is speaking. This is compared to the assumed noise energy value. In this way, the SNR provides a good measure of how loud the speech of the user is, compared to the background noise.

Finally, for the third case, when some interactions of the user result in something that the system was not expecting, the speech system fails and the robot asks to repeat the interaction or paraphrase it. In some more drastic cases the system abandons the action or the task. Table 2 shows some examples of the prompting messages used by the robot in the *Follow me* task (see RoboCup@Home [14]).

Table 2. Examples of prompting messages for Following the user task

could you repeat it
i can't hear you well, could you repeat
say follow me one more time
say follow me again please
sorry, i'm a little deaf, say follow me

6   Audio Setting and Calibration

Our robot system consists of a mobile platform with on-board microphones. Our strategy to guarantee a consistent performance of the speech recognizer is to perform a calibration of the audio setting at the location where the robot performs the task.

The audio setting of the robot consists of the following hardware[1]:

- 1 directional microphone
- 1 USB interface with 4 channels
- 2 speakers

The directional microphone is the source of sound for the speech recognition module. This implies that the user has to speak face to face to the robot in order to reach a good sound quality. From our experience, we have noticed that the directionality of the microphone provides a good quality speech signal. The two speakers are used to generate sound feedback to the user (e.g., such as synthesized voice or prompting signals).

The volume settings of the audio system are manually calibrated using a monitor. The monitor provides the energy magnitude of the directional microphone signal. The goal of the calibration procedure is to define a level for the background noise. Extensive tests carried out in several acoustic circumstances showed that the energy of this signal, when no user is speaking near the robot, should be close to −58 dB to provide a good balance between noise reduction and speech intelligibility.

Additionally, it was found that a SNR value around 20 dB provided a good speech recognition performance for the case of *LoudSystem* module. This is due to the assumption of a static speech energy value (−58 dB) throughout the interaction, a SNR value that is far from 20 dB implies that the user is either whispering, screaming or that a non-stationary noise has occurred. In the first two cases, the acoustic features of the voice are corrupted, which is a problem for speech recognition. For the last case, the module serves as a simple SNR-based filter.

7   Evaluation

We have evaluated the three strategies presented above. First, we have determined the improvement of the recognizer using the contextualized speech recognition. Second, we have measured the effect of the prompting strategies on the speech recognition or human-robot interaction. Finally, we have measured the effect of the performance of the speech recognition in alternative calibration settings.

---

[1] The specific equipment is: One RODE VideoMic microphone, one M-Audio Fast Track Ultra external sound interface and two generic speakers.

Table 3. *Robot Log* corpus statistics

Number of utterances/recordings	1,439	Number of tasks	11
Vocabulary size (token)	2,472	Number of contextualized tasks	9
Vocabulary size (type)	120	Number of contextualized LMs	14

Table 4. Performance for *full-based*, *task-based* and *contextualized* speech recognition (WER, the lower the better)

LM	Vocab. size	Utt No.	WER	LM	Vocab. size	Utt No.	WER
Unique LM				Contextualized Speech Recognition			
Total	198	1,439	53.84%	yes/no	3	588	6.66%
Task-based Speech Recognition				follow me	6	226	25.17%
Who is who	52	285	34.91%	products	69	139	55.40%
Shopping mall	80	262	36.94%	room	6	94	30.98%
Restaurants	73	244	14.50%	common names	21	63	31.34%
Follow me	10	219	30.25%	types of destinations	13	59	17.24%
GPSR-I	122	166	30.25%	drinks	22	50	28.07%
Clean-it-up	122	116	27.27%	restaurant order	54	41	14.81%
Pharmacy staff	11	97	15.79%	complex command	96	38	43.64%
Nurse	80	29	50.85%	medicine	9	35	12.50%
Cleaner	9	21	2.17%	start hosting party	9	33	4.17%
Total	-	1,439	28.28%	leave elevator	5	31	13.56%
				host party order	15	29	38.89%
				cleaner order	5	13	0.0%
				Total	-	1,439	23.42%

For the evaluations we use the *Robot Log* corpus[2]. This consists of a collection of one year logs of out robot *Golem-II+* performing different tasks related to the RoboCup@Home competition [3] [14] (2011 and 2012 rulebooks). This corpus is composed by the dialogue manager logs and the speech recordings from user interactions while the robot performed a task or was tested during the development process. Table 3 summarizes the main properties of this corpus. The users in the corpus range from members of our research group to members of the RoboCup@Home competitions, all of them adults. We have selected the 9 contextualized task for the evaluation[4]:

— Who is who: a party host.
— Shopping mall: companion while shopping.
— Restaurant: waitress in charge of bringing objects to the table.

---

[2] Available in http://golem.iimas.unam.mx/RobotLog
[3] Some videos of the robot in action are available at
http://www.youtube.com/user/golemiimas
[4] The task and language model lists and results will be ordered by the number of utterances, from larger to fewer.

- Follow me: following a user in a diverse environment.
- General Purpose Service Robot: execute complex commands.
- Clean-it-up: cleans a room of objects.
- Pharmacy staff: in charge of getting a prescription and delivering the medicine.
- Nurse: helps carrying objects.
- Cleaner: cleaning tables with a cloth.

The contextualized language models are:

- yes/no (e.g., *yes, no*).
- follow me (e.g., *follow me, come with me*).
- products (e.g., *coke, toy*).
- drinks (e.g., *orange juice, milk*).
- names (e.g., *mary, anthony*).
- types of destination (e.g., *table one, drinks*).
- restaurant order (e.g., *toy to table one, cookies to table two*).
- leave elevator (e.g., *leave, get out*).
- start hosting party (e.g., *start*).
- complex command (e.g., *go to the table introduce yourself and leave*).
- medicine (e.g., *vitamins, cough syrup*).
- host party order (e.g., *coke to john, sprite to emma*).
- cleaner order (e.g., *clean table one*).
- staff order (e.g., *i want an anti flu*).

For the evaluation, we only vary the language models in the speech recognizer. All language models were created using a bi-gram configuration. The speech recognition system used on the evaluation is based on PocketSphinx with the default setting and acoustic models (i.e., `hub4wsj_sc_8k`) which makes it a user-independent recognizer.

In order to evaluate contextualized speech recognition we compared the word error rate (WER, the lower the better) of the contextualized recognition versus the *unique* language model and the *task-based* strategies. Table 4 summarizes these results. On top of the table, we see the WER when using an unique language model, which is quite high. This is followed by the performance of the task-based speech recognition for each of the tasks which remember is the common strategy nowadays. Finally, the table enumerates the performance for the contextualized speech recognition. From these results, we can see that there is a large difference between using a unique language model versus one for each task. This provides an improvement in the reduction of error of 47.5%. Also notice that the contextualized speech recognition provides the best performance with an improvement of 4.9% points of the WER, which is equivalent to an improvement of 17.2% when compared with the *task-based* strategy.

Table 4 also illustrates some interesting facts for the language models. The most common utterances were *yes/no* answers. This can be explained by the strategy followed by the designers of the tasks in which the robot frequently asks for confirmation. Since the complexity of this language model is minimum

Table 5. Direct comparison for *task-based* and *contextualized* speech recognition (WER the lower the better)

Contextualized LMs				Contextualized LMs			
WER	LM	No. Utts	WER	WER	LM	No. Utts	WER
Who is who				GPSR-I			
34.91%	yes/no	121	3.28%	30.25	yes/no	118	4.20%
	names	56	28.33%		complex	38	43.64%
	drinks	46	30.00%		follow	5	20.00%
	orders	29	38.89%		names	5	40.00%
	hosting	33	4.17%		**total**	166	34.10%
	total	285	16.27%	Clean-it-up			
Shopping mall					room	94	30.98%
36.94%	products	139	55.40%	27.27	yes/no	22	16.00%
	yes/no	118	9.17%		**total**	116	29.19%
	follow	5	11.11%	Pharmacy staff			
	total	262	33.20%	15.79	yes/no	62	10.61%
Restaurant					medicine	35	12.50%
14.50%	yes/no	136	5.80%		**total**	97	11.40%
	label	59	17.24%	Nurse			
	order	41	14.81%	50.85%	follow	24	57.41%
	drink	4	14.29%		yes/no	3	0.0%
	follow	4	50.00%		names	2	100.00%
	total	244	12.75%		**total**	29	42.37%
Follow me				Cleaner			
30.25%	follow	188	22.73%	2.17%	order	13	0.0%
	elevator	31	13.568%		yes/no	8	12.50%
	total	219	21.48%		**total**	21	2.17%

(2 words) its performance is high (i.e., 6.66% WER). On the other hand, the language model *products* has the worst performance. This can be explained by the nature of the corpus in which this task did not reach a full cycle of development.

Table 5 presents a more direct comparison between the performance of the task-based and the contextualized strategy per task. For each task, the table presents the WER for a task-based strategy and its contextualized version. It also presents a total which is comparable with the task-based WER. For most cases, there is an improvement when using a contextualized speech recognition with an average gain of 3.8 WER points.

For the evaluation of the prompting strategies, we measured three aspects. For the two beeps approach we measured the performance of a speech recognizer with and without the inclusion of such strategy. Unfortunately, the data is not balanced, as the corpus has few examples recorded without the beep strategy. To overcome this problem, we compared the performance of the recogniser on those utterances with two sets of uttereances recorded using the beep strategy. The first set contains the same amount of utterances and correspond to the first 79 recorded utterances after introducing the strategy, the second set contains all

Table 6. Results of the prompting strategies

Two beeps		
Strategy	Utt No.	WER
Without beeps	79	55.86%
With beeps	79	39.75%
With beeps (full corpus)	1370	53.72%
LoudSystem		
Could be triggered		174
Times soft speech detected		21
Times loud speech detected		4
Repeat and paraphrase		
Could be triggered		504
Times activated		85

Table 7. WER performance of speech recognition of language models (the higher the SNR the less noise, the lower the WER the better)

LM	SNR						
	10	12	14	16	18	20	22
yes/no	6.66%	6.49%	6.66%	6.66%	6.66%	6.82%	6.82%
follow me	38.85%	36.20%	33.11%	31.35%	29.80%	28.48%	26.71%
products	61.87%	58.27%	55.40%	56.83%	53.96%	52.52%	53.96%
room	35.82%	32.84%	35.82%	32.84%	34.33%	32.84%	31.34%
names	35.82%	32.84%	35.82%	32.84%	34.33%	32.84%	31.34%
types of destination	20.69%	19.54%	19.54%	19.54%	20.69%	18.39%	14.94%
drinks	45.61%	35.09%	29.82%	28.07%	29.82%	28.07%	28.07%

the utterances that were recorded using the beeps. For all cases we measure the WER performance using the *unique* LM from the previous evaluation. As Table 6 shows, the cases which use the two beep strategy improve the performance.

Table 6 also presents the evaluation for the case of the *LoudSystem* and of asking to paraphrase or repeat. We noticed that both strategies were relatively seldom used (approx. 16% of the time). The *LoudSystem* could have been triggered 174 times from which only 25 prompted the user. In the case of asking to repeat from the 504 in which a repetition was possible only 85 were necessary. We notice that the *LoudSystem* is more sensitive to detect when the person is speaking softly, this could be for a variety of reasons, for instance the user does not speak in front of the microphone or is faraway the robot.

Finally, we measured the effect of alternative calibration settings to the chosen for our calibration. The settings were automatically generated using the methodology proposed by *Dean et. al.* ([16]). The generation consists on mixing recordings of a type of noise (e.g., street, food court noisie) and recordings of speech. The SNR level is controlled during such mixing. In particular, we used the food court type of noise[5], the Robot Log corpus as the speech source and

---

[5] Labelled as *CAFE-FOODCOURTB1* in the type noise corpus.

we tried various SNR levels (i.e., 10 to 22). For this, we measured speech performance of seven of the contextualized language models. The seven LMs where
chosen because they had more than 50 interactions in the corpus. For each language model we evaluate the WER for each setting. Table 7 summarizes the
findings. As expected, a noisier environment worsens speech recognition. However, we can notice that if we did not specify to 20 dB as our base SNR, the
performance would have been reduced. It is important to notice as well that the
achieved performance is as good as the performance reached in original settings
(see Table 4).

8   Conclusions

In this work, we have presented three strategies that improve practical speech
recognition in a service robot. These strategies are: 1) contextualized speech
recognition, 2) the use of prompting strategies, and 3) *in situ* calibration of
our audio hardware. In the case of contextualized speech recognition we use the
context of the task to direct the speech recognition process through the use of
specific language models. In the case of the prompting strategies, the goal is to
communicate the context of what the robot is expecting to the user so he/she
knows when, how and what to say. And for the calibration setting strategy, we
take advantage of the environmental context in which the robot performs the
task.

The strategies were evaluated with the Robot Log corpus. We found that the
use of the contextualized speech recognition improves the performance in the
recognition module. We also found that the prompting strategies have a positive
effect on the interaction. In particular, we found evidence that the strategy of
letting know the user when to speak with a couple beeps improves the speech
recognition performance. We also found evidence that calibrating our system has
had a positive effect on the type of speech signal we obtain and on recognition
rates.

These strategies were implemented in the Golem-II+ robot at different stages
of its development. As we incorporated and tuned them we found these provided
a good base for a speech recognition module in a service robot using an out of the
box recognizer. At the core of the strategies is to take advantage of the context. It
is his exploitation and the combination of the strategies which has made possible
to improve the performance of the speech recognition in our service robot.

References

1. Paliwal, K.K., Yao, K.: Robust speech recognition under noisy ambient conditions.
   In: Human-Centric Interfaces for Ambient Intelligence, ch. 6, pp. 135–162. Academic Press, Elsevier (2009)
2. Iocchi, I., Ruiz-del-Solar, J., van der Zant, T.: Domestic Service Robots in the Real
   World. Intelligent & Robotic Systems 66, 183–186 (2012)
3. Kanda, T., Shiomi, M., Miyashita, Z., Ishiguro, H., Hagita, N.: A Communication
   Robot in a Shopping Mall. IEEE Transctions on Robotics 26(5), 897–913 (2010)

4. Doostdar, M., Schiffer, S., Lakemeyer, G.: A Robust Speech Recognition System for Service-Robotics Applications. In: Iocchi, L., Matsubara, H., Weitzenfeld, A., Zhou, C. (eds.) RoboCup 2008. LNCS, vol. 5399, pp. 1–12. Springer, Heidelberg (2009)
5. Heinrich, S., Wermter, S.: Towards Robust Speech Recognition for Human-Robot Interaction In. In: Proc. IROS 2011 Workshop on Cognitive Neuroscience Robotics, pp. 29–34 (2011)
6. Ishi, C.T., Matsuda, S., Kanda, T., Jitsuhiro, T., Ishiguro, H., Nakamura, S., Hagita, N.: Robust speech recognition system for communication robots in real environments. In: Proceedings of IEEE International Conference on Humanoid Robots (Humanoids 2006), pp. 340–345 (2006)
7. Shiomi, M., Sakamoto, D., Kanda, T., Ishi, C., Ishiguro, H., Hagita, N.: A semi-autonomous Communication Robot - A field Trail ar a Train Station. In: Proc. ACM/IEEE Int. Conference on Human Robot Interaction, pp. 380–389 (2008)
8. Pineda, L., Meza, I., Avilés, H., Gershenson, C., Rascón, C., Alvarado, M., Salinas, L.: IOCA: Interaction-Oriented Cognitive Architecture Research in Computer Science, vol. 54, pp. 273–284 (2011)
9. Bharatheesha, M., Rudinac, M., Chandarr, A., Gaisser, F., Pons, S., Küpers, B., Driessen, S., Bruinink, M., Wisse, M., Jonker, P.: Delf+ Robotics RoboCup@Home 2012 team Description Paper. In: Proccedings of RoboCup 2012 (2012)
10. Lemon, O., Gruenstein, A.: Multithreaded context for robust conversational interfaces: context-sensitive speech recognition and interpretation of corrective fragments. ACM Transactions on Computer-Human Interaction (ACM TOCHI) 11(3), 241–267 (2004)
11. Galescu, L., Allen, J., Ferguson, G., Quinn, J., Swift, M.: Speech Recognition in a Dialog System for Patient Health Monitoring. In: Proceedings of the IEEE International Conference on Bioinformatics and Biomedicine (BIBM 2009) Workshop on NLP Approaches (2009)
12. Ruiz-del-Solar, J., Correa, M., Smith, F., Loncomilla, P., Pairo, W., Verschae, R.: UChile HomeBreakers 2012 Team Description Paper. In: Proceedings of RoboCup 2012 (2012)
13. Hegger, F., Müller, C., Jin, Z., Álvarez, J., Giorgana, G., Hochgeschwender, N., Reckhaus, M., Paulus, J., Ploeger, P., Kraetzschmar, G.: The b-it-bots RoboCup@Home 2011 Team Description Paper. In: Proceedings of RoboCup 2011 (2011)
14. van der Zant, T., Wisspeintner, T.: RoboCup X: A proposal for a new league where roboCup goes real world. In: Bredenfeld, A., Jacoff, A., Noda, I., Takahashi, Y. (eds.) RoboCup 2005. LNCS (LNAI), vol. 4020, pp. 166–172. Springer, Heidelberg (2006)
15. Huggins-Dainesi, D., Kumar, M., Chan, A., Black, A.W., Ravishankar, M., Rudnicky, A.I.: PocketSphinx: A Free, Real-Time Continuous Speech Recognition System for Hand-Held Devices. In: Proc. of ICASSP 2006 (2006)
16. Dean, D., Sridharan, S., Vogt, R., Mason, M.: The QUT-NOISE-TIMIT corpus for the evaluation of voice activity detection algorithms. In: Proceedings of INTER-SPEECH 2010, pp. 3110–3113 (2010)

Using Monte Carlo Tree Search to Solve Planning Problems in Transportation Domains

Otakar Trunda and Roman Barták

Charles University in Prague, Faculty of Mathematics and Physics
Malostranské náměstí 25, Praha, Czech Republic
otaTrunda@gmail.com, bartak@ktiml.mff.cuni.cz

Abstract. Monte Carlo Tree Search (MCTS) techniques brought fresh breeze to the area of computer games where they significantly improved solving algorithms for games such as Go. MCTS also worked well when solving a real-life planning problem of the Petrobras company brought by the Fourth International Competition on Knowledge Engineering Techniques for Planning and Scheduling. In this paper we generalize the ideas of using MCTS techniques in planning, in particular for transportation problems. We highlight the difficulties of applying MCTS in planning, we show possible approaches to overcome these difficulties, and we propose a particular method for solving transportation problems.

Keywords: planning, search, Monte Carlo, logistic, transportation.

1 Introduction

Planning deals with problems of selection and causally ordering of actions to achieve a given goal from a known initial situation. Planning algorithms assume a description of possible actions and attributes of the world states in some modeling language such as Planning Domain Description Language (PDDL) as its input. This makes the planning algorithms general and applicable to any planning problem starting from building blocks to towers and finishing with planning transport of goods between warehouses. Currently, the most efficient approach to solve planning problems is heuristic forward search. The paper [13] showed that classical planners are not competitive when solving a real-life transportation planning problem of the Petrobras company [15]. The paper proposed an ad-hoc Monte Carlo Tree Search (MCTS) algorithm that beat the winning classical planner SGPlan in terms of problems solved and solution quality. This brought us to the idea of generalizing the MCTS algorithm to a wider class of planning problems. A sampling based approach has already been investigated in the field of planning [17] (in a simplified form). The Arvand planner [9] proved that the idea of using random-walks to evaluate states in deterministic planning is viable.

Monte Carlo Tree Search algorithm is a stochastic method originally proposed for computer games. MCTS was modified for a single-player games and it is also applicable to optimization problems. However, there are still difficulties when applying to planning problems, namely existence of infinite sequences of

F. Castro, A. Gelbukh, and M. González (Eds.): MICAI 2013, Part II, LNAI 8266, pp. 435–440, 2013.
© Springer-Verlag Berlin Heidelberg 2013

actions and dead-ends. In this paper we identify these difficulties and we discuss possible ways to overcome them. We then show how to modify the MCTS algorithm to be applicable to a planning problem specification enhanced by so called meta-actions. We demonstrate this idea using transportation problems which are natural generalizations of the Petrobras domain [15].

The paper is organized as follows. We will first give a short background on planning and Monte Carlo Tree Search techniques and we will highlight possible problems when applying MCTS in planning including a discussion how to resolve these problems. We will then characterize the transportation planning domains and show how to identify them automatically. After that we will describe the modifications necessary to apply MCTS to solve planning problems in transportation (and possible other) domains. The paper will be concluded by experimental comparison of our approach with the LPG planner [6].

2   Background

2.1   Planning

In this paper we deal with classical planning problems, that is, with finding a sequence of actions transferring the world from a given initial state to a state satisfying certain goal condition [5]. *World states* are represented as sets of predicates that are true in the state (all other predicates are false in the state). For example the predicate $at(r1, l1)$ represents information that some object $r1$ is at location $l1$. *Actions* describe how the world state can be changed. Each action a is defined by a set of predicates $prec(a)$ as its precondition and two disjoint sets of predicates $eff^+(a)$ and $eff^-(a)$ as its positive and negative effects. Action a is applicable to state s if $prec(a) \subseteq s$ holds. If action a is applicable to state s then a new state $\gamma(a, s)$ defines the state after application of a as

$$\gamma(a, s) = (s \cup eff^+(a)) - eff^-(a)$$

Otherwise, the state $\gamma(a, s)$ is undefined. The goal g is usually defined as a set of predicates that must be true in the goal state. Hence the state s is a *goal state* if and only if $g \subseteq s$.

The *satisficing planning task* is formulated as follows: given a description of the initial state s_0, a set A of available actions, and a goal condition g, is there a sequence of actions $(a_1, \ldots, a_n)$, called a *solution plan*, such that $a_i \in A$, a_1 is applicable to state s_0, each a_i s.t. $i > 1$ is applicable to state $\gamma(a_{i-1}, \ldots \gamma(a_1, s_0))$, and $g \subseteq \gamma(a_n, \gamma(a_{n-1}, \ldots \gamma(a_1, s_0)))$?

Assume that each action a has some cost $c(a)$. An *optimal planning task* is about finding a solution plan such that the sum of costs of actions in the plan is minimized. Formally, the task is to find a sequence of actions $(a_1, \ldots, a_n)$, called an *optimal plan*, minimizing $\sum_{i=1}^{n} c(a_i)$ under the condition $g \subseteq \gamma(a_n, \gamma(a_{n-1}, \ldots \gamma(a_1, s_0)))$. In this paper we deal only with the optimal planning task so for brevity we will be talking about planning while we will mean optimal planning.

In practice, the planning problem is typically specified in two components: a planning domain and a planning problem itself. The *planning domain* specifies the names of predicates used to describe world states. For example, *at(?movable, ?location)* means that we can use relations *at* between movable objects and locations (typing is used to classify objects/constants). Similarly, instead of actions the planning domain describes so called *operators* that are templates for actions. A particular action is obtained by substituting particular objects (constants) to the operator. We will give examples of operators specified in the PDDL language later in the text. The *planning problem* then specifies a particular goal condition and an initial state and hence it also gives the names of used objects (constants).

2.2   Monte Carlo Tree Search

Monte Carlo Tree Search (MCTS) is a stochastic optimization algorithm that combines classical tree search with random sampling of the search space. The algorithm was originally used in the field of game playing where it became very popular, especially for games Go and Hex. A single player variant has been developed by Schadd et al. [11] which is designed specifically for single-player games and can also be applied to optimization problems. The MCTS algorithm successively builds an asymmetric tree to represent the search space by repeatedly performing the following four steps:

1. *Selection* – The tree built so far is traversed from the root to a leaf using some criterion (called *tree policy*) to select the most urgent leaf.
2. *Expansion* – All applicable actions for the selected leaf node are applied and the resulting states are added to the tree as successors of the selected node (sometimes different strategies are used).
3. *Simulation* – A pseudo-random simulation is run from the selected node until some final state is reached (a state that has no successors). During the simulation the actions are selected by a *simulation policy*,
4. *Update/Back-propagation* – The result of the simulation is propagated back in the tree from the selected node to the root and statistics of the nodes on this path are updated according to the result.

The core schema of MCTS is shown at Figure 1 from [3].

One of the most important parts of the algorithm is the *node selection criterion* (a tree policy). It determines which node will be expanded and therefore it affects the shape of the search tree. The purpose of the tree policy is to solve the exploration vs. exploitation dilemma.

Commonly used policies are based on a so called *bandit problem* and *Upper Confidence Bounds for Trees* [1,7] which provide a theoretical background to measure quality of policies. We will present here the tree policy for the single-player variant of MCTS (SP-MCTS) due to Schadd et al. [11] that is appropriate for planning problems (planning can be seen as a single-player game where moves correspond to action selection).

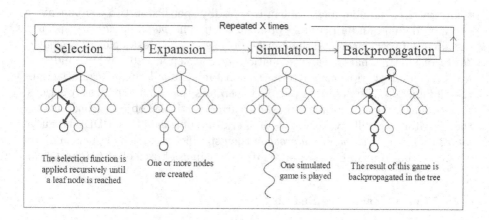

Fig. 1. Basic schema of MCTS [3]

Let $t(N)$ be the number of simulations/samples passing the node N, $v_i(N)$ be the value of i-th simulation passing the node N, and $\bar{v}(N)$ be the average value of all simulations passing the node N:

$$\bar{v}(N) = \frac{\sum_{i=1}^{t(N)} v_i(N)}{t(N)}$$

The SP-MCTS tree policy suggests to select the children node N_j of node N maximizing the following function:

$$\bar{v}(N_j) + C \cdot \sqrt{\frac{2\ln(t(N))}{t(N_j)}} + \sqrt{\frac{\sum_{i=1}^{t(N_j)} v_i(N_j)^2 - t(N_j) \cdot \bar{v}(N_j)^2}{t(N_j)}}$$

The first component of the above formula is a so called *Expectation* and it describes an expected value of the path going through a given node. This supports exploitation of accumulated knowledge about quality of paths. The second component is a *Bias*. The Bias component of a node N_j slowly increases every time the sibling of N_j is selected (that is every time the node enters the competition for being selected but it is defeated by another node) and rapidly decreases every time the node N_j is selected, that is the policy prefers nodes that have not been selected for a long time. This supports exploration of unknown parts of the search tree. *Bias* is weighted by a constant C that determines the *exploration vs. exploitation* ratio. Its value depends on the domain and on other modifications to the algorithm. For example in computer Go the usual value is about 0.2. When solving optimization problems, the range of values for the *Expectation* component is unknown opposite to computer games, where *Expectation* is between 0 (loss) and 1 (win). Nevertheless it is possible to use an adaptive technique for adjusting the parameter C in order to keep the components in the formula (*Expectation* and *Bias*) of the same magnitude [2]. The last component of the evaluation formula is a standard deviation and it was added by Schadd et al. [11] to improve efficiency for single-player games (puzzles).

3   MCTS for Planning

The planning task can be seen as the problem of finding a shortest path in an implicitly given state space, where transitions/moves between the states are defined by the actions. The reason why classical path-finding techniques cannot be applied there is that the state space is enormous. From this point of view planning is very close to single-player games though there are some notable differences.

3.1   Cycles in the State-Space

MCTS uses simulations to evaluate the states. Hence, from the planning perspective, we need to generate solution plans – valid sequences of actions leading to a goal state. Unlike the SameGame and other game applications of MCTS, planning problems allow infinite paths in the state-space (even though the state-space is finite) and this is quite usual in practice since the planning actions are typically reversible. This is a serious problem for the MCTS algorithm since it causes the expected length of the simulations to be very large and therefore only a few simulations can be carried out within a given time limit. There are several ways how to solve this problem.

1. *Modifying the state-space* so that it does not contain infinite paths. In general this is a hard problem itself as it involves solving the underlying satisficing planning problem, which is intractable.
2. *Using a simulation heuristic* which would guarantee that the simulation will be finite and short. Such a heuristic is always a contribution to the MCTS algorithm since it makes the simulations more precise. Obtaining this heuristic may require a domain-dependent knowledge, but there exist generally applicable planning heuristics.
3. *Setting an upper bound* on the length of simulations. This approach has two disadvantages: the upper bound has to be set large enough so that it would not cut off the proper simulations. Still if most of the simulations end on the cut-off limit, then every one of them would take a long time to carry out which would have a bad impact on the performance. Furthermore it is not clear how to evaluate the cut-off simulations.

3.2   Dead-Ends

The other problem is existence of plans that do not lead to a goal state. We use the term *dead-end* to denote a state such that no action is applicable to this state and the state is not a goal state. Note that dead-ends do not occur in any game domain since in games any state that does not have successors is considered a goal state and has a corresponding evaluation assigned to it (like Win, Loss, or Draw in case of Chess or Hex, or a numerical value in case of SameGame for example). In planning, however, the evaluation function is usually defined only for the solution plans leading to goal states. A plan that cannot be extended doesn't necessarily have to be a solution plan and it is not clear how to evaluate the simulation that ended in a dead-end. Possible ways to solve this issue are:

1. *Modifying the state-space* so that it would not contain dead-ends.
2. *Using a simulation heuristic* which would guarantee that the simulation never encounters a dead-end state.
3. *Ignoring the simulations* that ended in dead-end states. If the simulation should end in a dead-end we just forget it and run another simulation (hoping that it would end in a goal state and gets properly evaluated). This approach might be effective if dead-ends are sparse in the search space. Otherwise we could be waiting very long until some successful simulation occurs.
4. Finding a way to *evaluate the dead-end states.*

3.3   Dead Components

A *dead component* is a combination of both previous problems – it is a strongly connected component in the state-space that does not contain any goal state. This is similar to the dead-ends problem except that we can easily detect a dead-end (since there are no applicable actions there) but it is much more difficult to detect a dead component since we would have to store all visited states (and search among them every time) which would make the simulation process much slower and the algorithm less effective.

4   Transportation Domains

As we mentioned earlier, modifying the planning domain so that its state-space wouldn't contain infinite paths and dead-end states requires to actually *solve* the underlying satisficing problem. The MCTS algorithm has been used to solve satisficing problems such as Sudoku however the method is much better suited for optimization problems. Since the problem of satisficing planning is difficult and in general intractable we have decided to restrict the class of domains which our planner addresses. Based on good results with the Petrobras domain [13], we chose to work with the transportation domains. This kind of domains seems to be well suited for the MCTS method since:

1. it is naturally of an optimization type (typically fuel and time consumption are to be minimized),
2. the underlying satisficing problem is usually not difficult,
3. transportation problems frequently occur in practice.

Knowing that the domain is of the transportation type we can use *domain analysis techniques* to gather more information about the domain structure and dynamics. This higher level information is then exploited during the planning process/simulation (as described in the next chapter).

We introduce the term *Transportation component* denoting a part of the planning domain that has a typical *transportation structure*. The transportation component describes some *vehicles*, *locations*, and *cargo* and specifies actions for *moving* the vehicles between the locations and for transporting the cargo by *loading* and *unloading* it by the vehicles. We also assume that the goal is to deliver cargo to specific destinations. We have created a template that describes such a structure – the template describes *relations* between the *symbols* that are typical for the transportation domains. By *symbols* we mean names of the predicates, types of the constants, and names of the operators.

For example consider the following two operators (specified in PDDL) originating from two different planning domains:

```
(:action load
    :parameters   (?a - airplane ?p - person
                   ?l - location)
    :precondition (and (at ?a ?l) (at ?p ?l))
    :effect       (and (not (at ?p ?l))
         (in ?p ?a)))
```

```
(:action get
    :parameters   (?v - vehicle ?c - cargo
                   ?d - destination)
    :precondition (and (isCargoAt ?c ?d)
         (isVehicleAt ?v ?d))
    :effect       (and (not (isCargoAt ?c ?d))
         (isInside ?c ?v))))
```

Even though these operators use different predicates, relations between the symbols *(get, vehicle, cargo, destination, isCargoAt, isVehicleAt, isInside)* are exactly the same as the relations between *(load, airplane, person, location, at, at, in)*.

The example shows that the *structure* of the domain (which is what we want to capture) does not depend on the symbols used but only on the relations between the symbols. This gives us means to define a *generic transportation structure* and then we can check whether some given domain *matches* this predefined structure. For example, the action *get* in the above example can be seen as a *template of loading* and we can say that the action *load* matches this template.

A *transportation component* is defined by the names of operators for loading (denoted *Op-L*), unloading (*Op-U*) and moving (*Op-M*) actions, the names of predicates describing positions of the vehicles (denoted *Veh-At*) and of the cargo (*Carg-At*, *Carg-In*), as well as the types of constants that represent vehicles (*Type-Veh*), cargo (*Type-Carg*) and locations (*Type-Loc*). Moreover there has to be a certain relationship between these symbols. Operator *Op-L* has to have a predicate with the name *Cargo-At* among its positive preconditions and negative effects and a predicate with the name *Cargo-In* among its positive effects. Both these predicates has to share some variable that has to have a type *Type-Cargo*. Also it has to have a predicate with the name *Veh-At* in its positive preconditions and this predicate has to share some variable with the predicate *Cargo-In* mentioned above. This variable has to have a type *Type-Veh*. Finally the two predicates with names *Veh-At* and *Cargo-At* in the operator definition have to share some variable that has a type *Type-Loc*. In the above example of two loading operators, we have the following matchings:

Op-L	load	get
Veh-At	at	isVehicleAt
Cargo-At	at	isCargoAt
Cargo-In	in	isInside
Type-Veh	airplane	vehicle
Type-Carg	person	cargo
Type-Loc	location	destination

The reader can easily verify that the required relations between the symbols hold. In a similar way we can define the templates for *unloading* and *moving* operators. A complete description of all the variables and constraints of the templates as well as more examples of transportation components can be found in [14].

We say that a planning domain contains a transportation component if it is possible to substitute symbols from the domain description (names of the operators, predicates, and types) to all three operator templates such that all the constraints hold. It is possible that the domain contains more types of vehicles or cargo or more operators for loading, unloading, and moving. For example in the Zeno-Travel domain [10] the planes can travel at two different speeds – the domain contains two different operators for moving - *Fly* and *Fly-Fast*. In these cases we say that the domain contains more than one transportation component. It is also possible that the transportation component is embedded within a more complex structure in the planning domain. For example we may assume that *hoist* is necessary to load cargo to a vehicle. Then the predicates may have arity larger than two (*hoist* holds *cargo* at given *location*), the operators may have more than three parameters (hoist is included), and they may have more preconditions (vehicle is empty) and effects (hoist will be empty after the action, while the vehicle will be full). Such operators can still fit the template as we do not require the domain to be *isomorphic* to the template but rather only to *match* the template.

Notice that the transportation component is defined by the values of some variables which have to satisfy certain constraints defined by the template. Hence, we can search for the components automatically in the domain description using constraint programming (CP) techniques [4]. The names of operators (like *Op-L* or *Op-M*), the names of the predicates (like *Veh-At* or *Carg-In*) and the types (like *Type-Loc*) in the definition of the transportation component can be seen as CP variables. The domains of these variables are derived from the planning domain description. For example the domain of the variable *Op-L* is a set of all names of operators defined in the planning domain, the domain of the variable *Type-Veh* is a set of all types used in the planning domain and so on. Finding all the transportation components is equivalent to finding all the solutions of this Constraint Satisfaction Problem. This step might be computationally demanding but it is done only once as preprocessing before the actual planning starts. The transportation component is defined by relations between symbols including types. Therefore this domain analysis technique can only be used on domains that support typing. This however is not a restriction since the types can be automatically derived from the domain description even if they are not given explicitly [16].

5   MCTS in Planning for Transportation Domains

Recall that one of the main components of the MCTS algorithm is simulation – looking for a solution plan from a given state. As these simulations are run frequently to evaluate the states, it is critical to make the simulations short (i.e. with low expected number of steps/actions) and to ensure that most of the simulations will reach the goal (i.e. low probability of reaching a dead-end or a dead component) so that the sampling would be fast and effective. We achieve this by modifying the state space based on the analysis of the planning domain.

We modify the planning domain by replacing the given action model with so called meta-actions (will be explained later). Meta-actions are learned during planning and their purpose is to rid the domain of cycles and dead-ends. The proposed model of meta-actions is theoretically applicable to all types of domains however in our planner we only use it for a specific type of planning domains where the learning technique is reasonably fast.

5.1   Meta-actions

Meta-actions (or composite actions) consist of sequences of original actions. The purpose of using Meta-actions instead of the original actions is to prevent some paths in the state-space from being visited during the simulation phase of the MCTS algorithm. The original action model allows *every* possible path in the search space to be explored by the planner though many paths are formed of meaningless combinations of actions which do not lead to the goal. For example the sequence *load − unload − load − unload − . . .* is a valid plan, but does not bring us closer to the goal. If the simulation visits such a path, it might spend a lot of time in cycles or end up in a dead-end. We use the meta-actions to eliminate as many meaningless paths as possible which makes the Monte-Carlo sampling process efficient enough to be worth using.

Each meta-action represents a sequence of original actions. If we want to apply the meta-action, we apply all the actions in the sequence successively. If we represent the state-space as a directed graph where vertices represent states and edges represent actions then the meta-actions correspond to paths in this graph. Our modification of the state-space can be seen as follows:

1. Identify important paths in the graph (learn the meta-actions).
2. Remove all original edges from the graph (we no longer use the original actions once we learned the meta-actions).
3. Add new edges to the graph. Edge is added from u to v if there exists a meta-action A such that $v = \gamma(A, u)$.

The planning/simulation is then performed on this new search space. Notice that by removing the original actions, we may effectively remove some valid plans from being assumed. Our goal is to create the meta-actions in such a way that the important paths in the state-space would be preserved (especially paths representing optimal solutions should be preserved) and paths leading to cycles or dead-ends would be eliminated.

5.2 Example of the Meta-actions Model

We will first give examples of two meta-actions constructed for the Zeno-Travel Domain [10]. The original domain description contains actions *Fly*, *Load* and *Unload*. The following two meta-actions were learned by the planner (the learning method will be described later).

```
(:action fly+load
 :parameters    (?a - airplane ?p - person
        ?from ?to - location)
 :precondition  (and (at ?a ?from)
          (at ?p ?to))
 :effect (and (not (at ?a ?from))
    (not (at ?p ?to)) (at ?a ?to)
    (in ?p ?a)))

(:action fly+unload
 :parameters (?a - airplane ?p - person
        ?from ?to - location)
 :precondition  (and (at ?a ?from)
          (in ?p ?a))
 :effect (and (not (at ?a ?from))
    (at ?a ?to) (not (in ?p ?a))
    (at ?p ?to)))
```

In this example the original state-space contains many infinite paths – for example performing action *fly* without ever loading anything or repeatedly performing actions *load-unload*. The modified state-space which uses meta-actions doesn't contain these paths. It still contains some infinite paths but their number is greatly reduced.

5.3 Learning the Meta-actions

Let us suppose that we have already found the transportation components in the planning domain. Every meta-action we create belongs to some transportation component and we shall describe the learning algorithm using the terms from the definition of a transportation component. In particular, we will use terms such as *vehicle*, *cargo*, *loaded cargo*, *operator Move* and so on even though we do not know the exact symbols that play these roles in the particular planning domain (for example *Move* can be called *fly* in the particular domain). The operators, types, and predicates might have different names in each particular transportation planning domain but their meaning is still the same. The term *operator Load* for example refers to the operator that *plays the role of loading* in the particular domain. We can use this assumption since we have already assigned meaning to these symbols by identifying the transportation components.

To recognize the important paths we use a landmark-based approach where we first find the state landmarks in the domain (*landmark* is a set of states such that every solution plan has to visit at least one of these states) and then we find paths between the nearest landmarks. These paths will be stored in a form of meta-operators and used during the simulation phase of MCTS (instantiated to meta-actions).

Assuming the transportation domains where the goal is to deliver some cargo simplifies the process of identifying landmarks. Basically, we have two types of landmarks. In order to deliver cargo, it has to be loaded in some vehicle and then unloaded. For every cargo that has not yet been delivered the set of all states where this cargo is loaded in some vehicle represents a state landmark of the problem. Similarly for a cargo that is loaded the set of all states where this cargo is not loaded represents a state landmark. We create the meta-actions by finding the shortest paths between two consecutive landmarks. For finding the shortest paths we use an exhaustive search where we assume that the domain is simple enough for this process to be tractable - i.e. the paths between the landmarks are short and simple. Having the sequence of actions, we do lifting to obtain a sequence of operators that then define the meta-operator.

Let us summarize the whole learning technique. Suppose that during the simulation phase the MCTS algorithm visits a state where no known meta-action is applicable. Then the learning procedure is initiated which works as follow.

1. select some transportation component randomly
2. select some not delivered cargo from this component randomly
3. if this cargo is not loaded, find the shortest path (paths) to some state where it is loaded; otherwise (i.e. if it is already loaded) find the shortest path to some state where it is not loaded. These paths consist of original actions.
4. create meta-actions from these sequences, lift them to meta-operators, and store them for future use.

In the Zeno-Travel domain these shortest paths only contained two actions and the meta-actions were fly+load and fly+unload. In the Petrobras domain however the paths might be longer. In this case meta-actions of a length up to four were found, namely *undock+navigate+dock+load* and *undock+navigate+dock+unload*.

The method of exploiting meta-actions can be described as follows. We find optimal sub-plans for sub-goals that need to be achieved to reach the expected "big" goal (for example load yet-unloaded cargo by first flying to the cargo location and then loading it), we encapsulate these sub-plans into meta-actions and generalize the meta-actions to meta-operators by lifting, and finally we use these meta-operators when planning for the "big" goal. This can be in principle done for any planning domain, but identifying the landmarks and finding sub-plans is in general a hard problem.

6   Experimental Results

We have compared our technique with the LPG planner [6] – a state-of-the-art domain-independent optimal planner for PDDL2.2 domains and the top performer at IPC4 in plan quality. We used two domains for comparison: the *Zeno-Travel domain* as an example of an artificial IPC domain – one of the simplest transportation domains possible, and the *simplified Petrobras domain*, which is much closer to real practical problems. The simplified Petrobras domain is similar to the originally proposed Petrobras domain [15] with the difference that the cargo no longer has any weight assigned to it, loading and unloading takes a fixed amount of time (no longer depends on the weight) and the ships can hold arbitrarily many cargo (no longer have a capacity limit). Also the plan quality is only measured by the fuel consumption and makespan (the original domain used several other vaguely defined criteria).

We have generated 40 random problems from both domains with the increasing size of the problems. The LPG planner optimized the fuel consumption while the MCTS planner optimized weighted sum of both fuel consumption and makespan. Every problem had a time limit assigned according to its size. The smallest problems had the time limit of 5 minutes, the largest ones had a limit of 40 minutes. The best solutions found within the time limit are reported. The experiments were conducted on the same computer – Asus A8N-VM CSM with processor AMD Opteron (UP) 144 @ 1800 MHz (8 cores) and 1024MB of physical memory.

6.1   Zeno-Travel Domain

The results of the experiments with the Zeno-Travel domain are shown in Figure 2. Both planners were able to solve all the problems. In plan quality the LPG planner outperformed the MCTS planner by approximately 10 percent overall (measured by the sum of fuel consumption and makespan).

6.2   Simplified Petrobras

In the case of simplified Petrobras domain both planners were again able to solve all the problems within the given time limit. The results of experiments are shown in Figures 3(a), 3(b) and 4.

The LPG planner outperformed the MCTS in fuel consumption as Figure 3(a) shows. The MCTS planner on the contrary outperformed LPG in makespan

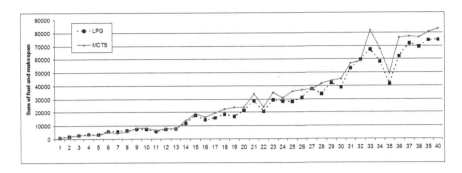

Fig. 2. Results of the experiments in the Zeno-Travel domain

(see Figure 3(b)). Figure 4 shows the results according to the weighted sum of both these criteria. We used the combined objective function $1 * fuel + 4 * makespan$ so that both criteria are comparable and equally important in the sum. In this case MCTS slightly outperformed the LPG by approximately 5 percent overall.

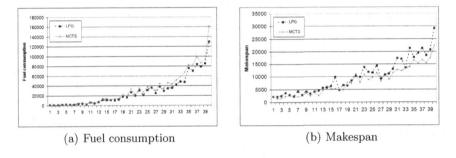

(a) Fuel consumption   (b) Makespan

Fig. 3. Results of the experiments in the simplified Petrobras domain

6.3 Discussion

The preliminary experimental results show that the simple MCTS planner is competitive with the complex LPG planner. The LPG planner found simpler plans with less parallelism and less vehicles used. Therefore it had better fuel consumption but worse makespan. The MCTS planner on the contrary found more sophisticated plans using more vehicles and more actions.

The MCTS planner performed better on the more complicated domain (compared to LPG) which we believe is caused by the use of meta-actions. Meta-actions can capture complex paths in the state-space and allow to use these paths again during the planning. In the Zeno-Travel domain the planner only learned 2 meta-operators while in the simplified Petrobras the number of learned meta-operators was 12.

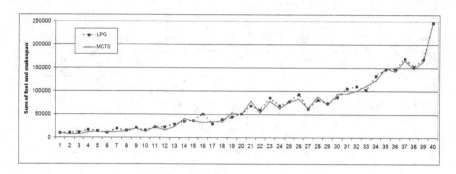

Fig. 4. Results of the experiments in the simplified Petrobras domain - weighted sum of makespan and fuel consumption

The MCTS technique combined with the learning of meta-actions proved to be competitive with standard planning software even though it is still only a prototype and still has a potential for further improvement. We believe that by efficient implementation, integration of other techniques [12] or by hybridization with other algorithms [8] the performance can be further increased.

7   Conclusions

In this paper we showed that an ad-hoc MCTS planner from [13] can be generalized to a wider range of planning domains while keeping its efficiency. We characterized transportation planning domains using templates of three typical operations (loading, moving, unloading), we showed how to automatically identify these operations in the description of any planning domain and how to exploit the structure found for learning macro-operations that speed-up MCTS simulations. The resulting MCTS planner is already competitive with the state-of-the-art planner LPG thought the implementation of the MCTS planner is not fine-tuned. Due to space limit, the paper focused on explaining the main concepts of the method, the formal technical details can be found in [14].

A universal MCTS planner would require a fast technique for solving the underlying satisficing problem which does not seem possible for arbitrary planning domain. It can however be used in the domains where the underlying problem is easy to solve and a complex objective function is used in the optimization problem. Transportation domains are a good example of such domains. We believe that there are many more planning domains that have this property (especially those that are practically motivated) and therefore MCTS techniques may become a new and efficient way to address such problems.

Acknowledgment. Research is supported by the Czech Science Foundation under the project no. P103-10-1287.

References

1. Auer, P., Cesa-Bianchi, N., Fischer, P.: Finite-time Analysis of the Multiarmed Bandit Problem. Machine Learning 47(2-3), 235–256 (2002)
2. Baudiš, P.: Balancing MCTS by Dynamically Adjusting Komi Value. ICGA Journal 34, 131–139 (2011)
3. Chaslot, G., Bakkes, S., Szita, I., Spronck, P.: Monte-Carlo Tree Search: A New Framework for Game AI. In: Proceedings of the 4th Artificial Intelligence for Interactive Digital Entertainment conference (AIIDE), pp. 216–217. AAAI Press (2008)
4. Dechter, R.: Constraint Processing. Morgan Kaufmann Publishers Inc. (2003)
5. Ghallab, M., Nau, D.S., Traverso, P.: Automated Planning: Theory and Practice. Elsiever Morgan Kaufmann, Amsterdam (2004)
6. Gerevini, A., Saetti, A., Serina, I.: Planning in PDDL2.2 Domains with LPG-TD. In: International Planning Competition, 14th International Conference on Automated Planning and Scheduling (IPC at ICAPS) (2004)
7. Kocsis, L., Szepesvári, C.: Bandit Based Monte-Carlo Planning. In: Fürnkranz, J., Scheffer, T., Spiliopoulou, M. (eds.) ECML 2006. LNCS (LNAI), vol. 4212, pp. 282–293. Springer, Heidelberg (2006)
8. Loth, M., Sebag, M., Hamadi, Y., Schoenauer, M., Schulte, C.: Hybridizing Constraint Programming and Monte-Carlo Tree Search: Application to the Job Shop Problem (unpublished)
9. Nakhost, H., Müller, M.: Monte-Carlo exploration for deterministic planning. In: Proceedings of the International Joint Conference on Artificial Intelligence (IJCAI), pp. 1766–1771 (2009)
10. Olaya, A., López, C., Jiménez, S.: International Planning Competition (2011), http://ipc.icaps-conference.org/ (retrieved)
11. Schadd, M.P.D., Winands, M.H.M., van den Herik, H.J., Chaslot, G.M.J.B., Uiterwijk, J.W.H.M.: Single-player Monte-Carlo tree search. In: van den Herik, H.J., Xu, X., Ma, Z., Winands, M.H.M. (eds.) CG 2008. LNCS, vol. 5131, pp. 1–12. Springer, Heidelberg (2008)
12. Schadd, M.P.D., Winands, M.H.M., van den Herik, H.J., Aldewereld, H.: Addressing NP-Complete Puzzles with Monte-Carlo Methods. In: Proceedings of the AISB 2008 Symposium on Logic and the Simulation of Interaction and Reasoning vol. 9, (2008)
13. Toropila, D., Dvořák, F., Trunda, O., Hanes, M., Barták, R.: Three Approaches to Solve the Petrobras Challenge: Exploiting Planning Techniques for Solving Real-Life Logistics Problems. In: Proceedings of ICTAI 2012, pp. 191–198. IEEE Conference Publishing Services (2012)
14. Trunda, O.: Monte Carlo Techniques in Planning. Master's thesis. Faculty of Mathematics and Physics, Charles University in Prague (2013)
15. Vaquero, T.S., Costa, G., Tonidandel, F., Igreja, H., Silva, J.R., Beck, C.: Planning and scheduling ship operations on petroleum ports and platform. In: Proceedings of the ICAPS Scheduling and Planning Applications Workshop, pp. 8–16 (2012)
16. Wickler, G.: Using planning domain features to facilitate knowledge engineering. In: Proceedings of the Workshop on Knowledge Engineering for Planning and Scheduling (KEPS 2011), pp. 39–46 (2011)
17. Xie, F., Nakhost, H., Müller, M.: A Local Monte Carlo Tree Search Approach in Deterministic Planning. In: Proceedings of the AAAI Conference on Artificial Intelligence (AAAI 2011), pp. 1832–1833 (2011)

An Approach Based on an Interactive Procedure for Multiple Objective Optimisation Problems

Alejandra Duenas[1], Christine Di Martinelly[2], and Isabelle Fagnot[1]

[1] IESEG, School of Management (LEM-CNRS), Socle de la Grande Arche,
1 Parvis de La Défense, 92044 Paris, France
[2] IESEG, School of Management (LEM-CNRS), 3 rue de la Digue, 59000 Lille, France
{a.duenas,c.dimartinelly,i.fagnot}@ieseg.fr

Abstract. In this paper the Interactive Procedure for Multiple Objective Optimisation Problems (IPMOOP) is presented as a tool used for the solution of multiple objective optimisation problems. The first step of this procedure is the definition of a decision-making process group (DMPG) unit, where the decision maker (DM) and the analytic programmer actively interact throughout the solution of the problem. The DMPG is responsible for providing the information about the problem's nature and features. The main characteristic of IPMOOP is the definition of a surrogate objective function to represent the different objectives. The objectives are transformed into goals and the DM is asked to define aspiration levels which include his preferences. In each iteration, the solutions are presented to the DM who decides whether to modify the aspiration levels or not. This allows the DM to find a satisfactory solution in a progressive manner. In order to demonstrate the applicability of this approach an activity allocation problem was solved using a genetic algorithm since the surrogate function can act as the fitness function. The solutions found were satisfactory from the DM's point of view since they achieved all the goals, aspiration levels and met all the constraints.

Keywords: multiple objective problems, genetic algorithms, interactive methods.

1 Introduction

Multiple objective problems (MOP) arise in various fields and numerous papers have been published either on the development of new techniques to solve MOPs [1, 2] or on the application of multiple objective techniques to solve particular problems [3, 4].

The purpose of solving a multiple objective optimisation problem is to optimise the decision maker's (DM) utility or preference function [5]. Because the objective functions are conflicting with one another, an optimal solution that simultaneously maximises or minimises all the objective functions does not usually exist. Therefore, it is necessary to identify non-dominated solutions or efficient solutions. It is important to bear in mind that all non-dominated solutions can be considered equally appropriate and consequently the DM may have to identify the most preferred [6].

F. Castro, A. Gelbukh, and M. González (Eds.): MICAI 2013, Part II, LNAI 8266, pp. 450–465, 2013.

MOPs can be classified according to the DM's preferences. A number of techniques consider the DM's preferences a-priori, where the objectives are transformed into a single objective function, together with some preference information expressed as weights. The main drawback of those techniques is that an evident assumption is made about the ability of the DM to give detailed and precise information [7]. A-posteriori methods are concerned with finding all or most of the efficient solutions to a problem without first asking the DM about preferences. As a result, these methods take a lot of computation time and the DM ends with too much information to choose from [8].

Interactive methods, however, require a progressive articulation of the DM preferences. The emphasis is on finding a compromise solution [9]. The main advantage of these methods is that, in comparison with a-posteriori methods, they require a much shorter computation time since only the solutions that the decision makers are interested in are generated. Also, the DM can learn about the problem during the process, understand the relationship between the objective functions and have more realistic goals [8]. Gardiner and Steuer [10] suggested a framework that can accommodate the different interactive methods, that are based on either a reference point, a classification, a marginal rate of substitution or a surrogate value for trade-offs. Luque et al. [6] concluded that the same efficient solutions were found regardless of which interactive method was used in any iteration as long as the same information (results) was presented to the DM.

The objective of this paper is to present a framework to solve multiple objective optimisation problems following an interactive procedure. The framework is generic and can be used with any optimisation method. The partial information about the DM's preferences are obtained interactively in several steps of the framework. This information is used to define a surrogate function. It gives the DM more insight into the problem and helps to identify the objectives to be satisfied.

2   Method Definition

The main purpose of a general multi-objective problem (MOP) is defined as finding the maximal/minimal solution, having a decision variable vector x of dimension n and k objectives:

$$max/min\ [f_1(x), f_2(x), \dots, f_k(x)] \tag{1}$$

subject to:

$$g_i(x) \le 0, \quad i = 1, 2, \dots, m \tag{2}$$

where m is the number of constraints [11].

A non-dominated solution exists where it is not possible to improve one objective without decreasing the other objectives. In a formal way x^* is a non-dominated solution if and only if there is not any $x \in X$ (where X is the feasible set of variables that satisfies the constraints) such that $f_i(x^*) \le f_i(x)$ for all i, and $f_j(x^*) < f_j(x)$ for at least one j [11]. The members of the solution set that are non-dominated constitute the Pareto optimal set.

As stated by Churchman et al. [12] there are two main actors in the solution of a decision problem: the DM and the researcher (analytic programmer). It is important to bear in mind that the DM could be one person or a group of people. The DM and the researcher have to be in continuous communication. Therefore, they will be considered as a unit called a *decision-making process group* (DMPG). The main purpose of this unit is to consider the DM and the researcher as one entity that will work together throughout the solution of the problem.

Saaty [13] stated that to make a decision it is necessary to have "knowledge, information and technical data" such as details about the problem, the people involved, objectives and policies, constraints and time horizons. The IPMOOP proposed in this paper includes all the elements defined by Saaty [13]. This procedure is divided into two phases.

2.1   Phase 1

1. The DM Identification. This is a vital aspect of the process because the DM is one of the most important elements in the application of this kind of method. The DM is the individual or group of people that recognises the problem, sets the objectives and selects the decision to be made by defining its preferences in an interactive way. The DM can be one individual or a group of individuals.

2. Objective Definition.   Keeney and Raiffa [14] define an objective as the element that gives the direction to follow in order to achieve a better outcome. Hwang and Masud [11] and Keeney and Raiffa [14], define an objective as the direction in which it is expected "to do better" but they also include the DM's perception. In other words, the definition of objective considered for purposes of this research will be the direction to follow to find a better outcome as perceived by the DM or a group of experts.

3. Decision Variables Definition. The DM defines the decision variables which are used to describe the objective and choose among the solution alternatives to the problem.

4. Constraint Equations Formulation
Goals and aspiration levels definition. The goal levels are defined as "conditions imposed on the DM by external forces" and the aspiration levels are "attainment levels of the objectives which the DM personally desires to achieve" [15]. A goal is something desired by the DM that helps to clearly identify a level of achievement or a target. To determine this definition both Keeney and Raiffa [14] and Hwang and Masud [11] were considered. The DM participates in an interview or answers a questionnaire developed by the researcher. The main purpose of this questionnaire or interview is to gather as much quantitative information as possible from the DM to be used in the goals and aspiration levels definition.

   (a) Goal equations formulation. Two vectors U and V are defined as having the maximum and minimum values of the objective functions respectively. This means that vector U has the values of the maximisation of each objective separately (e.g. max $z_1(x)$, max $z_2(x)$, max $z_3(x)$, max $z_4(x)$, max $z_5(x)$), subject to constraints $g_i(x) \leq 0$. In addition vector V has the minimum values found following the same procedure, in other words, minimising each objective separately subject to the constraints. This is to know the ranges of objective vectors in the non-dominated set [16].

(b) Aspiration levels definition. The aspiration levels are directly related to the decision-maker's preferences. Simon [17] concluded that aspiration levels specify the conditions for satisfaction. He considered satisfying models have a better performance than optimising models. The satisfying model offers the DM the possibility of searching for new alternatives of action. Finally, Simon [17] stated that most entrepreneurs want to achieve a satisfactory alternative of action rather than the optimal.

As mentioned before, this process is completely focused on the introduction of the DM's preferences and also the DM is part of the DMPG unit definition.

2.2   Phase 2

Phase 2 is a process which is cycling until a satisfactory solution is obtained. The solutions found in each iteration are used in the assessment process in which the DM makes a decision about changes prior to the next iteration. In this way, the process is interactive because it takes into account the DM's preferences.

1. Surrogate Function Formulation. The decision problem has k goals, n decision variables, and a constraint set X. Each goal is connected to an objective function, so for k goals there will be k objective functions. These functions are represented in a set $z = (z_1, z_2, ..., z_k)$ and will be used to evaluate how well the goals have been accomplished. It is necessary that the set of constraints X be continuous, and the constraint and objective functions be at least first order differentiable [18]. The goals are transformed into a function $d(x)$ in the real positive set. If $d < 1$ the goal is satisfied. Each goal function will be compared to its correspondent aspiration level AL and will be transformed into a d function as follows:

At most:

$$z_i(\mathbf{x}) \leq AL_i; \quad d_i = \frac{z_i(\mathbf{x})}{AL_i} \tag{3}$$

At least:

$$z_i(\mathbf{x}) \geq AL_i; \quad d_i = \frac{AL_i}{z_i(\mathbf{x})} \tag{4}$$

Equal:

$$z_i(\mathbf{x}) = AL_i; \quad d_i = \frac{1}{2}\left[\frac{AL_i}{z_i(\mathbf{x})} + \frac{z_i(\mathbf{x})}{AL_i}\right] \tag{5}$$

Within an interval:

$$AL_{iL} \leq z_i(\mathbf{x}) \leq AL_{iU}$$

$$d_i = \left[\frac{AL_{iU}}{AL_{iL} + AL_{iU}} \right] \left[\frac{AL_{iL}}{z_i(\mathbf{x})} + \frac{z_i(\mathbf{x})}{AL_{iU}} \right]$$

(6)

These equations are based on Monarchi et al. [18] method. The surrogate function s used will be defined as:

$$s = \sum_{i=1}^{P} d_i$$

(7)

subject to

$$\mathbf{x} \in \mathbf{X}$$

2. Surrogate Function Optimisation and Solution Technique Selection. Having defined the surrogate function, the next step is the surrogate function optimisation, in other words, its maximisation or minimisation. The problem solution involves making a decision on which analytic, numerical or simulation [12] technique to use. The selection of this technique depends on the problem's characteristics.

3. Possible Solutions Analysis. The solutions found are presented to the DM.

4. DM's Preferences. In this method the DM's preferences are expressed in the form of aspiration levels.

5. Solution Technique Selection. The solution technique selected in this paper is genetic algorithms (GA). IPMOOP includes the use of a surrogate function that can be directly understood as the objective function and mapped as the GA's fitness function. The selection operator to be used in this binary GA is tournament selection where a group of chromosomes is chosen randomly. These chromosomes participate in a tournament where the one with the best fitness value wins. The winner is inserted in the next population. In order to obtain the new population this process is repeated v times. This selection procedure could be implemented in a polynomial time complexity $O(v)$, and scaling and translation do not affect it.

- Initial population: $P(t) = \{p_1, p_2, p_3, \ldots, p_n\}$; $P(t) \in I^v$
- Tournament size: $r \in \{1, 2, \ldots, v\}$
- Population after selection: $P'(t) = \{p'_1, p'_2, p'_3, \ldots, p'_v\}$

For the recombination operator a probability of crossover p_x is defined. A one-point crossover with a uniform distribution is used to select a random position in the two chromosomes (parents). The segments to the right hand side of the position selected are swapped generating two new individuals (offspring).

The mutation operator is defined with a probability of mutation p_m (small) where all positions in the parent (chromosome) have the same probability of being chosen.

- Selected parent: $p = (a_1, ..., a_w) \in I^w = \{0,1\}^w$
- Probability of mutation: p_m is the probability of independently inverting each a_i (gene) and $i \in \{1,...,w\}$
- New individual: $p' = m(p)$

3   Problem Formulation

An academic department at a university provides a range of undergraduate and post-graduate degree courses, five separate courses, each of which can lead to a Bachelor degree. The five courses are: Computer Systems Engineering, Systems and Control Engineering, Electronic, Control and Systems Engineering, Mechanical Systems Engineering, and Medical Systems Engineering.

In this department, every semester or every year a resource allocation problem is solved. This problem consists of allocating different activities to the academic staff. The main purpose is to achieve the objectives of the university and the department in the best way possible. In this section, this problem using the IPMOOP is solved. It can be considered as an overall objective "to improve the activities allocation of the academic staff in the department".

The department counts five professors, three readers, six senior lecturers and three lecturers. This makes a total of 17 members of the academic staff to be considered in the allocation. Each member of the academic staff has to work 37 hours a week.

The academic staff activities are divided into three areas: research, lectures and administrative work. Lectures are divided into two areas: undergraduate and graduate. The graduate programmes are an MSc and PhD research and taught programmes. It is important to bear in mind that the academic year is divided into two semesters: spring and autumn.

3.1   Phase 1

1. The DM Identification. The first step is the DM identification. For this problem the DM identified is the Assistant Head of Department. The second step of the procedure is the data collection. For this reason as much information as possible has to be gathered about the department and its academic activities.

Each academic staff member has to be considered as an individual with different preferences and skills. For this reason, it is necessary to formulate a final problem that considers other aspects of the problem outlined by the DM. The number of modules offered by the department a year is 30 for undergraduates and 16 for graduates, this makes a total of 46 modules. It is important to bear in mind that more than one lecturer gives some of these modules. Additionally, it is also important to take into consideration that the modules that involve the development of a project are not considered in the total number of modules because they require another kind of supervision rather than giving a lecture.

Table 1 presents the number of modules taught by each academic staff member representing the current teaching allocation needed to cover all courses offered. The modules are measured in terms of credits and one aspect to be aware of is that some modules do not have integer numbers. This occurs because some modules are given by more than one member of the academic staff and therefore the module's number of credits is divided by the number of academic staff members that are involved in it. An interesting aspect to consider is the arithmetical mean of the total of credits because it can yield information about the average of credits taught in the department by each member of academic staff. The arithmetic mean in this case is 32. In order to make the problem more understandable and easier to handle, the DMPG unit decided to assign values from 1 to 3 to each member of academic staff to classify them in terms of the rounded number of credits they taught.

The values assigned are as follows:

- from 0 to 29 credits a value of 1 is assigned;
- from 30 to 39 credits a value of 2 is assigned;
- from 40 to 60 credits a value of 3 is assigned.

In other words, an academic staff member who has been assigned a value of three is someone that dedicates most of his or her time to lecturing activities.

The total number of credits in the department is 545. This total number of credits can be used as a constraint in the final problem formulation.

Once the information about the lecturing activities is gathered, it is necessary to analyse the research activities. The term research activities will be understood as any activity related to research such as writing papers, attending conferences, research student supervision, and research projects.

The DM wants to allocate as many hours as possible to research activities. For this reason, it was decided to assign a value of 3 to the research activities of each academic staff member. This means, that each academic staff member is expected to have high levels in the research activity allocation in order to maintain high standards in the department research activities. The research activities will be measured in hours a week.

Table 2 presents the administrative roles of the department. From this table, it can be seen that the number of administrative work activities in the department is 38. The DM was asked to evaluate each activity using a scale from 1 to 5, where 1 represents activities that require low performance time and 5 represents activities that require high performance time. Consequently, the administrative work activities will be measured in points. The total of points assigned to the 38 different activities is 80.

Table 1 shows the total of points of administrative work activities assigned to each academic staff member. As in the research activities, the DM was asked to assign a value from 1 to 3 to each academic staff member. The DMPG unit decided to assign the values using the following rules:

- from 0 to 3 points a value of 1 is assigned;
- from 4 to 6 points a value of 2 is assigned;
- from 7 to 15 points a value of 3 is assigned.

Table 1. Credits taught by each academic staff member and total of points assigned to each academic staff member (teaching and administrative work)

Academic staff member		Credits Semester 1	Credits Semester 2	TOTAL	Assigned values Teaching	Total Points Admin work	Assigned Values Admin work
1	Professor and Head of Department	5	5	10	1	11	3
2	Professor	24	15	39	2	5	2
3	Professor	24.17	8.75	32.92	2	4	2
4	Professor	30.83	20	50.83	3	5	2
5	Professor	0	0	0	1	0	1
6	Reader	22.5	10	32.5	2	3	1
7	Reader	3.33	50	53.33	3	5	2
8	Reader	14	23.75	37.75	2	6	2
9	Senior Lecturer	10	35	45	3	4	2
10	Senior Lecturer	32.5	0	32.5	2	5	2
11	Senior Lecturer	3.33	35.42	38.75	2	5	2
12	Senior Lecturer	24	25	49	3	4	2
13	Senior Lecturer	10.67	36.67	47.34	3	9	3
14	Senior Lecturer	20.67	13.75	34.42	2	4	2
15	Lecturer	0	20	20	1	3	1
16	Lecturer	5	6.67	11.67	1	4	2
17	Lecturer	10	0	10	1	3	1
	Total credits			**545**			

2. Objectives Definition. The first objective is to maximise the overall number of research activities in the department. The second objective is to minimise the number of points of administrative work in the department. The third objective is to maximise the number of credits of the academic staff. The overall objective of this problem is to maintain a high level of fairness in the allocation results for each academic staff member.

3. Decision Variables Definition. As in the initial problem formulation, three decision variables will be considered, each of them representing one of the three main activities (research, lecturing and administrative work) of the academic staff. The research activities are represented by the decision variable xr_i, measured in hours/week, where $i = 1, 2, 3,..., n$ and n is the total number of academic staff members. The lecturing activities are represented by the decision variable xl_i, measured in credits/year, where $i = 1, 2, 3,..., n$ and n is the total number of academic staff members. The administrative work activities are represented by the decision variable xa_i, measured in hours/week, where $i = 1, 2, 3,..., n$ and n is the total number of academic staff members. It is expected that each member of the academic staff will have a different activities allocation according to his or her skills and preferences.

Table 2. DM's evaluation of administrative work activities

Administrative roles	Evaluation	Administrative roles	Evaluation
Chair, Health and Safety Committee	1	BEng Programme Leader	2
Chair, Research Committee	1	Chair, Teaching and Learning Committee	2
Demonstrator Co-ordinator	1	PGR Admissions Tutor	2
RTP Co-ordinator	1	Industrial Liaison Co-ordinator	2
Chair, Strategy Committee	1	Assistant Examinations Officer	2
Subject Review Co-ordinator	1	Chair, Policy Committee	3
Chair, Student Affairs Committee	1	Timetable Co-ordinator	3
ERASMUS/SOCRATES Co-ordinator	1	Chair, Computing Committee	3
Careers Co-ordinator	1	MTP/DLP Director	3
Assistant Chair, Teaching and Learning Committee	1	MSc Programme Leader	3
Library Co-ordinator	1	Project Co-ordinator (MSc & UG)	3
Deputy UUG Admissions Tutor	1	Examinations Officer	3
Schools Liaison Officer	1	Aerospace Tutor/Admissions	3
Seminar Co-ordinator	1	PACT Director	3
Schools Liaison Officer	1	MEng Programme Leader	4
Chair, Executive Committee	2	UG Admissions Tutor	4
PG(Taught) Admissions Tutor	2	Assistant Head of Department	5
Head of Web Team	2	Head of Department	5
Quality Assurance Co-ordinator	2	**Total of points**	**80**
Chair, Publicity Committee	2		

4. Constraints Equation Formulation. The constraints are defined as follows:

— Each academic staff member has to work a minimum of 10 hours a week on research.
— The total number of credits that the academic staff members have to teach is a minimum of 545.
— The total number of points of administrative work for the academic staff members is a minimum of 80.

5. Goals Definition

Goal equations formulation.

<u>Goal 1</u> Hours of research ($z_1 \geq t_r$)

$$z_1 = \sum_{i=1}^{n} xr_i \qquad (8)$$

<u>Goal 2</u> Credits of lecturing ($z_2 \geq t_l$)

$$z_2 = \sum_{i=1}^{n} xl_i \tag{9}$$

<u>Goal 3</u> Points of administrative work ($z_3 \le t_a$)

$$z_3 = \sum_{i=1}^{n} xa_i \tag{10}$$

The goals defined are:

- To raise the number of hours/week doing research to at least $t_r = 170$. This means at least 10 hours/week for each academic staff member.
- To maintain the number of credits lecturing above $t_l = 545$.
- To hold the number of points doing administrative work below $t_a = 90$.

Table 3. Activity allocation proposed by the DMPG unit

Academic staff Member	Assigned values (research)		Assigned values (lecturing)		Assigned values (administrative work)	
	Current	DMPG	Current	DMPG	Current	DMPG
1	3	3	1	1	3	3
2	3	3	2	2	2	2
3	3	3	2	2	2	2
4	3	3	3	3	2	1
5	3	3	1	2	1	1
6	3	3	2	2	1	1
7	3	3	3	3	2	1
8	3	3	2	2	2	2
9	3	3	3	3	2	1
10	3	3	2	2	2	2
11	3	3	2	2	2	2
12	3	3	3	3	2	1
13	3	3	3	2	3	3
14	3	3	2	2	2	2
15	3	3	1	3	1	1
16	3	3	1	1	2	2
17	3	3	1	2	1	2

Aspiration levels definition. The aspiration levels for each academic staff were defined as follows:

- $AL_1 = 20$ hrs/week (research).

In the lecturing case three aspiration levels were assigned, each level corresponds to the value assigned by the DMPG unit.

- value = 1, $AL_2 \leq 19$ credits (lecturing);
- value = 2, $20 \leq AL_2 \leq 39$ credits (lecturing);
- value = 3, $AL_2 \geq 40$ credits (lecturing).

In the administrative work case three aspiration levels were assigned, each level corresponds to the value assigned by the DMPG unit.

- value = 1, $AL_3 \leq 3$ points (administrative work);
- value = 2, $4 \leq AL_3 \leq 6$ points (administrative work);
- value = 3, $AL_3 \geq 7$ points (administrative work).

Table 3 presents the activity allocation in the department and the new activity allocation proposed by the DMPG unit in terms of assigned values form 1 to 3. The new activity allocation will be used as the programme's input data.

3.2   Phase 2

1. Surrogate Function Formulation. A surrogate function is defined for each academic staff member. Following the formulations defined in equations 3 to 6, the function d is calculated as follows:

<u>Goal 1</u> Hours of research a week ($z_1 \geq AL_1$)

$$d_1 = \frac{AL_1}{z_1} = \frac{20}{z_1} \tag{11}$$

<u>Goal 2</u> Credits of lecturing

$$\text{value}=1 \ (z_2 \leq AL_2); d_2 = \frac{z_2}{AL_2} = \frac{z_2}{19}$$

$$\text{value}=2 \ (AL_{L2} \leq z_2 \leq AL_{U2}); d_2 = \left[\frac{AL_{U2}}{AL_{L2}+AL_{U2}} \right]\left[\frac{AL_{L2}}{z_2} + \frac{z_2}{AL_{U2}} \right] = \left[\frac{39}{20+39} \right]\left[\frac{20}{z_2} + \frac{z_2}{39} \right]$$

$$\text{value}=3 \ (z_2 \geq AL_2); d_2 = \frac{AL_2}{z_2} = \frac{40}{z_2} \tag{12}$$

<u>Goal 3</u> Points of administrative work ($z_3 \leq AL_{T3}$)

$$\text{value}=1 \ (z_3 \leq AL_3); d_3 = \frac{z_3}{AL_3} = \frac{z_3}{3}$$

$$\text{value}=2 \ (AL_{L3} \leq z_3 \leq AL_{U3}); d_3 = \left[\frac{AL_{U3}}{AL_{L3}+AL_{U3}} \right]\left[\frac{AL_{L3}}{z_3} + \frac{z_3}{AL_{U3}} \right] = \left[\frac{6}{4+6} \right]\left[\frac{4}{z_3} + \frac{z_3}{6} \right]$$

$$\text{value}=3 \ (z_3 \geq AL_3); d_3 = \frac{AL_3}{z_3} = \frac{40}{z_3} \tag{13}$$

The surrogate function for each academic staff member is defined as follows:

$$s_i = d_{1i} + d_{2i} + d_{3i} \tag{14}$$

Non-dominated solutions are generated and evaluated for each member of staff to obtain the individual surrogate function. Then the global surrogate function is optimised.

2. Surrogate Function Optimisation. After the surrogate function is formulated, the GA will be performed minimising the surrogate function defined as follows:

$$\min s_T = \sum_{i=1}^{n} s_i \tag{15}$$

3. Solution Technique Selection. It was decided to programme a binary GA with tournament selection and single-point crossover. The initial population size is 1360 and the probabilities of crossover and mutation are 0.50 and 0.15 respectively and the GA is run 50 cycles. The GA is defined considering two fitness functions: one for each academic member of staff and another for the entire allocation. The genotype is then defined a matrix of size n x 3; where n is the total number of members of staff and 3 is the number of decision variables xr_i, xl_i, xa_i. It also includes s_i, d_{1i}, d_{2i}, d_{3i} and S_T which are represented as floating point vectors. The chromosomes are randomly generated subject to the research constraint of working a minimum of 10 hours a week and the overall matrix is subject to the teaching and administrative points' constraints of minimum 545 credits and minimum 80 points respectively.

Academic staff member	Research	Lecturing	Administrative	d_1	d_2	d_3	s
1	x_{r1}	x_{l1}	x_{a1}	d_{11}	d_{21}	d_{31}	s_1
2	x_{r2}	x_{l2}	x_{a2}	d_{12}	d_{22}	d_{32}	s_2
...	...	...	...	...	...	...	...
n	x_{rn}	x_{ln}	x_{an}	d_{13}	d_{23}	d_{33}	s_3
Total	T_{rh}	T_{lh}	T_{ah}				S_T

4. Possible Solutions Analysis. In order to find the final problem's possible solutions, the GA has to be run minimising the total surrogate function. This is performed in such way to be able to handle each academic staff member individually. It is important to bear in mind that the goals are achieved if the values of the d functions are smaller than one.

The solutions found after running the GA are presented in Table 4. From this table, it is possible to see that only for academic staff member number 1 the research aspiration level is not achieved. The rest of the allocation results are appropriate and achieve their correspondent aspiration levels. It can also be seen that the constraints such as "each academic staff member has to work a minimum of 10 hours/week doing research", "the total number of credits that the academic staff members have to teach is a minimum of 545" and "the total number of points of administrative work for the academic staff members is a minimum of 80" have been met. In other words, each academic staff member has been allocated more than 10 hours/week for research activities, the total number of credits to teach is greater than 545 (598) and the number of points of administrative work is greater than 80 (82). Therefore, it could be concluded that the allocation results are appropriate. However, the fact that for one academic staff member the research aspiration level is not achieved makes the DMPG unit generate a new activity allocation.

The DMPG unit decided not to modify the whole allocation results; instead the allocation for member 1 has been calculated again, obtaining the following results:

— Research activities 20 hrs/week;
— Lecturing activities 9 credits a year;
— Administrative work activities 13 points.

Table 4. First allocation results

Academic staff member	Research (hrs/week)	Lecturing (credits/year)	Administrative work (points)	d_1	d_2	d_3	s
1	19	7	15	1.052632	0.368421	0.466667	1.887719
2	20	29	5	1.000000	0.945942	0.980000	2.925942
3	20	36	4	1.000000	0.975897	1.000000	2.975897
4	20	49	2	1.000000	0.816327	0.666667	2.482993
5	22	27	1	0.909091	0.945812	0.333333	2.188236
6	22	30	2	0.909091	0.947692	0.666667	2.523450
7	20	59	2	1.000000	0.677966	0.666667	2.344633
8	23	27	4	0.869565	0.945812	1.000000	2.815377
9	20	57	1	1.000000	0.701754	0.333333	2.035088
10	24	37	6	0.833333	0.982911	1.000000	2.816244
11	20	28	6	1.000000	0.945275	1.000000	2.945275
12	24	57	3	0.833333	0.701754	1.000000	2.535088
13	24	37	14	0.833333	0.982911	0.500000	2.316244
14	22	27	4	0.909091	0.945812	1.000000	2.854903
15	26	52	3	0.769231	0.769231	1.000000	2.538462
16	23	8	4	0.869565	0.421053	1.000000	2.290618
17	27	31	6	0.740741	0.950422	1.000000	2.691163
Total	376	598	82				

It can be seen that in these allocation results all the individual aspiration levels are achieved. Therefore, the DMPG unit decided to include it in the complete activity allocation. The results are presented in Table 5 where it can be seen that the constraints are met. The DMPG unit decided to run the GA once more to see if it is possible to find an allocation that does not have to be modified. Table 6 presents the new allocation results.

Finally, the DM has to decide which of the solutions found satisfies most of his or her preferences. The main conclusion, after applying the IPMOOP for the solution of this activity allocation problem, is that this procedure is very effective in the solution of these kinds of optimisation problems and that the use of GAs allows the DMPG unit to find satisfactory solutions. It has been demonstrated that the IPMOOP is capable of handling the interaction between the DM and the analytic programmer in a very smooth way. Finally, the use of hybrid approaches provides the necessary tools for the solution of multiple objective optimisation problems.

Table 5. Second allocation results

Academic staff member	Research (hrs/week)	Lecturing (credits/year)	Administrative work (points)	d_1	d_2	d_3	s
1	20	9	13	1.052632	0.368421	0.466667	1.887719
2	20	29	5	1.000000	0.945942	0.980000	2.925942
3	20	36	4	1.000000	0.975897	1.000000	2.975897
4	20	49	2	1.000000	0.816327	0.666667	2.482993
5	22	27	1	0.909091	0.945812	0.333333	2.188236
6	22	30	2	0.909091	0.947692	0.666667	2.523450
7	20	59	2	1.000000	0.677966	0.666667	2.344633
8	23	27	4	0.869565	0.945812	1.000000	2.815377
9	20	57	1	1.000000	0.701754	0.333333	2.035088
10	24	37	6	0.833333	0.982911	1.000000	2.816244
11	20	28	6	1.000000	0.945275	1.000000	2.945275
12	24	57	3	0.833333	0.701754	1.000000	2.535088
13	24	37	14	0.833333	0.982911	0.500000	2.316244
14	22	27	4	0.909091	0.945812	1.000000	2.854903
15	26	52	3	0.769231	0.769231	1.000000	2.538462
16	23	8	4	0.869565	0.421053	1.000000	2.290618
17	27	31	6	0.740741	0.950422	1.000000	2.691163
Total	377	600	80				

Table 6. Third allocation results

Academic staff member	Research (hrs/week)	Lecturing (credits/year)	Administrative work (points)	d_1	d_2	d_3	s
1	23	8	11	0.869565	0.421053	0.636364	1.926981
2	27	30	5	0.740741	0.947692	0.980000	2.668433
3	23	27	5	0.869565	0.945812	0.980000	2.795377
4	23	47	3	0.869565	0.851064	1.000000	2.720629
5	20	29	2	1.000000	0.945942	0.666667	2.612608
6	23	27	2	0.869565	0.945812	0.666667	2.482044
7	23	47	2	0.869565	0.851064	0.666667	2.387296
8	20	33	5	1.000000	0.958462	0.980000	2.938462
9	22	47	1	0.909091	0.851064	0.333333	2.093488
10	20	33	5	1.000000	0.958462	0.980000	2.938462
11	26	31	6	0.769231	0.950422	1.000000	2.719653
12	24	57	3	0.833333	0.701754	1.000000	2.535088
13	26	31	13	0.769231	0.950422	0.538462	2.258114
14	20	38	5	1.000000	0.990445	0.980000	2.970445
15	26	52	3	0.769231	0.769231	1.000000	2.538462
16	27	12	6	0.740741	0.631579	1.000000	2.372320
17	22	30	5	0.909091	0.947692	0.980000	2.836783
Total	395	579	82				

From Table 6, it can be seen that all the allocation results are appropriate and achieve their correspondent aspiration level. It can also be concluded that the constraints such as "each academic staff member has to work a minimum of 10 hours/week doing research", "the total number of credits that the academic staff members have to teach is a minimum of 545" and "the total number of points of administrative work for the academic staff members is a minimum of 80" have been met. In other words, each academic staff member has been allocated with more than 10 hours/week for research activities, the total number of credits to teach is greater than 545 (579) and the number of points of administrative work are greater than 80 (82). Consequently, it can be concluded that the allocation results are appropriate.

4   Conclusions

The IPMOOP's first step is the definition of a unit called *decision-making process group* (DMPG), where the DM and the researcher continuously interact during the solution of the problem, the formulation and solution of an initial problem, the use of surrogate functions, the use of different techniques in the solution of the problem and the formulation and solution of a final problem.

The method presented in this paper is similar to the synchronous approach in interactive multiple objective optimization method presented by Miettinen [8]. The main difference is that the classification used in this paper is simpler than the five classes presented in [8] where upper bounds corresponding to the classification are necessary. When IPMOOP is compared to an interactive reference point based method [20] it can be seen that there is no need of weight generation to reflect the DM's preference information. Therefore, the ideal and the nadir objective vectors do not have to be generated making the process faster and easier for the DM to incorporate his preferences.

An activity allocation for the academic staff members in a department at a university was solved using the IPMOOP. The final problem formulation consisted of the definition of more general objectives and the activities were measured as follows: research (hours/week), lecturing (credits/year) and administrative work (points). A binary GA performed the optimisation, making the interactive process more efficient (faster). The solutions found were satisfactory from the DM's point of view. The allocation results found in the final problem allow the DM to visualise each academic staff member as an individual with different preferences and skills.

It can be concluded that the IPMOOP is effective in the solution of multiple objective optimisation problems because it is capable of handling the interaction between the DM and the researcher (DMPG unit). It considers that it is not always the first problem formulation that takes into account all the problem's characteristics, objectives and constraints. For this reason the use of a final problem makes the IPMOOP a desirable tool for the solution of MCDM problems. Also, the use of a surrogate function allows local improvement (for each individual) without weakening the global solution. In terms of computation time, it means improving the problem's solution without solving it entirely again.

References

1. Miettinen, K.: Nonlinear multiobjective optimization, vol. 12. Springer (1999)
2. Vira, C., Haimes, Y.Y.: Multiobjective decision making: theory and methodology. North-Holland (1983)
3. Van den Bergh, J., et al.: Personnel scheduling: A literature review. European Journal of Operational Research 226(3), 367–385 (2013)
4. Melo, M.T., Nickel, S., Saldanha-Da-Gama, F.: Facility location and supply chain management–A review. European Journal of Operational Research 196(2), 401–412 (2009)

5. Shin, W.-S., Ravindran, A.: An interactive method for multiple-objective mathematical programming problems. Journal of Optimization Theory and Applications 68(3), 539–561 (1991)
6. Luque, M., et al.: Equivalent Information for Multiobjective Interactive Procedures. Management Science 53(1), 125–134 (2007)
7. Mavrotas, G., Diakoulaki, D.: Multi-criteria branch and bound: A vector maximization algorithm for Mixed 0-1 Multiple Objective Linear Programming. Applied Mathematics and Computation 171(1), 53–71 (2005)
8. Miettinen, K., Mäkelä, M.M.: Synchronous approach in interactive multiobjective optimization. European Journal of Operational Research 170(3), 909–922 (2006)
9. Evans, G.W.: An Overview of Techniques for Solving Multiobjective Mathematical Programs. Management Science 30(11), 1268–1282 (1984)
10. Gardiner, L.R., Steuer, R.E.: Unified Interactive Multiple Objective Programming: An Open Architecture for Accommodating New Procedures. The Journal of the Operational Research Society 45(12), 1456–1466 (1994)
11. Hwang, C.L., Masud, A.S.M., Paidy, S.R.: Multiple objective decision making, methods and applications: a state-of-the-art survey. Springer, Berlin (1979)
12. Churchman, C.W., Ackoff, R.L., Arnoff, E.L.: Introduction to Operations Research. Wiley International Edition, John Wiley and Sons, Inc. (1957)
13. Saaty, T.L.: Fundamentals of Decision Making and Priority Theory with the Analytic Hierarchy Proces. RWS Publications (1994)
14. Keeney, R., Raiffa, H.: Decisions with Multiple Objective: Preferences and Value Tradeoffs. Series in probability and mathematical statistics. John Wiley and Sons (1976)
15. Goicoechea, A., Hansen, D., Duckstein, L.: Multiobjective decision analysis with engineering and business applications. John Wiley & Sons, Inc. (1982)
16. Luque, M., et al.: Incorporating preference information in interactive reference point methods for multiobjective optimization. Omega 37(2), 450–462 (2009)
17. Simon, H.A.: Theories of Decision-Making in Economics and Behavioral-Science. American Economic Review 49(3), 253–283 (1959)
18. Monarchi, D.E., Kisiel, C.C., Duckstei, L.: Interactive Multiobjective Programming in Water-Resources - Case Study. Water Resources Research 9(4), 837–850 (1973)
19. Zimmermann, H.-J.: Fuzzy Set Theory and its Applications, 3rd edn. Kluwer Academic Publishers, Dordrecht (1996)
20. Luque, M., et al.: Incorporating preference information in interactive reference point methods for multiobjective optimization. Omega-International Journal of Management Science 37(2), 450–462 (2009)

On Modeling Planning Problems:
Experience from the Petrobras Challenge

Roman Barták[1] and Neng-Fa Zhou[2]

[1] Charles University in Prague,
Faculty of Mathematics and Physics
bartak@ktiml.mff.cuni.cz
[2] The City University of New York,
Brooklyn College
nzhou@acm.org

Abstract. The International Planning Competitions have led to development of
a standard modeling framework for describing planning domains and problems
– Planning Domain Description Language (PDDL). The majority of planning
research is done around problems modeled in PDDL though there are only a
few applications adopting PDDL. The planning model of independent actions
connected only via causal relations is very flexible, but it also makes plans less
predictable (plans look different than expected by the users) and it is probably
also one of the reasons of bad practical efficiency of current planners ("visibly"
wrong plans are blindly explored by the planners). In this paper we argue that
grouping actions into flexible sub-plans is a way to overcome the efficiency
problems. The idea is that instead of seeing actions as independent entities that
are causally connected via preconditions and effects, we suggest using a form of
finite state automaton (FSA) to describe the expected sequences of actions. Arcs
in FSA are annotated by conditions guiding the planner to explore only "proper" paths in the automaton. The second idea is composing primitive actions into
meta-actions, which decreases the size of a FSA and makes planning much
faster. The main motivation is to give users more control over the action
sequencing with two primary goals: obtaining more predictable plans and improving efficiency of planning. The presented ideas originate from solving the
Petrobras logistic problem, where this technique outperformed classical
planning models.

Keywords: planning, modeling, transportation, tabling.

1   Introduction

Recent research in the area of planning is centered on the representation of problems
in the Planning Domain Description Language introduced for International Planning
Competitions [2]. Having a standard modeling language accelerated research in the
area of planning and led to development of many benchmark problems that are used
to experimentally evaluate and compare various solving approaches. On the other
hand, PDDL is based on the original STRIPS idea of having actions that are causally
connected via their preconditions and effects. This makes planning very flexible but

F. Castro, A. Gelbukh, and M. González (Eds.): MICAI 2013, Part II, LNAI 8266, pp. 466–477, 2013.
© Springer-Verlag Berlin Heidelberg 2013

also introduces some undesirable behaviors. For example, an action for unloading an item can be planned immediately after an action that loaded the item. This is causally correct (unloading requires the item to be loaded which is achieved by the loading action) though from a human perspective such action sequences are not desirable (the state after unloading will be identical to the state before loading). It is possible to forbid such situations by changing the model in such a way that, for example, a transportation action is planned between loading and unloading[1]. However, such enhanced models are less natural and less readable by humans, and flaws can be easily introduced in the models if more such modifications are required. It seems more natural, if a human modeler prescribes possible (reasonable) action sequences. There exist two modeling approaches based on this idea, *hierarchical task networks* (HTNs) [9] and *timelines* [13]. While HTN uses the notion of task that decomposes into sub-tasks until primitive activities are obtained, timelines focus on modeling allowed time evolutions of state variables and synchronizations between the state variables.

In this paper we study a modeling framework positioned half way between timelines and HTNs. Similarly to [4] we propose to use a *finite state automaton* (FSA) describing allowed sequences of actions. A FSA plays the role of effects and conditions from classical planning as it says which actions may follow a given action. A FSA can be accompanied by additional constraints restricting when some transitions between the actions may occur. These conditions are different from classical action preconditions as they involve information about the goal (*Pickup* cargo only when there is some cargo to deliver). This is much closer to *control rules* [7], but rather than specifying control rules separately from the description of the planning domain, we suggest integrating them in the domain. This is an original idea of this paper.

We have found that the above modeling approach is not sufficient enough when solving real-life problems and we suggest additional extensions motivated by the Petrobras challenge. The Petrobras challenge is a logistic problem [15] of transporting cargo items between ports and oil platforms using vessels with limited capacity. The paper [14] studied three approaches to solve this problem. The winning technique was based on Monte Carlo Tree Search (MCTS) where the search was done over sequences of meta-actions. Each meta-action was then decomposed to primitive actions based on the situation. In this paper we use a very similar idea where we take "reasonable" sub-plans (sequences of actions) and encode them as a single meta-action. The FSA is then defined over these meta-actions. During planning the selected meta-action decomposes into a sequence of primitive actions depending on the current situation. There already exists a concept of *macro-actions* in planning [5]. However, while a macro-action decomposes to a fixed sequence of primitive actions, a meta-action may decompose to different sequences of primitive actions based on the situation. The concept of meta-actions is closer to HTNs, though we use only one level of decompositions – from a meta-action to a sequence of primitive actions. Also, planning in our framework is based on action sequencing rather than on task decomposition.

This paper shows that action grouping and prescribed action sequencing are very important for the Petrobras challenge. Instead of sophisticated MCTS method, we use backtracking accompanied by tabling [16] to solve the problem. As we shall experi-

---

[1] The action *unload* may use some new proposition – a semaphore – as its precondition, and this proposition is removed by the *load* action while added by the *transport* actions.

mentally show the resulting method achieves very similar performance to the MCTS algorithm. Hence we believe the presented modeling concepts are important for solving real-life planning problems and may bring significant efficiency boost.

The paper is organized as follows. We will first briefly introduce the Petrobras challenge, highlight some of its important components, and describe the three techniques already applied to this problem. Then we will present the proposed modeling framework based on finite state automata, explain the solving technique, and show how actions can be grouped to meta-actions. After that we will experimentally compare our method with the current best methods using the Petrobras benchmarks from [14]. Description of possible future directions of research will conclude the paper.

2   The Petrobras Challenge

2.1   Problem Formulation

International Competition on Knowledge Engineering for Planning and Scheduling (ICKEPS 2012) brought several real-life motivated modeling and solving challenges including the Petrobras problem. The Petrobras problem [15] deals with planning deliveries of cargo items between ports and platforms while respecting the capacity limits of vessels, ports, and platforms. The ports and platforms can serve a limited number of vessels at the same time; the vessels can transport limited weight of cargo items, vessels' load influences vessels' speeds and fuel consumption, and the limited capacity of fuel tanks must also be assumed when planning transport (refueling is possible). Given a set of cargo items to deliver (including cargo weights and initial ports), the problem is to find a feasible plan that guarantees the delivery of all cargo items to given destinations (platforms) and respects the constraints on the vessel, port, and platform capacities. The vessels should leave a waiting area, perform their mission and go back to one of the waiting areas. Loading and unloading of cargo items are done at ports and platforms and require some time. The vessels can be refueled at ports and certain platforms and each vessel must always have enough fuel to go to the nearest refueling station. We will describe the particular primitive actions, which can be assumed during planning, later in the text.

2.2   Techniques Used to Solve the Challenge

So far there was only one attempt to solve the full Petrobras challenge. Toropila et al. [14] applied classical planning, temporal planning, and Monte Carle Tree Search (MCTS) to solve the Petrobras challenge.

The **classical planning approach** modeled the problem in PDDL 3.0 [10] with numerical fluents describing the restricted resource capacities (fuel tank, cargo capacity, ports/platforms docks). This model used actions as specified in the problem formulation, namely: *navigate-empty-vessel, navigate-nonempty-vessel, load-cargo, unload-cargo, refuel-vessel-platform, refuel-vessel-port, dock-vessel, undock-vessel.* SGPlan 6.0 [11] was used to solve the problem while optimizing fuel consumption (other planners have been tried but were not able to process the domain description). Action duration was added to the solution in the post-processing stage.

The **temporal planning approach** modeled the problem in PDDL 3.1 [12] with fluents and durative actions. Basically the same set of actions with durations was used. This model supports concurrency of actions directly. The Filuta planner [8] was used to solve the problem while optimizing makespan. Filuta uses ad-hoc solvers to handle resources, namely unary, consumable, and reservoir resources are supported.

The last approach exploited **Monte Carlo Tree Search** (MCTS) techniques that become recently popular in computer Go [6]. To allow using MCTS, a different action model was applied to obtain finite plans in search branches. This model is based on four abstract actions: *Load, Unload, Refuel, GoToWaitingArea*. These actions describe "intentions" and they are decomposed to particular actions based on situation (state). For example, the action *Unload* assumes that cargo is loaded and vessel is either in a port or a platform. This action is decomposed in the following way. If the current location of the vessel is the same as the target location of the cargo then only a single underlying action *unload-cargo* is performed, otherwise the abstract action is translated to the following sequence of the original actions: *undock-vessel, navigate-nonempty-vessel, dock-vessel, unload-cargo*.

The experiments with the challenge data and randomly generated data, where the number of vessels and cargo items varied (3-10 vessels, 1-15 cargo items), showed that the classical planning approach is not viable as it cannot solve problems with more (7+) cargo items. The MCTS was the clear winner, followed by Filuta that can solve all problems, but the quality of plans was significantly lower (30% for makespan, 130% for fuel consumption).

3   The Novel Modeling Approach

The approaches from the Petrobras challenge inspired us to explore the reasons of success of the MCTS technique (and partly Filuta). In particular we focused on the "predefined" action sequences that are hidden in the abstract actions of the MCTS approach and partly also in the special resource solvers in the Filuta planner. Another motivation for our research went from the efficient model of the Sokoban game implemented in B-Prolog [17]. This model was also based on grouping actions into specific sequences. Our hypothesis is that even a simple search algorithm, for example depth-first search with tabling [16], can solve complex planning problems provided that the model itself guides the solver by describing expected action sequences rather than giving only independent actions connected via causal relations.

3.1   Model Based on Finite State Automata

Let us first describe the possible plans of each vessel in the Petrobras challenge as a finite state automaton. Finite state automata (FSA) were shown to significantly improve efficiency of constraint-based planners [4] and they represent a natural model to describe allowed action sequences. FSAs are also used in the Filuta planner to describe allowed state transitions. Figure 1 shows the FSA that models all possible actions and transitions between the actions for a single vessel in the Petrobras domain.

We already use some abstract actions there, for example the action *navigate* means *navigate-empty-vessel*, if the vessel is empty, or *navigate-nonempty-vessel*, if some cargo is loaded to the vessel. Similarly the action *refuel* means either *refuel-vessel-platform* or *refuel-vessel-port* depending on whether the vessel is docked in a platform or in a port. Notice also that the presented FSA restricts some action sequences. In particular, it is not possible to dock immediately after undocking – there is no practical reason for such a sequence of actions though the classical PDDL model allows it. Similarly, refueling is done only after loading/unloading – this removes symmetrical sequences of actions with an identical overall effect (the vessel is loaded/unloaded and refueled). Finally, during one stop at the port or platform, the FSA allows either loading of cargo or unloading of cargo, but not both operations together. This is motivated by the particular problem to be solved – we need to move cargo from ports to platforms. Hence, there is no need to unload a cargo (at some platform) and load another cargo at the same location. In principle, it might be possible to move cargo to some intermediate location where it will be picked up by another vessel. However such flexible plans were not found necessary in the Petrobras challenge. Note finally that all these sequencing restrictions are naturally modeled using the transitions in the FSA. If more flexible plans are desirable then the corresponding transitions can be added to the FSA. We also use another mechanism to restrict sequencing by putting constraints on the transitions. These constraints describe situations when the transition is allowed. We will describe these constraints in more detail later in the text. The classical planning model with action preconditions and effects makes expressing such allowed action sequences much more complicated and not very natural (see the footnote 1 in the Introduction).

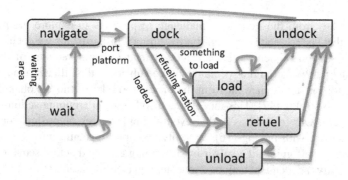

Fig. 1. Finite state automaton describing actions and allowed transitions (with some conditions) between the actions in the Petrobras challenge

Actions in the model have specific durations that are given by action parameters (such as locations and current load for the navigation actions). Hence, in the planning terminology we should rather talk about *planning operators* and actions are obtained by setting values of the parameters. The capacity of the vessel is modeled in the action, for example, the transition to a loading action is allowed only if there is enough capacity in the vessel.

So far we discussed plans for a single vessel, but if there are more vessels in the problem, their plans interact. For example at most two vessels can be docked at the port at the same time. We check these synchronization constraints when adding a new action to the plan as described in the next section.

3.2   Solving Approach

The solving algorithm uses the round-robin approach, where an action is selected for each vessel provided that the last action for that vessel finished before the rolling horizon. Figure 2 demonstrates the left-to-right round-robing solving approach that combines planning (action selection) with scheduling (allocation to time and resources). At the beginning all vessels are waiting so in the first step, we select an action for each vessel. There is only one exception of this process – if a vessel is waiting and a new waiting action is selected, we only prolong the existing waiting action for that vessel. Waiting action is the only action with arbitrary duration so it is possible to set its duration to any time. Action selection represents the choice point of the search algorithm. The only "heuristic" for action selection is the fixed order of actions in the model specification, where for example *unloading* is before *loading* which is before *refueling* for a docked vessel. There are also "control rules" encoded in the action descriptions – for example, the navigation action for an empty vessel goes only to a port with some remaining cargo, or to a refueling station, or to a waiting area.

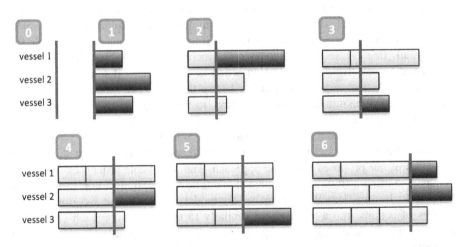

Fig. 2. Illustration of the left-to-right integrated planning and scheduling approach with a rolling horizon (vertical line). Newly added actions are displayed as black rectangles; x-axis represents time.

We have implemented the above solving approach in B-Prolog using tabling [1]. It means that we use depth-first search with remembering visited states – the state is represented by current states of vessels and a list of cargo items to be still delivered. In each step, we select an action for each vessel and move the time horizon. The core idea of this "planning" algorithm can be described using the following abstract code (this is actually an executable code in Picat [3] the follower of B-Prolog):

```
table (+,-,min)
plan(S,Plan,Cost),final(S) =>
    Plan=[],Cost=0.
plan(S,Plan,Cost) =>
    action(Action,S,S1,ActionCost),
    plan(S1,Plan1,Cost1),
    Plan = [Action|Plan1],
    Cost = Cost1+ActionCost.
```

As the reader can see, the search procedure is very simple. The real power of the solving approach is hidden in the action model and in the tabling mechanism. Tabling is important to save visited states so they are not re-explored. In the above code, for each state S the tabling mechanism stores the found Plan while minimizing the Cost of the plan (the cost is measured by makespan in the Petrobras problem). It is a form of a branch-and-bound procedure.

3.3   Meta-actions

Though the presented action model already included some sequencing restrictions, we have found experimentally that the model did not scale up well. In fact, it worked only for a single vessel with a few cargo items to deliver. By exploring the generated plans we noticed two types of erratic behavior. If more cargo items were available for delivery, all "free" vessels headed to the port, where cargo was located. This behavior was caused by preferring the navigation action to other actions if some cargo should be delivered. As the cargo was available before the first vessel loaded it, the other vessels "believed" that there is still some cargo to deliver and so transport to the port was planned for them. The second problematic behavior was that vessels left the waiting area just to refuel and then returned back to the waiting area.

Though the naïve model was not competitive to solve the problem, it showed the core ideas of our proposed modeling approach. The reasonable sequences of actions are modeled using a finite state automaton. To follow some transition a specific condition must be satisfied. We can make this model more efficient by grouping sequences of actions into a meta-action similarly to the MCTS approach [14]. Each meta-action may be a sequence of primitive actions with possible alternatives. We propose a model using four meta-actions with more specific conditions to apply the actions. Figure 3 shows the resulting finite state automaton including the transition conditions. Each meta-action decomposes into primitive actions while applying additional conditions on the actions. For example, the *Deliver* action starts with the *navigate* action but the destination is selected only from the destinations of loaded cargo items (a choice point). The next action in the sequence is *docking* followed by *unloading* and, if possible *refueling* done in parallel with *unloading*. We always unload all cargo items for a given destination and we always refuel the full tank (deterministic choice). The last action in the sequence is *undocking*. The *Deliver* action can only be used if some cargo is loaded to the vessel. Similarly, the *Pickup* action is applicable only if the vessel is empty and there is some cargo to deliver. We select the port where cargo is available (choice point) and pre-allocate some cargo items to the vessel (choice point). These conditions ensure that vessels are moving only when necessary. The *Pickup* action then decomposes to *navigate, docking, loading* and *refueling,* and *undocking* actions. Note that there could be more *loading* actions if more cargo items are loaded. As the order of loaded items is not important, only a single sequence of loading actions is explored during the decomposition (based on the fixed order of cargo items). This further reduces the search space – equivalent permutations of *loading* actions are not explored (similarly for *unloading* actions). The last two actions are *Waiting* and *Go2Wait* that are applicable if the vessel is empty and it is in the waiting area (then *Waiting*) or elsewhere (*Go2Wait*). The *Go2Wait* action decomposes to the *navigate* action, but if there would not be enough fuel then the vessel navigates to a refueling station before navigating to the waiting area. The three actions that include transport – *Pickup, Delivery, Go2Wait* – force the vessels to do only "reasonable" moves. If the vessel is empty, it can either go to a waiting area or to some port to pickup cargo, if any cargo is available. No other movement is allowed. Similarly, if the vessel is loaded, it can go only to some platform where some loaded cargo should be delivered.

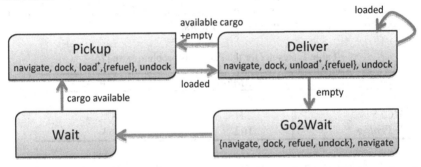

Fig. 3. Meta-actions and allowed transitions between meta-action in the Petrobras domain

The meta-actions allow users to specify expected sub-plans with conditions when to apply the sub-plans and non-determinism to be resolved by the planner (what cargo by which vessel). The user has better control about how the plans look like while leaving some decisions to the solver. The major caveat is some loss of flexibility. By specifying the sub-plans we may omit possible plans that were not assumed by the user. For example, in our model, we do not allow to pickup new cargo while some cargo is still loaded to the vessel. Also the cargo is only unloaded at its final destination. In particular, it is not possible to deliver the cargo "half-way" and using another vessel to deliver it to the final destination. These restrictions were intentional to reduce exploration of "unwanted" plans.

4   Experimental Results

To evaluate the proposed modeling and solving techniques we compare them with the best approaches from [14], namely the Filuta planner and the MCTS approach. We do not include SGPlan as its results were poor compared to other approaches. The Filuta planner minimized makespan identically to our method, while the MCTS planner used a manually tuned ad-hoc objective function that combined makespan, the number of actions, and fuel consumption: $usedFuel+10*numActions+5*makespan$. We re-use here the results reported in [14] where the experiments were run on the Ubuntu Linux machine equipped with Intel® Core™ i7-2600 CPU @ 3.40GHz and 4GB of memory and the planners were allowed to use approximately 10 minutes of runtime. Our method was implemented in B-Prolog, we run the experiments on the MacOS X 10.7.5 (Lion) machine with 1.8 GHz Intel® Core™ i7 CPU and 4GB of memory, and we report the best results found within one minute of runtime (we did not observe any further improvement when running B-Prolog longer).

We will first present the results for the original Petrobras problem described in [15], which consisted of 10 vessels and 15 cargo items to deliver, with the original fuel tank capacity for all vessels set to 600 liters. Table 1 shows the comparison of makespan and fuel consumption that were two major objectives in the Petrobras challenge. We can see that our approach is significantly better than the Filuta planner in both objectives and it also beats the best so-far approach based on MCTS in the makespan though the total fuel consumption is worse.

Table 1. Results for the Petrobras problem from [15]

Planner	Makespan	Fuel
Filuta	263 (1.62x)	1989 (2.24x)
MCTS	204 (1.26x)	**887** (1.00x)
B-Prolog	**162** (1.00x)	1263 (1.42x)

To compare the approaches in more detail, the paper [14] proposed several random benchmarks based on the Petrobras domain, where the number of cargo items to deliver and the number of available vessels varied. They also varied the fuel tank capacity, but according to the experiments this had a limited impact of performance so we kept the fuel tank capacity at 600 liters. We used two scenarios from [14] with 3 vessels and 10 vessels (called Group A and Group B in [14]), and we varied the number of cargo items from 1 to 15. Figure 4 shows the comparison of makespan for all three planners. We can observe that our approach is better for problems with the smaller number of cargo items, while the MCTS method takes lead when the number of cargo items increases. In fact, for the first six problems in each group, our system found (and proved) makespan-optimal plans, while the other two planners are suboptimal only. We were also consistently better than the Filuta planner.

Regarding the fuel consumption (Figure 5), our planner is closer to the Filuta planner; we are mostly better but there were problems on which Filuta found plans with less fuel consumption. The MCTS method was consistently the best planner regarding fuel consumption, though this is not surprising as the other two planners optimized makespan only.

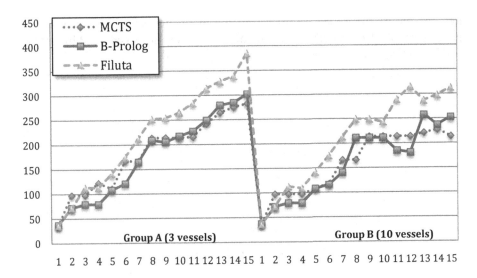

Fig. 4. Comparison of makespan for problems with different numbers of cargo items

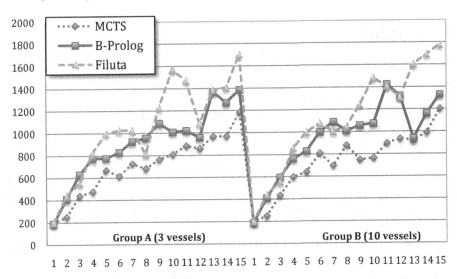

Fig. 5. Comparison of fuel consumption for problems with different numbers of cargo items

In the final experiment, we looked at the behavior of our planner when exploring the feasible plans. Recall that our method mimics the branch-and-bound algorithm in the sense that it starts with the first feasible plan and then outputs only better plans. Figure 6 shows the evolution of makespan and fuel consumption for the original Petrobras problem (so the order of solutions is from right to left as the makespan decreases). The figure shows a bit surprising "jumps" of fuel consumption when the makespan is decreasing. It may seem that this can be explained by increasing the number of vessels as the makespan decreases, but adding one more vessel to the plan does not always correspond with the increased fuel consumption. This behavior requires more detailed study that can also uncover why the plans generated by our method have larger fuel consumption than the MCTS method.

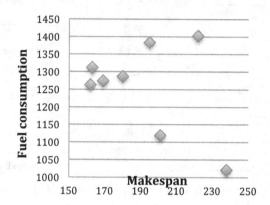

Fig. 6. Makespan and fuel consumption in plans found for the Petrobras challenge

5   Conclusions

We proposed a novel framework for describing planning problems that is based on meta-actions and transitions between them accompanied by conditions when the transitions can be used. Each meta-action decomposes into primitive actions; again specific conditions can be imposed on the parameters of these actions and also on their composition. The main motivation was to give users more control over action sequencing with two primary goals: obtaining more predictable plans and improving efficiency of planning. We demonstrated the modeling principles using a single domain – the Petrobras challenge – and using a single solving approach – B-Prolog with tabling. Though the solving technique is very simple, the proposed approach was shown to be competitive with the leading technique for the Petrobras problem in terms of plan quality (our technique was also faster).

The next step is to decouple the modeling approach from the solving mechanism and applying it to other planning problems. We sketched the modeling principles informally; a formal description in the form of a modeling language is necessary for more general applicability. The presented approach can also drive further research in the tabling methods applied to optimization problems. Other solving techniques may also be applied, we are not aware of any current planner supporting all three presented features: meta-actions, predefined action sequencing, and control rules. It would be interesting to study how these three modeling techniques contribute to plan efficiency. Our preliminary experiments showed that their combination helped to successfully solve the Petrobras challenge.

Acknowledgements. Roman Barták is supported by the Czech Science Foundation under the project KnowSched (P202-10-1188).

References

1. B-Prolog, http://www.probp.com
2. International Planning Competitions, http://ipc.icaps-conference.org
3. Picat, http://www.picat-lang.org
4. Barták, R.: On Constraint Models for Parallel Planning: The Novel Transition Scheme. In: Proceedings of SCAI 2011. Frontiers of Artificial Intelligence, vol. 227, pp. 50–59. IOS Press (2011)
5. Botea, A., Enzenberger, M., Muller, M., Schaeffer, J.: Macro-FF: Improving AI planning with automatically learned macro-operators. Journal of Artificial Intelligence Research 24, 581–621 (2005)
6. Chaslot, G., Bakkes, S., Szita, I., Spronck, P.: Monte-Carlo tree search: A new framework for game AI. In: Proceedings of the Fourth Artificial Intelligence and Interactive Digital Entertainment Conference. The AAAI Press (2008)
7. Doherty, P., Kvarnström, J.: TALplanner: An empirical investigation of a temporal logic-based forward chaining planner. In: Proceedings of the Sixth International Workshop on Temporal Representation and Reasoning (TIME 1999), pp. 47–54. IEEE Computer Society Press, Orlando (1999)
8. Dvořák, F., Barták, R.: Integrating time and resources into planning. In: Proceedings of ICTAI 2010, vol. 2, pp. 71–78. IEEE Computer Society (2010)
9. Erol, K., Hendler, J., Nau, D.: HTN Planning: Complexity and Expressivity. In: Proceedings of AAAI 1994, pp. 1123–1128 (1994)
10. Gerevini, A., Long, D.: BNF description of PDDL 3.0 (2005), http://cs-www.cs.yale.edu/homes/dvm/papers/pddl-bnf.pdf
11. Hsu, C., Wah, B.W.: The SGPlan planning system in IPC-6 (2008), http://wah.cse.cuhk.edu.hk/wah/Wah/papers/C168/C168.pdf
12. Kovacs, D.L.: BNF definition of PDDL 3.1 (2011), http://www.plg.inf.uc3m.es/ipc2011-deterministic/OtherContributions?action=AttachFile&do=view&target=kovacs-pddl-3.1-2011.pdf
13. Muscettola, N.: HSTS: Integrating Planning and Scheduling. In: Intelligent Scheduling. Morgan Kaufmann (1994)
14. Toropila, D., Dvořák, F., Trunda, O., Hanes, M., Barták, R.: Three Approaches to Solve the Petrobras Challenge: Exploiting Planning Techniques for Solving Real-Life Logistics Problems. In: Proceedings of ICTAI 2012, pp. 191–198. IEEE Conference Publishing Services (2012)
15. Vaquero, T.S., Costa, G., Tonidandel, F., Igreja, H., Silva, J.R., Beck, C.: Planning and scheduling ship operations on petroleum ports and platform. In: Proceedings of the Scheduling and Planning Applications Workshop, pp. 8–16 (2012)
16. Warren, D.S.: Memoing for Logic Programs. CACM 35(3), 93–111 (1992)
17. Zhou, N.-F., Dovier, A.: A Tabled Prolog Program for Solving Sokoban. In: Proceedings of the 26th Italian Conference on Computational Logic (CILC 2011), pp. 215–228 (2011)

An Introduction
to Concept-Level Sentiment Analysis

Erik Cambria

Temasek Laboratories, National University of Singapore
cambria@nus.edu.sg
http://sentic.net

Abstract. The ways people express their opinions and sentiments have radically changed in the past few years thanks to the advent of social networks, web communities, blogs, wikis, and other online collaborative media. The distillation of knowledge from the huge amount of unstructured information on the Web can be a key factor for marketers who want to create an image or identity in the minds of their customers for their product or brand. These online social data, however, remain hardly accessible to computers, as they are specifically meant for human consumption. The automatic analysis of online opinions, in fact, involves a deep understanding of natural language text by machines, from which we are still very far. To this end, concept-level sentiment analysis aims to go beyond a mere word-level analysis of text and provide novel approaches to opinion mining and sentiment analysis that enable a more efficient passage from (unstructured) textual information to (structured) machine-processable data, in potentially any domain.

Keywords: AI, NLP, concept-level sentiment analysis, big social data analysis.

1 Introduction

Hitherto, online information retrieval has been mainly based on algorithms relying on the textual representation of web pages. Such algorithms are very good at retrieving texts, splitting them into parts, checking the spelling, and counting their words. But when it comes to interpreting sentences and extracting meaningful information, their capabilities are known to be very limited.

Early works aimed to classify entire documents as containing overall positive or negative polarity, or rating scores of reviews. Such systems were mainly based on supervised approaches relying on manually labeled samples, such as movie or product reviews where the opinionist's overall positive or negative attitude was explicitly indicated. However, opinions and sentiments do not occur only at document-level, nor they are limited to a single valence or target. Contrary or complementary attitudes toward the same topic or multiple topics can be present across the span of a document.

Later works adopted a segment-level opinion analysis aiming to distinguish sentimental from non-sentimental sections, e.g., by using graph-based techniques for segmenting sections of a document on the basis of their subjectivity, or by performing a classification based on some fixed syntactic phrases that are likely to be used to express opinions.

F. Castro, A. Gelbukh, and M. González (Eds.): MICAI 2013, Part II, LNAI 8266, pp. 478–483, 2013.

In more recent works, text analysis granularity has been taken down to sentence-level, e.g., by using presence of opinion-bearing lexical items (single words or n-grams) to detect subjective sentences, or by exploiting association rule mining for a feature-based analysis of product reviews. These approaches, however, are still far from being able to infer the cognitive and affective information associated with natural language as they mainly rely on knowledge bases that are still too limited to efficiently process text at sentence-level. Moreover, such text analysis granularity might still not be enough as a single sentence may contain different opinions about different facets of the same product or service.

2   Main Approaches to Sentiment Analysis

Existing approaches to sentiment analysis can be grouped into three main categories: keyword spotting, lexical affinity, and statistical methods. Keyword spotting is the most naive approach and probably also the most popular because of its accessibility and economy. Text is classified into affect categories based on the presence of fairly un-ambiguous affect words like 'happy', 'sad', 'afraid', and 'bored'. The weaknesses of this approach lie in two areas: poor recognition of affect when negation is involved and reliance on surface features. About its first weakness, while the approach can correctly classify the sentence "today was a happy day" as being happy, it is likely to fail on a sentence like "today wasn't a happy day at all". About its second weakness, the approach relies on the presence of obvious affect words that are only surface features of the prose. In practice, a lot of sentences convey affect through underlying meaning rather than affect adjectives. For example, the text "My husband just filed for divorce and he wants to take custody of my children away from me" certainly evokes strong emotions, but uses no affect keywords, and therefore, cannot be classified using a keyword spotting approach.

Lexical affinity is slightly more sophisticated than keyword spotting as, rather than simply detecting obvious affect words, it assigns arbitrary words a probabilistic 'affin-ity' for a particular emotion. For example, 'accident' might be assigned a 75% prob-ability of being indicating a negative affect, as in 'car accident' or 'hurt by accident'. These probabilities are usually trained from linguistic corpora. Though often outper-forming pure keyword spotting, there are two main problems with the approach. First, lexical affinity, operating solely on the word-level, can easily be tricked by sentences like "I avoided an accident" (negation) and "I met my girlfriend by accident" (other word senses). Second, lexical affinity probabilities are often biased toward text of a par-ticular genre, dictated by the source of the linguistic corpora. This makes it difficult to develop a reusable, domain-independent model.

Statistical methods, such as Bayesian inference and support vector machines, have been popular for affect classification of texts. By feeding a machine learning algorithm a large training corpus of affectively annotated texts, it is possible for the system to not only learn the affective valence of affect keywords (as in the keyword spotting approach), but also to take into account the valence of other arbitrary keywords (like lexical affinity), punctuation, and word co-occurrence frequencies. However, traditional statistical methods are generally semantically weak, meaning that, with the exception of obvious affect keywords, other lexical or co-occurrence elements in a statistical model have little predictive value individually. As a result, statistical text classifiers only work with acceptable accuracy when given a sufficiently large text input. So, while these methods may be able to affectively classify user's text on the page- or paragraph- level, they do not work well on smaller text units such as sentences or clauses.

3   Concept-Level Sentiment Analysis

Concept-based approaches to sentiment analysis focus on a semantic analysis of text through the use of web ontologies or semantic networks, which allow the aggregation of conceptual and affective information associated with natural language opinions. By relying on large semantic knowledge bases, such approaches step away from blind use of keywords and word co-occurrence count, but rather rely on the implicit features associated with natural language concepts. Unlike purely syntactical techniques, concept-based approaches are able to detect also sentiments that are expressed in a subtle manner, e.g., through the analysis of concepts that do not explicitly convey any emotion, but which are implicitly linked to other concepts that do so.

The analysis at concept-level is intended to infer the semantic and affective information associated with natural language opinions and, hence, to enable a comparative fine-grained feature-based sentiment analysis. Rather than gathering isolated opinions about a whole item (e.g., iPhone5), users are generally more interested in comparing different products according to their specific features (e.g., iPhone5's vs Galaxy S3's touchscreen), or even sub-features (e.g., fragility of iPhone5's vs Galaxy S3's touchscreen). In this context, the construction of comprehensive common and common-sense knowledge bases is key for feature-spotting and polarity detection, respectively [1]. Common-sense, in particular, is necessary to properly deconstruct natural language text into sentiments— for example, to appraise the concept "small room" as negative for a hotel review and "small queue" as positive for a post office, or the concept "go read the book" as positive for a book review but negative for a movie review [2].

Current approaches to concept-level sentiment analysis mainly leverage on existing affective knowledge bases such as ANEW [3], WordNet-Affect [4], ISEAR [5], Senti-WordNet [6], and SenticNet [7]. In [8], for example, a concept-level sentiment dictionary is built through a two-step method combining iterative regression and random walk with in-link normalization. ANEW and SenticNet are exploited for propagating sentiment values based on the assumption that semantically related concepts share common sentiment. Moreover, polarity accuracy, Kendall distance, and average-maximum ratio are used, in stead of mean error, to better evaluate sentiment dictionaries. A similar approach is adopted in [9], which presents a methodology for enriching SenticNet concepts with affective information by assigning an emotion label to them. Authors use various features extracted from ISEAR, as well as similarity measures that rely on the polarity data provided in SenticNet (those based on WordNet-Affect) and ISEAR distance-based measures, including point-wise mutual information, and emotional affinity. Another recent work that builds upon an existing affective knowledge base is [10], which proposes the re-evaluation of objective words in SentiWordNet by assessing the sentimental relevance of such words and their associated sentiment sentences. Two sampling strategies are proposed and integrated with support vector machines for sentiment classification. According to the experiments, the proposed approach significantly outperforms the traditional sentiment mining approach, which ignores the importance of objective words in SentiWordNet. In [11], the main issues related to the development of a corpus for opinion mining and sentiment analysis are discussed both by surveying the existing works in this area and presenting, as a case study, an ongoing project for Italian, called Senti–TUT, where a corpus for the investigation of irony about politics in social media is developed.

Other works explore the ensemble application of knowledge bases and statistical methods. In [12], for example, a hybrid approach to combine lexical analysis and machine learning is proposed in order to cope with ambiguity and integrate the context of sentiment terms. The context-aware method identifies ambiguous terms that vary in polarity depending on the context and stores them in contextualized sentiment lexicons. In conjunction with semantic knowledge bases, these lexicons help ground ambiguous sentiment terms to concepts that correspond to their polarity. More machine-learning based works include [13], which introduces a new methodology for the retrieval of product features and opinions from a collection of free-text customer reviews about a product or service. Such a methodology relies on a language-modeling framework that can be applied to reviews in any domain and language provided with a seed set of opinion words. The methodology combines both a kernel-based model of opinion words (learned from the seed set of opinion words) and a statistical mapping between words to approximate a model of product features from which the retrieval is carried out.

Other recent works in the context of concept-level sentiment analysis include tasks such as domain adaptation [14], opinion summarization [15], and multimodal sentiment analysis [16,17]. In the problem of domain adaptation, there are two distinct needs, namely labeling adaptation and instance adaptation. However, most of current research focuses on the former attribute, while neglects the latter one. In [14], a comprehensive approach, named feature ensemble plus sample selection (SS-FE), is proposed. SS-FE takes both types of adaptation into account: a feature ensemble (FE) model is first adopted to learn a new labeling function in a feature re-weighting manner, and a PCA-based sample selection (PCA-SS) method is then used as an aid to FE. A first step towards concept-level summarization is done by STARLET [15], a novel approach to extractive multi-document summarization for evaluative text that considers aspect rating distributions and language modeling as summarization features. Such features encourage the inclusion of sentences in the summary that preserve the overall opinion distribution expressed across the original reviews and whose language best reflects the language of reviews. The proposed method offers improvements over traditional summarization techniques and other approaches to multi-document summarization of evaluative text.

A sub-field of sentiment analysis that is becoming increasingly popular is multimodal sentiment analysis. [16], for example, considers multimodal sentiment analysis based on linguistic, audio, and visual features. A database of 105 Spanish videos of 2 to 8 minutes length containing 21 male and 84 female speakers was collected randomly from the social media website YouTube and annotated by two labellers for ternary sentiment. This led to 550 utterances and approximately 10,000 words. The authors state that the data is available per request. The joint use of the three feature types leads to a significant improvement over the use of each single modality. This is further confirmed on another set of English videos. In [17], instead, authors introduce the ICT-MMMO database of personal movie reviews collected from YouTube (308 clips) and ExpoTV (78 clips). The final set contains 370 of these 1-3 minutes English clips in ternary sentiment annotation by one to two coders. The feature basis is formed by 2 k audio features, 20 video features, and different textual features for selection. Then, different levels of domain-dependence are considered: in-domain analysis, cross-domain analysis based on the 100 k textual Metacritic movie review corpus for training, and use of on-line knowledge sources. This shows that cross-corpus training works sufficiently well, and language-independent audiovisual analysis to be competitive with linguistic analysis.

4 Conclusion

Between the dawn of civilization through 2003, there were just a few dozens exabytes of information on the Web. Today, that much information is created weekly. The advent of the Social Web has provided people with new tools for creating and sharing, in a time and cost efficient way, their own contents, ideas, and opinions with virtually the millions of people connected to the World Wide Web. The opportunity to capture the opinions of the general public about social events, political movements, company strategies, marketing campaigns, and product preferences has raised increasing interest both in the scientific community, for the exciting open challenges, and in the business world, for the remarkable fallouts in marketing and financial market prediction. This huge amount of useful information, however, is mainly unstructured as specifically produced for human consumption and, hence, it is not directly machine-processable.

Concept-level sentiment analysis can help with this in which, unlike other word-based approaches, it focuses on a semantic analysis of text through the use of web ontologies or semantic networks, which allow the aggregation of conceptual and affective information associated with natural language opinions. The validity of concept-based approaches, however, depends on the depth and breadth of the employed knowledge bases. Without a comprehensive resource that encompasses human knowledge, it is not easy for an opinion mining system to grasp the semantics associated with natural language text. Another limitation of semantic approaches is in the typicality of their knowledge bases. Knowledge representation, in fact, is usually strictly defined and does not allow different concept nuances to be handled, as the inference of semantic and affective features associated with concepts is bounded by the fixed, flat representation. In the big social data context, finally, semantic parsing techniques will be key in quickly identifying natural language concepts from free text without requiring time-consuming phrase structure analysis [18].

References

1. Cambria, E., Song, Y., Wang, H., Howard, N.: Semantic multi-dimensional scaling for open-domain sentiment analysis. IEEE Intelligent Systems (2013), doi:10.1109/MIS.2012.118
2. Cambria, E., Schuller, B., Xia, Y., Havasi, C.: New avenues in opinion mining and sentiment analysis. IEEE Intelligent Systems 28(2), 15–21 (2013)

3. Bradley, M., Lang, P.: Affective norms for english words (ANEW): Stimuli, instruction manual and affective ratings. Technical report, The Center for Research in Psychophysiology, University of Florida (1999)
4. Strapparava, C., Valitutti, A.: WordNet-Affect: An affective extension of WordNet. In: LREC, Lisbon, pp. 1083–1086 (2004)
5. Bazzanella, C.: Emotions, language and context. In: Weigand, E. (ed.) Emotion in Dialogic Interaction. Advances in the complex, pp. 59–76, Benjamins, Amsterdam (2004)
6. Esuli, A., Sebastiani, F.: SentiWordNet: A publicly available lexical resource for opinion mining. In: LREC (2006)
7. Cambria, E., Havasi, C., Hussain, A.: SenticNet 2: A semantic and affective resource for opinion mining and sentiment analysis. In: FLAIRS, Marco Island, pp. 202–207 (2012)
8. Tsai, A., Tsai, R., Hsu, J.: Building a concept-level sentiment dictionary based on common-sense knowledge. IEEE Intelligent Systems 28(2), 22–30 (2013)
9. Poria, S., Gelbukh, A., Hussain, A., Das, D., Bandyopadhyay, S.: Enhanced SenticNet with affective labels for concept-based opinion mining. IEEE Intelligent Systems 28(2), 31–30 (2013)
10. Hung, C., Lin, H.K.: Using objective words in SentiWordNet to improve sentiment classification for word of mouth. IEEE Intelligent Systems 28(2), 47–54 (2013)
11. Bosco, C., Patti, V., Bolioli, A.: Developing corpora for sentiment analysis and opinion mining: A survey and the Senti-TUT case study. IEEE Intelligent Systems 28(2), 55–63 (2013)
12. Weichselbraun, A., Gindl, S., Scharl, A.: Extracting and grounding context-aware sentiment lexicons. IEEE Intelligent Systems 28(2), 39–46 (2013)
13. García-Moya, L., Anaya-Sanchez, H., Berlanga-Llavori, R.: A language model approach for retrieving product features and opinions from customer reviews. IEEE Intelligent Systems 28(3), 19–27 (2013)
14. Xia, R., Zong, C., Hu, X., Cambria, E.: Feature ensemble plus sample selection: A comprehensive approach to domain adaptation for sentiment classification. IEEE Intelligent Systems 28(3), 10–18 (2013)
15. Di Fabbrizio, G., Aker, A., Gaizauskas, R.: Summarizing on-line product and service reviews using aspect rating distributions and language modeling. IEEE Intelligent Systems 28(3), 28–37 (2013)
16. Perez-Rosas, V., Mihalcea, R., Morency, L.P.: Multimodal sentiment analysis of Spanish online videos. IEEE Intelligent Systems 28(3), 38–45 (2013)
17. Wollmer, M., Weninger, F., Knaup, T., Schuller, B., Congkai, S., Sagae, K., Morency, L.P.: YouTube movie reviews: In, cross, and open-domain sentiment analysis in an audiovisual context. IEEE Intelligent Systems 28(3), 46–53 (2013)
18. Cambria, E., Rajagopal, D., Olsher, D., Das, D.: Big social data analysis. In: Akerkar, R. (ed.) Big Data Computing, pp. 401–414. Chapman and Hall/CRC (2013)

Common Sense Knowledge Based Personality Recognition from Text

Soujanya Poria[1], Alexandar Gelbukh[2,3], Basant Agarwal[4],
Erik Cambria[1], and Newton Howard[5]

[1] Nanyang Technological University, Singapore and Jadavpur University, India
[2] CIC, Instituto Politecnico Nacional, 07738 DF, Mexico
[3] Institute for Modern Linguistic Research,
"Sholokhov" Moscow State University for Humanities, Moscow, Russia
[4] Malaviya National Institute of Technology, Jaipur 302017, India
[5] Massachusetts Institute of Technology, USA
soujanya.poria@ieee.org, thebasant@gmail.com,
cambria@nus.edu.sg, nhmit@mit.edu
www.gelbukh.com

Abstract. Past works on personality detection has shown that psycho-linguistic features, frequency based analysis at lexical level, emotive words and other lexical clues such as number of first person or second person words carry major role to identify personality associated with the text. In this work, we propose a new architecture for the same task using common sense knowledge with associated sentiment polarity and affective labels. To extract the common sense knowledge with sentiment polarity scores and affective labels we used Senticnet which is one of the most useful resources for opinion mining and sentiment analysis. In particular, we combined common sense knowledge based features with phyco-linguistic features and frequency based features and later the features were employed in supervised classifiers. We designed five SMO based supervised classifiers for five personality traits. We observe that the use of common sense knowledge with affective and sentiment information enhances the accuracy of the existing frameworks which use only psycho-linguistic features and frequency based analysis at lexical level.

Keywords: personality detection, common sense knowledge, affective and sentiment information.

1 Introduction

The existence of various personality types and its connection with the different patterns of human behavior has been discussed since the times of Aristotle [21]. The computer era has made it possible to access and analyze large amounts of text samples in order to automatically identify personality types of authors and predict potential reactions and behaviors. The discipline of the Computational Psychology [10] has experienced a tremendous boost having roots in artificial intelligence, traditional psychology and natural language processing.

F. Castro, A. Gelbukh, and M. González (Eds.): MICAI 2013, Part II, LNAI 8266, pp. 484–496, 2013.
© Springer-Verlag Berlin Heidelberg 2013

The rapid development of Web 2.0, the appearance of Social Media tools, and the interest to Social network analysis brought a necessity of modeling personality of the main agent of online interactions. Recent studies show that the connection between personality and user behavior online preserves [9]. Earlier researchers have also found correlations between personality and success at work, in personal relationships and general feeling of happiness in life [16].

The computer-based Personality Recognition (PT) discipline studies the approaches for constructing personality models of Social Web participants, their evaluation and application for the needs of electronic social services.

Personality Recognition from Text (a sub-disciplinary of PT) focuses on the analysis of textual samples. Various researchers found correlations between linguistic features and personality characteristics (first-person singular pronouns correlate with depression levels [24], anger and swearing words correlate with [20]).

The further development of the discipline is beneficial for many activities that are performed by means of online facilities on a daily basis (customer support, recommendation of services and products, etc.). Recruiters of the HR department analyze hundreds of job applications working hard to map them to the required characteristics the future stuff should have [18]. At the same time the developers of the e-commerce resources are constantly improving the personification algorithms to help the customers obtain products and services that match the needs more precisely and present the information in a more appealing way to increase sales [8]. All these tasks will eventually involve a crucial step of implicit (mental) or explicit (through a user profile) modeling of the user personality.

In our present work we extracted common sense knowledge [2] available in text and further using sentic computing [7] we enhance the accuracy of the PRT system. We show that how personality is inferred by common sense knowledge concepts used by a person and sentic computing uses the affective information and sentiment information of these concepts along with psycholinguistic information from LIWC as the features to train the personality classifier.

The paper is organized as follows. In Section 2 we give an overview of the related work done in the Personality Recognition from Text field. In Section 3 we provide a description of the proposed algorithm followed by its evaluation in Section 4. We conclude with the discussion of the results and future work.

2   Background

2.1   Personality Estimation

The definition of the personality has been among one of the vague and philosophical questions. Modern trait theory is trying to model personality through fixing of a number of classification dimensions (usually following a lexical approach) and construction of the questionnaire to measure them [21].

Researchers use various schemes for personality modeling such as 16PF [12], EPQ-R [15], MBTI [11]. Apart from Myers-Briggs classification [22] one of the most widely exploited schemes for Personality Recognition from Text is the Big Five (BF)

[19]. It shows consistency across age and gender, and its validity remains the same when using different tests and languages [16]. The model provides the following five descriptive dimensions abbreviated as OCEAN:

- *Openness to experience* (tendency to non-conventional, abstract, symbolic thinking vs preference of non-ambiguous, familiar and non-complex things)
- *Conscientiousness* (tendency to hold to long-term plans vs impulsive and spontaneous behavior)
- *Extraversion* (active participation in the world around vs concentration on one's own feelings)
- *Agreeableness* (eagerness to cooperate and help vs self-interest)
- *Neuroticism* (tendency to experience negative feelings and being overemotional vs emotional stability and calmness)

2.2   Related Work

The general procedure for Personality Recognition from Text (PRT) involves collecting the dataset labeled with personality scores gathered through questionnaires, selection of particular linguistic features, construction of the recognition algorithm and its evaluation over a gold standard.

Pioneers in PRT showed that individual words usage can reveal personality. Even a small set of extracted features based on bi-grams and tri-grams has a correlation with particular traits [23] Features based on linguistic (LIWC) and psycholinguistic (MRC) categories also reflect personality types [20, 27, 28]. In [24], authors used lexical categories from Linguistic Inquiry and Word Count (LIWC) to identify the impact of linguistic features on personality. Their study revealed that the fewer use of articles and frequent use of positive emotion words actually support agreeability but neuroticism actually supported by the frequent use of negative emotion words and first person pronouns.

In [13], authors adapted 22 features exploited by authors in [20] to construct the PRT algorithm over the Italian **FriendFeed** dataset [13] with 1065 user posts. Their system did not require a dataset to be annotated as they were using previously published correlations between the features and personality traits. For each of those 22 features the mean, standard deviation, minimum, and maximum values were calculated based on a sample of 500 posts. The overall score for a particular feature was calculated in the following way: if the frequency of the feature was *higher* than the previously estimated *mean value plus standard deviation* and:

1. the feature for in a particular sentence correlates *positively* with the specific trait then the score of the trait was *incremented*.
2. the feature for in a particular sentence correlates *negatively* with the specific trait then the score of the trait was *decremented*.

Then the resulting score was substituted with "y" (if it is positive), "n" (if it is negative) or "o" (if it is zero). Finally, the majority score per each trait was treated as a personality model of the particular user. It is interesting to note that people who produced the largest amount of posts were extravert, insecure, friendly, not very precise and unimaginative while the average user was extravert, insecure, agreeable, organized and unimaginative.

Some researchers answer specific questions about personality while concentrating only at a subset of the Big Five traits. Tomlinson et al. [25] studied the Conscientiousness trait to detect goal, motivation, and the way the author perceives control over the described situations. They performed the analysis of event structures of textual user status updates in a Facebook dataset. The features under consideration were event-based verbs graded by their objectivity and specificity (calculated using WordNet[1]). Less objectivity and greater specificity are suggested to have connection with more control and stronger goal orientation. Also two thematic roles or relations (agent and patient) were taken into account (annotated using Propbank[2] corpus). The accuracy of predicting the score of the Conscientiousness trait being above or below the median (3.5) was 58.13%.

Golbeck et al. [16] concentrated on the analysis of Facebook profiles through the processing of 161 statistics of 167 users including personal information (name, birthday, gender, etc.), list of interests (music, movies, etc.), language features of status updates and "About Me" section, and internal statistics (userID, time of the last profile update, etc.). They found that the extracted features had the largest number of correlations with the Conscientiousness trait. The authors concluded that conscious people use fewer words that describe perceptive information (something they see or feel) and tend to discuss other people more.

In [26], authors used various emotion lexicons like NRC hash tag emotion lexicon and NRC emotion lexicon for the personality detection and found key improvement in the accuracy of the PRT system. In particular, this work of Mohammad et al. motivated us to use common sense knowledge and sentic computing to infer personality associated with the text.

3   Resources

To detect personality associated with the texts, information related to the language and the properties of individual words of concepts was used. Specifically, we used the following lexical resources. As the aim of this research is to improve the accuracy of the personality framework using emotional features carried by the common sense knowledge exist in the text, we use senticnet as a sentiment polarity dataset, emosenticnet as an emotion lexicon and emosenticspace and conceptnet as common sense knowledge base. In the other hand, LIWC and MRC were used as a psycholinguistic lexicon to extract linguistic features.

The SenticNet dataset As an a priori polarity lexicon of concepts, we used the SenticNet 2.0 [1], a lexical resource that contains more than 14,000 concepts along with their polarity scores in the range from −1.0 to +1.0. Among these concepts, 7,600 are multiword concepts. SenticNet 2.0 contains all WordNet Affect concepts as well. The first 20 SenticNet concepts in the lexicographic order along with the corresponding polarities are shown in Table 1.

---

[1] http://wordnet.princeton.edu/
[2] http://verbs.colorado.edu/~mpalmer/projects/ace.html

Table 1. A sample of SenticNet data

a lot	+0.970	*Abhorrent*	−0.396
a lot sex	+0.981	*able read*	+0.964
a way of	+0.303	*able run*	+0.960
Abandon	−0.858	*able use*	+0.941
Abase	−0.145	*abominably*	−0.396
Abash	−0.130	*abominate*	−0.376
abashed	−0.135	*abomination*	−0.376
abashment	−0.118	*Abortion*	−0.116
Abhor	−0.376	*Abroad*	+0.960
abhorrence	−0.376	*Absolute*	+0.495

3.1   The ConceptNet

The ConceptNet [2] represents the information from the Open Mind corpus as a directed graph, in which the nodes are concepts and the labeled edges are common-sense assertions that interconnect them. For example, given the two concepts *person* and *cook*, an assertion between them is CapableOf, i.e. *a person is capable of cooking*; see Figure 1 [2].

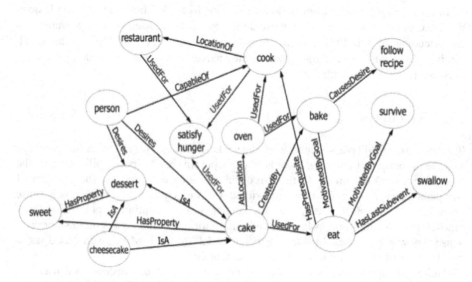

Fig. 1. Labelling facial images in the sequence as neutral or carrying a specific emotion

3.2   The EmoSenticNet

The Emosenticnet [3] contains about 5,700 common-sense knowledge concepts, including those concepts that exist in Wordnet Affect list, along with their affective labels in the set {anger, joy, disgust, sadness, surprise, fear}.

3.3   EmoSenticSpace

In order to build a suitable knowledge base for emotive reasoning, we applied the blending technique to ConceptNet and EmoSenticNet. Blending is a technique that performs inference over multiple sources of data simultaneously, taking advantage of the overlap between them [4]. Basically, it linearly combines two sparse matrices into a single matrix, in which the information between the two initial sources is shared.

Before doing the blending, we represented EmoSenticNet as a directed graph similarly to ConceptNet. For example, the concept *birthday party* is assigned an emotion *joy*. We took them as two nodes, and added the assertion HasProperty on the edge directed from the node *birthday party* to the node *joy*.

Then, we converted the graphs to sparse matrices in order to blend them. After blending the two matrices, we performed the Truncated Singular Value Decomposition (TSVD) on the resulted matrix to discard those components representing relatively small variations in the data. We discarded all of them keeping only 100 components of the blended matrix to obtain a good approximation of the original matrix. The number 100 was selected empirically: the original matrix could be best approximated using 100 components.

3.4   LIWC (Linguistic Inquiry and Word Count)

LIWC [3] is a text analysis tool that counts and sorts words according to the psychological and linguistic categories defined in the program dictionaries [24]. It processes the text word by word to establish the category of each of them and calculate the overall percentage of words in the discovered categories. Appendix A shows the list of LIWC categories and examples of words [24].

3.5   MRC (Medical Research Council)

MRC [4] database of psycholinguistic categories is an online service (since version 1) [14] and a machine usable dictionary (since version 2) that can be freely utilized for the purposes of natural language processing and artificial intelligence tasks. Appendix B shows the full list of MRC categories and the explanation of each of them [17].

4   Algorithm

We use essays dataset by [24] which contains 2400 essays labelled manually with personality scores for five different personality traits. Later, the data was tuned by Fabio Celli who manually converted the regression scores into class labels of five

---

[3] http://www.liwc.net
[4] http://websites.psychology.uwa.edu.au/school/MRCDatabase/ uwa_mrc.htm

different traits. In our case, we extracted several features from the text using LIWC (Appendix A), MRC (Appendix B) and combine them with the common sense knowledge based features extracted by sentic computing techniques. Later, we employed these features into five different classifiers (each for five traits) to build the model for personality prediction.

4.1   LIWC Features

Below we show the features extracted from text using LIWC dictionary, along with a definition or examples. Total 81 features were extracted related to the frequency of word count, number of words which have different emotions according to Ekman's model, the number of verbs in the future tense etc.

Linguistic processes

Word count	
Words per sentence	
Dictionary words	Percentage of all words captured by the program
Words having more than 6 letters	Percentage of all the words longer than 6 letters
First-person singular	*I, me, mine*
First-person plural	*We, us, our*
Second person	*You, your*
Third person singular	*She, her, him*
Third person plural	*They, their, they'd*
Indefinite pronouns	*It, it's, those*
Articles	*A, an, the*
Common verbs	*Walk, went, see*
Auxiliary verbs	*Am, will, have*
Past tense	*Went, ran, had*
Present tense	*Is, does, hear*
Future tense	*Will, gonna*
Adverbs	*Very, really, quickly*
Prepositions	*To, with, above*
Conjunctions	*And, but, whereas*
Negations	*No, not, never*
Quantifiers	*Few, many, much*
Numbers	*Second, thousand*
Swear words	*Damn, piss, fuck*

Psychological processes

Social processes

Family	*Daughter, husband*
Friends	*Buddy, friend*
Humans	*Adult, baby, boy*

Affective processes

Positive emotion	*Love, nice, sweet*
Negative emotion	*Hurt, ugly, nasty*
Anxiety	*Worried, nervous*
Anger	*Hate, kill, annoyed*
Sadness	*Crying, grief, sad*

Cognitive processes

Insight	*Think, know*
Causation	*Because, effect, hence*
Discrepancy	*Should, would, could*
Tentative	*Maybe, perhaps*
Certainty	*Always, never*
Inhibition	*Block, constrain*
Inclusive	*And, with, include*
Exclusive	*But, without*

Perceptual processes

See	*View, saw, seen*
Hear	*Listen, hearing*
Feel	*Feels, touch*

Biological processes

Body	*Cheek, hands, spit*
Health	*Clinic, flu, pill*
Sexual	*Horny, love, incest*
Ingestion	*Dish, eat, pizza*

Relativity

Motion	*Arrive, car, go*
Space	*Down, in, thin*
Time	*End, until, season*

Personal concerns

Work	*Job, majors, Xerox*
Achievement	*Earn, hero, win*
Leisure	*Cook, chat, movie*
Home	*Apartment, kitchen*
Money	*Audit, cash, owe*
Religion	*Altar, church, mosque*
Death	*Bury, coffin, kill*

Spoken categories

Assent	*Agree, OK, yes*
Nonfluencies	*Er, hm, umm*
Fillers	*Blah, Imean, yaknow*

4.2   MRC Features

Below we present the features extracted using MRC. These are mainly linguistic features, such as the number of syllables and phonemes in the word.

NLET	Number of letters in the word
NPHON	Number of phonemes in the word
NSYL	Number of syllables in the word
K-F-FREQ	Kucera and Francis written frequency
K-F-NCATS	Kucera and Francis number of categories
K-F-NSAMP	Kucera and Francis number of samples
T-L-FREQ	Thorndike-Lorge frequency
BROWN-FREQ	Brown verbal frequency
FAM	Familiarity
CONC	Concreteness
IMAG	Imagery
MEANC	Mean Colorado Meaningfulness
MEANP	Mean Paivio Meaningfulness
AOA	Age of Acquisition
TQ2	Type (for example, shows whether the word is a derivational variant of another word or ends in letter "R" that is not pronounced)
WTYPE	Part of Speech (10 categories)
PDWTYPE	PD Part of Speech (only 4 categories: noun, verb, adjective and other)
ALPHSYL	Shows whether the word is an abbreviation or a suffix, or a prefix, or is hyphenated, or is a multi-word phrasal unit or none of these
STATUS	Status
VAR	Variant Phoneme
CAP	Written Capitalised
IRREG	Irregular Plural
WORD	the actual word
PHON	Phonetic Transcription
DPHON	Edited Phonetic Transcription
STRESS	Stress pattern

4.3   Sentic Based Emotional Features

In our present research we show how emotional clues can help to detect personality from the text. We used emotional features in the personality engine is to find out the role of emotional features to detect personality from text. Below we first discuss the major difficulties associated with the detection of emotion from text and then discuss the features to grasp emotion from text. All of these emotional features described below were used as the features of personality detection engine.

Identifying emotions in text is a challenging task, because of ambiguity of words in the text, complexity of meaning and interplay of various factors such as irony, politeness, writing style, as well as variability of language from person to person and from culture to culture. In this work, we followed the sentic computing paradigm developed by Cambria and his collaborators, which considers the text as expressing both semantics and sentics [6]. We used a novel approach for identifying the emotions in the text by extracting the following key features using our new resource, EmoSenticnetSpace, described in Section 3.3. Later, we use these following features (which are recognized as emotional features) for the personality detection classifier.

4.4 Bag of Concepts

For each concept in the text, we obtained a 100-dimensional feature vector from the EmoSenticSpace. Then we aggregated the individual concept vectors into one document vector by coordinate-wise summation:

$$x_i = \sum_{i=1}^{N} x_{ij},$$

where xi is the i-th coordinate of the document's feature vector, xij is the i-th coordinate of its j-th concept's vector, and N is the number of concepts in the document. We have also experimented with averaging instead of summation:

$$x_i = \frac{1}{N} \sum_{i=1}^{N} x_{ij},$$

but contrary to our expectation and in contrast to our past experience with Facebook data, summation gave better results than averaging.

4.5 Sentic Feature

The polarity scores of each concept extracted from the text were obtained from the SenticNet and summed up to produce one scalar feature.

4.6 Negation

As we mentioned earlier, negations [5] can change the meaning of a statement. We followed the approach of [5] to identify the negation and reverse the polarity of the sentic feature corresponding to the concept that followed the negation marker.

5   Evaluation Results and Discussions

The primary goal of the proposed approach is to investigate the impact of common sense knowledge with affective and sentiment information in personality recognition. To evaluate the proposed methods, feature vector is constructed using LIWC features, MRC features, Sentic based emotional features, and Sentic features, further these features are used to build the learning model using Sequential Minimal Optimization (SMO) classifier. We trained five different classifiers, one for each trait. Performance evaluation is performed using 10 fold cross validation. All the results in for all these classifiers for every trait are reported in Table 2.

For the trait 1, openness the F-score is 0.662 which is highest among the other traits it shows that it is easiest to identity the openness trait in the text over other traits. Similarly, Agreeableness trait gives the minimum F-score of 0.615 as shown in Table 2. It shows the most difficult trait to identify among all other traits. For other traits, our model produces the F-score of 0.633, 0.634 and 0.637 respectively for Conscientiousness, Extraversion and Neuroticism trait.

Table 2. Results for five traits with SVM classifier

Trait	Precision	Recall	F-score
Openness	0.662	0.662	0.661
Conscientiousness	0.634	0.634	0.633
Extraversion	0.636	0.636	0.634
Agreeableness	0.622	0.622	0.615
Neuroticism	0.637	0.637	0.637

Proposed method performs much better than previously reported state-of-art methods on the same dataset as shown in Table 2. Mohammad et al. (2012) [26] investigated with various feature sets and achieved the best accuracy by incorporating the emotion features. However, their reported best accuracy is quite low as compared to our proposed method as shown in Table 3.

In [20], authors extracted various linguistic features which were able to incorporate the syntactic and semantic information. Our method could give better performance as compared to previous methods due to incorporation of more important information for personality detection in form of common sense knowledge with affective and sentiment information.

Table 3. performance comparison with state-of-art methods

	Extra-version	Neuro-ticism	Agree-ableness	Conscien-tiouness	Open-ness
[26]	0.546	0.557	0.540	0.564	0.604
[20]	0.549	0.573	0.557	0.552	0.621
Proposed method	**0.634**	**0.637**	**0.615**	**0.633**	**0.661**

6   Conclusion

The task of personality recognition from the text has been very important. In this paper, a new approach is proposed for this task that is based on incorporating the sentiment, affective and common sense knowledge from the text using resources viz. SenticNet, ConceptNet, EmoSenticNet and EmoSenticSpace. In the proposed approach, we combined common sense knowledge with phycho-linguistic features to get the feature vector. Further, this feature vector is used by five SMO based supervised classifier for five personality traits. Experimental results show the effectiveness of the proposed approach. The main reason for this observation is the use of common sense knowledge with affective and sentiment information unlike other state-of-art approaches those were based on mostly on psycho-linguistic features and frequency based analysis at lexical level.

Acknowledgments. The second author recognizes the support from the Instituto Politécnico Nacional grants SIP-IPN 20131702 and 20131441, CONACYT grant 50206-H, and CONACYT-DST India grant 122030 *Answer Validation through Textual Entailment*. We thank Prof. Dr. Anton Zimmerling (MSUH) for the valuable discussions during the development of this work.

References

1. Cambria, E., Havasi, C., Hussain, A.: SenticNet 2: A semantic and affective resource for opinion mining and sentiment analysis. In: Proceedings of FLAIRS, Marco Island, pp. 202–207 (2012)
2. Havasi, C., Speer, R., Alonso, J.: ConceptNet 3: A Flexible, Multilingual Semantic Network for Common Sense Knowledge. In: RANLP (2007)
3. Poria, S., Gelbukh, A., Hussain, A., Das, D., Bandyopadhyay, S.: Enhanced SenticNet with Affective Labels for Concept-based Opinion Mining. IEEE Intelligent Systems 28(2), 31–38 (2013), doi:10.1109/MIS.2013.4
4. Havasi, C., Speer, R., Pustejovsky, J.: Automatically Suggesting Semantic Structure for a Generative Lexicon Ontology. In: Generative Lexicon (2009)
5. Lapponi, E., Read, J., Ovrelid, L.: Representing and resolving negation for sentiment analysis. In: ICDM SENTIRE, Brussels, pp. 687–692 (2012)
6. Cambria, E., Hussain, A.: Sentic Computing: Techniques, Tools, and Applications. Springer, Dordrecht (2012)
7. Cambria, E., Speer, R., Havasi, C., Hussain, A.: SenticNet: A publicly available semantic resource for opinion mining. In: AAAI CSK, Arlington, pp. 14–18 (2010)
8. Alghamdi, A., Aldabbas, H., Alshehri, M., Nusir, M.: Adopting User-Centered Development Approach For Arabic E-Commerce Websites. International Journal of Web & Semantic Technology, IJWesT (2012)
9. Amichai-Hamburger, Y., Vinitzky, G.: Social network use and personality. Computers in Human Behavior 26(6), 1289–1295 (2010)
10. Boden, M., Mellor, D.H.: What Is Computational Psychology? Proceedings of the Aristotelian Society, Supplementary Volumes 58, 37–53 (1984)
11. Briggs Myers, I., McCaulley, M.H., Quenk, N., Hammer, A.: MBTI Handbook: A Guide to the development and use of the Myers-Briggs Type Indicator, 3rd edn. Consulting Psychologists Press (1998)
12. Cattell, H.E.P., Mead, A.D.: The Sixteen Personality Factor Questionnaire (16PF): SAGE Knowledge. In: The SAGE Handbook of Personality Theory and Assessment (2008), http://people.wku.edu/richard.miller/520%2016PF%20Cattell%20and%20Mead.pdf (retrieved May 27, 2013)
13. Celli, F.: Unsupervised Personality Recognition for Social Network Sites. In: The Sixth International Conference on Digital Society, ICDS 2012 (c), pp. 59–62 (2012)

14. Coltheart, M.: The MRC Psycholinguistic Database. Quarterly Journal of Experimental Psychology 33A(4), 497–505 (1981)
15. Eysenck, H.J., Eysenck, S.B.: Manual for the EPQ-R. EdITS, San Diego (1991)
16. Golbeck, J., Robles, C., Turner, K.: Predicting personality with social media. In: CHI Extended Abstracts, pp. 253–262 (2011)
17. Wilson, M.: MRC Psycholinguistic Database: Machine Usable Dictionary, Version 2.00 (1987), http://citeseerx.ist.psu.edu/viewdoc/ summary?doi=10.1.1.52.6928 (retrieved)
18. Isaacson, K., Peacey, S.: Human resources and social media (2012)
19. John, O.P., Naumann, L.P., Soto, C.J.: Paradigm shift to the integrative Big Five trait taxonomy: History, measurement, and conceptual issues. In: Handbook of Personality Theory and Research, pp. 114–158 (2008)
20. Mairesse, F., Walker, M.A., Mehl, M.R., Moore, R.K.: Using Linguistic Cues for the Automatic Recognition of Personality in Conversation and Text. Journal of Artificial Intelligence Research 30(1), 457–500 (2007)
21. Matthews, G., Deary, I.J., Whiteman, M.C.: Personality Traits, Cambridge, UK, pp. 23–26 (2009)
22. Noecker, J., Ryan, M., Juola, P.: Psychological profiling through textual analysis. Literary and Linguistic Computing (2013)
23. Oberlander, J., Nowson, S.: Whose thumb is it anyway? Classifying author personality from weblog text. Computational Linguistics, 627–634 (2006)
24. Tausczik, Y.R., Pennebaker, J.W.: The Psychological Meaning of Words: LIWC and Computerized Text Analysis Methods. Journal of Language and Social Psychology 29(1), 24–54 (2009)
25. Tomlinson, M.T., Hinote, D., Bracewell, D.B.: Predicting Conscientiousness through Semantic Analysis of Facebook Posts. In: Proceedings of WCPR 2013, Workshop on Computational Personality Recognition at ICWSM 2013 (7th International AAAI Conference on Weblogs and Social Media) (2013)
26. Mohammad, S.M., Kiritchenko, S.: Using Nuances of Emotion to Identify Personality (2012)
27. Sidorov, G., Castro-Sánchez, N.A.: Automatic emotional personality description using linguistic data. Research in Computing Science 20, 89–94 (2006)
28. Sidorov, G., Castro-Sánchez, N.A.: System for linguistically-based evaluation of psychological profiles. In: Dialogue 2006, Russia, pp. 464–467 (2006)

Implementing Fuzzy Subtractive Clustering to Build a Personality Fuzzy Model Based on Big Five Patterns for Engineers

Luis G. Martínez[1], Juan Ramón Castro[1], Guillermo Licea[1],
Antonio Rodríguez-Díaz[1], and Reynaldo Salas[2]

[1] Universidad Autónoma de Baja California
Calzada Universidad 14418, Mesa de Otay 22300 Tijuana B.C., México
{luisgmo,jrcastro,glicea,ardiaz}@uabc.edu.mx
[2] Tijuana Institute of Technology
Calzada Tecnológico, Frac. Tomás Aquino 22370 Tijuana B.C., México
reynaldo.salas@tectijuana.edu.mx

Abstract. Data mining has become an essential component in various fields of human life including business, education, medical and scientific. Cluster analysis is an important data mining technique used to find data segmentation and pattern recognition. This paper proposes the application of Fuzzy Subtractive Clustering (FSC) technique as an approach to define Big Five Patterns (B5P) using psychometric tests for students in engineering programs. In comparison with an ANFIS Learning Approach, FSC gives us a better and broader relationship of the behavioral pattern between B5 traits and careers. This will help students find a better way to choose a career and relate their personality with career planning or for job advice; and school counselors as a tool to guide their students in career counseling.

Keywords: Fuzzy Logic, Fuzzy Clustering, Big Five Personality Test.

1 Introduction

Integration of fuzzy logic with data mining techniques has become one of the key constituents of soft computing in handling the challenges posed by massive collections of natural data [1]. The central idea in fuzzy clustering is the non-unique partitioning of the data into a collection of clusters.

The data points are assigned membership values for each of the clusters and the fuzzy clustering algorithms allow the clusters to grow into their natural shapes [2].

Data mining tools scour databases for hidden patterns, finding predictive information that experts may miss since such knowledge lies outside their expectations. Data mining is an interdisciplinary field that uses sophisticated data search capabilities and statistical algorithms to discover patterns and correlations in large preexisting databases [3]. A number of machine learning, knowledge engineering, and probabilistic based methods have been proposed to analyze the data

F. Castro, A. Gelbukh, and M. González (Eds.): MICAI 2013, Part II, LNAI 8266, pp. 497–508, 2013.

and extract information. The most popular methods include regression analysis, neural network algorithms, clustering algorithms, genetic algorithms, decision trees and support vector machines [4] [5] [6].

Data mining has been widely applied in various domains; however, limited studies have been done into discovering hidden knowledge from factual data about selected groups of people with special characteristics. Trend in mine data about such group of individuals lately [7] has been to extract insightful knowledge that could lead to a better understanding of their personalities, in addition to further sociological conclusions.

Aim of our research is to discover the relationship between those special characteristics of students, their personality traits, and the engineering career program they are studying. Personality tests are based on interpretation, therefore a Fuzzy Inference System (FIS) type model is the appropriate way to represent and identify behavioral patterns for these engineers.

This paper presents the application of Fuzzy Subtractive Clustering (FSC) technique as an approach to define B5P using psychometric tests to find common features and relations among traits of students and their different engineering careers, therefore discovering behavioral patterns between Big Five (B5) traits and careers.

The rest of the paper is organized as follows: section 2 is a brief background of personality and careers in engineering relationship, and clustering techniques applied to personality behavior. Section 3 defines the methodology towards defining our Fuzzy Model. Section 4 displays results of the big five personality test, the big five patterns and implementation of FSC technique, concluding in section 5 with observations and discussion of our case study.

2   Background

Many studies have found personality to be related to academic performance, choice of electives, completing university education, and choice of career [8][9].The question of which personality variables are relevant to career choice and job satisfaction has been considered by several personality theories. Rosati's research [10] at the University of Western Ontario provided insightful perspective on the personality preferences of different groups on engineering students and their progress through the engineering program using the Myers-Briggs Type Indicator (MBTI) personality test instrument based on Jung's theory of psychological types.

Udoudoh [11] researched personality traits of Information Scientists in Federal University of Technology at Nigeria, defining him as enterprising and investigative; information scientists see themselves as managers of people and information resources, contrary to the traditional assumptions of being introverts and individuals who prefer to work independently.

Lounsbury and colleagues [12] related personality traits and career satisfaction of human resource professionals, defining that optimism, emotional resilience, assertiveness and extraversion are powerful traits of managers or human resource professionals. Those with low levels of these traits were recommended to be coached to develop optimism-enhancing, to learn defensive pessimism strategies or engage in counseling or stress management programs. Another of his study [13] among adolescents in middle and high school indicates that B5 personality traits are related to career decidedness, being conscientiousness the most related, proposing the use of B5 personality test to be used by counselors or school psychologist to predict career decidedness and help them plan and respond proactively to their future.

Rubinstein [14] study in Tel-Aviv University offers support claiming that personality patterns may play a part in vocational decision making processes, his study used the B5 scale to study personality traits students of natural sciences, law, social sciences, and art. He found art students to be more neurotic; social science, art and law students to be more extraverted; art student to be more open; law students and natural sciences more agreeable and conscientious.

The engineering profession is one area of human endeavor in which there is a very high consistency in human character traits, we can say that an "engineering personality" exist [15]. The engineer's most obvious characteristics are his precision, his meticulousness, his attention to detail and accuracy, in other words his perfectionism.

Nagarjuna's [16] study comparing engineers with commerce students, shows that engineering students are more self-reliant, realistic, responsible and emotionally tough. Engineering students are more socially aware, controlled, self-disciplined and perfectionists as compared to the commerce background students. The curriculum for engineering course is more technical and focused and demands more perfection to be successful and also due to the fact that the engineering students spend more years with their classmates they tend to become tougher minded and focused as they are given lot of team assignments in their curriculum as compared to the commerce graduates.

In 1980 a consortium of eight universities and the Center for Applications of Psychological Type was formed to study the role of personality type in engineering education. Introverts, intuitors, and judgers generally outperformed their extraverted, sensing, and perceiving counterparts in the population studied [17]. Wankat and Oreovicz [18] observe that if memorization and recall are important, sensing types should perform better, while if analysis is required, intuitive students should have an advantage. Rosati [19] also observed that introverts, thinkers, and judgers were more likely than extraverts, feelers, and perceivers to graduate in engineering after four years, but sensors were more likely than intuitors to do so.

From previous research we can see that commonly held opinions about the relationship between some occupations and character traits have considerable validity; for engineering careers we tend to see a pattern of traits, skills and therefore personality style. Continuous research and additional inputs of these characteristics gives insight to counselors in job advising, career planning, and career counseling, shaping overall personality of the students so they can choose appropriately and wisely to fare better in the corporate world once graduated.

This paper specifically analyzes results of internet's free Big Five Test applied in a case study of students of engineering programs to find B5P for these careers.

3   Methodology

At the University of Baja California, Tijuana, Mexico we took a sample of 200 students from different engineering programs applying the Big Five Test to the group. Big Five personality tests claim to measure your intensities in relation to the "Big Five" factors [20]. The structure of the tests requires selecting options from multiple choice questionnaires. These big five personality tests equate your personality to your collective degrees of behavior in five factors.

The Big Five factors are Openness, Conscientiousness, Extroversion, Agreeableness, and Neuroticism (OCEAN). The Neuroticism factor is sometimes referred to as Emotional Stability. And Openness factor sometimes is referred to as Intellect. Openness (O) is a disposition to be imaginative, inventive, curious, unconventional and autonomous, has an appreciation for art, emotion, adventure, unusual ideas, curiosity and variety of experience. Conscientiousness (C) comprises of two related facets achievement and dependability, has a tendency to show self-discipline, be efficient, organized, act dutifully and aim for achievement, plans rather than behave spontaneously.

Extroversion (E) represents tendency to be sociable, outgoing and assertive, experiences positive affect such as energy, passion and excitement. Agreeableness (A) is a tendency to be trusting, friendly, compassionate, cooperative, compliant, caring and gentle. Neuroticism (N) represents tendency to exhibit poor emotional adjustment and experience negative or unpleasant emotions easily, such as anxiety, insecurity, depression and hostility, opposite of this trait is Emotional Stability (ES), as out big five test throws us a value of ES instead of N, we are considering ES as a linguistic variable and representing it with a label of N-1.

Because of uncertainty of personality traits, a fuzzy based approach is considered to provide an integrated quantity measure for abilities of engineering careers which incorporates all aspects of personality traits involved in each engineering program. Recent studies are incorporating fuzzy approaches to personnel selection and job selection relating traits with careers [21] [22] [23].

Cluster analysis is a technique for grouping data and finding structures in data [24]. The most common application of clustering methods is to partition a data set into clusters or classes, where similar data are assigned to the same cluster whereas dissimilar data should belong to different clusters. In real world applications there is very often no clear boundary between clusters, so that fuzzy clustering is often a good alternative to use.

Pattern recognition techniques can be classified into two broad categories: unsupervised techniques and supervised techniques. Unsupervised techniques do not use a given set of unclassified data points, whereas a supervised technique uses a data set with known classifications.

Unsupervised clustering techniques have been applied to criminology using Data Mining techniques to identify patterns from data and to examine the existence of criminal types [3]. These criminal types have emerged from psychological or social theories and remain much in dispute over how to identify them, the challenge is to use data mining techniques to address reliable patterns of criminal offenders and replicate substantive criminal profiles as good as criminological experts can.

Data mining has been used for education extracting meaningful information from an educational environment trying to help teachers to reduce dropout ratio and improve student performance [25]. Ladas and colleagues [26] presented a method to extract Behavioral Groups demonstrating that it is possible to extract information regarding the personality of individuals from similar datasets by using simple clustering techniques (Clara and K-means).

In 2004 a cluster analysis was performed on PCI data collected from 259 astronaut applicants, suggesting three distinct subgroups, or clusters, in this population; characteristics of each subgroup appear consistent with commercial pilots [27] and military cadets [28]. McFadden and colleagues [29] found that astronauts with higher levels of Instrumentality and Expressivity tended to outperform their peers of other personality types. Musson research group [30] concluded in previous study that data suggested a certain degree of uniformity among test individuals, and the lack of discernable differences between clusters, and pointed out that some unidentified aspect of personality not assessed by the instruments used may have had a role in final selection.

Data mining techniques have been applied also in recruitment of fresh graduates for IT industry. The selection process uses different criteria that comprise the average of their semester marks, marks obtained in the aptitude, programming and technical tests conducted by the company, group discussion, technical and HR interviews. Sivaram and Ramar [31] have applied clustering and classification algorithms to recruitment data of an IT industry, using K-means and fuzzy C-means clustering and decision tree classification algorithms; they observed that Fuzzy C-means and K-means clustering techniques were not suitable for this type of data distribution but C4.5 decision tree construction algorithm has better accuracy than the rest.

Clustering partitions a data set into several groups such that the similarity within a group is larger than that among groups [32]. Achieving such a partitioning requires a similarity metrics that takes two input vectors and returns a value reflecting their similarity.

This paper implements Subtractive Clustering proposed by Chiu [33], in which data points are considered as the candidates for cluster centers. By using this method, cluster computation is simply proportional to the number of data points and independent of the dimension of the problem under consideration.

Considering a collection of n data points $\{x_1, ..., x_n\}$ in a M-dimensional space, a density measure at data point x_i is defined as:

$$D_i = \sum_{j=1}^{n} \exp\left(-\frac{\|x_i - x_j\|^2}{\left(\frac{r_a}{2}\right)^2}\right) \tag{1}$$

where r_a is the radius defining a neighborhood and is a positive constant. Hence, a data point will have a high density value if it has many neighboring data points. Data points outside this radius contribute only slightly to the density measure. After the density measure of each data point has been calculated, the data point with the highest density measure is selected as the first cluster center. Being x_{c1} the point selected and D_{c1} its density measure, the density measure for each data point x_1 is revised by the formula:

$$D_i = D_i - D_{c_1} \exp\left(-\frac{\|x_i - x_{c_1}\|^2}{\left(\frac{r_b}{2}\right)^2} \right) \qquad (2)$$

After the density measure for each data point is revised, the next cluster center x_{c2} is selected and all of the density measures for data points are revised again. This process is repeated until a sufficient number of cluster centers are generated.

Applying subtractive clustering to a set of input-output data, each of the cluster centers represents a prototype that exhibits certain characteristics of the system to be modeled. These cluster centers would be used as centers to generate fuzzy rules' antecedents and consequents to be evaluated by recursive least square (RLS) method in a first-order Sugeno fuzzy model. The center c_i can be decomposed into two component vectors p_i and q_i, where p_i is the input part containing the first N elements of c_i, q_i is the output part and it contains the last $M\text{-}N$ elements of c_i.

The degree to which fuzzy rule i is fulfilled is defined by:

$$\mu_i = \exp\left(-\frac{\|x_i - p_i\|^2}{\left(\frac{r_a}{2}\right)^2} \right) \qquad (3)$$

Our subtractive clustering approach employed leads to produce a Takagi-Sugeno-Kang Fuzzy Inference System (TSK FIS). With OCEAN traits as input linguistic variables and Engineering Programs (EP) as an output linguistic variable the TSK FIS type model was developed using MatLab's Editor GUI [34]. The primary idea is to cluster the attributes of the OCEAN personality traits, generating the IF-THEN product rules applying the FSC technique. Figure 1 is an abstract visualization of the rules generated by the model, whereas the number of clusters is the number of rules for each input-output considered.

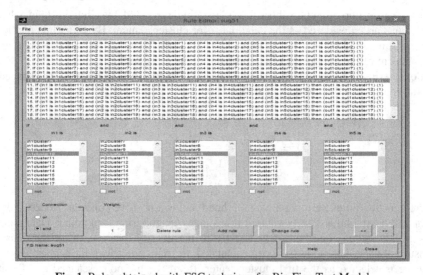

Fig. 1. Rules obtained with FSC technique for Big Five Test Model

4   Results

Work of our case study consisted of 200 engineering students from a lot of 700, distributed as follows: 22 aerospace engineers (AE), 16 bioengineers (BI), 52 computer engineers (CE), 18 chemical engineers (CH), 25 electronic engineers (EE) and 50 industrial engineers (IE) and 17 mechatronic engineers (ME).

Table 1. Results of OCEAN test for Engineering Programs

	O	C	E	A	N-1
AE	62.45	57.09	44.73	52.45	59.27
BI	58.25	54.63	53.13	46.06	54.75
CE	54.88	62.77	44.42	51.58	54.75
CH	56.33	59.67	52.56	49.67	56.22
EE	53.04	57.68	43.76	49.28	55.04
IE	49.64	60.48	53.46	48.32	58.72
ME	58.94	57.41	53.53	49.18	61.53
AE = aerospace engineers, BI= bioengineers, CE= computer engineers, CH= chemical engineers, EE= electronic engineers, IE= industrial engineers, ME=mechatronic engineers. O=Openness, C=Conscientiousness, E=Extroversion, A=Agreeableness, N-1=Emotional Stability					

Big Five personality test results are presented in Table 1 showing the means of each trait value result related to every engineering program. Each table row is a personality vector unique for each engineering program student type; no two rows have exactly the same values for every attribute, giving a significant difference between each program student type distinguishing patterns based on the Big Five Personality Test.

There are two ways to evaluate this data; first we can analyze the Trait Personality Vector Ev for extroversion trait with values Ev = {44.73, 53.13, 44.42, 52.56, 43.76, 53.46, 53.53}, meaning that considering a high score on this trait it is possible to recommend that person to be a Bioengineer, if it's a low score then we can recommend this person to study electronic engineering. A second way is to consider the Engineering Program Vector for example EEv for electronic engineer with values EEv = {53.04, 57.68, 43.76, 49.28, 55.04}, meaning that an EE program can be recommended for a person with high scores in (C) Conscientiousness and low score of (E) Extroversion.

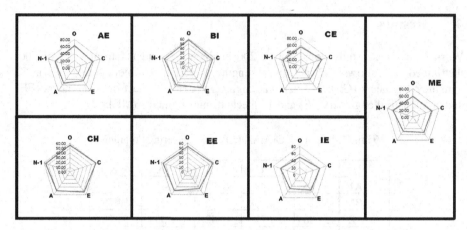

Fig. 2. Student Type Educational Program's Big Five Patterns

To see a broader picture these results can be displayed relating them with a center point using a radar chart type, obtaining Big Five Patterns (B5P) for Engineering Programs, these patterns are shown in figure 2.

There are significant differences between each type of student. For example an Aerospace Engineer has highest values for traits (O) and (A) compared to an Industrial Engineer that has lowest values for these same traits. This comparison can give us a glimpse of specific traits for particular type of engineers, as always we should know that one trait does not define the personality of a type of engineer, but a personality vector with all traits involved can give us differences between types of student engineers.

These data was used for our TSK FIS model using FSC technique obtaining figure 4 where it shows Input Trait and Output Engineering Program (EP) Relationships of this model. Whereas numeric values for linguistic variable EP were (1) Aerospace Engineer, (2) Bioengineer, (3) Computer Engineer, (4) Chemical Engineer, (5) Electonic Engineer, (6) Industrial Engineer and (7) Mechatronic Engineer.

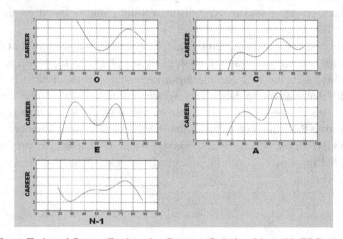

Fig. 3. Input Trait and Output Engineering Program Relationships with FSC approach

The Fuzzy Model relates each trait with each EP, analizing data, range of trait means are from 40 to 60, we will consider low degree around 20-40 and high degree around 60-80 based on standard deviation. With these results and ranges we can assertain that a high degree of trait values for (C) and (N-1) we are talking about EP students of BI or CE, they are emotionally stable, efficient, organized, aim for achievement. For a low degree of trait values (O) and (A) we are talking about EP students of II and EE, they are less creative, less trustworthy, less cooperative.

Previous research was used with an ANFIS Learning Approach [35] obtaining similar B5P, figure 5 shows these Input Trait and Output Engineering Program relationships; while figure 6 is the comparative between both graphics of each technique implemented.

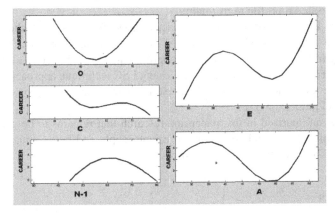

Fig. 4. Input Trait and Output Engineering Program Relationships with ANFIS Learning Approach

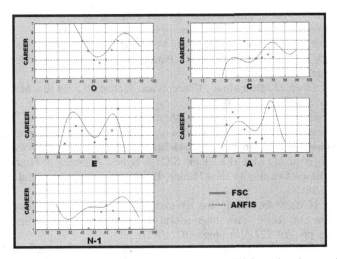

Fig. 5. Comparative Relationships with FSC and ANFIS Learning Approach

Comparing these B5P graphics we observe high similarity between each trait of the OCEAN personality model. Although using the FSC technique gives us a better approximation of the relationships between traits and EPs, as we can see a broader range of trait input values and a broader range of output EPs related in the FCS graphics than in the ANFIS results.

5   Conclusions

Our case study results have shed insight on a pattern of personality traits in relationship with engineering careers, there are significant differences between each EP vector, which is why we can only analyze our results viewing a student/professional profile in its totality.

The TSK FIS obtained with the subtractive clustering technique showed a better performance than the ANFIS model. FSC uses the data points as cluster centers instead of grid points, clusters generated approximate with a better similarity between data as this technique optimizes the rules. Using FSC technique approach is helping to better define the relationship between personality traits and EPs providing a simple and powerful model for B5P.

Research summarized in this paper and research that remains to be done will help students, professionals and counselors to orient people and better situate themselves for a better job occupation and career success.

References

1. Mitra, S., Pal, S.K., Mitra, P.: Data Mining in Soft Computing Framework: A Survey. IEEE Transactions on Neural Networks 13(1), 3–14 (2002)
2. Gath, I., Geva, A.B.: Unsupervised Optimal Fuzzy Clustering. IEEE Transactions on Pattern Analysis and Machine Intelligence 11(7), 773–781 (1989)
3. Breitenbach, M., Brennan, T., Dieterich, W., Grudic, G.Z.: Clustering of Psychological Personality Tests of Criminal Offenders. Practical Data Mining: Applications, Experiences and Challenges 84 (2006)
4. Han, J., Kamber, M.: Data Mining Concepts and Techniques, 2nd edn. Morgan Kaufmann Publishers, San Francisco (2006)
5. Agrawal, R., Arning, A., Bollinger, T., Mehta, M., Shafer, J., Srikant, R.: The Quest Data Mining System, in Proc.2nd Int'l Conference on Knowledge Discovery in Databases and Data Mining, Portland, Oregon, USA 244-249 (1996)
6. Shin, C.K., Yun, U., Kim, H.K., Park, S.C.: A Hybrid Approach of Neural Network and Memory Based Learning to Data Mining. IEEE Transactions on Neural Network 11(3), 637–646 (2000)
7. Al-Naimi, N.M., Shaban, K.B.: The 100 most influential persons in history: a data mining perspective. In: IEEE 11th International Conference on Data Mining Workshops (ICDMW), pp. 719–724. Vancouver, BC (2011)
8. Tett, R.P., Jackson, D.M., Rothstein, M.: Personality measures as predictors of job performance; a meta analytic review. Personnel Psychology 44, 703–742 (1991)

9. Song, Z., Wu, Q., Zhao, F.: Academic achievement and personality of college students. Chinese Mental Health Journal 16, 121–123 (2002)
10. Rosati, P.: Academic Progress of Canadian Engineering Students in terms of MBTI Personality Type. Int. J. Engineering 14(5), 322–327 (1998)
11. Udoudoh, S.J.: Impacts of personality traits on career choice of Information Scientists in Federal University of Technology, Minna, Niger State, Nigeria. Int. J. of Library and Information Science 4(4), 57–70 (2012)
12. Lounsbury, J.W., Steel, R.P., Gibson, L.W., Drost, A.W.: Personality traits and career satisfaction of human resource professionals. Human Resource Development International 11(4), 351–366 (2008)
13. Lounsbury, J.W., Hutchens, T., Loveland, J.M.: An Investigation of Big Five Personality traits and Career Decidedness among Early and Middle Adolescents. Journal of Career Assessment 13(1), 25–39 (2005)
14. Rubinstein, G.: The big five among male and female students of different faculties. Personality and Individual Differences 38, 1495–1503 (2005)
15. Goshen, C.E.: The Engineer Personality. The Bent of Tau Beta Pi, pp. 15–20. The engineering Honor Society (1954)
16. Nagarjuna, V.L., Mamidenna, S.: Personality Characteristics of Commerce and Engineering Graduates – A Comparative Study. Journal of the Indian Academy of Applied Psychology 34(2), 303–308 (2008)
17. McCaulley, M.H., Godleski, E.S., Yokomoto, C.F., Harrisberger, L., Sloan, E.D.: Applications of Psychological Type in Engineering Education. Engineering Education 73, 394–400 (1983)
18. Wankat, P., Oreovicz, F.: Teaching Engineering. McGraw-Hill, New York (1993)
19. Rosati, P.: A Personality Type Perspective of Canadian Engineering Students. In: Proceedings of the Annual Conference of the Canadian Society of Civil Engineering, CSCE, vol. 4, pp. 11–12 (1999)
20. Costa Jr., P.T., McCrae, R.R.: Revised NEO Personality Inventory (NEO-PI-R) and NEO Five-Factor Inventory (NEO-FFI) manual. Psychological Assessment Resources, Odessa (1992)
21. Selcuk, H., Cevikcan, E.: Job selection based on fuzzy AHP: An investigation including the students of Istanbul Technical University Management Faculty. Int. Journal of Business and Management Studies 3(1), 173–182 (2011)
22. Dereli, T., Durmusoglu, A., Ulusam, S.S., Avlanmaz, N.: A fuzzy approach for personnel selection process. TJFS: Turkish Journal of Fuzzy Systems 1(2), 126–140 (2010)
23. Nobari, S., Jabrailova, Z., Nobari, A.: Design a Fuzzy Model for Decision Support Systems in the Selection and Recruitment. In: Int. Conference on Innovation and Information Management, IPCSIT, vol. 36, pp. 195–200. IACSIT Press, Singapore (2012)
24. Melin, P., Castillo, O.: Clustering with Intelligent Techniques. In: Hybrid Intelligent Systems for Pattern Recognition using Soft Computing. STUDFUZZ, vol. 172, pp. 169–184. Springer, Heidelberg (2005)
25. Ayesha, S., Mustafa, T., Sattar, A.R., Khan, M.I.: Data Mining Model for Higher Education System. European Journal of Scientific Research 43(1), 24–31 (2010)
26. Ladas, A., Aickelin, U., Garibaldi, J., Ferguson, E.: Using Clustering to extract Personality Information from socio economic data. In: 12th Annual Workshop on Computational Intelligence, UKCI 2012, Heriot-Watt University, Edinburgh, UK (2012)

27. Gregorich, S.E., Helmreich, R.L., Wilhelm, J.A., Chidester, T.: Personality based clusters as predictors of aviator attitudes and performance. In: Jensen, R.S. (ed.) Proceedings of the 5th International Symposium on Aviation Psychology, Columbus, OH, USA, vol. 2, pp. 686–691 (1989)

28. Sandal, G.M., Gronningsaeter, H., Eriksen, H.R.: Personality and endocrine activation in military stress situations. Mil. Psychol. 70, 45–61 (1998)

29. McFadden, T.J., Helmreich, R.L., Rose, R.M., Fogg, L.F.: Predicting astronaut effectiveness: a multivariate approach. Aviat. Space Environ. Med. 65(10), 904–909 (1994)

30. Musson, D.M., Sandal, G.M., Helmreich, R.L.: Personality Characteristics and Trait Clusters in Final Stage Astronaut Selection. Aviation, Space and Environmental Medicine 75(4), 342–349 (2004)

31. Sivaram, N., Ramar, K.: Applicability of Clustering and Classification Algorithms for Recruitment Data Mining. International Journal of Computer Applications 4(5), 23–28 (2010)

32. Jang, J.S.R., Sun, C.T., Mizutani, E.: Neuro-Fuzzy and Soft Computing. Prentice Hall, NJ (1997)

33. Chiu, S.L.: Fuzzy model identification based on cluster estimation. Journal of Intelligent and Fuzzy Systems 2(3) (1994)

34. Fuzzy Logic Toolbox: User's Guide of Matlab. The Mathworks, Inc. (1995-2009)

35. Martínez, L.G., Castro, J.R., Licea, G., Rodríguez-Díaz, A., Salas, R.: Towards a Personality Fuzzy Model Based on Big Five Patterns for Engineers Using an ANFIS Learning Approach. In: Batyrshin, I., Mendoza, M.G. (eds.) MICAI 2012, Part II. LNCS (LNAI), vol. 7630, pp. 456–466. Springer, Heidelberg (2013)

Finding Opinion Strength Using Rule-Based Parsing for Arabic Sentiment Analysis

Shereen Oraby[1], Yasser El-Sonbaty[2], and Mohamad Abou El-Nasr[1]

[1] Departments of Computer Engineering
[2] Computer Science
Arab Academy for Science and Technology
Alexandria, Egypt
{shereen.oraby,yasser,mnasr}@aast.edu

Abstract. With increasing interest in sentiment analysis research and opinionated web content always on the rise, focus on analysis of text in various domains and different languages is a relevant and important task. This paper explores the problems of sentiment analysis and opinion strength measurement using a rule-based approach tailored to the Arabic language. The approach takes into account language-specific traits that are valuable to syntactically segment a text, and allow for closer analysis of opinion-bearing language queues. By using an adapted sentiment lexicon along with sets of opinion indicators, a rule-based methodology for opinion-phrase extraction is introduced, followed by a method to rate the parsed opinions and offer a measure of opinion strength for the text under analysis. The proposed method, even with a small set of rules, shows potential for a simple and scalable opinion-rating system, which is of particular interest for morphologically-rich languages such as Arabic.

1 Introduction

The tasks of opinion mining and sentiment analysis have become essential points of research in recent years, particularly due to the wide array of applications and industrial potential involved in gathering informative statistics on the polarity of opinions expressed in various settings, ranging from social, to political, to commercial. The need for efficient, reliable, and scalable automatic classification systems is on the rise, in order to take advantage of the abundance of available opinionated web data for classification and analysis.

While much work is available regarding the sentiment analysis tasks under various approaches in English, research is more limited for morphologically-rich languages such as Arabic, particularly with respect to rule-based approaches that attempt to determine syntactic patterns in the language to aid in the analysis tasks. This paper focuses on the task of sentiment analysis in Arabic through a rule-based approached using sentiment lexicons and modifying words lists to determine document sentiment on a standard opinion movie-review corpus. The considered documents are compared based on their sentiment strength (as compared to ratings given in the text), as opposed to a simple, crisp classification, thus offering a more detailed measure of opinion *strength*.

F. Castro, A. Gelbukh, and M. González (Eds.): MICAI 2013, Part II, LNAI 8266, pp. 509–520, 2013.
© Springer-Verlag Berlin Heidelberg 2013

A survey of related work is detailed in Section 2, followed by introduction to the syntax of the Arabic language and the intuition behind a rule-based approach for rating in Arabic in Section 3. The proposed rule-based classification algorithm is introduced in Section 4, with results and evaluation presented in Section 5 and conclusions and future research points discussed in Section 6.

2   Related Work

The standard two-class problem of sentiment classification into *positive* and *negative* sets was addressed early on by Pang et al. (2002) for English movie reviews from the Internet Movie Database (IMDB) corpus, developing a baseline for the task employing machine learning techniques [1]. Yu et Hatzivassiloglou (2003) improved on the feature selection problem for the machine learning task by adopting N-gram based features and a polarity lexicon on the Wall Street Journal (WSJ) corpus [2], while Bruce and Wiebe (1999) employ additional lexical, part-of-speech (POS) and structural features to the same corpus, demonstrating variations in feature selection and optimization [3].

While supervised learning techniques often employ the use of classifiers such as Naive Bayes or Support Vector Machines (SVMs) to perform classification on sets of test samples given a tagged training set and rich feature sets for various tasks [4], such methods are often very accurate on the domain in which they are trained, and the most successful features reported are often simple unigrams, with performance often faltering when tested on different domains [5].

Because sentiment-bearing words and phrases have proven to be the "dominating factor" [6] in sentiment classification systems in general, samples of approaches focusing in on these features in particular are frequent in the literature. Turney (2002) uses fixed opinion-bearing patterns based on part-of-speech information to perform classification [6] by measuring the *semantic orientation* between terms [7]. For document-level classification dictionaries of sentiment words and phrases categorized by polarity and strength are employed with negations and intensifiers by Taboada (2011) to compute document-level sentiment scores [6], as compared to sentence and word level analysis. Kar and Mandal (2011) analyze product reviews by mining product features, extracting opinion-bearing phrases in the reviews, and measuring the strength of the extracted opinion-phrases to determine overall product ranking [8].

Although research and corpora are more limited for more morphologically-rich languages such as Arabic, some interesting work in lexicon and rule-based classification does exist. An example of Chinese sentence-level sentiment classification presented by Fu and Wang (2010) takes advantage of very language-specific traits in Chinese to tailor the opinion-phrase extraction and score assignment task closely to the distinctive structure of the language, where words are segmented into their respective component sentiment-bearing morphemes, in a "fine-to-coarse grained" methodology [9]. Another notable contribution to lexicon-based sentiment analysis is the work of Syed et al. (2010) in Urdu, where shallow-parsing methods and a developed sentiment-annotated lexicon are used for the task, as a baseline development in a language which differs greatly from English in its scripture, syntactic formation, and morphological features [10].

With respect to the task of Arabic sentiment analysis in particular, Abdul-Mageed et al. (2011) present a manually-annotated corpus of Modern Standard Arabic (MSA) from the newswire domain, together with a tailored wide-scale polarity lexicon, to show the effects of using language-specific features with an SVM classifier on morphologically-rich languages, achieving results of 57.84% F and up to 95.52% F with a domain-specific lexicon [11]. Likewise, Abbasi et al. (2008) use an "Entropy Weighted Genetic Algorithm (EWGA)" that incorporates both syntactic and stylistic features, as well as the information-gain heuristic, to classify document-level text from Middle-Eastern web forums to a reported 93.6% accuracy, also using machine learning classifiers [12]. Rushdi-Saleh et al. (2011) introduce the Opinion Corpus for Arabic (OCA), which consists of movie reviews compiled from various Arabic web pages, and use combinations of N-grams, stemming, and stop-word removal pre-processing under both Naive Bayes and SVM classifiers, achieving a best result of 90% accuracy under SVM [13].

In comparison to the discussed work, the proposed method utilizes the OCA movie review corpus [13] to explore syntactic patterns specific to Arabic to develop a set of rules that are used in conjunction with a polarity lexicon and sets of fixed grammatical units to extract sentiment phrases from opinionated documents, and calculate opinion scores and ratings for each of them. This methodology attempts to take advantage of opinion-bearing language patterns in Arabic for a simple approach that can scale appropriately to different contexts and domains depending on the lexicons utilized, without the need to re-learn data features as with supervised learning methods, and in turn provides a means of determining the respective *strength* of the classified text.

3   Background Information

The complexity of syntax and structure in morphologically-rich languages makes the task of language modeling and representation a challenging one for natural language processing systems. In particular, the effect of a language's morphology on its overall syntax is significant: in Arabic, the language's rich morphology allows for a greater degree of freedom for word order and syntactic structure, as the morphology itself defines many aspects of the language's syntax, and is an important consideration for language modeling [14].

3.1   Basic Descriptive Sentence Structure in Arabic

In Arabic, the most basic sentences used to describe a subject are nominal, consisting of a definite noun, proper noun, or pronoun subject, with an indefinite noun, proper noun, or adjective predicate agreeing with the subject (in number and gender) [15]. For example, the sentence الكتاب جديد (*alkitāb ğadyd*, meaning *"The book is new."*) consists of a simple definite noun, الكتاب (*alkitāb*, meaning "*book*"), with a simple adjective, جديد (*ǧadyd*, meaning "*new*"), and constructs a full sentence in this sense [14].

Arabic adjectives in particular have a structured position in basic sentences: adjectives follow the nouns they modify, and agree with them in gender and number [14]. A particular exception to this rule is found with adjectives that modify plural irrational nouns, which are always feminine singular [14]. Still, the placement of the adjective with respect to the noun it describes is an important detail of descriptive sentence structuring [15].

3.2   Other Morphological Components of Syntax

Not all Arabic part-of-speech units are distinct, independent word forms; rather, several grammatical units are more related to the morphology of word forms they are attached to than separate entities [15]. Clitics, or morphemes that syntactically define words but are often bound to other base words, serve to change the meaning of the inflections they attach to.

For example, conjunctions are cliticization morphemes, such as و (*wāw*, signifying "*and*") and ف (*fā*, indicating "*in*"), that can attach to any part-of-speech. Negations can attach to various parts-of-speech, or they can be independent words or morphemes, as well, such as لم (*lam*, signifying "*did not*"), while adverbs of degree, such as كثيرا (*ktyrā*, signifying "*a lot*") and قليلا (*qalylā*, signifying "*a little*"), can modify verbs, adjectives, other adverbs, and more complex phrases, and usually come after the modified word.

3.3   Intuition Behind the Rule-Based Method for Sentiment Analysis

The basic word forms and simple sentence structures described can be used to derive a simple system for a set of rules focused around descriptive sentences in Arabic. Because some of the most basic and essential units governing the existence of descriptive opinion-detail in sentences revolve around adjectives and their modifiers, including negations, conjunctions, and adverbial intensifiers, these basic units offer a simple structure to map out sentiment-bearing phrases and sentences, as is proposed and modeled in this paper.

The motivation behind a rule-based method for Arabic sentiment analysis lies in the ability to use the basic rules introduced to score documents (and more particularly, reviews) based on the opinion-bearing units within them. While standard machine-learning algorithms can serve to classify documents based on rich sets of word features, the simple proposed method offers a way to capture the *level* of positive or negative sentiment within the analyzed text, and therefore rank the text *within* the observed classes, rather than declaring a strict membership to one or the other.

4   Proposed Algorithm

The proposed rule-based opinion-strength calculation algorithm is presented in the following sections, which detail the system design, dataset, tools, derived rule-set and score calculation scheme utilized.

4.1   System Design

The experiments conducted on the dataset are carried out in a number of steps, as shown in Figure 1 and described in the following sections.

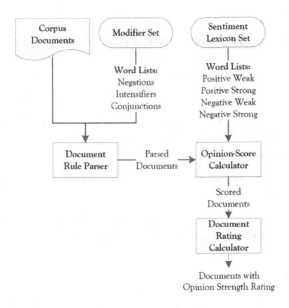

Fig. 1. Experimental system block diagram

Initially, the corpus documents and derived set of modifier word lists (negations, intensifiers, and conjunctions) are parsed using a set of developed grammar rules, mapping the documents into patterns of words and modifiers that are to be used to match with polar word sets. These polar word sets compose the four sentiment lexicons (weak and strong word sets for both the positive and negative classes), which are used to match words in the already rule-parsed documents in the opinion-score calculation phase. Each document receives both a positive and negative score, according to a scoring scheme based on the number of polar units and modifiers in each sentence of the document. Each of the documents is then given a document rating, depending on a measure of the ratio of polar items within them, resulting in a strength rating for each of the documents, which can be compared to the actual review rating for validation, and used to find system accuracy and other assessment metrics.

4.2   Opinion Corpus

The dataset chosen for system implementation was the Opinion Corpus for Arabic (OCA) movie-review corpus [13], particularly for its highly subjective content and review rating scale, which was necessary to validate the proposed opinion-strength rating scheme. The corpus consists of 500 Arabic movie reviews, 250 positive and 250 negative, collected from 15 different Arabic web sites. Each of the written reviews are sets of text detailing the movie and author's commentary, with most reviews followed by an overall numerical rating of the movie to supplement the written review.

To prepare the corpus for analysis, considering the non-uniform nature of the different reviews, a process involving tokenization, basic stop-word, special character, and punctuation removal, and light stemming were performed. Additionally, considering that each site utilizes a different rating scheme to allow the author to give an overall numeric rating of the movie under review, normalization of the rating schemes (rating out of five versus rating out of ten, for example) was performed [13]. For the purposes of the rating-strength assessment conducted using the proposed algorithm, only documents with a review rating were considered for the opinion-strength rating task (to establish a means of validation), and so the actual number of documents used were 483 (250 positive, and 233 negative), with 17 negative reviews excluded due to unavailable ratings.

4.3   Resources and Tools

Several resources and tools were employed in the algorithm implementation to prepare the text and aid in the rule-based rating task.

Sentiment Lexicons and Modifier Lists: As mentioned in the literature, sentiment-bearing words and phrases are the most crucial components for opinion-related tasks [6], considering that the overall semantic meaning of the sentences is ultimately reliant on the collection of the individual polar units within it. This features lends to the use of a set of sentiment lexicons and modifier lists adapted for various natural language processing systems [16].

Sentiment Lexicons: The applied set of four sentiment lexicons were adapted from the Mutli-Perspective Question Answering (MPQA) Subjectivity Lexicon [17], an English set of subjective words that are part of the OpinionFinder project [18], used to identify various aspects of subjectivity in document sets. The words are divided into four sets, {*positive weak, positive strong, negative weak, negative strong*}, with additional "subjectivity queues", such as part-of-speech tags, that could be relevant to usage. As described by Riloff and Wiebe (2003), the sets were collected from both manually and automatically-tagged sources [19].

In order to use the wide-scale lexicon set for the presented Arabic analysis task, a translated version of the lexicon, the Arabic MPQA Subjectivity Lexicon [20] was adapted for use in the proposed system. Because of the scale of the lexicon, problems with the relevance of many translated terms appropriated the task of manual filtering of the set for irrelevant terms, post-translation.

Modifier Lists: In addition to the sentiment lexicons used, a set of Arabic-specific modifiers was also utilized to help define the rules applied for document parsing, as input to the opinion-scoring phase of the algorithm with the sentiment words. The modifier set consists of three word lists, {*negations, intensifiers, conjunctions*}, which represent either full Arabic words or clitic prefixes for polarity inversion, incrementing or decrementing adverbs, and connective conjunctions.

The effects of each of the modifier types are articulated in the derived rule sets, with the general intuition that at the most basic form negations serve to flip (or, at least diminish) the polarity of the following word or set of words, intensifiers update the polarity of the *preceding* word, and conjunctions carry polarity over to the connected set of words.

4.4 Document-Parsing Rule Set

As detailed in set of rules derived for document parsing presented in Figure 2, the top-most classification of a document is a group of one or more terminating (ending with a terminal punctuation) sentences, which are composed of one or more phrases. A phrase may consist of one or more expressions, which may include a negated phrase (simply defined as a basic phrase prefixed with a negation from the negations modifier list). These phrase-forming expressions, in turn, are more basic building-blocks containing conjunction groups (defined as strings of words connected with a conjunction from the modifier list), incremented words (single words preceded or followed by an incremented from the modifier list), or simply single-word units (which are later interpreted as either polar or not, depending on whether they exist in the sentiment lexicons). Each of the terminals are either entries in one of the modifier lists, basic punctuation, or word units.

The document rule-parsing phase works by tokenizing each entering corpus document into its respective grammar units, in accordance with the components defined. The parser then reduces each set of tokenized groups using the grammar rule set, such that each level of granularity within the document (word, conjunction and negation groups, expressions, phrases, and sentences) are clearly and uniquely defined, and the parse tree for each document can be traced back to each of its distinct components, resulting in a single parse per sentence that is ready to be mapped for polarity queues. Sample parse trees for two corpus sentences [13] are shown in Table 1, to be mapped for sentiment words in the subsequent interpretation and score-calculation phases.

4.5 Opinion-Score and Rating Calculations

Given a rule-parsed document, the opinion-score calculation algorithm can be applied to find a polarity score for both positive and negative sentiment, followed by subsequent rating calculations on the derived opinion scores.

Rule Set

⟨document⟩	::= {⟨sentence⟩ PUNCTERM}+
⟨sentence⟩	::= ⟨phrase⟩ {PUNCINT ⟨phrase⟩}+
⟨phrase⟩	::= {⟨expression⟩}+ {⟨negated_phrase⟩}?
	| ⟨negated_phrase⟩
⟨negated_phrase⟩	::= NEG ⟨phrase⟩
⟨expression⟩	::= ⟨conjunction_group⟩
	| ⟨incremented⟩
	| ⟨word⟩
⟨conjunction_group⟩	::= ⟨expression⟩ CONJ ⟨expression⟩
⟨incremented⟩	::= WORD INC
	| INC WORD

Terminal Descriptors

PUNCTERM	::= *terminal punctuation*
PUNCINT	::= *intermediate punctuation*
NEG	::= *an entry in the Negations modifier list*
CONJ	::= *an entry in the Conjunctions modifier list*
INC	::= *a word in the Intensifiers modifier list*
WORD	::= *any word unit*

Fig. 2. Derived rule set for document parsing

Opinion-Score Calculation The basic positive and negative opinion score points are determined when the parsed documents are interpreted by attempting to match each of the terminal words with words from the four adapted sentiment lexicons. Likewise, as dictated by the rule set, each of the individual modifier terminals serve to affect the score of the polar words they operate on.

Negations: A negation can invert the polarity of the word it modifies or decrease its polarity in the same class, just as ليس جيد (*lays ğayd*, meaning *"not good"*) does not necessarily mean سيء (*syʾ*, meaning *"bad"*), but rather a diminished form of جيد (*ğayd*, meaning *"good"*). More particularly because of the less predictable sentence structure of Arabic (where the negations may be further off from the modified polar word), negation words in the algorithm serve to halve the score of the phrase that they precede, where this phrase could be either a single negated word, or a longer negated phrase.

Intensifiers: Intensifiers (in the most general case, "incrementers", or words that intensify the polarity of the word they modify) double the score of the polarity word they operate on in the algorithm, which can appear either before or after the modifier. The scope of the simple grammar only handles the case of a direct intensifier attached to the modified polar word, such as the case of ليس جيد جدا (*lays ğayd ğdā*, meaning *"not very good"*).

Table 1. Sample parse trees for two OCA corpus sentences [13] using the rule-based parser

Sentence 1 with Parse Tree	Sentence 2 with Parse Tree
القصه طريفه للغايه ومسليه	لم يكن ظاهرا بقوه في فيلمه
alqsh ṭryfh lilġāyh wamosaleyh	lm ykon ẓāhrā bqowh fy fylmah
"The story is very funny and entertaining."	"[It] was not powerfully present in his film."

("phrase",
[("WORD", "القصه"),
  ("conjunction_group",
   [("incremented",
     ("WORD", "طريفه"),
     ("INC", "للغايه")),
    ("CONJ", "و"),
    ("WORD", "مسليه")])]])
	("negated",
	  ("NEG", "لم"),
	  ("phrase",
	   [("WORD", "يكن"),
	    ("incremented",
	     ("WORD", "ظاهرا"),
	     ("INC", "بقوه")),
	    ("WORD", "في"),
	    ("WORD", "فيلمه"),
	    ("WORD", "الاخير")]))

Conjunctions: In the simple grammar presented, conjunction groups are defined as sets of expressions (which can be larger conjunction groups, or single words) connected by a conjunction word, such as جيد و مهم (ǧayd wa mohim, meaning *"good and important"*). In the case of conjunction groups containing only similar-polarity words with neutral intermediate words, the algorithm calculates the score of the conjunction as the combined count of all the similar-polarity connected words in the group (thus, "passing the polarity" through the group).

Review Rating Calculation: By interpreting each of the parsed documents with the basic counting scheme proposed, a final positive and negative score is calculated for each of the documents. These scores are calculated as the word scores from the sentiment lexicons, with a single point for a weak lexicon words, and double points for strong lexicon words, along with the updates to the scores based on the surrounding modifiers, according to grammar rules described.

pos_score: count of the positive polar words, with modifier updates
neg_score: count of the negative polar words, with modifier updates

From these two document polarity scores, the overall document rating, as shown in Equation (1), is calculated by taking the positive polarity score over the total document polarity score (for both positive and negative), to give an estimate of the document's polarity score as a ratio of polar units.

$$doc\_rating = \frac{pos\_score}{(pos\_score + neg\_score)} \tag{1}$$

This rating is then compared to the actual numerical rating given in the review to give a sense of the polarity strength of opinions in the document, measured by the average absolute difference between actual and calculated ratings.

5   Results and Evaluation

The results of the review-rating experiments conducted on the 483 rated documents in the Opinion Corpus for Arabic (OCA) dataset [13] under the proposed rule-based algorithm are presented in the following section.

Based on Equation (1), the absolute difference between the actual document review and the predicted document rating was found for all of the documents. Figure 3 shows a frequency distribution of the absolute difference in points between actual and predicated ratings for the *full set* of documents.

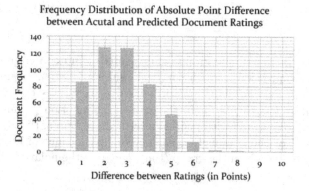

Fig. 3. Frequency of absolute difference in rating points between actual and predicted ratings versus the number of documents with that rating difference

For example, a positive document with an actual rating of 9/10 and given a predicted rating of 7.5/10 and would get a difference score of 1.5 points. The graph shows the highest frequency in the 2-3 difference point bin, with a drop in frequency in either point direction in the range of a 0-10 point-scale difference.

An average difference of 2.1 and 2.5 points (and standard deviation of 1.3 and 1.4) was found for the positive and negative reviews, respectively, giving an average of 2.3 point difference between the ratings for both classes, as compared to the ratings given in the reviews. This gives an indication of how closely the document opinion score matches the actual rating (in ratio between positive and negative scores) and reflects the existence of significant polar items in the document under consideration. As a novel approach, the results give good evidence of the potential of using a rule-based method for the Arabic opinion-rating task.

6   Conclusions

Due to the morphological complexity of languages such as Arabic, rule-based schemes for modeling and parsing the language are often considered difficult tasks. The proposed algorithm, which offers basic decomposition and modeling of Arabic grammar structure as focused around simple opinion-phrase units, including polar words and basic negation, intensifier, and conjunction modifiers, shows that using these simple rules and adapted word lists achieve promising results in sentiment rating tasks.

For further enhancement of the approach, the word lists and rules themselves can be expanded and more thoroughly modeled to the intricacies of the language. Likewise, the task of using more semantic information and modeling of *relationships* between words in the text is important for further research.

The great variance of the semantic meaning of words even in the same polarity class makes the task of measuring opinion strength very relevant. The proposed system uses the polar scores derived from the rule-based method to determine an overall document polarity rating, which coincides to a high degree with the actual document rating given by the author. With this extra classification information, documents can be also be ranked according to their sentiment strength.

The proposed rule-based classifier and novel opinion-strength calculation scheme for Arabic reviews thus provide a scalable approach to sentiment analysis to help further the possibilities of text classification and rating schemes for more complex languages, helping to model sentiment and opinion more closely and correctly.

References

1. Pang, B., Lee, L., Vaithyanathan, S.: Thumbs up?: sentiment classification using machine learning techniques. In: Proceedings of the ACL 2002 Conference on Empirical Methods in Natural Language Processing, EMNLP 2002, vol. 10, pp. 79–86. Association for Computational Linguistics, Stroudsburg (2002)
2. Yu, H., Hatzivassiloglou, V.: Towards answering opinion questions: separating facts from opinions and identifying the polarity of opinion sentences. In: Proceedings of the 2003 Conference on Empirical Methods in Natural Language Processing, EMNLP 2003. Association for Computational Linguistics, Stroudsburg (2003)
3. Bruce, R., Wiebe, J.: Recognizing subjectivity: a case study in manual tagging. Nat. Lang. Eng. 5, 187–205 (1999)
4. Saleh, S., El-Sonbaty, Y.: A feature selection algorithm with redundancy reduction for text classification. In: 22nd International Symposium on Computer and Information Sciences, Turkey (2007)
5. Taboada, M., Brooke, J., Tofiloski, M., Voll, K., Stede, M.: Lexicon-based methods for sentiment analysis. Comput. Linguist. 37, 267–307 (2011)
6. Liu, B.: Sentiment Analysis and Opinion Mining. Morgan & Claypool Publishers (2012)
7. Turney, P.: Thumbs up or thumbs down? Semantic orientation applied to unsupervised classification of reviews. In: Proceedings of the 40th Annual Meeting of the Association of Computational Linguistics, Philadelphia, Pennsylvania (2002)

8. Kar, A., Mandal, D.: Finding opinion strength using fuzzy logic or web reviews. International Journal of Engineering and Industries 2(1) (2011)

9. Fu, G., Wang, X.: Chinese sentence-level sentiment classification based on fuzzy sets. In: Proceedings of the 23rd International Conference on Computational Linguistics: Posters, COLING 2010, pp. 312–319. Association for Computational Linguistics, Stroudsburg (2010)

10. Syed, A.Z., Aslam, M., Martinez-Enriquez, A.M.: Lexicon based sentiment analysis of urdu text using sentiunits. In: Sidorov, G., Hernández Aguirre, A., Reyes García, C.A. (eds.) MICAI 2010, Part I. LNCS, vol. 6437, pp. 32–43. Springer, Heidelberg (2010)

11. Abdul-Mageed, M., Diab, M., Korayem, M.: Subjectivity and sentiment analysis of modern standard arabic. In: Proceedings of the 49th Annual Meeting of the Association for Computational Linguistics: Human Language Technologies: Short Papers, HLT 2011, vol. 2. Association for Computational Linguistics, Stroudsburg, pp. 587–591 (2011)

12. Abbasi, A., Chen, H., Salem, A.: Sentiment analysis in multiple languages: Feature selection for opinion classification in web forums. ACM Trans. Inf. Syst. 26 (2008)

13. Rushdi-Saleh, M., Martin-Valdivia, M., Urena-Lopez, L., Perea-Ortega, J.: Oca: Opinion corpus for arabic. J. Am. Soc. Inf. Sci. Technol. 62, 2045–2054 (2011)

14. Habash, N.: Introduction to Arabic Natural Language Processing. Synthesis Lectures on Human Language Technologies. Morgan & Claypool Publishers (2008)

15. Ryding, K.: A Reference Grammar of Modern Standard Arabic. Reference Grammars. Cambridge University Press, New York (2006)

16. Ezzeldin, A.M., Kholief, M.H., El-Sonbaty, Y.: ALQASIM: Arabic language question answer selection in machines. In: Forner, P., Müller, H., Paredes, R., Rosso, P., Stein, B. (eds.) CLEF 2013. LNCS, vol. 8138, pp. 100–103. Springer, Heidelberg (2013)

17. Wilson, T., Wiebe, J., Hoffmann, P.: Recognizing contextual polarity in phrase-level sentiment analysis. In: Proceedings of the Conference on Human Language Technology and Empirical Methods in Natural Language Processing, HLT 2005, pp. 347–354. Association for Computational Linguistics, Stroudsburg (2005)

18. Wilson, T., Hoffmann, P., Somasundaran, S., Kessler, J., Wiebe, J., Choi, Y., Cardie, C., Riloff, E., Patwardhan, S.: Opinionfinder: a system for subjectivity analysis. In: Proceedings of HLT/EMNLP on Interactive Demonstrations, HLT-Demo 2005, pp. 34–35. Association for Computational Linguistics, Stroudsburg (2005)

19. Riloff, E., Wiebe, J.: Learning extraction patterns for subjective expressions. In: Proceedings of the 2003 Conference on Empirical Methods in Natural Language Processing, EMNLP 2003, pp. 105–112. Association for Computational Linguistics, Stroudsburg (2003)

20. ALTEC: Arabic mpqa subjective lexicon (2012), http://www.altec-center.org/

Emotion Based Features of Bird Singing
for *Turdus migratorius* Identification

Toaki Esaú Villareal Olvera[1,*], Caleb Rascón[2], and Ivan Vladimir Meza Ruiz[2]

[1] Facultad de Estudios Superiores Zaragoza (FES Zaragoza)
[2] Instituto de Investigaciones en Matemticas Aplicadas y en Sistemas (IIMAS)
Universidad Nacional Autnoma de Mxico (UNAM)
Mexico City, DF, Mxico
{esau.villarreal,ivanvladimir}@turing.iimas.unam.mx,
caleb.rascon@iimas.unam.mx
http://www.unam.mx

Abstract. A possible solution for the current rate of animal extinction in the world is the use of new technologies in their monitoring in order to tackle problems in the reduction of their populations in a timely manner. In this work we present a system for the identification of the *Turdus migratorius* bird species based on their singing. The core of the system is based on turn-level features extracted from the audio signal of the bird songs. These features were adapted from the recognition of human emotion in speech, which are based on Support Vector Machines. The resulting system is a prototype module of acoustic identification of birds which goal is to monitor birds in their environment, and, in the future, estimate their populations.

1 Introduction

Birds are the most diverse class of terrestrial vertebrate animals. Based on the morphology of the animals *Mayr (1942)* [6] estimated approximately 8,200 species. More recent classifications from *Sibley and Monroe (1990)* and calculations from *Burnie (2003)* and *Perrrins (2011)* have estimated 9,672, 9,720 or 9,845 species respectively [23, 4, 3]. In particular, Mexico is home of 10% of the worlds' avifauna with 1,076 species [20] from which 104 live exclusively in Mexico [7]. However, this richness of biodiversity is in danger: *Birdlife International (2011)* estimates 103 bird species have become extinct since 1600, of which 24 were located in Mexico [15]. The problem has become acute with respect to endangered species, which are 12% of the bird species. In Mexico, there are 40 species in danger of becoming extinct, and the Mexican government has classified 373 species at some kind of risk [5].

In face of this situation, the monitoring of bird populations are part of a more general scheme which helps determine actions to prevent the extinction of

* We thank the Golem Group and from Laidetec, Hernando Hortega, for their feedback while developing this research and prototype.

F. Castro, A. Gelbukh, and M. González (Eds.): MICAI 2013, Part II, LNAI 8266, pp. 521–530, 2013.

species. Current methodologies are quite intrusive, as they require the capture of birds specimens and/or tagging them with devices [16]. Less intrusive techniques are being explored, among which, machine learning Bio-acoustic methodologies are an attractive option [9]. In particular, the identification of bird species through their singing has several advantages: it does not require to capture the specimen, it can capture multiple birds and species at once, and audio capture devices does not invade their natural environments.

In this work, we explore the bird species identification task. Specifically, we focus on the *Turdus Migratorius* species (also know as *Common Robin*). This species is distributed throughout North America, from Canada to Mexico. Although the status of this species is not of concern, its availability and singing characteristics made it a good candidate to test our approach[1]. We explore the use of acoustic features at the syllable level of the bird song inspired by methodologies used by Human Emotion Recognition [22]. We use these features to label the species in offline recordings or live audio capture using our prototype module of acoustic identification of birds.

The outline of this work is as follows. Section 2 presents previous and related work. Section 3 explains in detail our approach. Section 4 presents the acoustic features used. Section 5 lists the audio resources used in our development and evaluation. It also presents the prototype for live audio capture and identification. Section 6 explains our experiments and results. Finally, Section 7 presents our main findings and future work.

2   Previous Work

Bird singing is divided in three levels: song, syllable and notes. With respect to human speech these correspond to: sentences/utterances, words and phonemes. Figure 1 illustrates such levels in a segment of singing of a *Turdus migratorius*. At the note level, *Graciarena et. al (2011)* [11] uses a note model based on Gaussian Mixture Models (GMM), in combination with n-gram models for the sequence of notes to reach a song level. In addition, Hidden Markov Models (HMM) are a popular approach for sequencing syllables [17].

Most of the research has focused at the syllable level using different machine learning techniques and feature representations. Multivariate and Hypersignal [18], distance statistics and syllables sinusoidals [13], GMM and Mel-Frequency Cepstral Coefficients (MFCCs) [12], GMM correlations and histograms [24], Linear Discriminant Analysis (LDA) using Linear Prediction Cepstral Coefficients (LPCCs) and MFCCs [14], Support Vector machines (SVM) and MFCCs [8], MFCCs and Manifolds [2]. From these examples, we want to distinguish the approaches which automatically segments audio into syllables [24, 14], for the practicality of the application, since they do not requiere human tagging.

In the work of *Trifa et. al. (2008)* [25], where Mexican native species (specifically *antbirds* species from the Mexican rainforest) where studied for species

---

[1] A recording of a *Turdus Migratorius* specimen can be found in *Anonymous*.

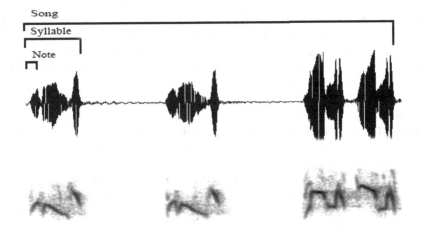

Fig. 1. Acoustic levels of a bird song

recognition, they used a HMM setting which reached high accuracy with manually-segmented song recordings (2 − 4 seconds).

In this work, we focus on the *Turdus Migratorius* which inhabits Mexico. The features we use are MFCC representations commonly used in the Human Emotion Recognition field. In addition, our system automatically identifies the syllables in offline recording or live audio capture.

3   The System

Figure 2 illustrates our approach. The first stage syllabifies the audio signal, the result of which are segments of audio to be classified. The second phase classifies such segments into two classes: a part of a song of a *Turdus Migratorius* or not[2].

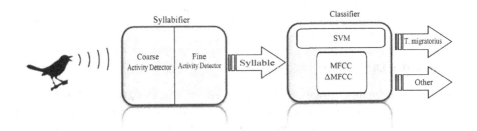

Fig. 2. Stages for the identification of species

---

[2] The source code can be obtained from: *Anonymous.*

The *syllabifier* consists of two phases for live audio capture: a) a coarse activity detector which identifies segments of activity, b) a fine-grained activity detector. The coarse activity detector is an energy-based Voice Activity Detector (VAD) [19] which uses an adaptive threshold depending on the energy of n previous frames. Then, the detected segment is processed by the fine grained activity detector using the signal energy of the whole segment to identify a threshold [21]. The result of the fine grained phase is a segment of activity that has been further segmented into a set of syllables.

If the identification is carried out via an offline recording, only the fine grained phase is carried out, using the whole recording as one segment of activity.

The classifier is a straight forward Support Vector Machine (SVM) with a Radial Basis Function (RBFs), where we have defined two classes: the *Turdus migratorius* and *other*. The classifier uses MFCC-based features (explained in more detail in the following section) extracted at the syllable level [1] to attribute a label to the segment of activity.

4 Acoustic Features

In our approach, we use two feature groups as our source of features: MFCCs and ΔMFCCs. These features have been inspired by the emotion detection field [26, 22]. Over each syllabified segment, we extract the two features groups (one set of features per syllable), and for each group we calculate nine functionals: *mean, standard deviation, quartile* 1, 2 and 3, *minimum, maximum, skweness* and *kustosis* metrics.

In particular, the MFCCs we used are optimized for bird songs. Table 1 compares the parameters used with the commonly used for human speech.

Table 1. Comparison of MFCC parameters between birds songs and humans speech

Parameter	Birds songs	Human speech[3]
Coefficients	16	13
Bank filter	40	40
Up frequency	4, 000Hz	6, 855.49Hz
Low frequency	0Hz	133.33Hz
Sample rate	16, 000	16, 000

5 Audio Libraries

For our experiments the main source of recordings was the *Maculay Library*. For the *Turdus migratorius* label we used samples from the *Biblioteca de la Facultad de Ciencias* [10] and our own recordings carried out in the enviroments where we expect our system to help to monitor the species. For the *other* label we used recordings of the *Turdus accidentalis, Myadestes occidentalis, Thryomanes bewickii, Cardinalis cardinalis* and *Toxostoma curvirostre*, as well as the silences detected on all recordings. Table 2 summarizes the information from which we obtained the recordings.

Table 2. Description of audio sources

Species	Source	Total time	Total recordings
Turdus migratorius	Maculay Library Facultad de Ciencias Own recording⁴.	1h 53m	59
Turdus rufopalliatus	Maculay Library	16m	11
Myadestes occidentalis	Maculay Library	36m	4
Thryomanes bewickii	Maculay Library	24m	3
Cardinalis cardinalis	Maculay Library	21m	5
Toxostoma curvirostre	Maculay Library	36m	4

5.1   The Prototype

The prototype is a teleoperated static robot with capabilities of audio capture, for which it has two shotgun microphones which can be pointed with an angle with respect to the ground (to consider foliage). It can also capture temperature, humidity, and global position coordinates. All this under the control of an operator.

It is designed to work live with a module of acoustic identification of birds, the main purpose of which is to record the ambient audio and to identify the presence of the *Turdus migratorius* species.

Figure 3 shows a scheme of the prototype and some of their components.

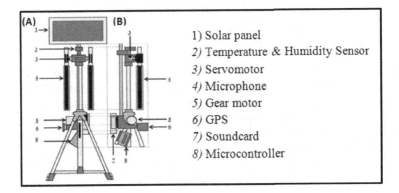

1) Solar panel
2) Temperature & Humidity Sensor
3) Servomotor
4) Microphone
5) Gear motor
6) GPS
7) Soundcard
8) Microcontroller

Fig. 3. Module of acoustic identification of birds (a) front view (b) sideview

6   Experiments

First we evaluate the fine-grained syllabifier by manually labelling the recordings corresponding to the *Turdus migratorius* and comparing the automatic versus

Table 3. Syllabifier performance for *Turdus migratorius* recordings

Measure	Value
Precision	87.49%
Recall	75.15%
F1-measure	78.30%

the manual segmentation. For this purpose, we use a turn based evaluation based on the midpoint of the manual transcription [27], using a 10-fold cross-validation over the recordings (so that features from the recorded environment could be learnt by the classifier). Table 3 summarizes the results, which show that if the recording is of a *Turdus migratorius*, the syllabifier will recall approximately 75% of its syllables.

In a similar manner we evaluate the performance of the classifier stage. In this case, we perform two evaluations over the manually labelled and automatic syllabified recordings. Table 4 summarizes the performance of the classifier over the syllables.

Table 4. Classification performance of *manual* and *automatic* segmented syllables of *Turdus migratorius* and the *other* class

Measure	Manual (only *Turdus migratorius*)	Automatic
Precision	73.94%	83.26%
Recall	64.64%	83.26%
F1-score	67.34%	83.26%

The *manual* results represent the classification of the *Turdus migratorius* species on the recordings with only this species. As it can be seen, once we eliminate the certainty that the recording is of a certain species, the system has a lower performance as it attempts to classify the erroneous sillabified segments.

The *automatic* results show the accuracy of the system over both *Turdus migratorius* species and the *other* category. As it can be seen, the module can identify correctly 83% of the syllables. However, it is important to remember that some of the syllables from the syllabifier stage were not passed into the classifier stage and, thus, were not considered in the performance metric.

In order to illustrate the performance of the classifier Figure 4 shows the Receiver Operating Characteristic (ROC) curve, which shows the discriminative power of the classifier. In addition, the ROC curves for a classifier with only

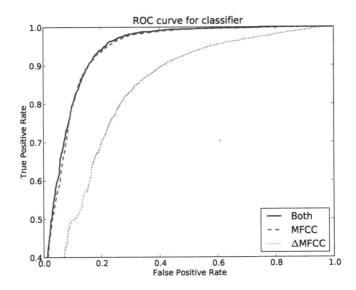

Fig. 4. ROC curves for classifier with both MFCC and ΔMFCC group features, only MFCC and only ΔMFCC

Table 5. Performance of the classifier with only MFCC and only ΔMFCC group of features

Measure	Only MFCC	Only ΔMFCC
F1-score	83.63%	79.26%

MFCC and only ΔMFCC features are also shown. As it can be seen, the MFCC features are the most helpful to perform the task of identifying the species. The classifier base only on those features is as good as the combined classifier. Table 5 list the performance results of only MFCC and ΔMFCC, since these results were calculated over the automatic segmentation, the metrics *precision, recall* and $f1 - score$ have the same value.

Finally, Figure 5 shows the learning curve for the task if we add recordings to the classifier. For this evaluation, we split the *Turdus migratorius* in training (35 recordings) and testing (24 recordings), we only vary the amount of *Turdus Migratorius* recordings during training. For the *other* samples we split in half of the recordings for each species into the training and testing. In this Figure, we can notice a good performance was reached with 20 recordings which are approximately $40min$. When reached 35 the performance is getting stable.

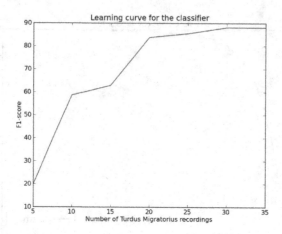

Fig. 5. Learning curve for the task of *Turdus migratorius* identification

7   Conclusion

We have presented a system for the identification of the *Turdus migratorius* bird species. Our approach relies on features inspired by the recognition of human emotion in speech. Our system recalls 75% of the syllables and classifies 83% of them correctly as *Turdus migratorius* or *other*. We showed that MFCC group of features is the most helpful for the classification. Finally, we show 35 of recordings can be enough to reach similar results to ours. Our current system is part of module of acoustic identification of birds prototype (*MIAA* for its initials in Spanish.) which is designed to be used to monitor birds in their natural environment.

Future work will focus into improve the identification rates and consider more species. We are looking into how to relate the monitored data with the estimated population of the birds, so we can follow the population of birds during a great period of time and provide measurements of their population, migratory behaviour and future plans of conservation.

References

[1] Bogert, B., Healy, M., Tukey, J.: The quefrency alanysis of time series for echoes: Cepstrum, pseudo-autocovariance, cross-cepstrum, and saphe-cracking. In: Rosenblatt, E.M. (ed.) Symposium on Time Series Analysis, ch. 15, pp. 209–243 (1963)

[2] Briggs, F., Raich, R., Fern, X.Z.: Audio classification of bird species: A statistical manifold approach. In: Ninth IEEE International Conference on Data Mining, ICDM 2009, pp. 51–60 (2009)

[3] Perrins, C.: The new encyclopedia of birds (2011)

[4] Burnie, D.: Animal (2003)

[5] Semarnat. Secretaría de Medio Ambiente y Recursos Naturales. Norma oficial mexicana nom-059-semarnat-2010 (2010)

[6] Mayr, E.: The number of species of birds, vol. 63 (1946)

[7] González, G.F., Gómez de Silva, H.: Especies endmicas: riqueza, patrones de distribucin y retos para su conservacin, p. 150 (2003)

[8] Fagerlund, S.: Bird species recognition using support vector machines. EURASIP J. Appl. Signal Process. (1), 64 (2007)

[9] Glotin, H., Clark, C., Lecun, Y., Dugan, P., Halkais, X., Seuer, J. (eds.): The1st Ingternational Workshop on Machine Learning for Bioacoustics (2013)

[10] Sosa-López, J.R., Gordillo-Martínez, A.: Digitalización de la biblioteca de sonidos naturales del museo de zoología, facultad de ciencias. Universidad nacional autnoma de México (2010)

[11] Graciarena, M., Delplanche, M., Shriberg, E., Stolcke, A.: Bird species recognition combining acoustic and sequence modeling. In: 2011 IEEE International Conference on Acoustics, Speech and Signal Processing (ICASSP), pp. 341–344 (2011)

[12] Graciarena, M., Delplanche, M., Shriberg, E., Stolcke, A., Ferrer, L.: Acoustic front-end optimization for bird species recognition. In: Proceedings of the IEEE International Conference on Acoustics, Speech, and Signal Processing, ICASSP 2010, pp. 293–296 (2010)

[13] Harma, A.: Automatic identification of bird species based on sinusoidal modeling of syllables. In: Proceedings of the IEEE International Conference on Acoustics, Speech, and Signal Processing (ICASSP 2003), vol. 5, pp. 545–548 (2003)

[14] Lee, C.H., Lee, Y.K., Huang, R.Z.: Automatic recognition of bird songs using cepstral coefficients. Journal of Information Technology and Applications (1), 17–23 (2006)

[15] BirdLife International. Threantened birds of the world. Lynx Editions y Birdlife International (2000)

[16] Ralph, C.J., Geupel, G.R., Pyle, P., Martin, T.E., DeSante, D.F., Milan, B.: Manual de métodos para el monitoreo de aves terrestres, vol. (45). Pacific Aouthwest Research Stattion, Forest Service, U.S. Departament of Agriculture (1996)

[17] Kwan, C., Mei, G., Zhao, X., Ren, Z., Xu, R., Stanford, V., Rochet, C., Aube, J., Ho, K.C.: Bird classification algorithms: theory and experimental results. In: Proceedings of the IEEE International Conference on Acoustics, Speech, and Signal Processing, ICASSP 2004, pp. 289–292 (2004)

[18] McIlraith, A.L., Card, H.C.: Birdsong recognition using backpropagation and multivariate statistics. IEEE Transactions on Signal Processing 45(11), 2740–2748 (1997)

[19] Milanovic, S., Lukac, Z., Domazetovic, A.: One solution of speech activity detection. In: Conference on Telecommunications ETRAN (1999)

[20] Navarro-Singüenza, Sánchez-González, L.: La diversidad de Aves, vol. (24-56). CIPAMEX/CONABIO/NFWF (2003)

[21] Pikrakis, A., Giannakopoulos, T., Theodoridis, S.: An overview of speech/music discrimination techniques in the context of audio recordings. In: Tsihrintzis, G.A., Jain, L.C. (eds.) Multimedia Services in Intelligent Environments. SCI, vol. 120, pp. 81–102. Springer, Heidelberg (2008)

[22] Schuller, B.: Voice and speech analysis in search of states and traits. In: Gevers, T., Salah, A.A. (eds.) Computer Analysis of Human Behavior, pp. 227–253 (2011)

[23] Sibley, C.G., Monroe Jr., B.L.: Distribution and taxonomy of the birds of the world. Yale University Press (1990)

[24] Somervuo, P., Harma, A.: Bird song recognition based on syllable pair histograms. In: Proceedings of the IEEE International Conference on Acoustics, Speech, and Signal Processing (ICASSP 2004), vol. 5, pp. 825–828 (2004)

[25] Trifa, V., Kirschel, A., Taylor, C.E., Vallejo, E.E.: Automated species recognition of antbirds in a mexican rainforest using hidden markov models. Journal of the Acoustical Society of America 123(4), 2424–2431 (2008)

[26] Vlasenko, B., Schuller, B., Wendemuth, A., Rigoll, G.: Frame vs. turn-level: Emotion recognition from speech considering static and dynamic processing. In: Paiva, A.C.R., Prada, R., Picard, R.W. (eds.) ACII 2007. LNCS, vol. 4738, pp. 139–147. Springer, Heidelberg (2007)

[27] Ward, J.A., Lukowicz, P., Gellersen, H.W.: Performance metrics for activity recognition. ACM Trans. Intell. Syst. Technol. 2(1), 6:1–6:23 (2011)

Author Index